GENE THERAPY - DEVELOPMENTS AND FUTURE PERSPECTIVES

Edited by **Chunsheng Kang**

Gene Therapy - Developments and Future Perspectives
Edited by Chunsheng Kang

Published by InTech
Janeza Trdine 9, 51000 Rijeka, Croatia

Publishing Process Manager Romina Krebel

Technical Editor Teodora Smiljanic

Cover Designer InTech Design Team

Additional hard copies can be obtained from orders@intechopen.com

Gene Therapy - Developments and Future Perspectives, Edited by Chunsheng Kang
p. cm.
ISBN 978-953-307-617-1

For EU product safety concerns:
IN TECH d.o.o., Prolaz Marije Krucifikse Kozulić 3, 51000 Rijeka, Croatia,
info@intechopen.com or visit our website at intechopen.com.

Meet the editor

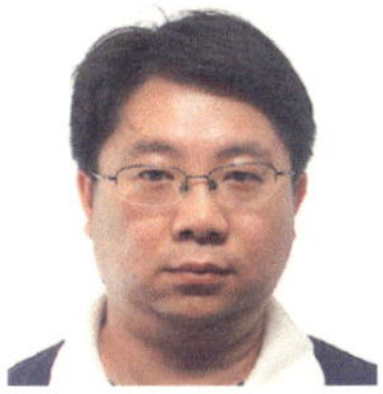

Dr. Chunsheng Kang is Professor and Vice-director at Lab of Neuro-oncology, Tianjin Neurological Institute, Department of neurosurgery, Tianjin Medical University General Hospital, P. R. China. He is a member of many professional societies, including American Association for Cancer Research and Chinese Neurosurgical Society. He is also a vice board chairman of Tianjin Genetics Society. Dr. Kang received his bachelor degree in medicine from Tianjin Medical University, P. R. China in 1993 and his Ph.D. in neurosurgery from Tianjin Medical University General Hospital, Tianjin, P. R. China in 2003. He specializes in RNAi in cancer, microRNA and signaling pathway in cancer, high-throughput analysis in cancer, nonviral gene delivery system. His research has received sustained funding from the Chinese Natural Science Foundation, "Program for New Century Excellent Talents in University" of Ministry of Education, Natural Science Foundation of Tianjin Municipal Science and Technology Commission and other foundations. Dr. Kang has supervised the research efforts of over 30 postdoctoral associates, doctoral candidates and master's level graduate students in the past 8 years.

Contents

Preface

We are delighted to be offered the opportunity to help construct a book dealing with important issues of development and future perspectives in gene therapy.

The goal of our work on this project is to provide a means, via the contributions of many collaborating authors, to make our doctors become comfortable with the common problems of gene therapy in a single accessible book.

The current volume aims at providing an up-to-date report on the field of the development and future perspectives in gene therapy. Contributions consist of basic and translational research, as well as clinical experiences, and they outline functional mechanisms, predictive approaches, patient-related studies, and upcoming challenges in this stimulating but also controversial field of gene therapy research.

We hope that our efforts and those of our collaborators will well present our specialty and may, perhaps, inspire others to delve a bit more deeply into a topic of interest.

Dr. Chunsheng Kang
Professor at Lab of Neuro-oncology
Tianjin Neurological Institute
China

Part 1

Approach of Gene Therapy

1

New Vectors for Stable and Safe Gene Modification

Francisco Martín, Karim Benabdellah, Marién Cobo, Pilar Muñoz, Per Anderson and Miguel G. Toscano
Andalusian Stem Cell Bank, Granada University, Spain

1. Introduction

Stable gene modification without affecting normal cellular function is a main goal both for basic and applied science. Current strategies to achieve stable gene modification are either very inefficient (homologous recombination) or very genotoxic (retroviral gene transfer). Retroviral vectors derived from oncoretroviruses (murine leukaemia virus - MLV) were the first to be widely used for stable gene modifications for gene therapy strategies. They are efficient, poorly immunogenic and derived from a non-pathogenic virus. MLV-based vectors were also the first ones to show real therapeutic effect by correcting the immune system of about 50 patients with four different severe immunodeficiencies X-linked Severe Combined Immunodeficiency (SCID-X1), SCID-Adenosine Deaminase Deficiency (SCID-ADA), Wiskott-Aldrich Syndrome (WAS) and Chronic Granulomatous Disease (CGD)(Fischer *et al.*). However, for most applications therapeutic efficacy were incomplete or come together with serious adverse effects such as cell transformation(Neven *et al.*, 2009). Different studies have demonstrated that the enhancer elements present in the old generation retroviral vectors are important in cell transformation(Montini *et al.*, 2009). Therefore, safer integrative vectors are required to replace MLV-based retroviral vectors when stable gene modification is required. New vectors for stable expression must consider three aspects: 1- efficiency, 2- ectopic or unregulated expression of the transgene and 3- genotoxicity (genomic alterations due to vector integrations).
Probably the most important feature for a vector to reach clinic is efficiency. Gene Therapy vectors must be able to efficiently transduce their target cells in order to reach therapeutic benefits. High efficiency is especially relevant when the therapeutic protein does not confer any positive advantage to the target cells. It is therefore important to keep in mind that very safe vectors are of no use if the efficiency does not reach a minimum. We can say that, at least for some applications, efficiency is no longer a limitation, and that safety is now the main concern.
The ectopic or unregulated expression of the transgene is other aspect to take into consideration. As conventional therapeutic agents, transgenes have a window where and when to exert their function. In many diseases, the expression of the affected gene is restricted to a particular tissue, to a particular stage of the development and/or in response to environmental conditions. The expression of the transgene in non-target cells as well as the expression of non-physiological transgene levels may cause toxic or deleterious effects.

Therefore, an important safety issue concerning gene therapy is to achieve regulated and/or physiological expression of the transgene(reviewed in Toscano *et al.* 2011).
Genotoxicity can be defined as harmful actions on the integrity of the genetic material. Genotoxic substances are potentially mutagenic or carcinogenic. Integrative vectors are genotoxic due to their ability to integrate into the host DNA since vector integration can result in alteration of gene expression. In the worst scenario, genotoxicity can cause cell transformation and tumor development. Several factors influence vector genotoxicity (Baum *et al.*, 2003) such as integration site preference, presence of strong enhancers in the vector, weak polyadenylation sites or the integration mechanism. To minimize or eliminate genotoxicity problems of integrative vectors we can use safer integration sites (safe harbor), block the effect of the vector on the surrounding chromatin (using insulators) or gene correction strategies (Figure 1).
In this chapter we will discuss the most promising strategies that tackle these issues: 1- improving safety of retroviral-based vectors, 2- novel non-viral systems to achieve efficient transgene integrations, 3- site-specific integrative vector systems and 4- gene correction by enhanced homologous recombination.

2. Improving safety of retroviral-based vectors

There are two alternative means of improving safety of retroviral-based gene delivery; 1- by using alternative retroviruses for vector development and 2-by improving the properties of existing retroviral vectors.

2.1 Alternative retroviral vectors

One way to improve the safety of stable gene expression is the search for retroviral vectors other than the original Moloney-murine-leukemia-virus (MoMLV)-based vectors. Retroviruses from two different genus from the retroviridae family have been the main focus for the development of new integrative vectors: lentivirus and spumavirus

2.1.1 Lentiviral-based vectors (LV)

Lentiviruses are part of the retrovirus family that includes the human immunodeficiency virus-1 (HIV-1). Viral vectors are useful vehicles for the delivery of genes into target cells and retroviral vectors have become popular because of their ability to integrate into the host cell genome and maintain persistent gene expression. Also, the ability to stably transduce non-dividing cells has made them one of the best platforms for vector development(Ikeda *et al.*, 2003; Cockrell and Kafri, 2007). Lentiviral vectors (LV) offer several advantages over gammaretroviral vectors (GVs) (reviewed in Chang and Sadelain, 2007): 1- Transduction with LV does not require preactivation of non-dividing cells. They are very efficient for stable gene modification of most primary stem cells including neurons, hematopoietic, mesenchymal and embryonic stem cells. 2- LV are more resistant to silencing and different regulatory elements can be incorporated to minimize influence from neighbouring chromatin without substantially affecting vector titre(Ramezani and Hawley, 2010). The modifications include utilization of strong internal enhancer-promoter sequences, addition of scaffold/matrix attachment regions and flanking the transcriptional unit with chromatin domain insulators. 3- The integration "pattern" of LVs is less genotoxic than GVs. Contrary to GVs, LVs do not have a preferential insertion next to transcriptional start sites and regulatory gene regions. Modlich et al. found(Modlich *et al.*, 2009) that the LVs insertion

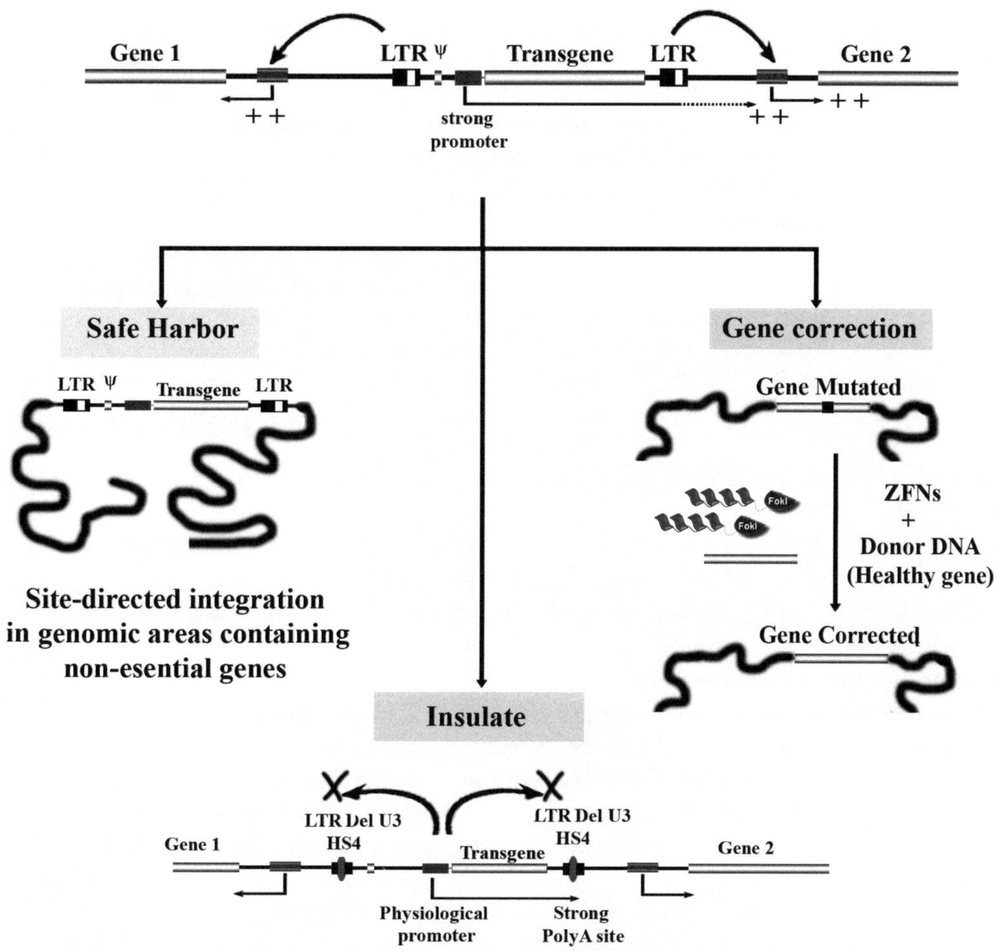

Fig. 1. Main strategies to achieve safer stable genetic modification for gene therapy applications. First generation gammaretroviral vectors (top) contained strong enhancer sequences in their LTR backbones that can influence genes located upstream (Gene 1) or downstream (Gene 2) of the insertion site. In addition, the promoter activity of the LTR (U3 region) or that of a strong internal promoter, can also influence activity of downstream genes by 3′ readthrough (dashed lines) during the transcription of the transgene. There are three main strategies to avoid the potential deleterious effects of stable genetic modification: 1- Safe harbor. In this direction scientists search for vector systems that integrate in safer locations than gammaretroviral vectors. 2- Insulate. Another strategy is to modify the integrative vectors by eliminating enhancers from the Long Terminal Repeats (LTRs), by using physiological promoters and by the introduction of insulator boundaries that block the potential residual effects of the internal promoters on the nearby genes. 3- Gene Correction. Recently, a new possibility has come thanks to technologies that dramatically increase the efficiency of homologous recombination for gene editing. It is now feasible to restore the correct version of almost any mutated gene by the use of zinc finger nucleases or meganucleases together with the correct version of the gene.

pattern was approximately threefold less likely than the GVs to trigger transformation of primary hematopoietic cells. 4- The LVs backbone is more flexible to modifications and insertions.

Of all LVs, HIV-1-based are by far the most used for gene therapy strategies. Other lentiviruses commonly used are equine infectious anaemia virus (EIAV), Simian immunodeficiency virus(SIV), Feline immunodeficiency virus(FIV) and Bovine immunodeficiency virus (BIV):

Human Immunodeficiency Virus-1 (HIV-1) based vectors. Latest generation LVs are devoid of any HIV coding sequences from the original virus (the most commonly used is HIV-1). Proteins needed for particle formation and enzymatic activities are supplied in trans by separate plasmids encoding *Gag, Pol, Env, Tat* and *Rev* proteins (Figure 2). The transactivator *Tat* (generally used in *trans* to allow vector genome production in producer cells) is also dispensable for the generation of fully efficient LV vector particles. In these vectors, the *Tat*-dependent U3 promoter has been replaced by promoters such as the cytomegalovirus immediate-early enhancer and promoter (CMVp), resulting in *Tat*-independent transcription with no decrease in viral titers(Miyoshi *et al.*, 1998; Delenda, 2004).

HIV-1 based LVs efficiently transduce the most important target cells for gene therapists (neurons, hepatocytes, dendritic cells). They are probably the most efficient vectors for stem cells transduction. They are also safer than other integrative vector systems because they do not have integration preference for transcriptional start sites, although they do integrate semi-randomly in transcriptionally active areas (Montini *et al.*, 2006). In fact several studies have recently demonstrated the lower genotoxicity of LVs compared to oncoretroviral-based vectors(Montini *et al.*, 2006; Gonzalez-Murillo *et al.*, 2008). These characteristics have prompted scientists to propose LVs as one of the most interesting vectors for gene therapy strategies when stable gene expression is required. There are at the moment 29 approved clinical trials using lentiviral vectors (http:// www.wiley.com /legacy /wileychi /genmed /clinical/) for the treatment of primary immunodeficiencies, adrenoleukodystrophy, Parkinson disease, beta-thalasemia, sickle cell disease, Fanconi anemia, AIDS and cancer.

Since HIV-1 is a highly infectious agent for humans, several groups have though that equivalent vectors derived from lentiviruses that are not pathogens for humans could be of interest. Vectors based on non-human primates (simian) and non-primates (feline, equine and bovine) lentiviruses would theoretically be safer than HIV-1-based vectors, minimizing the risk of generating replication-competent virus:

Simian immunodeficiency virus (SIV)-based vectors. LVs derived from the Simian immunodeficiency virus (SIV) have been developed by several groups(Mangeot *et al.*, 2000; Hanawa *et al.*, 2004), with safety issues similar to HIV-1 based vectors. They have been used for efficient transduction of simian and human hematopoietic stem cells (HSCs)(Sandrin *et al.*, 2002). In addition, SIV vectors have been used for correction of CGD in animal models(Naumann *et al.*, 2007). They have also demonstrated to facilitate safe and efficient retinal gene transfer(Murakami *et al.*2010) and for the respiratory epithelium (for cystic fibrosis treatment) when pseudotyped with the envelope protein of the Sendai virus(Mitomo *et al.*2010). Interestingly, integration site studies have demonstrated that while MLV-based vectors integrate predominantly around transcription start sites, SIV integrants strongly favoured transcription units and gene-dense regions of the genome without a preference for transcription start sites(Hematti *et al.*, 2004).

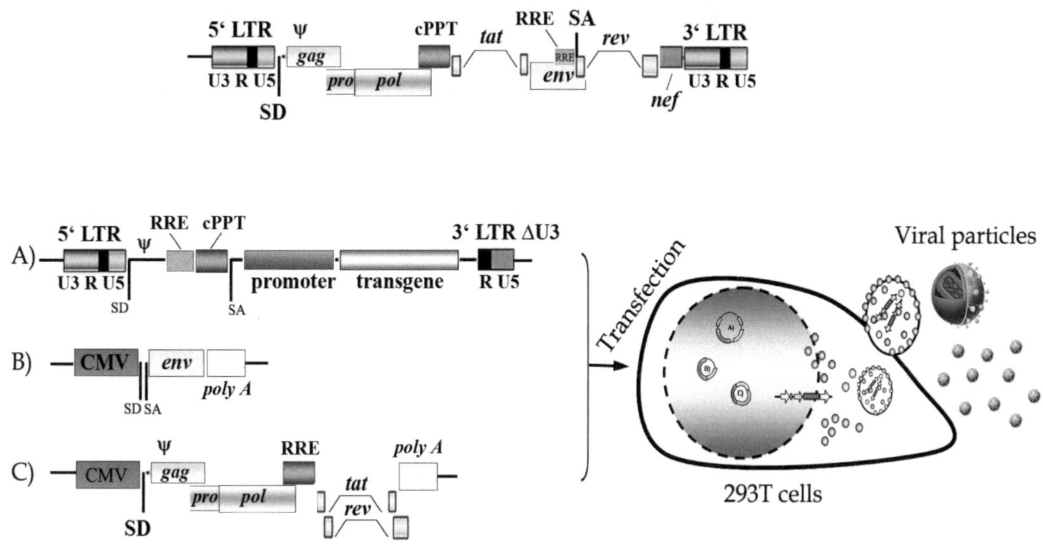

Fig. 2. Schematic representation of HIV-1 provirus DNA and HIV-1 based vector system. In the HIV-1 genome (top), the coding regions are flanked by LTRs (5´and 3´) and other *cis*-acting elements such as the Primer Binding Site (PBS), the *Rev* responsive element (RRE) and the packaging signal (Ψ). The vector genome (A) does not contain any gene from the original virus and the structural and enzymatic proteins required for particle formation, cell entry, reverse transcription and integration are supplied by other plasmid constructs (B and C) to allow the formation of a functional particle. In the majority of the vector constructs, the removed viral genes are substituted by an expression cassette consisting of an internal promoter driving the expression of a relevant transgene. To produce the viral particles, a set of three or four plasmids coding for the viral genome (A), the *env* gene (B) and the *gag-pol-rev* genes (C) are transfected into a cell line (a packaging cell line) that will be use as a vector factory. After transfection, the vector plasmid will produce the vector genome (RNA) and the other plasmids will drive the expression and synthesis of the *Env, Rev* and *Gag-Pol* proteins required for particle formation. *Abbreviations*: LTR, viral long terminal repeat; U3, LTR 3′ unique element; U5, LTR 5′ unique element; R, repeat element; SA, splice acceptor site; SD, splice donor site; ψ, viral RNA packaging signal; ΔU3, self-inactivating deletion in U3 region of 3' LTR, cPPT, central polypurine tract; RRE, Rev response element; polyA, polyadenylation signal; HEK 293T, human embryonic kidney 293T cells

Equine infectious anaemia virus (EIAV)-based vectors. Other groups have focused their attention to equine infectious anaemia virus (EIAV) based vectors(Mitrophanous *et al.*, 1999). Although EIAV-based vectors are about 10-fold less efficient in several human cell lines than HIV-1 based vectors(Ikeda *et al.*, 2002), they have demonstrated good efficiency for treatment of neuromuscular pathologies in animal models(Azzouz *et al.*, 2004; Yip *et al.*, 2006). In addition, they are able to transduce human HSCs(Siapati *et al.*, 2005) and are very efficient *in vivo*. Several groups have demonstrated their potential applicability for gene therapy applications using animal models of neurological disorders, macular dystrophy and choroidal neovascularisation. There is at the moment a Phase I/II study using EIAV vectors for the treatment of Parkinson disease (Prosavin) developed by Oxford BioMedica. The authors observed an average improvement in motor function of 26%(Trial ID: FR-0041)

Feline immunodeficiency virus(SIV)-based vectors. Feline immunodeficiency virus has been a good choice to develop LVs(Poeschla *et al.*, 1998) as demonstrated by their success in several fields (reviewed in Barraza and Poeschla, 2008). However FIV-based vectors are very inefficient expressing transgenes in human primary cells due to unknown elements that inhibit expression(Price *et al.*, 2002). This low level of transgene expression has hindered the wide use of FIV-based vectors for gene therapy strategies. In spite of this, several groups have demonstrated the potential of FIV-based vectors in animal models. Grinshpun et al. were able to attenuate disease symptoms in a murine model of glycogen storage diseases type I (GSD-Ia) by a double neonatal administration protocol(Grinshpun *et al.*2010). The authors extended survival, improved body weight, and decreased the accumulation of liver glycogen. Finally, several groups have also demonstrated that FIV integration favoured actively transcribed genes (as all retroviral vectors) but the integration preferences were more similar to those of primate lentiviruses and distinct from those of moloney murine leukemia virus, avian sarcoma leukosis virus, and foamy virus(Kang *et al.*, 2006).

Bovine immunodeficiency virus based vectors. Another alternative to HIV-1 based vectors are the LVs based on bovine immunodeficiency virus (BIV)(Berkowitz *et al.*, 2001; Matukonis *et al.*, 2002). BIV-based vectors also transduced a wide panel of gene therapy primary targets including unstimulated human HSCs. However, in spite of the generation of safer packaging cell lines for BIV-based vectors a few groups have followed these LVs as an alternative for gene therapy strategies.

In summary, the use of non-human LVs is a field of intensive research with some promising results in gene therapy. However, based on the published data it is clear that HIV-based vectors are still the vector of choice for most applications since they are more efficient and have at least the same safety profiles than non-HIV-1 based vectors. In fact, there is not a single study demonstrating that non-human LVs are safer than HIV-based LVs.

2.1.2 Foamy viral vectors (FVV)

Foamy viruses (FV) share with other retroviruses the principal genetic order of LTR, *gag–pol–env–accessory genes*–LTR, as well as the reverse transcription and integration processes. However they complete the reverse transcription process before budding from the cell membrane. Another interesting property is the stability of the resulting DNA genome that could be the reason for the excellent capability of FV vectors (FVV) to transduce rarely dividing cells, such as HSCs. Other important feature is that the viral envelope mediates access to virtually any cell type, although the viral receptor is still unknown. The viral genome is complex, as it contains not only the *gag, pol* and *env* genes, but also genes that encode proteins that are not incorporated into the viral particle (*bel-1* (*tas*) and *bet*).

FVV were developed over fifteen years ago(Schmidt and Rethwilm, 1995). The majority of FVV are based on human foamy virus (HFV) which was derived by a rare zoonotic infection of humans by a chimpanzee spumavirus (CFV)(reviewed in Williams, 2008). FVV are highly efficient for HSCs transduction, they have a favourable integration profile, can deliver large DNA fragments and are derived from a non-pathogenic virus. These properties make them a very attractive tool for gene therapy. Novel FVV vectors are devoid of the *env* gene and the internal promoter (Bel1/Tas-independent vectors) and the expression is directed by a heterologous human promoter(Trobridge *et al.*, 2002; Bastone *et al.*, 2007).

For a long time, the low FVV titers have been a major hurdle for FVV clinical applications. However, this problem has been overcome and vector titers above 10^7 per ml are routinely produced in different laboratories. Bauer et al(Bauer *et al.*, 2008) described the first successful use of a FVV to treat a genetic disease. The authors used FVV to treat canine leukocyte adhesion deficiency (CLAD). Four out of five dogs that received infusion of HSCs transduced by a FVV expressing CD18 had complete reversal of the CLAD phenotype for more than 2 years. Integration site analysis showed polyclonality of transduced cells and a decreased risk of integration near oncogenes as compared to GVs. More recently, Park et al. used FFV for conditional expression of short interfering RNAs (siRNAs) in HIV infected cells(Park *et al.*, 2009) and their results showed inhibition of HIV replication by more than 98%.

2.2 Improvements of first generation retroviral vectors

In addition to searching for new viruses for vector development, gene therapists are continuously trying to improve safety and efficiency of old (MLV-based) and new (HIV-1 based) retroviral vectors. Below we described the main strategies to achieve better safety profiles:

2.2.1 Self-inactivating (SIN) vectors

One of the major drawbacks of first generation retroviral vectors has been the use of the viral LTR U3 region to drive the expression of the transgene. The U3 contains a strong viral promoter and enhancer sequences that have been responsible for the activation of downstream host genes leading to transformation and leukemia-like diseases upon insertion in hematopoietic stem cells(Baum *et al.*, 2003; Modlich *et al.*, 2009). Therefore, one way to improve safety of retroviral vectors is to eliminate the U3 region from the 5′ LTR and to use alternative promoters to drive the expression of the transgene. Different authors have included different deletions at the U3 region in the 3′ LTR of GVs(Yu *et al.*, 1986; Olson *et al.*, 1994) and LVs(Miyoshi *et al.*, 1998; Zufferey *et al.*, 1998). During the transduction process, reverse transcription transfer this deletion also to the 5′LTR of the proviral DNA. Since the U3 region harbor the promoter and enhancer regions required for RNA transcription, this mutation not only abrogates potential mobilization of the vector but also reduces genotoxicity due to promoter/enhancer interference(Modlich *et al.*, 2006; Modlich *et al.*, 2009).

In oncoretroviruses like MVL or SNV, SIN vector development was compromised since the U3 from the 3′ LTR is partially involved in the polyadenylation of the viral RNA. Therefore, most MLV-derived SIN vectors carry a deletion that still maintain significant transcriptional activity in their long terminal repeats (LTRs). Attempts to mutate the TATA box dramatically decreased vector titers, presumably due to weak polyadenylation. However in LVs, the polyadenylation site is located just upstream of the R region of the LTR and therefore tolerate large U3 deletions without functional loss. This has facilitated the use of SIN LVs over SIN GVs counterparts.

2.2.2 Insulators

Limitations derived from randomly genome insertion of retroviral vectors have two sides, 1- possible deleterious effects of vector enhancer elements in host cell gene expression (as mentioned above) 2- the effect of chromosomal position in vector expression such as transcriptional silencing. Therefore a main goal of gene therapists has been to isolate integrative vectors from the host chromatin in such a way that 1- enhancers present in the vector can not influence expression of cellular host genes and 2- that regulatory sequences present in the host chromatin can not influence vector expression (Figure 3).

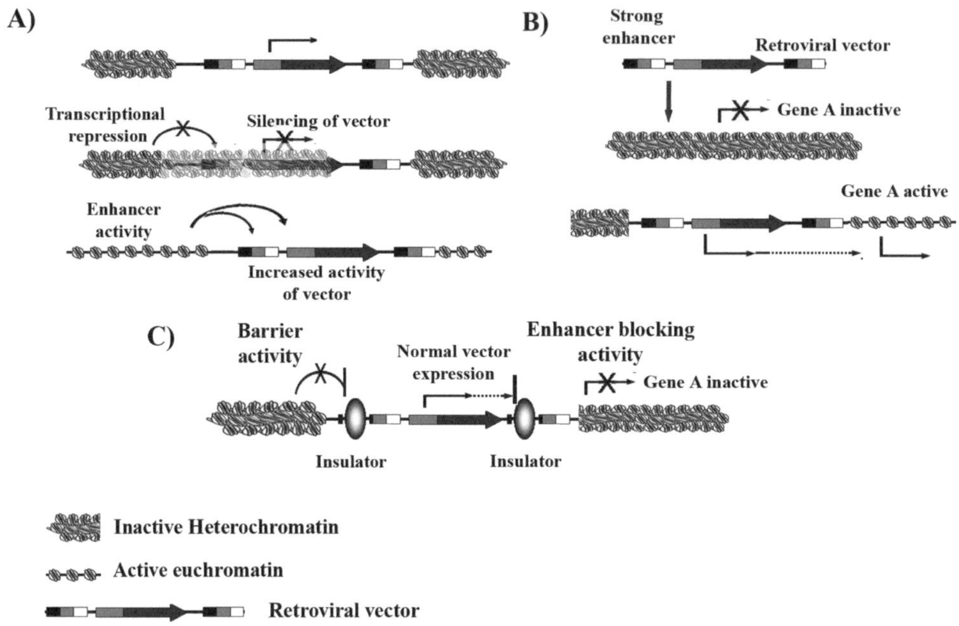

Fig. 3. Insulator functions in vector development. A) Vector expression can be enhanced or silenced if integrated in a transcriptionally active site or near heterochromatin respectively. B) Retroviral vectors can produce the activation or upregulation of poorly active or silent genes. This can lead to cell transformation. C). Retroviral vectors can be modified to reduce both effects by including insulators boundaries such as HS4 in the backbone. These insulators should have two activities; 1- a barrier activity to avoid vector silencing and a 2- enhancer blocking activity to block both the effect of chromatin enhancers on vector expression and the influence of vectors enhancer on nearby chromosomal genes.

Insulators are genetic elements near chromatin domain boundaries that function as barriers against repressive effects of neighbouring heterochromatin or preventing inappropriate activation of a promoter by nearby heterologous enhancers(Bell *et al.*, 2001). The best studied vertebrate element is a 1.2-kilobase (kb) fragment containing the chicken β-globin 5´ DNase I hypersensitive site 4 (5´HS4) (Bell *et al.*, 1999). This element can protect against position effects and also provide enhancer blocking function, two important and separable characteristics for an insulator. In addition of HS4, there are several other chromosomal elements that function as insulators in different organisms (Gaszner and Felsenfeld, 2006). Neff et al.(Neff *et al.*, 1997) hypothesized that the incorporation of chromatin insulator in gene therapy vectors should lead to improved safety and expression of therapeutic transgenes. However the incorporation of insulator elements may also have undesirable consequences such as reduction in viral titre that need to be solved(Hanawa *et al.*, 2009).
Different insulators have been used to improve safety and expression of various GVs and LVs (Emery *et al.*, 2000; Hino *et al.*, 2004; Ramezani *et al.*, 2008). Some authors have combined two different elements such as HS4 and BEAD-1 with good results(Ramezani *et al.*, 2008). The introduction of these elements into the vector backbone has been shown to decrease

genotoxicity and gene silencing(Emery *et al.*, 2000; Hino *et al.*, 2004; Arumugam *et al.*, 2007; Robert-Richard *et al.*, 2007; Ramezani *et al.*, 2008; Li *et al.*, 2009). Nienhuis and colleagues demonstrated that the inclusion of the insulator in the retroviral construct suppressed cellular transformation(Evans-Galea *et al.*, 2007). These important results have pushed gene therapists to incorporate these elements into therapeutic vectors, especially when the strategy involves gene transfer into stem cells.

2.2.3 Improved polyadenylation signal

Although long distance enhancer interactions are the most frequent form of retroviral insertional mutagenesis, read-through transcripts (not stopping at the polyadenylation site contained in the vector) could be, theoretically, an important safety problem. In retroviruses, the polyA motif is contained within the R region of the LTRs and is therefore present in both ends of the transcript. To avoid premature termination and polyadenylation in the 5´R region, retroviruses have developed weak polyA sites and additional mechanisms of 5 ´polyA site suppression. In addition, SIN vectors lack the majority of the U3 region and this increases the probability of read-through. The insufficient termination causes read-through of randomly integrated retroviral sequences into cellular genes and contribute to the up-regulation of cellular proto-oncogenes, potentially triggering malignant transformation (Almarza *et al.*; Schambach *et al.*, 2007). Some groups have shown that the inclusion of upstream polyadenylation enhancer elements improves the efficiency of 3' end mRNA processing in GV and LV SIN vectors(Schambach *et al.*, 2007; Hager *et al.*, 2008). The resulting vectors not only have improved titer and transgene expression in target cells but they also displayed a lower rate of vector mobilization(Koldej and Anson, 2009). Still, whether stronger polyA signals in retroviral vectors will result in an improvement of biosafety must be further analyzed in animal models.

3. Novel non-viral systems to achieve efficient transgene integrations

Although most gene therapy approaches use viral-based vectors to obtain stable integration, new non-viral systems may offer some advantages: 1- Viral vector preparations, in particular those for clinical use, are very expensive and time consuming. Non-viral vectors are less expensive and easy to manufacture. 2- Viral vectors need packaging cell lines for their production whereas other non-viral vectors rely on cell free systems with defined components. 3- Non-viral vectors are less immunogenic than viral systems(Yant *et al.*, 2000). 4- Finally, integrative viral vectors have a limited packaging capacity whereas non-viral systems can deliver larger DNA fragments (Zayed *et al.*, 2004; Ding *et al.*, 2005). The use of non-viral vectors has been limited due to the low efficiency, low rate of integration and silencing issues. However there have been important advances in the field in recent years. Two main strategies using non-viral systems, transposons and zinc-finger nuleases, are having a mayor impact in the area:

3.1 Transposons

Transposons (in particular the *Sleeping Beauty* (SB)) are becoming serious players as gene delivery tools. Transposons are DNA sequences that can move from one chromosomal location to another utilizing an enzyme named transposase which recognizes two sequences flanking the transposon. Any sequence included between the two flanking regions can also be mobilized and this characteristic makes the transposons attractive as a gene therapy tools to achieve stable transgene integrations (Figure 4). The mechanism involved behind the mobilization of transposons is described elsewhere(Izsvak *et al.*, 2000). Briefly, the inverted terminal repeats (ITR) flanking the transposon are recognized by the transposase which excises the transposon from the genome (or from a donor plasmid). The transposon is inserted into TA sequences in the genome with no preference for genes or intergenic regions. This characteristic makes the transposon integration semi-random. It seems that they induce low epigenetic changes and no adverse effects have been reported yet(Zhu *et al.*2010). To avoid further transposition events, the expression of the transposase must be transient in the target cell. To increase the safety level of transposition, three different ways to target SB transposition have been proposed based in the addition of particular DNA binding domains to the SB transposase (reviewed in Izsvak *et al.*2010).

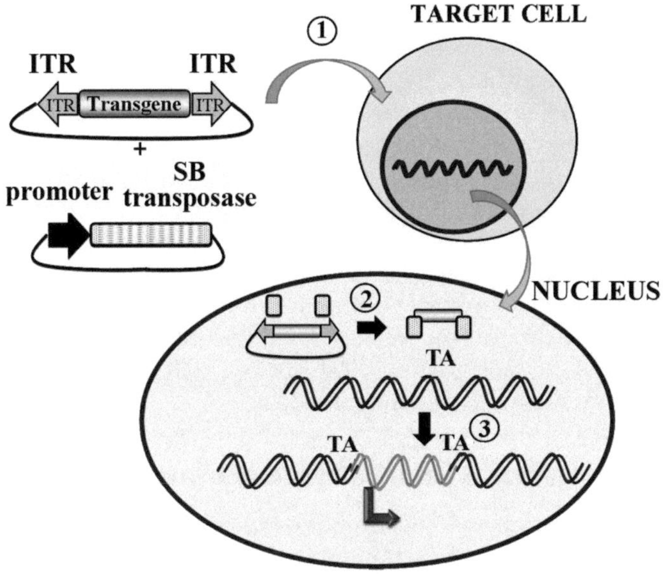

ITR: Inverted Terminal Repeats; SB: Sleeping Beauty Transposase.

Fig. 4. Transposition mechanism of Sleeping Beauty transposon: 1) Delivery of both the SB transposon (containing the genetic material to be integrated) and the SB transposase (expressed under the control of a constitutive promoter) into the nucleus of the target cell. The transposon is flanked by the ITR. 2) In the nucleus, the SB transposase cleaves the transposon at the ITR sites. 3) The SB transposase integrates the transgene into any accessible TA site in the host genome.

The development of transposases with higher activity (Sleeping Beauty transposase, SB10 or SB100)(Izsvak *et al.*, 2000; Mates *et al.*, 2009) and the new delivery techniques such as lipofection, PEI-complexes, hydrodynamic injection, nucleofection or electroporation have achieved efficient integration of large fragments of DNA into hard to modify cells, as hESCs (Wilber *et al.*, 2007; Mates *et al.*, 2009) or HSCs (Mates *et al.*, 2009). These improvements have allowed the use of SB as a real alternative for therapeutic strategies for diseases such as junctional epidermolysis bullosa, haemophilia A and B, pulmonary hypertension, glioblastoma, inherited tyrosinemia, mucopolysaccharidosis, lung transplantation-associated complications and B-lymphoid malignancies(Izsvak *et al.*2010). Indeed, three clinical trials have been approved for the treatment of CD19+ B cell malignancies (Trials ID: US-0922, US-1003 and US-1022) using SB transposons.

4. Site-specific integrative vector systems

Although the systems mentioned above can reduce genotoxicity of first generation integrative MLV-based vectors, they still integrate randomly and have therefore potential genotoxicity consequences. Therefore, several groups have dedicated much effort to achieve site-specific integration to safer genomic areas. This strategy allows the selection of areas that are less rich in genes involved in tumorogenicity and are therefore less likely to cause serious side effects. However as we will see in this section, the low efficacy and/or poor integration specificity of most site-specific integrative systems have been mayor drawbacks of this strategy.

4.1 Adeno-associated viruses (AAV)

Adeno-associated virus (AAV) are nonpathogenic, nonenveloped DNA virus that belong to the parvovirus family. AAV virions contain a single-stranded DNA genome of only 4,680 bases, which is flanked by two inverted terminal repeats (ITRs). AAV can replicate in cell culture only in the presence of a co-infection by a helper virus, either adenovirus (Ad) or herpesvirus (HV). Infection of human cells with wild-type AAV results in site-specific integration into the AAVS1 region of chromosome 19 (Kotin et A., 1990). Recombinant AAV (rAAV) vectors have an excellent safety record with demonstrated efficiency and safety in preclinical studies in thousands of animal studies. AAV have been very successful for human gene therapy strategies in liver, muscle and eye (reviewed in Rolling, 2010; Tang *et al.*, 2010); van der Laan *et al.*, 2011), however, the therapeutic benefits did not correlate with site-specific vector integration. Expression of *Rep78* or *Rep68* is necessary for targeted integration of AAV-derived DNA and, in its absence, AAV genome is kept as episomal DNA or integrates by nonhomologous recombination at random locations. The limited DNA cargo capacity of AAV particles and the need to maintain the *rep* ORF, precludes the use of AAV itself as a site-specific integration vector. It is now well established that the rAAV vector genomes exist in a predominantly episomal form and that transduced dividing cells lose expression with time (Miao *et al.*, 1998). However, the non-specific integration of rAAV vectors allow stable expression in several cell types, including hematopoietic stem cells (Maina *et al.*, 2008) and germ line stem cells (Honaramooz *et al.*, 2008). AAV vectors have been used in preclinic studies of immunodeficiencies like CGD, a heterogeneous group of disorders arising from molecular lesions in the genes encoding a phagocyte-specific enzyme system, the NADPH-oxidase. Vectors based on AAV with a functional copy of the p47phox gene have been used to transduce EBV-immortalized B cells derived from patients with CGD, achieving a stable expression of protein and restoration of NADPH-oxidase function in these cells for 3 months without selection (Thrasher *et al.*, 1995). In summary, although rAAV can achieve stable integration in certain cell types, this integration is random as for retroviral vectors and can cause mutations (Nakai *et al.*, 2003) and tumor development (Donsante *et al.*, 2007). Therefore, although AAV vectors can achieve stable gene expression, they are not safer than other integrative systems such as GVs or LVs.

4.2 AAV Hybrid vectors

AAV hybrid viral vectors utilize the cis- (ITRs) and trans- (*Rep68/78*) acting components of AAV viruses to specifically target transgenes into the AAVS1 integration site at chromosome 19. This technology has opened the possibility of integrating large DNA sequences in a site specific fashion with the aim of minimizing genotoxicity. AAV-Hybrid vectors based on plasmids, baculovirus, Ad and HSV can potentially accommodate genetic material of more than 30.000 base pairs (Smith, 2008). Two factors are limiting in this system, the first one is the delivery efficiency of the transgene flanked by the AAV ITRs and the *Rep68/78* to the target cells and the second is the *Rep68/78* protein toxicity. In fact, *Rep* proteins down-regulate the expression c-H-*ras*, c-*fos*, c-*myc*, and c-*sis* and can inhibit the proliferation of some cell lines. In addition *Rep*-mediated integration at AAVS1 can lead to nonspecific genomic rearrangements at the same locus. The frequency and severity of these undesired effects might be attenuated or suppressed by setting a time limit to the activity of *Rep* proteins in target cells. This has been achieved by trasfecting *Rep* proteins or *rep* mRNA directly, by using inducible promoters or by construction of regulated *Rep* chimeras.

4.2.1 Plasmid/AAV

Based on data obtained from AAV integration process, several groups have designed a site-specific integration system based in two plasmids: an integrating plasmid containing AAV ITRs and the second providing the AAV Rep proteins. Co-transfection of both plasmids in 293T cells achieved site-specific integration in the AAVS1 integration site. This system has achieved stable expression in several cell lines including hematopoietic cells(Howden *et al.*, 2008). However the low plasmid transfection efficiency in primary cells has limited its use in gene therapy applications. New gene delivery technologies will certainly improve the results obtained with this system.

4.2.2 Baculovirus/AAV

The baculoviruses are a family of large, double stranded DNA (80-180kb), enveloped viruses that infects only invertebrates. The baculovirus *Autographa californica multiple nucleopolyhedrovirus* (AcMNPV)-based vectors have recently been developed as a new tool for gene therapy (reviewed in Hu *et al.* 2010). Latest generation of baculovirus vectors systems are safe, easy to use and amenable to scale up. Baculovirus vectors are able to transduce a wide range of human cell lines, including primary cells such as bone marrow fibroblasts, neural cells, hepatocytes and mesenchymal stem cells. Zeng and co-workers(Zeng *et al.*, 2007) have demonstrated their ability to transduce human embryonic stem cells without altering their characteristics. The hybrid vectors contained three promoters, one driving the expression of the complete baculovirus genome, the second expressing *eGFP* and the third (AAVp5) driving the expression of *Rep78*. However, in spite of their potential, the usefulness of this technology for stable integrations of transgenes into stem cells has not yet been achieved.

4.2.3 Adenovirus/AAV

Adenoviruses (Ad) are non-enveloped non-integrative viruses composed of a nucleocapsid and a double-stranded linear DNA genome. There are 51 immunologically distinct human Ad serotypes, however, the subgroup C serotypes 2 or 5 are the most used for vector development. The wild type Ad genome is approximately 35 kb of which up to 34 kb can be replaced with foreign DNA in the helper dependent (HD) Ad gutless vector. Ad vectors can mediate high level of transduction in a wide variety of both quiescent (post-mitotic cells) and proliferating cells. However, since they are non-integrating, transgene expression in dividing cells is progressively lost. The development of Ad/AAV hybrid vectors(Lieber *et al.*, 1999; Recchia *et al.*, 1999) aim to increase the integration efficiency. Clearly, a vector that combines the advantages of Ad (high titer, high infectivity, and large capacity) with the integration capability of AAV would be advantageous for gene therapy. The Ad/AAV hybrid vectors system requires two Ad vectors; one containing the Ad-ITRs, the Ad packaging signal and the AAV-ITRs flanking the DNA of interest and a second one expressing the AAV *Rep68/78* protein (Figure 5).

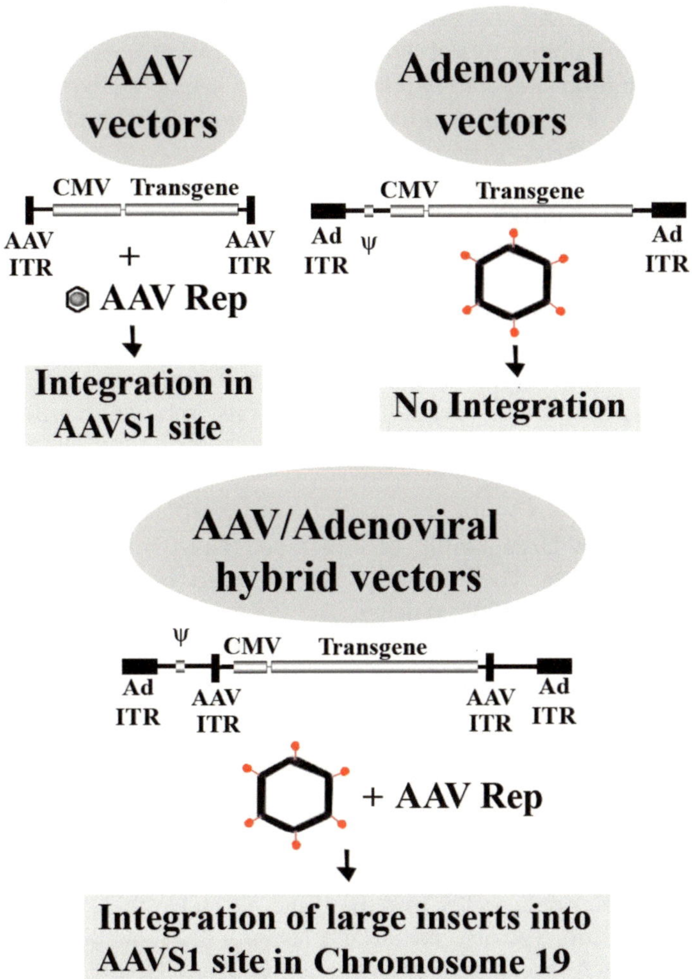

Fig. 5. *AAV/Adenoviral hybrid vectors.* The AAV/Ad hybrid vectors combine the large packaging capacity of Ad with the site-specific integration potential of AAV vectors. Either AAV *Rep68* or *Rep78* proteins are sufficient to mediate insertion of AAV-ITR-containing DNA into the AAVS1 on chromosome 19. By including the AAV-ITR into the adenoviral backbone and expressing *Rep68* or *Rep78* we can achieve integration of the adenoviral vector into the AAVS1 site. Only DNA sequences flanked by the AAV-ITR will be integrated into the chromosome 19. The most efficient systems use an additional adenoviral vector to produce the *Rep68/78* proteins required for specific integration.

Although Ad vectors harboring transgenes flanked by AAV-ITRs can be produced easily, the production of Ad expressing *Rep68/78* is more complicated due to the *Rep68/78* inhibition of Ad replication. Recchia and co-workers (Recchia *et al.*, 1999) tackled this problem by expressing Rep78 gene under the control of promoters with low activity in the packaging cells. Another relevant issue is that transduction of stem cells with first generation Ad vectors is associated with toxicity due to viral gene expression. Therefore helper dependent (HD) Ad vectors depleted of all viral genes should be used for stem cells transduction. In fact most Ad/AAV hybrid systems are based on HD Ad vectors which have demonstrated their ability to stably express several transgenes by specific integration into the AAVS1 integration site, both *in vitro* and *in vivo* achieving expression of therapeutic levels of *Factor VIII* in hemophilia A mice (Gnatenko *et al.*, 2004) and of *dystrophin* in mdx mice (Goncalves *et al.*, 2005).

Although the Ad/AAV hybrid system has achieved specific integration into the AAVA1 site, the efficiency is far from 100%. Recently Wang et al(Wang and Lieber, 2006) demonstrated that Ad/AAV can achieve up to 30% efficiency of stable expression (30% of the cloned cells have stable expression of the transgene). In addition only 30% of these clones stably expressing the transgene were integrated at the AAVA1 site while in the other 70% the stable expression was a consequence of homologous recombination or random insertion. Further knowledge of the mechanism involved in site specific integration into the AAVA1 site and the processes involving homologous recombination will certainly increase the potential of these vectors.

4.2.4 Herpesvirus/AAV

Herpesvirus (HSV) are a large family of enveloped DNA virus that cause diseases in animals, including humans. Their genome is composed of large (over 150kb) double stranded linear DNA encoding 100-200 genes. The DNA is packed by an icosahedral protein structure or capsid that is surrounded by a lipid bilayer membrane (envelope). HSV-1 have several characteristics that make them a promising gene delivery vector such as their capacity to package large amounts of heterologous DNA (over 100kb), their ability to establish persistent, lifelong infections and a broad range of cell tropism including dividing and non-dividing cells (reviewed in Berto *et al.*, 2005)). An important property of HSV-1-based vectors is the ability to deliver a complete genomic locus, in which the native promoter and regulatory regions drive and control expression of the transgene. However first and second generation HSV-1 based vectors require the expression of regulatory viral proteins that hinder their applicability into the clinic. To tackle this problem several authors developed HSV amplicon vectors, bacterial plasmids that contain only the origin of replication and the DNA packaging/cleavage signal from HSV-1. These HSV amplicon vectors are dependent on helper virus function to provide the replication machinery and structural proteins necessary for packaging the amplicon vector DNA into viral particles. Helper packaging function is provided by a replication-defective virus or by packaging methods using a set of 5 overlapping cosmids or bacterial artificial chromosomes (BAC) that encode the entire HSV genome.

The HSV/AAV hybrid vectors combine the high efficiency and large transgene capacity of HSV-1 amplicon vectors with the potential for site-specific chromosomal integration of AAV vectors. The hybrid HSV/AAV vectors contain the origin of DNA replication and the DNA cleavage/packaging signal of HSV-1 and a transgene (ie *lacZ* reporter gene) under the control of a desired promoter flanked by AAV inverted terminal repeat (ITR) sequences. HSV/AAA hybrid vectors are relatively inefficient in achieving stable expression of the trasngene (2-20% depending of the cell line and the vector system), however they are one of the most efficient systems to direct site-specific integration (50-70% of stably-expressing cells). One of the main advantages of HSV/AAV hybrid vectors is their capability to achieve site-specific integration of up to 100kb in a significant proportion of transduced cells. Although HSV/AAV vectors have been successful in animal models of Ataxia-Telangiectasia(Cortes *et al.*, 2003; Cortes *et al.*, 2008) they still have some safety concerns such as the low efficiency in important target cells (HSCs) and the random integrations observed in over 40% of stably expressing cells.

4.3 Site-specific integrases

Another alternative used by gene therapists to achieve site-specific integration of therapeutic genes is based on naturally occurring site-specific integrases recognizing specific target in the human genome. One of such enzymes is the *Streptomyces bacteriophage* derived *phiC31* integrase, which mediates site-specific integration of plasmid DNA (pDNA) into mammalian host genomes(Thyagarajan *et al.*, 2001; Olivares *et al.*, 2002). This integrase can insert large DNA elements (over ten kilobases in size) containing an *attB* sequence into genomes containing *attP* sites. Importantly, this integrase recognizes sequences in the mammalian genome termed pseudo-*attP* sites(Sclimenti *et al.*, 2001). These pseudo attP sites are also present in the human genome and can mediate efficient *phiC31* -integrase-mediated integration (Figure 6). In addition, directed evolution has rendered new integrases specific for pseudo attP sites located at human chromosome 8(Sclimenti *et al.*, 2001). Using this technology several authors have shown the potential of the *phiC31* integrase system for the treatment of lung diseases(Aneja *et al.*, 2007) and human skin diseases(Ortiz-Urda *et al.*, 2002). Others have shown long-term transgene expression in liver(Olivares *et al.*, 2002) and retina(Chalberg *et al.*, 2005) .

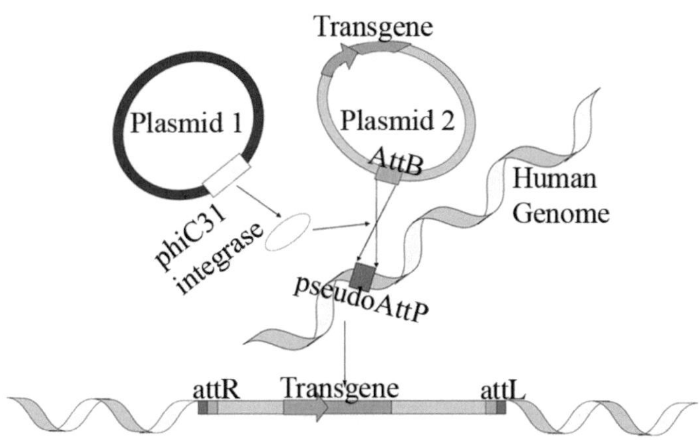

Fig. 6. Site specific integration of *phi*C31 integrase in the human genome. *Phi*C31 integrase mediates the integration of a plasmid containing an *attB* site and the transgene into *pseudo-attP* sites at the human genome. Once integrated the donor sequence is flanked by attR and attL sequences.

However safety of *phiC31* integrase-mediated integration has not yet been studied in detail. Several authors have found imprecise integrations into pseudo-attP sites resulting in DNA deletions(Thyagarajan *et al.*, 2001; Ehrhardt *et al.*, 2005) and others have found that the *phiC31* integrase may cause chromosomal instability(Held *et al.*, 2005; Chalberg *et al.*, 2006; Liu *et al.*, 2006). In any case, no serious adverse events have occurred so far in animal models and therefore further studies are required to assess the safety of this vector system.

4.4 Zinc-finger DNA binding domains-transposases chimeras

Other attempts to target DNA integration to specific sites have used transposases from sleaping beauty (SB)(Wilson *et al.*, 2005) or *piggyback(Wu et al., 2006)* transposons. SB-based vector systems have been successful in several preclinical models(reviewed in Izsvak *et al.*, 2010). However, first generation transposons have two major limitations; the low rate of integration compared to viral-based vectors and the nonspecific integration of the transgene. The incorporation of DNA-binding domains into the transposase can potentially increase efficiency and result in site-specific integration. SB transposase fused to the *Sp1* zinc finger DNA binding domain has achieved specific integration in *sp1*(Wilson *et al.*, 2005). Similarly, Wu et al*(Wu et al., 2006)* demonstrated targeted integration to *gal4* sites by coupling *Gal4* DNA-binding domain to piggyback transposase. As proof-of-principle, these results are promising while further work is needed to provide more information about non-desired integrations and to target other integration sites. Targeting *sp1* or *gal4* sites is not, in principle, the most appropriate strategy for most gene therapy applications since they could affect gene expression of a wide range of relevant genes.

4.5 Zinc-Finger Nucleases for site directed integration

In addition to the use of ZFN for gene repair (see below in point 5), ZFN can be use to introduce expression cassettes specifically into already identified "safe harbors", which are particular locations in the genome where the insertion of exogenous DNA is theoretically less genotoxic. This is the case for the adeno-associated visus integration site (AAVS1) locus in human or the ROSA26 locus in mouse. This strategy has already been utilized by some groups(DeKelver *et al.*; Hockemeyer *et al.*, 2009) and tested in cell lines including hESC. This strategy overcomes the need to develop ZFNs for a particular mutation for each particular disease, which nowadays is an expensive, cumbersome and time consuming process.

5. Gene correction by enhanced homologous recombination

Gene correction aims to repair a defective gene directly in the cellular genome by gene targeting, a process in which a DNA molecule introduced into a cell replaces the corresponding chromosomal segment by homologous recombination. This is certainly the more logic way to cure primary immunodeficiencies since the *"in situ"* correction of the mutation(s) will restore normal physiological gene function and therefore will warrant sustained and regulated expression of the repaired gene through its endogenous promoter. However, site-specific engineering of the human genome has been limited by the low frequency of homologous recombination (HR), by the requirement of sophisticated targeting vectors and by the use of drug selection. Recently, improvements in DNA-delivery technology and in the development of customized zinc-finger-nucleases (ZFN)(reviewed in Cathomen and Joung, 2008) have awaken new interest in this technology for its use in gene therapy approaches.

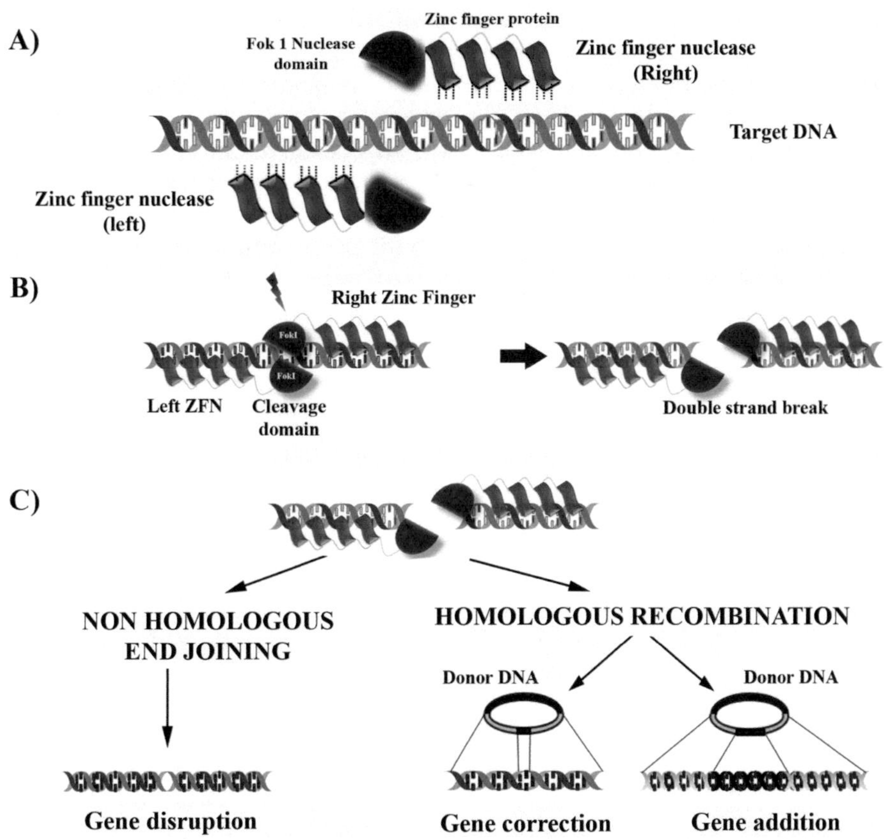

Fig. 7. Gene targeting using zinc finger nucleases. A) Zinc finger nucleases are chimeric proteins containing a zinc finger domain specific for a 9-12 nucleotide sequences and a Fok 1 nuclease domain that requires dimerization to cut DNA. For targeting specific DNA sequences the system require two ZFNs (right and left) each recognizing a 12 nucleotide sequence separate by a 4-6 nucleotide sequence. B) Once the zinc finger binds to its targets, the nuclease cleaves the DNA creating a double strand break C) The double strand break induces the own cell repair mechanisms to resolve the damage. The two main processes are non-homologous end joining (NHEJ) and homologous recombination directed repair. If a donor DNA (with homologous sequences) is not available the break is repaired by NHEJ yielding small deletions or additions. This process can be harnessed to induce gene disruption. When a homologous DNA sequence is present, the cell can repair the break by homologous recombination. The transfection of donor DNA with homologous regions together with the zinc finger nucleases allows gene editing by including the desired sequences inside the homologous regions. This system can be used to introduce small changes for gene repair or bigger changes to promote gene addition.

Zinc finger nucleases can be considered custom-designed molecular scissors. ZFNs combine the non-specific cleavage of an endonuclease (*FokI*) with the specific recognition properties of zinc finger proteins (ZFPs) to cut at the desired chromosomal locus inside the cells(Ashworth *et al.,* 2006)(Figure 7). A single zinc finger domain recognizes three consecutive nucleotides. The ZFN is composed by a ZFP containing three to four zinc finger domains, which recognize a 9 to 12 nucleotide sequence, and the FokI domain. The DNA cleavage by *FokI* requires dimerization(Miller *et al.*, 2007) and therefore two different ZFPs must properly bind to the DNA side-to-side from the breaking point. Once the target DNA has been cut, the cells´ own repair machinery resolves the break by non homologous end joining (NHEJ) or homologous recombination (HR) depending on the absence or presence of a donor DNA (Figure 7). When not present, the DNA break is repaired by NHEJ and when a donor DNA is present HR is the main mechanism.

Using this principle, ZFNs have proven invaluable for stimulating homology-directed gene repair in a variety of cell types. The accuracy and high efficiency of the HR process combined with the ability to design ZFNs that target most DNA sequences make this technology a powerful tool for gene correction. Recent results have shown that ZFNs can be used to create targeting frequencies from 5-50% in the absence of selection in several cell lines(Urnov *et al.*, 2005; Miller *et al.*, 2007) including primary T cells(Perez *et al.*, 2008), hematopoietic stem cells(Lombardo *et al.*, 2007), mesenchymal stem cells(Benabdallah *et al.*) and embryonic stem cells(Hockemeyer *et al.*, 2009).

Recently, ZFNs have shown *in vivo* correction of a humanized mouse model of hemophilia B (Hojun *et al.*, 2010). In this work, in vivo administration of AAV expressing the ZFNs achieved cleavage of the target site in up to 45% of the hepatocytes. When co-administered together with donor plasmids containing the correct version of the gene the authors achieved circulating F.IX levels 2-7% of normal which was enough to obtain phenotypic correction of the defect of clot formation.

The ZFNs have also been used in clinic not to correct a mutated gene but to disrupt the expression of a disease-causing-gene. Several clinical trials have been approved to use ZFNs with this aims: Reik et al have proposed the use of Zinc finger nucleases targeting the *glucocorticoid receptor* of allogenic transgenic Il13-expressing CTLs with idea to make them resistant to glucocorticoids for the treatment of glioblastoma (ClinicalTrials.gov Identifier: NCT01082926). Other two groups have targeted *CCR5* for the treatment of HIV, used as a co-receptor for HIV entrance (Holt *et al.*; Perez *et al.*, 2008) (ClinicalTrials.gov Identifier: NCT00842634 and NCT01044654).

6. Conclusion

Stable gene modification without affecting normal cellular function is a main goal both for basic and applied science. Most gene therapy targets, such as inherited, infectious and degenerative diseases will benefit from a safe and efficient integrative system. Old strategies to achieve stable gene medication are either very inefficient (homologous recombination) or very genotoxic (gammaretroviral gene transfer). Retroviral vectors derived from gammaretroviruses (the most widely used vectors for gene therapy studies) were the only alternative for stable gene modification for years. They were the first vectors to show real therapeutic effect but they also showed a high risk of cellular transformation, producing leukaemia in several patients. As we have seen in this chapter, a variety of different strategies are under development aiming to achieve efficient and stable gene modification with minor or undetected genomic alterations. Although exciting new non-viral technologies have been developed that efficiently integrate the genome into safe harbors in the genome, we are still investigating the real safety benefits of these technologies. By taking together efficiency and safety we can, at this moment, argue in favour of improved viral technologies as the better tools for clinical use. New viral vectors are more efficient and safer than first generation gammaretroviral vectors used in previous clinical trials. In particular, latest generation of lentiviral vectors have seen a major boost and we are convinced that new exciting clinical results will be coming in the next few years.

7. Acknowledgments

This work has been supported by the Fondo de Investigaciones Sanitarias (FIS) grant PS09/00340 and Junta de Andalucia grants P09-CTS-04532 and PI0001/2009 to Francisco Martín. Pilar Muñoz (Sara Borrel Contract) and Per Anderson (Miguel Servet Contract) are financed by the FIS. Karim Benabdellah is financed by the Consejería de Innovación y Ciencia (Junta de Andalucía). Marién Cobo is financed by the Fundación Publica Andaluza Progreso y Salud (Consejería de Salud-Junta de Andalucía).

8. References

Almarza, D., Bussadori, G., Navarro, M., Mavilio, F., Larcher, F., and Murillas, R. (2011) Risk assessment in skin gene therapy: viral-cellular fusion transcripts generated by proviral transcriptional read-through in keratinocytes transduced with self-inactivating lentiviral vectors. *Gene Ther*(Mar 3), ISSN:1476-5462 (Electronic) 0969-7128 (Linking)

Aneja, M.K., Imker, R., and Rudolph, C. (2007). Phage phiC31 integrase-mediated genomic integration and long-term gene expression in the lung after nonviral gene delivery. *J Gene Med* 9,11, (Nov),967-975, ISSN:1099-498X (Print)

Arumugam, P.I., Scholes, J., Perelman, N., Xia, P., Yee, J.K., and Malik, P. (2007). Improved human beta-globin expression from self-inactivating lentiviral vectors carrying the chicken hypersensitive site-4 (cHS4) insulator element. *Mol Ther* 15,10, (Oct),1863-1871, ISSN:1525-0016 (Print)

Ashworth, J., Havranek, J.J., Duarte, C.M., Sussman, D., Monnat, R.J., Jr., Stoddard, B.L., and Baker, D. (2006). Computational redesign of endonuclease DNA binding and cleavage specificity. *Nature* 441,7093, (Jun 1), 656-659, ISSN:1476-4687 (Electronic)

Azzouz, M., Le, T., Ralph, G.S., Walmsley, L., Monani, U.R., Lee, D.C., Wilkes, F., Mitrophanous, K.A., Kingsman, S.M., Burghes, A.H., and Mazarakis, N.D. (2004). Lentivector-mediated SMN replacement in a mouse model of spinal muscular atrophy. *J Clin Invest* 114,12, (Dec), 1726-1731, ISSN:0021-9738 (Print)

Barraza, R.A., and Poeschla, E.M. (2008). Human gene therapy vectors derived from feline lentiviruses. *Vet Immunol Immunopathol* 123,1-2, (May 15), 23-31, ISSN:0165-2427 (Print) 0165-2427 (Linking)

Bastone, P., Romen, F., Liu, W., Wirtz, R., Koch, U., Josephson, N., Langbein, S., and Lochelt, M. (2007). Construction and characterization of efficient, stable and safe replication-deficient foamy virus vectors. *Gene Ther* 14,7, (Apr), 613-620, ISSN:0969-7128 (Print)

Bauer, T.R., Jr., Allen, J.M., Hai, M., Tuschong, L.M., Khan, I.F., Olson, E.M., Adler, R.L., Burkholder, T.H., Gu, Y.C., Russell, D.W., and Hickstein, D.D. (2008). Successful treatment of canine leukocyte adhesion deficiency by foamy virus vectors. *Nat Med* 14,1, (Jan), 93-97, ISSN:1546-170X (Electronic)

Baum, C., Dullmann, J., Li, Z., Fehse, B., Meyer, J., Williams, D.A., and Von Kalle, C. (2003). Side effects of retroviral gene transfer into hematopoietic stem cells. *Blood* 101,6, (Mar 15), 2099-2114,

Bell, A.C., West, A.G., and Felsenfeld, G. (1999). The protein CTCF is required for the enhancer blocking activity of vertebrate insulators. *Cell* 98,3, (Aug 6), 387-396, ISSN:0092-8674 (Print)

Bell, A.C., West, A.G., and Felsenfeld, G. (2001). Insulators and boundaries: versatile regulatory elements in the eukaryotic. *Science* 291,5503, (Jan 19), 447-450, ISSN:0036-8075 (Print)

Benabdallah, B.F., Allard, E., Yao, S., Friedman, G., Gregory, P.D., Eliopoulos, N., Fradette, J., Spees, J.L., Haddad, E., Holmes, M.C., and Beausejour, C.M. Targeted gene addition to human mesenchymal stromal cells as a cell-based plasma-soluble protein delivery platform. *Cytotherapy* 12,3, (May), 394-399, ISSN:1477-2566 (Electronic)1465-3249 (Linking)

Berkowitz, R., Ilves, H., Lin, W.Y., Eckert, K., Coward, A., Tamaki, S., Veres, G., and Plavec, I. (2001). Construction and molecular analysis of gene transfer systems derived from bovine immunodeficiency virus. *J Virol* 75,7, 3371-3382.,

Berto, E., Bozac, A., and Marconi, P. (2005). Development and application of replication-incompetent HSV-1-based vectors. *Gene Ther* 12 Suppl 1(Oct), S98-102, ISSN:0969-7128 (Print)

Cathomen, T., and Joung, J.K. (2008). Zinc-finger nucleases: the next generation emerges. *Mol Ther* 16,7, (Jul), 1200-1207, ISSN:1525-0024 (Electronic)

Cockrell, A.S., and Kafri, T. (2007). Gene delivery by lentivirus vectors. *Mol Biotechnol* 36,3, (Jul), 184-204, ISSN:1073-6085 (Print) 1073-6085 (Linking)

Cortes, M.L., Bakkenist, C.J., Di Maria, M.V., Kastan, M.B., and Breakefield, X.O. (2003). HSV-1 amplicon vector-mediated expression of ATM cDNA and correction of the ataxia-telangiectasia cellular phenotype. *Gene Ther* 10,16, (Aug), 1321-1327,

Cortes, M.L., Oehmig, A., Saydam, O., Sanford, J.D., Perry, K.F., Fraefel, C., and Breakefield, X.O. (2008). Targeted integration of functional human ATM cDNA into genome mediated by HSV/AAV hybrid amplicon vector. *Mol Ther* 16,1, (Jan), 81-88, ISSN:1525-0024 (Electronic)

Chalberg, T.W., Genise, H.L., Vollrath, D., and Calos, M.P. (2005). phiC31 integrase confers genomic integration and long-term transgene expression in rat retina. *Invest Ophthalmol Vis Sci* 46,6, (Jun), 2140-2146, ISSN:0146-0404 (Print)

Chalberg, T.W., Portlock, J.L., Olivares, E.C., Thyagarajan, B., Kirby, P.J., Hillman, R.T., Hoelters, J., and Calos, M.P. (2006). Integration specificity of phage phiC31 integrase in the human genome. *J Mol Biol* 357,1, (Mar 17), 28-48, ISSN:0022-2836 (Print)

Chang, A.H., and Sadelain, M. (2007). The genetic engineering of hematopoietic stem cells: the rise of lentiviral vectors, the conundrum of the ltr, and the promise of lineage-restricted vectors. *Mol Ther* 15,3, (Mar), 445-456, ISSN:1525-0024 (Electronic)

Dekelver, R.C., Choi, V.M., Moehle, E.A., Paschon, D.E., Hockemeyer, D., Meijsing, S.H., Sancak, Y., Cui, X., Steine, E.J., Miller, J.C., Tam, P., Bartsevich, V.V., Meng, X., Rupniewski, I., Gopalan, S.M., Sun, H.C., Pitz, K.J., Rock, J.M., Zhang, L., Davis, G.D., Rebar, E.J., Cheeseman, I.M., Yamamoto, K.R., Sabatini, D.M., Jaenisch, R., Gregory, P.D., and Urnov, F.D. Functional genomics, proteomics, and regulatory DNA analysis in isogenic settings using zinc finger nuclease-driven transgenesis into a safe harbor locus in the human genome. *Genome Res* 20,8, (Aug), 1133-1142, ISSN:1549-5469 (Electronic)1088-9051 (Linking)

Delenda, C. (2004). Lentiviral vectors: optimization of packaging, transduction and gene expression. *J Gene Med* 6 Suppl 1(Feb), S125-138, ISSN:1099-498X (Print)

Ding, S., Wu, X., Li, G., Han, M., Zhuang, Y., and Xu, T. (2005). Efficient transposition of the piggyBac (PB) transposon in mammalian cells and mice. *Cell* 122,3, (Aug 12), 473-483, ISSN:0092-8674 (Print)0092-8674 (Linking)

Donsante, A., Miller, D.G., Li, Y., Vogler, C., Brunt, E.M., Russell, D.W., and Sands, M.S. (2007). AAV vector integration sites in mouse hepatocellular carcinoma. *Science* 317,5837, (Jul 27), 477, ISSN:1095-9203 (Electronic)

Ehrhardt, A., Xu, H., Huang, Z., Engler, J.A., and Kay, M.A. (2005). A direct comparison of two nonviral gene therapy vectors for somatic integration: in vivo evaluation of the bacteriophage integrase phiC31 and the Sleeping Beauty transposase. *Mol Ther* 11,5, (May), 695-706, ISSN:1525-0016 (Print)

Emery, D.W., Yannaki, E., Tubb, J., and Stamatoyannopoulos, G. (2000). A chromatin insulator protects retrovirus vectors from chromosomal position effects. *Proc Natl Acad Sci U S A* 97,16, ISSN:9150-9155.,

Evans-Galea, M.V., Wielgosz, M.M., Hanawa, H., Srivastava, D.K., and Nienhuis, A.W. (2007). Suppression of clonal dominance in cultured human lymphoid cells by addition of the cHS4 insulator to a lentiviral vector. *Mol Ther* 15,4, (Apr), 801-809, ISSN:1525-0016 (Print)

Fischer, A., Hacein-Bey-Abina, S., and Cavazanna-Calvo, M. Gene therapy for primary immunodeficiencies. *Immunol Allergy Clin North Am* 30,2, (May), 237-248, ISSN:1557-8607 (Electronic)0889-8561 (Linking)

Gaszner, M., and Felsenfeld, G. (2006). Insulators: exploiting transcriptional and epigenetic mechanisms. *Nat Rev Genet* 7,9, (Sep), 703-713, ISSN:1471-0056 (Print)

Gnatenko, D.V., Wu, Y., Jesty, J., Damon, A.L., Hearing, P., and Bahou, W.F. (2004). Expression of therapeutic levels of factor VIII in hemophilia A mice using a novel adeno/adeno-associated hybrid virus. *Thromb Haemost* 92,2, (Aug), 317-327, 0340-6245 (Print)

Goncalves, M.A., Van Nierop, G.P., Tijssen, M.R., Lefesvre, P., Knaan-Shanzer, S., Van Der Velde, I., Van Bekkum, D.W., Valerio, D., and De Vries, A.A. (2005). Transfer of the full-length dystrophin-coding sequence into muscle cells by a dual high-capacity hybrid viral vector with site-specific integration ability. *J Virol* 79,5, (Mar), 3146-3162, ISSN:0022-538X (Print)

Gonzalez-Murillo, A., Lozano, M.L., Montini, E., Bueren, J.A., and Guenechea, G. (2008). Unaltered repopulation properties of mouse hematopoietic stem cells transduced with lentiviral vectors. *Blood*(Aug 6), ISSN:1528-0020 (Electronic)

Grinshpun, A., Condiotti, R., Waddington, S.N., Peer, M., Zeig, E., Peretz, S., Simerzin, A., Chou, J., Pann, C.J., Giladi, H., and Galun, E. (2010) Neonatal gene therapy of glycogen storage disease type Ia using a feline immunodeficiency virus-based vector. *Mol Ther* 18,9, (Sep), 1592-1598, ISSN:1525-0024 (Electronic) 1525-0016 (Linking)

Hager, S., Frame, F.M., Collins, A.T., Burns, J.E., and Maitland, N.J. (2008). An internal polyadenylation signal substantially increases expression levels of lentivirus-delivered transgenes but has the potential to reduce viral titer in a promoter-dependent manner. *Hum Gene Ther* 19,8, (Aug), 840-850, ISSN:1557-7422 (Electronic)1043-0342 (Linking)

Hanawa, H., Hematti, P., Keyvanfar, K., Metzger, M.E., Krouse, A., Donahue, R.E., Kepes, S., Gray, J., Dunbar, C.E., Persons, D.A., and Nienhuis, A.W. (2004). Efficient gene transfer into rhesus repopulating hematopoietic stem cells using a simian immunodeficiency virus-based lentiviral vector system. *Blood* 103,11, (Jun 1), 4062-4069, ISSN:0006-4971 (Print)

Hanawa, H., Yamamoto, M., Zhao, H., Shimada, T., and Persons, D.A. (2009). Optimized lentiviral vector design improves titer and transgene expression of vectors containing the chicken beta-globin locus HS4 insulator element. *Mol Ther* 17,4, (Apr), 667-674, ISSN:1525-0024 (Electronic) 1525-0016 (Linking)

Held, P.K., Olivares, E.C., Aguilar, C.P., Finegold, M., Calos, M.P., and Grompe, M. (2005). In vivo correction of murine hereditary tyrosinemia type I by phiC31 integrase-mediated gene delivery. *Mol Ther* 11,3, (Mar), 399-408, ISSN:1525-0016 (Print)

Hematti, P., Hong, B.K., Ferguson, C., Adler, R., Hanawa, H., Sellers, S., Holt, I.E., Eckfeldt, C.E., Sharma, Y., Schmidt, M., Von Kalle, C., Persons, D.A., Billings, E.M., Verfaillie, C.M., Nienhuis, A.W., Wolfsberg, T.G., Dunbar, C.E., and Calmels, B. (2004). Distinct genomic integration of MLV and SIV vectors in primate hematopoietic stem and progenitor cells. *PLoS Biol* 2,12, (Dec), e423, ISSN:1545-7885 (Electronic)

Hino, S., Fan, J., Taguwa, S., Akasaka, K., and Matsuoka, M. (2004). Sea urchin insulator protects lentiviral vector from silencing by maintaining active chromatin structure. *Gene Ther* 11,10, (May), 819-828, ISSN:0969-7128 (Print)

Hockemeyer, D., Soldner, F., Beard, C., Gao, Q., Mitalipova, M., Dekelver, R.C., Katibah, G.E., Amora, R., Boydston, E.A., Zeitler, B., Meng, X., Miller, J.C., Zhang, L., Rebar, E.J., Gregory, P.D., Urnov, F.D., and Jaenisch, R. (2009). Efficient targeting of expressed and silent genes in human ESCs and iPSCs using zinc-finger nucleases. *Nat Biotechnol* 27,9, (Sep), 851-857, ISSN:1546-1696 (Electronic) 1546-1696 (Linking)

Hojun, L., Harigot, V., Doyon,Y., Li,J., Bhagwat, A., Wong,S., Anguela, X., Sharma, R., Ivanciu, L., Murphy, S., Zhou, S., Paschon, D., Rebar, E., Gregory F.D., Holmes M.C. and High K.A (2010). LBA-5 Phenotypic Correction of a Mouse Model of Hemophilia B by *in vivo Genetic* Correction of F9 gene American Society of Hematology Annual Meeting (December 10-13).

Holt, N., Wang, J., Kim, K., Friedman, G., Wang, X., Taupin, V., Crooks, G.M., Kohn, D.B., Gregory, P.D., Holmes, M.C., and Cannon, P.M. Human hematopoietic stem/progenitor cells modified by zinc-finger nucleases targeted to CCR5 control HIV-1 in vivo. *Nat Biotechnol* 28,8, (Aug), 839-847, ISSN:1546-1696 (Electronic) 1087-0156 (Linking)

Honaramooz, A., Megee, S., Zeng, W., Destrempes, M.M., Overton, S.A., Luo, J., Galantino-Homer, H., Modelski, M., Chen, F., Blash, S., Melican, D.T., Gavin, W.G., Ayres, S., Yang, F., Wang, P.J., Echelard, Y., and Dobrinski, I. (2008). Adeno-associated virus (AAV)-mediated transduction of male germ line stem cells results in transgene transmission after germ cell transplantation. *Faseb J* 22,2, (Feb), 374-382, ISSN:1530-6860 (Electronic)

Howden, S.E., Voullaire, L., Wardan, H., Williamson, R., and Vadolas, J. (2008). Site-specific, Rep-mediated integration of the intact beta-globin locus in the human erythroleukaemic cell line K562. *Gene Ther* 15,20, (Oct), 1372-1383, ISSN:1476-5462 (Electronic) 0969-7128 (Linking)

Hu, Y.C. Baculovirus: a promising vector for gene therapy? (2010) *Curr Gene Ther* 10,3, (Jun), 167, ISSN:1875-5631 (Electronic)1566-5232 (Linking)

Ikeda, Y., Collins, M.K., Radcliffe, P.A., Mitrophanous, K.A., and Takeuchi, Y. (2002). Gene transduction efficiency in cells of different species by HIV and EIAV vectors. *Gene Ther* 9,14, (Jul), 932-938, ISSN:0969-7128 (Print)

Ikeda, Y., Takeuchi, Y., Martin, F., Cosset, F.L., Mitrophanous, K., and Collins, M. (2003). Continuous high-titer HIV-1 vector production. *Nat Biotechnol* 21,5, (May), 569-572,

Izsvak, Z., Hackett, P.B., Cooper, L.J., and Ivics, Z. Translating Sleeping Beauty transposition into cellular therapies: victories and challenges. *Bioessays* 32,9, (Sep), 756-767, ISSN:1521-1878 (Electronic) 0265-9247 (Linking)

Izsvak, Z., Ivics, Z., and Plasterk, R.H. (2000). Sleeping Beauty, a wide host-range transposon vector for genetic transformation in vertebrates. *J Mol Biol* 302,1, (Sep 8), 93-102, ISSN:0022-2836 (Print) 0022-2836 (Linking)

Kang, Y., Moressi, C.J., Scheetz, T.E., Xie, L., Tran, D.T., Casavant, T.L., Ak, P., Benham, C.J., Davidson, B.L., and Mccray, P.B., Jr. (2006). Integration site choice of a feline immunodeficiency virus vector. *J Virol* 80,17, (Sep), ISSN:8820-8823, 0022-538X (Print)

Koldej, R.M., and Anson, D.S. (2009). Refinement of lentiviral vector for improved RNA processing and reduced rates of self inactivation repair. *BMC Biotechnol* 986, ISSN:1472-6750 (Electronic) 1472-6750 (Linking)

Li, C.L., Xiong, D., Stamatoyannopoulos, G., and Emery, D.W. (2009). Genomic and functional assays demonstrate reduced gammaretroviral vector genotoxicity associated with use of the cHS4 chromatin insulator. *Mol Ther* 17,4, (Apr), 716-724, ISSN:1525-0024 (Electronic)

Lieber, A., Steinwaerder, D.S., Carlson, C.A., and Kay, M.A. (1999). Integrating adenovirus-adeno-associated virus hybrid vectors devoid of all viral genes. *J Virol* 73,11, (Nov), 9314-9324, ISSN:0022-538X (Print)

Liu, J., Jeppesen, I., Nielsen, K., and Jensen, T.G. (2006). Phi c31 integrase induces chromosomal aberrations in primary human fibroblasts. *Gene Ther* 13,15, (Aug), 1188-1190, 0969-7128 (Print)

Lombardo, A., Genovese, P., Beausejour, C.M., Colleoni, S., Lee, Y.L., Kim, K.A., Ando, D., Urnov, F.D., Galli, C., Gregory, P.D., Holmes, M.C., and Naldini, L. (2007). Gene editing in human stem cells using zinc finger nucleases and integrase-defective lentiviral vector delivery. *Nat Biotechnol* 25,11, (Nov), 1298-1306, ISSN:1087-0156 (Print)

Maina, N., Han, Z., Li, X., Hu, Z., Zhong, L., Bischof, D., Weigel-Van Aken, K.A., Slayton, W.B., Yoder, M.C., and Srivastava, A. (2008). Recombinant self-complementary adeno-associated virus serotype vector-mediated hematopoietic stem cell transduction and lineage-restricted, long-term transgene expression in a murine serial bone marrow transplantation model. *Hum Gene Ther* 19,4, (Apr), 376-383, ISSN:1043-0342 (Print)

Mangeot, P.E., Negre, D., Dubois, B., Winter, A.J., Leissner, P., Mehtali, M., Kaiserlian, D., Cosset, F.L., and Darlix, J.L. (2000). Development of minimal lentivirus vectors derived from simian immunodeficiency virus (SIVmac251) and their use for gene transfer into human dendritic cells. *J Virol* 74,18, 8307-8315.,

Mates, L., Chuah, M.K., Belay, E., Jerchow, B., Manoj, N., Acosta-Sanchez, A., Grzela, D.P., Schmitt, A., Becker, K., Matrai, J., Ma, L., Samara-Kuko, E., Gysemans, C., Pryputniewicz, D., Miskey, C., Fletcher, B., Vandendriessche, T., Ivics, Z., and Izsvak, Z. (2009). Molecular evolution of a novel hyperactive Sleeping Beauty transposase enables robust stable gene transfer in vertebrates. *Nat Genet* 41,6, (Jun), 753-761, ISSN:1546-1718 (Electronic) 1061-4036 (Linking)

Matukonis, M., Li, M., Molina, R.P., Paszkiet, B., Kaleko, M., and Luo, T. (2002). Development of second- and third-generation bovine immunodeficiency virus-based gene transfer systems. *Hum Gene Ther* 13,11, (Jul 20), 1293-1303, ISSN:1043-0342 (Print)

Miao, C.H., Snyder, R.O., Schowalter, D.B., Patijn, G.A., Donahue, B., Winther, B., and Kay, M.A. (1998). The kinetics of rAAV integration in the liver. *Nat Genet* 19,1, (May), 13-15, ISSN:1061-4036 (Print)

Miller, J.C., Holmes, M.C., Wang, J., Guschin, D.Y., Lee, Y.L., Rupniewski, I., Beausejour, C.M., Waite, A.J., Wang, N.S., Kim, K.A., Gregory, P.D., Pabo, C.O., and Rebar, E.J. (2007). An improved zinc-finger nuclease architecture for highly specific genome editing. *Nat Biotechnol* 25,7, (Jul), 778-785, ISSN:1087-0156 (Print)

Mitomo, K., Griesenbach, U., Inoue, M., Somerton, L., Meng, C., Akiba, E., Tabata, T., Ueda, Y., Frankel, G.M., Farley, R., Singh, C., Chan, M., Munkonge, F., Brum, A., Xenariou, S., Escudero-Garcia, S., Hasegawa, M., and Alton, E.W. (2010) Toward gene therapy for cystic fibrosis using a lentivirus pseudotyped with Sendai virus envelopes. *Mol Ther* 18,6, (Jun), 1173-1182, ISSN:1525-0024 (Electronic) 1525-0016 (Linking)

Mitrophanous, K., Yoon, S., Rohll, J., Patil, D., Wilkes, F., Kim, V., Kingsman, S., Kingsman, A., and Mazarakis, N. (1999). Stable gene transfer to the nervous system using a non-primate lentiviral vector. *Gene Ther* 6,11, 1808-1818.,

Miyoshi, H., Blomer, U., Takahashi, M., Gage, F.H., and Verma, I.M. (1998). Development of a self-inactivating lentivirus vector. *J Virol* 72,10, (Oct), 8150-8157, ISSN:0022-538X (Print)

Modlich, U., Bohne, J., Schmidt, M., Von Kalle, C., Knoss, S., Schambach, A., and Baum, C. (2006). Cell-culture assays reveal the importance of retroviral vector design for insertional genotoxicity. *Blood* 108,8, (Oct 15), 2545-2553, ISSN:0006-4971 (Print)

Modlich, U., Navarro, S., Zychlinski, D., Maetzig, T., Knoess, S., Brugman, M.H., Schambach, A., Charrier, S., Galy, A., Thrasher, A.J., Bueren, J., and Baum, C. (2009). Insertional transformation of hematopoietic cells by self-inactivating lentiviral and gammaretroviral vectors. *Mol Ther* 17,11, (Nov), 1919-1928, ISSN:1525-0024 (Electronic) 1525-0024 (Linking)

Montini, E., Cesana, D., Schmidt, M., Sanvito, F., Bartholomae, C.C., Ranzani, M., Benedicenti, F., Sergi, L.S., Ambrosi, A., Ponzoni, M., Doglioni, C., Di Serio, C., Von Kalle, C., and Naldini, L. (2009). The genotoxic potential of retroviral vectors is strongly modulated by vector design and integration site selection in a mouse model of HSC gene therapy. *J Clin Invest* 119,4, (Apr), 964-975, ISSN:1558-8238 (Electronic)

Montini, E., Cesana, D., Schmidt, M., Sanvito, F., Ponzoni, M., Bartholomae, C., Sergi, L.S., Benedicenti, F., Ambrosi, A., Di Serio, C., Doglioni, C., Von Kalle, C., and Naldini, L. (2006). Hematopoietic stem cell gene transfer in a tumor-prone mouse model uncovers low genotoxicity of lentiviral vector integration. *Nat Biotechnol* 24,6, (Jun), 687-696,

Mueller, C., and Flotte, T.R. (2008). Clinical gene therapy using recombinant adeno-associated virus vectors. *Gene Ther* 15,11, (Jun), 858-863, ISSN:1476-5462 (Electronic)

Murakami, Y., Ikeda, Y., Yonemitsu, Y., Miyazaki, M., Inoue, M., Hasegawa, M., Sueishi, K., and Ishibashi, T. (2010) Inhibition of choroidal neovascularization via brief subretinal exposure to a newly developed lentiviral vector pseudotyped with Sendai viral envelope proteins. *Hum Gene Ther* 21,2, (Feb), 199-209, ISSN:1557-7422 (Electronic) 1043-0342 (Linking)

Nakai, H., Montini, E., Fuess, S., Storm, T.A., Grompe, M., and Kay, M.A. (2003). AAV serotype 2 vectors preferentially integrate into active genes in mice. *Nat Genet* 34,3, (Jul), 297-302, ISSN:1061-4036 (Print)

Naumann, N., De Ravin, S.S., Choi, U., Moayeri, M., Whiting-Theobald, N., Linton, G.F., Ikeda, Y., and Malech, H.L. (2007). Simian immunodeficiency virus lentivector corrects human X-linked chronic granulomatous disease in the NOD/SCID mouse xenograft. *Gene Ther* 14,21, (Nov), 1513-1524, ISSN:0969-7128 (Print)

Neff, T., Shotkoski, F., and Stamatoyannopoulos, G. (1997). Stem cell gene therapy, position effects and chromatin insulators. *Stem Cells* 15 Suppl 1265-271, ISSN:1066-5099 (Print)

Neven, B., Leroy, S., Decaluwe, H., Le Deist, F., Picard, C., Moshous, D., Mahlaoui, N., Debre, M., Casanova, J.L., Dal Cortivo, L., Madec, Y., Hacein-Bey-Abina, S., De Saint Basile, G., De Villartay, J.P., Blanche, S., Cavazzana-Calvo, M., and Fischer, A. (2009). Long-term outcome after hematopoietic stem cell transplantation of a single-center cohort of 90 patients with severe combined immunodeficiency. *Blood* 113,17, (Apr 23), 4114-4124, ISSN:1528-0020 (Electronic)

Olivares, E.C., Hollis, R.P., Chalberg, T.W., Meuse, L., Kay, M.A., and Calos, M.P. (2002). Site-specific genomic integration produces therapeutic Factor IX levels in mice. *Nat Biotechnol* 20,11, (Nov), 1124-1128, ISSN:1087-0156 (Print)

Olson, P., Nelson, S., and Dornburg, R. (1994). Improved self-inactivating retroviral vectors derived from spleen necrosis virus. *J Virol* 68,11, (Nov), 7060-7066, ISSN:0022-538X (Print)

Ortiz-Urda, S., Thyagarajan, B., Keene, D.R., Lin, Q., Fang, M., Calos, M.P., and Khavari, P.A. (2002). Stable nonviral genetic correction of inherited human skin disease. *Nat Med* 8,10, (Oct), 1166-1170, ISSN:1078-8956 (Print)

Park, J., Nadeau, P.E., and Mergia, A. (2009). Activity of TAR in inducible inhibition of HIV replication by foamy virus vector expressing siRNAs under the control of HIV LTR. *Virus Res* 140,1-2, (Mar), 112-120, ISSN:0168-1702 (Print) 0168-1702 (Linking)

Perez, E.E., Wang, J., Miller, J.C., Jouvenot, Y., Kim, K.A., Liu, O., Wang, N., Lee, G., Bartsevich, V.V., Lee, Y.L., Guschin, D.Y., Rupniewski, I., Waite, A.J., Carpenito, C., Carroll, R.G., Orange, J.S., Urnov, F.D., Rebar, E.J., Ando, D., Gregory, P.D., Riley, J.L., Holmes, M.C., and June, C.H. (2008). Establishment of HIV-1 resistance in CD4+ T cells by genome editing using zinc-finger nucleases. *Nat Biotechnol* 26,7, (Jul), 808-816, ISSN:1546-1696 (Electronic)

Poeschla, E.M., Wong-Staal, F., and Looney, D.J. (1998). Efficient transduction of nondividing human cells by feline immunodeficiency virus lentiviral vectors. *Nat Med* 4,3, (Mar), 354-357, ISSN:1078-8956 (Print)

Price, M.A., Case, S.S., Carbonaro, D.A., Yu, X.J., Petersen, D., Sabo, K.M., Curran, M.A., Engel, B.C., Margarian, H., Abkowitz, J.L., Nolan, G.P., Kohn, D.B., and Crooks, G.M. (2002). Expression from second-generation feline immunodeficiency virus vectors is impaired in human hematopoietic cells. *Mol Ther* 6,5, (Nov), 645-652, ISSN:1525-0016 (Print)

Ramezani, A., and Hawley, R.G. Strategies to insulate lentiviral vector-expressed transgenes. (2010) *Methods Mol Biol* 614 77-100, ISSN:1940-6029 (Electronic) 1064-3745 (Linking)

Ramezani, A., Hawley, T.S., and Hawley, R.G. (2008). Combinatorial Incorporation of Enhancer Blocking Components of the Chicken {beta}-Globin 5'HS4 and Human T-Cell Receptor {alpha}/{delta} BEAD-1 Insulators in Self-Inactivating Retroviral Vectors Reduces their Genotoxic Potential. *Stem Cells*(Sep 11), ISSN:1549-4918 (Electronic)

Recchia, A., Parks, R.J., Lamartina, S., Toniatti, C., Pieroni, L., Palombo, F., Ciliberto, G., Graham, F.L., Cortese, R., La Monica, N., and Colloca, S. (1999). Site-specific integration mediated by a hybrid adenovirus/adeno-associated virus vector. *Proc Natl Acad Sci U S A* 96,6, (Mar 16), 2615-2620, ISSN:0027-8424 (Print)

Robert-Richard, E., Richard, E., Malik, P., Ged, C., De Verneuil, H., and Moreau-Gaudry, F. (2007). Murine Retroviral but not Human Cellular Promoters Induce In Vivo Erythroid-specific Deregulation that can be Partially Prevented by Insulators. *Mol Ther* 15,1, (Jan), 173-182,

Rolling, F. AAV-mediated gene therapy for the treatment of retinal diseases. (2010) *Curr Gene Ther* 10,5, (Oct 1), 318, ISSN:1875-5631 (Electronic) 1566-5232 (Linking)

Sandrin, V., Boson, B., Salmon, P., Gay, W., Negre, D., Le Grand, R., Trono, D., and Cosset, F.L. (2002). Lentiviral vectors pseudotyped with a modified RD114 envelope glycoprotein show increased stability in sera and augmented transduction of primary lymphocytes and CD34+ cells derived from human and nonhuman primates. *Blood* 100,3, (Aug 1), 823-832,

Sclimenti, C.R., Thyagarajan, B., and Calos, M.P. (2001). Directed evolution of a recombinase for improved genomic integration at a native human sequence. *Nucleic Acids Res* 29,24, (Dec 15), 5044-5051, ISSN:1362-4962 (Electronic)

Schambach, A., Galla, M., Maetzig, T., Loew, R., and Baum, C. (2007). Improving transcriptional termination of self-inactivating gamma-retroviral and lentiviral vectors. *Mol Ther* 15,6, (Jun), 1167-1173, ISSN:1525-0016 (Print)

Schmidt, M., and Rethwilm, A. (1995). Replicating foamy virus-based vectors directing high level expression of foreign genes. *Virology* 210,1, (Jun 20), 167-178, 0042-6822 (Print)

Siapati, E.K., Bigger, B.W., Miskin, J., Chipchase, D., Parsley, K.L., Mitrophanous, K., Themis, M., Thrasher, A.J., and Bonnet, D. (2005). Comparison of HIV- and EIAV-based vectors on their efficiency in transducing murine and human hematopoietic repopulating cells. *Mol Ther* 12,3, (Sep), 537-546,

Smith, R.H. (2008). Adeno-associated virus integration: virus versus vector. *Gene Ther* 15,11, (Jun), 817-822, ISSN:1476-5462 (Electronic)

Tang, Y., Cummins, J., Huard, J., and Wang, B. AAV-directed muscular dystrophy gene therapy. (2010) *Expert Opin Biol Ther* 10,3, (Mar), 395-408, ISSN:1744-7682 (Electronic) 1471-2598 (Linking)

Thrasher, A.J., De Alwis, M., Casimir, C.M., Kinnon, C., Page, K., Lebkowski, J., Segal, A.W., and Levinsky, R.J. (1995). Functional reconstitution of the NADPH-oxidase by adeno-associated virus gene transfer. *Blood* 86,2, (Jul 15), 761-765, ISSN:0006-4971 (Print)

Thyagarajan, B., Olivares, E.C., Hollis, R.P., Ginsburg, D.S., and Calos, M.P. (2001). Site-specific genomic integration in mammalian cells mediated by phage phiC31 integrase. *Mol Cell Biol* 21,12, (Jun), 3926-3934, ISSN:0270-7306 (Print)

Toscano, M.G., Frecha, C., Ortega, C., Santamaria, M., Martin, F., and Molina, I.J. (2004). Efficient lentiviral transduction of Herpesvirus saimiri immortalized T cells as a model for gene therapy in primary immunodeficiencies. *Gene Ther* 11,12, (Jun), 956-961,

Trobridge, G., Josephson, N., Vassilopoulos, G., Mac, J., and Russell, D.W. (2002). Improved foamy virus vectors with minimal viral sequences. *Mol Ther* 6,3, (Sep), 321-328, ISSN:1525-0016 (Print)

Urnov, F.D., Miller, J.C., Lee, Y.L., Beausejour, C.M., Rock, J.M., Augustus, S., Jamieson, A.C., Porteus, M.H., Gregory, P.D., and Holmes, M.C. (2005). Highly efficient endogenous human gene correction using designed zinc-finger nucleases. *Nature* 435,7042, (Jun 2), 646-651, ISSN:1476-4687 (Electronic)

Van Der Laan, L.J., Wang, Y., Tilanus, H.W., Janssen, H.L., and Pan, Q. AAV-mediated gene therapy for liver diseases: the prime candidate for clinical application? (2010)*Expert Opin Biol Ther* 11,3, (Mar), 315-327, ISSN:1744-7682 (Electronic) 1471-2598 (Linking)

Wang, H., and Lieber, A. (2006). A helper-dependent capsid-modified adenovirus vector expressing adeno-associated virus rep78 mediates site-specific integration of a 27-kilobase transgene cassette. *J Virol* 80,23, (Dec), 11699-11709, ISSN:0022-538X (Print)

Wilber, A., Linehan, J.L., Tian, X., Woll, P.S., Morris, J.K., Belur, L.R., Mcivor, R.S., and Kaufman, D.S. (2007). Efficient and stable transgene expression in human embryonic stem cells using transposon-mediated gene transfer. *Stem Cells* 25,11, (Nov), 2919-2927, ISSN:1549-4918 (Electronic)

Wilson, M.H., Kaminski, J.M., and George, A.L., Jr. (2005). Functional zinc finger/sleeping beauty transposase chimeras exhibit attenuated overproduction inhibition. *FEBS Lett* 579,27, (Nov 7), 6205-6209, ISSN:0014-5793 (Print)

Williams, D.A. (2008). Foamy virus vectors come of age. *Mol Ther* 16,4, (Apr), 635-636, 1525-0024 (Electronic)

Wu, S.C., Meir, Y.J., Coates, C.J., Handler, A.M., Pelczar, P., Moisyadi, S., and Kaminski, J.M. (2006). piggyBac is a flexible and highly active transposon as compared to sleeping beauty, Tol2, and Mos1 in mammalian cells. *Proc Natl Acad Sci U S A* 103,41, (Oct 10), 15008-15013, ISSN:0027-8424 (Print)

Yant, S.R., Meuse, L., Chiu, W., Ivics, Z., Izsvak, Z., and Kay, M.A. (2000). Somatic integration and long-term transgene expression in normal and haemophilic mice using a DNA transposon system. *Nat Genet* 25,1, (May), 35-41, ISSN:1061-4036 (Print) 1061-4036 (Linking)

Yip, P.K., Wong, L.F., Pattinson, D., Battaglia, A., Grist, J., Bradbury, E.J., Maden, M., Mcmahon, S.B., and Mazarakis, N.D. (2006). Lentiviral vector expressing retinoic acid receptor beta2 promotes recovery of function after corticospinal tract injury in the adult rat spinal cord. *Hum Mol Genet* 15,21, (Nov 1), 3107-3118, ISSN:0964-6906 (Print)

Yu, S.F., Von Ruden, T., Kantoff, P.W., Garber, C., Seiberg, M., Ruther, U., Anderson, W.F., Wagner, E.F., and Gilboa, E. (1986). Self-inactivating retroviral vectors designed for transfer of whole genes into mammalian cells. *Proc Natl Acad Sci U S A* 83,10, (May), 3194-3198, ISSN:0027-8424 (Print)

Zayed, H., Izsvak, Z., Walisko, O., and Ivics, Z. (2004). Development of hyperactive sleeping beauty transposon vectors by mutational analysis. *Mol Ther* 9,2, (Feb), 292-304, ISSN:1525-0016 (Print) 1525-0016 (Linking)

Zeng, J., Du, J., Zhao, Y., Palanisamy, N., and Wang, S. (2007). Baculoviral vector-mediated transient and stable transgene expression in human embryonic stem cells. *Stem Cells* 25,4, (Apr), 1055-1061, ISSN:1066-5099 (Print)

Zhu, J., Park, C.W., Sjeklocha, L., Kren, B.T., and Steer, C.J. (2010). High-level genomic integration, epigenetic changes, and expression of sleeping beauty transgene. *Biochemistry* 49,7, (Feb 23), 1507-1521, ISSN:1520-4995 (Electronic) 0006-2960 (Linking)

Zufferey, R., Dull, T., Mandel, R.J., Bukovsky, A., Quiroz, D., Naldini, L., and Trono, D. (1998). Self-inactivating lentivirus vector for safe and efficient in vivo gene delivery. *J Virol* 72,12, 9873-9880.,

2

Gene Therapy Using RNAi

Yu-Lin Yang, Wen-Teng Chang and Yuan-Wei Shih
Chung Hwa University of Medical Technology
Graduate Institute of Biomedical Science
Taiwan

1. Introduction

In the chapter, we hereby provide a brief review about RNA interference (RNAi) and elucidate its therapeutic applications. The enzymatic synthesis of double-stranded RNA in vitro will be discussed. We also describe how to design and select short interfering RNA (siRNA) sequences. In addition, we also introduce a DNA-directed RNAi (ddRNAi) system, which is designed for the generation of small hairpin RNAs in mammalian cells and is an efficient approach to allow fast and easy expression of hairpin oligonucleotides for therapeutic purpose. Moreover, various strategies for delivery of siRNA to target cells are discussed in this chapter. Under the consideration of distinct need of different diseases, use of transient or stable transfection onto living organism will be introduced. Finally, we will discuss the application of RNAi in clinical or preclinical trial. Some ongoing therapeutic models, efficacy or limitation for RNAi will be demonstrated and clarified.

1.1 Overview and mechanism about RNAi

Andrew Fire and Craig Mello published their break-through study on the mechanism of RNA interference in Nature in 1998 (Fire et al., 1998). RNA interference (RNAi) is a phenomenon in which double-stranded RNA (dsRNA) suppresses expression of a target protein by stimulating the specific degradation of the target mRNA (Fuchs et al. 2004). RNAi has been used to study loss of function for a variety of genes in several organisms including various plants, Caenorhabditis elegans and Drosophila, and permits loss-of-function genetic screens and rapid tests for genetic interactions in mammalian cells (Hannon, 2002; Williams et al., 2003). RNAi is generated by a multistep process (Figure 1). First of all, intracellular dsRNA is recognized by an RNase III (designated as "Dicer" in Drosophila) and cleaved into siRNAs of 21–23 nucleotides (Hammond et al. 2000). These siRNAs are then integrated in a complex (designated as "RISC", RNA-induced silencing complex). Each siRNA in RISC is specific and targeting to certain sequences of mRNAs, which is homologous to the integral siRNA followed by completely degradation of targeted mRNA. (Hammond et al., 2000; Bernstein et al., 2001). Actually, the target mRNA is cleaved in the center of the sequence complementary to the siRNA (Elbashir et al., 2001c). As a result, rapid degradation of the target mRNA and decreased protein expression was observed.
It is well-known that proteins are responsible for the physical and dynamic properties of a living cell, and defects in their function or regulation contribute to many diseases. In fact, the majority of drugs used at the present time are actually designed to inactive proteins.

Thus, gene therapy using RNAi should be effective in ablating protein function since mRNA is the template for the translation of multiple proteins. Much of the interest in RNAi is based on the fact that the RNAi mechanism operates upstream of protein production by eliminating the mRNAs coding for such proteins. Thus, scientists are eager to finds solutions for treating diseases of all kinds and sorts by using RNAi.

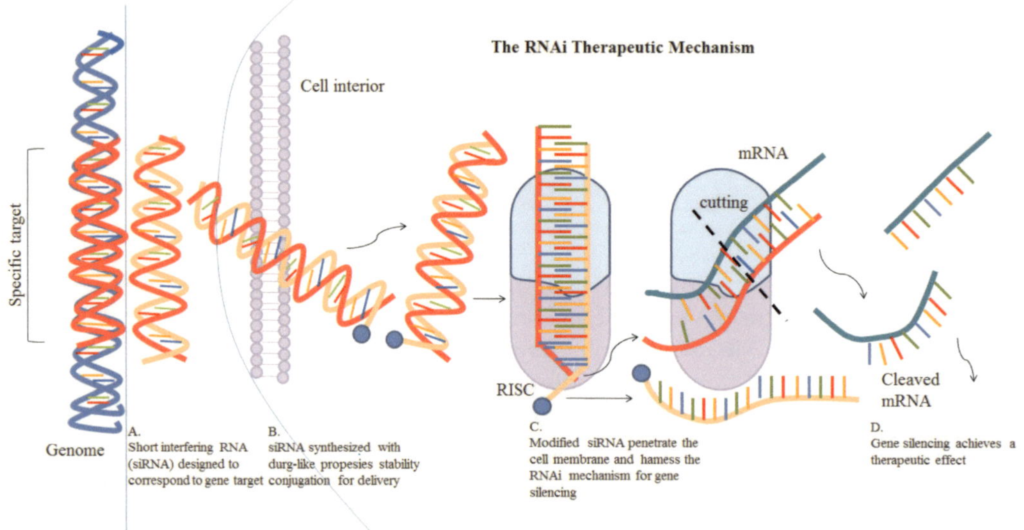

Fig. 1. Simplified schematic diagram of the proposed RNA interference mechanism. dsRNA processing proteins (RNase III-like enzymes) bind to and cleave dsRNA into siRNA. The siRNA forms a multicomponent nuclease complex, the RNA-induced silencing complex (RISC). The target mRNA recognized by RISC is cleaved in the center of the region complementary to the siRNA and quickly degraded.

1.2 siRNA design and optimization

Selecting an optimal target sequence is essential to the success of RNA interference. Since it is not possible to predict the optimal siRNA sequence for a given target, many siRNAs are usually required to be screened for optimal effects. Suggestions for the determination of sequences of siRNAs are usually being modified upon as knowledge of the RNAi continues to expand. The general recommendations are as follows: siRNA target sequences should be specific to the gene of interest and have GC content with about 20~50 percents (Henshel et al. 2004). According to Ui-Tei et al. (2004) and Elbashir et al., 2001a, siRNAs satisfying the following "RNAi target selection rules" are capable of effective gene silencing in mammalian cells: (1) Targeted regions on the cDNA sequence of a targeted gene should be located 50-100 nt downstream of the start codon (ATG). (2)Search for sequence motif AA(N19)TT or NA(N21), or NAR(N17)YNN, where N is any nucleotide, R is purine (A, G) and Y is pyrimidine (C, U). (3)Avoid targeting introns, since RNAi only works in the cytoplasm and not within the nucleus. (4)Avoid sequences with > 50% G+C content. (5)Avoid stretches of 4 or more nucleotide repeats. (6)Avoid 5URT and 3UTR, although siRNAs targeting UTRs have successfully induced gene inhibition.

Designing effective siRNAs is essential for effective RNAi knockdown. In addition to choosing the optimal sequence, other essential factors that affect the efficacy of siRNA should be as well considered. Once a siRNA sequence is selected using the above algorithm of choice, it is important to perform homology examination against all the other genes from the organism of your study. In addition, the homology test should be able to identify short regions of sequence identity since any siRNA displaying homology with the potential to cause mis-targeted effects should be excluded. Despite so many advances in siRNA design platforms showing highly likely to be functional, the only way to make sure if designed siRNA have the silencing effects in target gene is to validate in an actual experiment.

1.3 Enzymatic synthesis of siRNA

Several methods to generate siRNA have been developed. These include the preparation of siRNA mixtures using RNase III or Dicer enzymes to digest longer double-strand RNAs (dsRNAs) (Andrew et al., 2005; Myers et al., 2003). The short RNAs generated as a result of these digestions have been demonstrated to be efficient in RNAi study. siRNA synthesis in vitro provides an alternative approach instead of using the potentially expensive chemical synthesis of RNA. Take our study for example, which is published in Journal of Cellular Biochemistry (Yang et al., 2007). To analysis the effects of CD36 in renal tubule cells, CD36 siRNA was designed and synthesized. CD36 is an 88-kD integral-membrane glycoprotein that is present on renal tubular; however little is known about its actual biological function. We use LLC-PK1 cells to mimic proximal tubule cells. Cells were cultured in 10% fetal calf serum supplemented medium for 1 day. The cells were then transfected by 100 nM of synthetic CD36 siRNA (sense sequence: CUAAGUUGCUGAGACAAGGdTdT, anti-sense: CCUUGUCUCAGCAACUUAGdTdT), which was purchased from commercial biotech company. To make sure the silencing effects come from the siRNA introduced, scientists are required to make proper control experiments. Usually, we can design reverse sequence for a negative control for siRNA study. For example, we designed the reverse control for CD36 siRNA with sequence as following. Sense sequence is 5′-dTdTGGAACAGAGUCGUUGAAUC-3′ and anti-sense sequence is 5′-dTdTGAUUCAACGACUCUGUUCC-3′. Transfecting procedure was performed according to manufacturer's instructions. Cells were mixed with siRNA complex for 24 h and cultured in serum-free medium for 36 h. These results were shown in Figure 2.

1.4 DNA-directed RNAi

DNA-directed RNA interference (so called "ddRNAi") involves the introduction of DNA templates in cytoplasma and generation of siRNA in vivo. ddRNAi is dependent on RNA polymerase III for the production of siRNA which can silence specific gene of interest with the sequence related to that of siRNA (Brummelkamp et al. 2002; Novarino et al. 2004).Target sequences of si/shRNA can be generated by using PCR followed by cloning into selected vectors (Yu et al., 2002). Take pSUPER RNAi System for example, the pSUPER RNAi System (OligoEngine inc) can generates long-term silencing phenotypes in mammalian cell lines by vector system, along with a pair of oligo sequences specific to the target sequences that are ligated into the vector, to produce dsRNA and to provoke persistent synthesis of siRNA in cytoplasma as shown in Figure 3.

Vector-based RNA silencing strategy provides a way to induce stable, long-term inhibition of gene of interest by generating siRNAs in vivo. After specific gene silencing, the biochemical change in transfected cells can facilitate scientists to study the role of specific

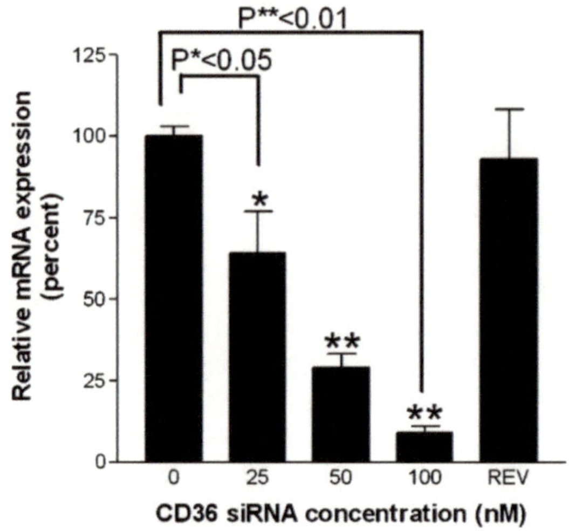

Fig. 2. CD36 mRNA is suppressed in LLC-PK1 using CD36 siRNA. CD36 mRNA was determined by quantitative real-time PCR in LLC-PK1 cell treated with CD36 siRNA (0, 25, 50, 100 nM) for 24 h following maintenance of cells in complete medium for 36 h. Bars represent mean +/- SEM of three experiments. It is evident that CD36 siRNA is a suitable approach applied in CD36 gene silencing. (Adapted from Yang et al., 2007)

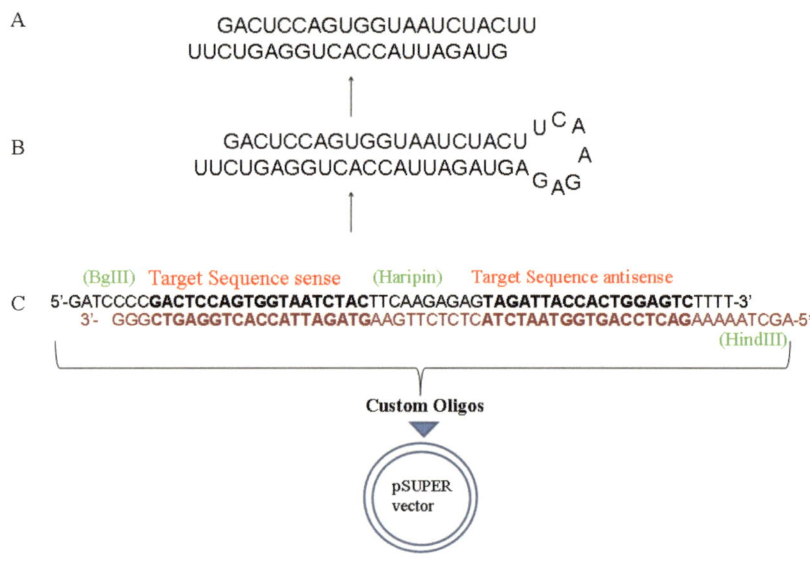

Fig. 3. (A) Demonstrating the sequence (sense strand) and its complement sequence (antisense strand) in the duplex form, with 3' UU overhang. (B) showing the same sequences along with hairpin loop. The loop is ready to be degraded by Dicer enzyme following RNA transcription. (C) Demonstrating the forward and reverse oligos in relative orientation. (Adapted from http://www.oligoengine.com/)

gene or protein. On the vectors, markers, such as puromycin or neomycin can be performed for long-term suppression of genes of interest. Usually, the silencing time period for synthetic siRNAs is between 48–72 hours. Thus, synthetic siRNAs is suitable for transient silencing purpose. However, vector-based RNA silencing can induce stable and long-term silencing of target gene. Furthermore, to obtain a successful ddRNAi, several parameters should be noted. First, well prepare the vectors containing full-length shRNA or siRNA sequences. Avoid contaminating endotoxin carried from prokaryotes host. Second, make sure of a successful delivery of those vectors into cells and induction of the expression of shRNA constructs. Third, properly select and clone siRNA target sequences into expression vectors. This sequence consists of two inverted repeats separated by a short spacer sequence (loop sequence). After transfection and transcription by RNA polymerase, the inverted repeats anneal and form a hairpin structure, which is then cleaved by Dicer to form siRNA. Taken together, DNA-Directed RNAi strategies provide another method for quickly and easily screening various targets (Yeager et al., 2005).

2. Therapeutic delivery of RNAi

There have been several reports on gene expression can be silenced by the targeted destruction of specific mRNA molecules in a highly conserved process known as RNAi. It is a form of post-transcriptional gene silencing that has been described in a number of plant, nematode, protozoan, and invertebrate species. In the recent years, RNAi has emerged as a major regulatory mechanism in eukaryotic gene expression. Also, RNAi is a powerful tool to silence gene expression in a sequence-specific manner and has the potential to treat diseases (ex. cancer therapeutics or in tissue regeneration) which can be corrected by the decreased expression of specific proteins (Izquierdo, 2005). A single strand of exogenously introduced double-stranded small interfering RNA (siRNA; 20-30 nucleotides) guides an RNA-inducing silencing protein complex to degrade the mRNA with the matching sequence; thus, translation into the target proteins is silenced (Elbashir et al., 2001b; Hannon & Rossi , 2004; Novina & Sharp, 2004). Theoretically, siRNA can interfere with the translation of almost any mRNA, as long as the mRNA has a distinctive sequence, whereas the targets of traditional drugs are limited by types of cellular receptors and enzymes (de Fougerolles et al., 2007). In designing a particular RNAi, it is important to identify the sense/antisense combination that provides the most potent suppression of the target mRNA, and several rules have been established to give > 90% gene expression inhibition. RNAi technology can be directed against cancer and various diseases using a variety of genetic therapeutic strategies. The RNAi delivery strategies are often exploited in experimental biology to study the function of genes in target cells or organisms. Successful RNAi experiments are dependent on both siRNA design and effective delivery of siRNA duplexes into cells.

2.1 Current challenges in RNAi *in vivo*

There are several challenges that currently limit the use of RNAi in the clinic. Methods that overcome these are being developed and are discussed below.

2.1.1 Design and delivery of chemically modified siRNA

Unmodified, naked siRNA are relatively unstable in blood circulation owing to its native form, though they are more stable than single-stranded RNA. siRNA are rapidly degraded by nucleases, renal clearance, and non-specific uptake by the reticuloendothelial system indicating that they have short half-lives in vivo. In order to enhance biological stability without affecting gene-silencing activity, chemical modifications have been introduced into the siRNA structure. Various chemical modifications to the backbone, base, and sugar of the siRNA for stability and activity against nuclease degradation have been reported. siRNA is an anionic macromolecule and does not readily enter cells by passive diffusion mechanisms. An appropriate siRNA delivery system enhances cellular uptake, protects its payload from enzymatic digestion and immune recognition, and improves the pharmacokinetics by avoiding excretion via the reticuloendothelial system and renal filtration (i.e. prolonged half-life in vivo) (Lorenz et al., 2004; Sioud & Sorensen, 2003; Sorensen et al., 2003). In addition, an appropriate delivery system localizes siRNA in the desired tissue, resulting in a reduction in the amount of siRNA required for efficient gene silencing in vivo, as well as minimized side effects. By these chemical modifications of siRNA, degradation of siRNA in blood and/or cells can be delayed from minutes to hours. Thus, gene-silencing activity in vivo can be sustained for several days in conjunction with an appropriate delivery system. Chemical modifications can also reduce off-target effects (Jackson et al., 2006) and alter thermal stability within the various critical sequence regions of the siRNA duplex for improved activity of siRNA (Khvorova et al., 2003; Reynolds et al., 2004; Schwarz et al., 2003). Also, this kind of backbone modification enhances the resistance of siRNA to enzymatic hydrolysis, immunogenicity and toxicology

2.1.2 Local versus systemic siRNA delivery

To achieve RNAi via siRNA delivery in vivo, it is critical for siRNA to be efficiently located in desired tissues/cells. The types of target tissues and cells dictate the optimum administration routes of local versus systemic delivery. For example, siRNA can be directly applied to the eye, skin or muscle via local delivery, whereas systemic siRNA delivery is the only way to reach metastatic and hematological cancer cells (Shim & Kwon, 2010). Recent study has indicated systemic siRNA delivery imposes several additional barriers compared with local delivery. Local delivery offers several advantages and makes achieving efficient RNAi over systemic delivery, such as low effective doses, simple formulation (e.g. no targeting moieties), low risk of inducing systemic side effects and facilitated site-specific delivery (Dykxhoorn et al., 2006). In other word, local administration is likely to be a more cost-efficient strategy for siRNA delivery in vivo than systemic administration. Generally, naked siRNA injected into the body has a very short half life, on the order of minutes, limiting its usefulness (Dykxhoorn & Lieberman, 2006). However, it has been found that some tissues are able to uptake naked siRNA to a much higher degree than other tissues (for instance the eye, central nervous system, and lung) making localized delivery by direct injection of siRNA to these sites a possibility. For example, initial clinical trials for RNAi-based treatment of age-related macular degeneration have exclusively used local injections of siRNA direct injection into the eye and central nervous system (Vives et al., 1997).

2.1.3 Nanotechnology platforms for gene therapeutics

The biomedical application of nanotechnology has been extensively used in drug or gene delivery system in the past few years. Nanotechnology is considered to be novel and potential technology that will have significant impact in all industrial sectors and across-the-board applications in gene therapeutics. Nanoshells are nanoparticle beads that consist of a silica core coated with a thin gold shell (1 nanoparticle). Nanoparticle carriers have the potential to overcome the challenges of intravascular degradation, and can provide safe and efficient delivery of synthetic dsRNAs. On entering the bloodstream, nanoparticles encounter a complex environment of plasma proteins and immune cells. Nanoparticle uptake by immune cells in blood circulation, such as monocytes, leukocytes, platelets and dendritic cells, occurs through various pathways and is facilitated by the adsorption of opsonins to the surface of the particle (Kim, 2007). Additionally, the application of nanotechnology significantly benefits clinical practice in cancer diagnosis, treatment, and management. Especially, nanotechnology offers a promise for the targeted delivery of drugs, genes, and proteins to tumor tissues and protect them from environmental factors which may degrade it and it typically uptake by cells with a higher efficiency (Loo et al., 2005).

3. Methods of siRNA delivery

Despite quite efficient and reliable gene silencing in vitro, only limited RNAi has been achieved in vivo because of rapid enzymatic degradation in combination with poor cellular uptake of siRNA (Kirchhoff, 2008). Therefore, novel delivery systems which enable prolonged naked siRNA and improve accessibility to target cells via clinically feasible administration routes and optimized cytosolic release of siRNA after efficient cellular uptake, are indispensably required (Grimm & Kay, 2007). There are several methods and major hurdles in siRNA delivery which overcome them and are discussed below:

3.1 Naked siRNA

"Naked" siRNA delivery is direct injection of a saline or excipient solution containing non-complexed siRNA sequences to a target site. Although naked siRNA was influenced by enzymes and rapid renal clearance, recent studies have also demonstrated the ability to deliver naked siRNA to target cells or tissues (for instance the eye, central nervous system, and lung) via local injection system delivery.

3.2 Microinjection

Microinjection offers a potentially powerful method for the analysis of the dynamics of expression because it enables real-time regulation of transient expression of multiple genes. Recent papers have provided a brief review of RNAi and discussion of the benefits and drawbacks of using long double-stranded RNA (dsRNA) into mouse oocytes and early embryos by microinjection and preparation and testing of constructs for transgenic RNAi based on long hairpin RNA expression. Furthermore, microinjection can provide a useful method for quantitative analysis of transient gene expression in single cells using RNAi.

3.3 Biolistics (gene gun)

The gene gun (also known as biolistic or bioballistic particle delivery) is the most novel physical transfection method. This technique is based on DNA (or RNA) become "sticky," adhering to biologically inert particles such as metal atoms (usually tungsten or gold), and then are accelerated to high velocity to get into target tissues or cells (Klein et al., 1992; Uchida et al., 2009). This approach allows DNA (or RNA) to penetrate directly through cell membranes into the cytoplasm or even the nucleus, and to bypass the endosomes, thus avoiding enzymatic degradation. Gene guns are so far mostly applied for plant cells.

However, there is much potential use in animals and humans as well. This technology was useful to transfection of cells and assessed by analyzing gene expression. Optimal transfection conditions were determined to be between 75 and 100 psi of helium pressure, 1.0 to 1.6 μm gold particle size and 0.5 mg of gold particle amount with a loading ratio of 4 μg DNA/mg gold particles (Uchida et al., 2009). These findings will be useful and suitable in the design of gene gun device, and bring further improvements to the in vivo transfection studies including gene therapy and vaccination.

3.4 Liposome

To increase the half-life of siRNA in vivo it can be encapsulated within liposomes or complex with cationic lipid to form siRNA-laden nanoparticles. Liposome are vesicles composed of phospholipids bilayer membranes that can enclose various substances, including DNA, siRNA, peptides, proteins, aptmers, chemicals, and drugs. Research on using liposomes to encapsulate and deliver chemotherapeutics has been performed since the late 1970s, and in the early 1980s they were extensively studied as potential vectors for gene therapy (Felgner et al., 1987). Recently, liposomes containing siRNA were modified with a peptide that targeted MCF-7 breast cancer cells, and were shown to effectively silence the expression of the PDMR14 gene that plays a role in breast cancer carcinogenesis, with minimal uptake and silencing effect in other non-cancerous cells (Bedi et al., 2011). Cationic liposomes can condense nucleic acids into a cationic particle when mixed together. This cationic lipid/nucleic acids complex (also called lipoplex) can protect nucleic acids from enzymatic degradation and deliver nucleic acids into cells by interacting with negatively charged cell membrane. Cationic liposomes have also been applied with substantial success for the in vitro as well as in vivo delivery of siRNA. Studies have been reported utilizing the advantage RNAi technology in vivo is successful knockdown of ApoB in nonhuman primates by systemically delivered siRNA in stable nucleic acid-lipid particles. The siRNA-lipid complexes showed significantly enhanced cellular internalization and endosomal escape of siRNA. Thus, the resulting ApoB siRNA-carrying liposome were stable during circulation in vivo after i.v. injection and reduced ApoB expression and serum cholesterol levels (Zimmermann et al., 2006).

3.5 Protein transduction domain-mediated siRNA

CPPs, also referred protein transduction domains (PTD) are short cationic peptide chains with a maximum of 30 amino acids. CPPs are able to penetrate biological membranes, to trigger the movement of various biomolecules across cell membranes into the cytoplasm and to improve their intracellular routing thereby facilitating interactions with the target. CPPs have been reported to deliver a wide variety of cargo (e.g. plasmid DNA, oligonucleotide, siRNA, protein, peptide, liposome, nanoparticle…), they are rapidly taken up into primary cells and most tissues by macropinocytosis in clinical trials. Most cellular uptake studies of PTD in the literature based on fluorescence microscopy of fixed cells and flow cytometry analysis report that internalization of PTD (Suzuki et al., 2002; Torchilin et al., 2001). As RNAi is one of the most promising strategies for gene therapy, further advances in CPP-based RNA delivery are expected in the near future.

3.6 Cationic polymers and polypeptide

Nucleic acids such as siRNA are easily complexed with synthetic cationic polymers e.g., polyethylenimine (PEI), biodegradable cationic polysaccharide (e.g. chitosan) and cationic polypeptides (e.g. atelocollagen, poly-L-lysine and protamine), via attractive electrostatic interactions. Polymer reduction can also allow for the release of nucleic acids into the cytoplasm. The use of reducible polymers and peptides is therefore a rapidly emerging strategy for enhanced transfection efficiency and cytoplasm-sensitive gene delivery. Various reduction-sensitive cationic polymers have been developed for gene delivery because they are highly stable in physiological conditions and rapidly reduced in the cytosol. For example, i.v. injection of siRNA-atelocollagen complexes silenced luciferase expression in germ cell tumor xenografted in mice and inhibited tumor growth (Minakuchi et al., 2004). In another study, the vascular endothelial growth factor (VEGF) siRNA-atelocollagen complexes successfully suppressed the secretion and expression of VEGF in human prostate PC-3 carcinoma cells, leading to the potent suppression of tumor growth in its xenograft model. This result clearly demonstrated that a novel VEGF blockade system by RNAi is valid as a therapeutic (Takei et al., 2004). Previous papers have demonstrated overexpression of RhoA in cancer indicates a poor prognosis, because of increased tumor cell proliferation and tumor angiogenesis. Furthermore, Pille´ et al showed that anti-RhoA siRNA inhibited aggressive breast cancer more effectively than conventional blockers of Rho-mediated signaling pathways. Likewise, the study has also demonstrated that intravenous administration of chitosan-RhoA siRNA complexes resulted in effective gene silencing in subcutaneously implanted breast cancer cells in nude mice (Pille et al., 2006). Tumor necrosis factor expression in systemic macrophages was silenced in mice after i.p. administration of chitosan/siRNA complexes, thus downregulating systemic and local inflammation (Howard et al., 2009).

3.6.1 Polyethylenimine

Polyethylenimine (PEI) is a synthetic polymer that can be either linear or branched, PEI is a well-known cationic polymer utilized as a non-viral vector because of its strong binding affinities to nucleic acids and proton buffering effect. In particular, 25 kDa PEI has been widely used in gene delivery. PEI with a high percentage of free amine groups which are positively charged and it is one of the most popularly investigated synthetic cationic polymers for nucleic acid delivery in vitro and in vivo. Paper has demonstrated that the noncovalent complexation of synthetic c-erbB2 / neu (HER-2) siRNA with low molecular weight polyethylenimine efficiently stabilizes siRNAs and delivers siRNAs into tumor cells via i.p. administration and results in a remarkable reduction of tumor growth, where where they display full bioactivity at completely nontoxic concentrations (Urban-Klein et al., 2005). Angiogenesis is the formation of new blood vessels from preexisting microvessels. In particular, tumor growth and metastasis were found to be dependent on angiogenesis. Thus, anti-angiogenic therapy has become an important route for cancer treatment (Cvetkovic et al., 2001; Lu et al., 2005). Likewise, a recent clinical trial examined the delivery of siRNA-laden polyethylenimine- based polymer modified with a targeting VEGF has been injected directly into subcutaneous tumors, and the silencing of VEGF and subsequent diminishment tumor growth was confirmed (Kim et al., 2008). For inhibition of VEGF expression, several gene therapeutic approaches using antisense oligonucleotide, ribozyme, and siRNA have been suggested as potential strategies for anti-cancer therapy (Lu et al., 2005; Rhee & Hoff, 2005; Takei et al., 2001). In another study, polyethylenimine-conjugated siRNA against secreted growth factor pleiotrophin (PTN) reduced tumor growth and cell proliferation without a measurable induction of siRNA-mediated immunostimulation after intracerebral or subcutaneous administration in an orthotopic glioblastoma nude mice model (Grzelinski et al., 2006). Overall, polyethylenimine seems to be a promising nonviral platform for siRNA delivery in vitro.

3.6.2 Chitosan

Chitosan, a linear and cationic polysaccharide composed of randomly distributed β-(1-4)-linked D-glucosamine (deacetylated unit) and N-acetyl-D-glucosamine (acetylated unit), is one of such biodegradable polymers, which has been extensively exploited for the preparation of nanoparticles for oral controlled delivery of several therapeutic agents. In recent years, the area of focus has shifted from chitosan to chitosan derivatized polymers, such as trimethylchitosan for the application of non-viral and non-toxic gene delivery. Paper has been shown quaternised chitosan transfect breast cancer cells; with the most efficient at gene delivery. In addition, chitosan's properties also allow it to be used in trans-dermal drug delivery.

3.6.3 Polypeptides

Polypeptides, such as poly-L-lysine and protamine, have also commonly been used to deliver siRNA. Poly-L-lysine (PLL) is a cationic polypeptide with the amino acid lysine as the repeating unit (Watanabe et al., 2009). PLL can be synthesized using various strategies leading to PLLs with different molecular weights (typically 1 kDa up to > 300 kDa), in linear conformation or as highly branched polypeptide (Garnett, 1999; Yoshida & Nagasawa, 2003). Also, protamine, a natural arginine-rich cationic polypeptide, condenses negatively charged nucleic acids and has been used as an efficient gene-delivery carrier (Vangasseri et al., 2005). Recent studies have investigated the low molecular mass protamine (LMWP)/VEGFsiRNA complex treatment, which possessed membrane translocating potency, the peptide could carry and localize siRNA inside tumors via i.p. administration and successfully inhibited the expression of VEGF, thereby suppressed the growth of hepatocarcinoma tumors in tumor-bearing mice (Choi et al., 2010). The data in this study clearly demonstrate that cell penetrating peptide-based systems not only enhance cellular uptake of siRNA, but also facilitate the suppression of VEGF expression without causing detectable systemic side effects. Furthermore, The LMWP is a potent transducible cell penetrating carrier for gene products including siRNA, and that potent growth inhibitory effects of the LMWP / VEGFsiRNA complex in vitro and in vivo. In addition, previous paper has also developed an efficient and low immunostimulatory nanoparticle formulation [liposomes-protamine-hyaluronic acid nanoparticle (LPH-NP)] for systemically delivering siRNA into the tumor (Chono et al., 2008). Overall, we expected that LMWP peptide and protamine could be used as a tool for siRNA delivery and may be applicable in an anti-angiogenic regulator to treat cancer in the future.

3.7 Electroporation

Electroporation, or electropermeabilization, is a popular in vitro technique for introducing siRNA or plasmid DNA into living cells. The application of electric pulses opens pores in the cell plasma membrane through which siRNA or DNA can pass and directly enter into the cytoplasm. Then, the pores close again and the DNA is trapped within the cell (Neumann et al., 1982). So, it is a significant increase in the electrical conductivity and permeability of the cell plasma membrane caused by an externally applied electrical field, and is usually used in molecular biology as a way of introducing some substance into a cell, such as loading it with a molecular probe, a drug that can change the cell's function, a piece of coding DNA or siRNA. Many research techniques in molecular biology require a foreign gene or protein material to be inserted into a host cell. Since the phospholipid bilayer of the plasma membrane has a hydrophilic exterior and a hydrophobic interior, any polar molecules, including DNA and protein, are unable to freely pass through the membrane (Hou, 2001). Electroporation is a dynamic phenomenon that depends on the local transmembrane voltage at each point on the cell membrane. It is generally accepted that for a given pulse duration and shape, a specific transmembrane voltage threshold exists for the manifestation of the electroporation phenomenon (from 0.5 V to 1 V). This leads to the definition of an electric field magnitude threshold for electroporation (Eth). That is, only the cells within areas where E≧Eth are electroporated. If a second threshold (Eir) is reached or surpassed, electroporation will compromise the viability of the cells, i.e., irreversible electroporation. This procedure is also highly efficient for the introduction of foreign genes in tissue culture cells, especially mammalian cells. For example, it is used in the process of producing knockout mice, as well as in tumor treatment, gene therapy, and cell-based therapy.

3.8 Calcium phosphate precipitation

A number of non-viral vectors have been explored till now. Some of these include cationic lipids, cationic polymers, peptides, other synthetic vectors, and precipitated calcium phosphate. Among these, the technique of calcium phosphate co-precipitation for in vitro transfection is used as a routine laboratory procedure. Calcium phosphate (CaP) is a well used non-viral vector for in vitro transfection of a wide variety of mammalian cells with little toxicity (Sokolova & Epple, 2008). Especially, DNA or siRNA-calcium phosphate coprecipitates have been used for many years as an efficient method to introduce genetic material in to cells, and the calcium phosphate particles have attracted much attention in gene therapy. Nucleic acids alone cannot penetrate the cell membrane, therefore special carriers like cationic polymers or inorganic nanoparticles are required. Single-shell and multi-shell calcium phosphate nanoparticles were prepared and functionalized with DNA and siRNA. The delivery activity is probably related to the fact that CaP rapidly dissolves in the acidic pH (Bisht et al., 2005). Endocytosed CaP is expected to deassemble in the endosomes and release its cargo into the cytoplasm. Many investigators have attempted to improve the manufacture of the CaP precipitate with limited success (Olton et al., 2007). In past study has reported that calcium ions play an important role in endosomal escape, cytosolic stability and enhanced nuclear uptake of siRNA through nuclear pore complexes. The siRNA encapsulated inside the nanoparticle is protected from the external RNase environment and could be used safely to transfer the encapsulated siRNA under in vivo conditions (Maitra, 2005). Thus, CaP precipitation is a dynamic and reversible process, and it can have multiple applications in gene function, regulation, and therapy and achieve its full potential in transfectional mammalian cells.

4. Application of RNAi

4.1 Clinical trials

There are many RNAi therapeutics approved by the U. S. Food and Drug Administration in various diseases in clinical trials (Table 1). Two *ex vivo* studies provided by City of Hope

Medical Center have designed for treating HIV infection through targeting on HIV tat and rev. IV transfer of in vivo lentiviral infected cells was used to treat patients with HIV infection. The expression of shRNA of tat and rev can knockdown the viral mRNA in T lymphocytes.
Four of these therapeutics for treating solid tumors are CALAA-01, siG12D LODER, ALN-VSP02, and Atu027. CALAA-01 provided by Calando Pharmaceuticals is a targeted therapeutic designed to inhibit tumor growth and/or reduce tumor size. It consists of a duplex siRNA to repress the expression of M2 subunit of ribonucleotide reductase. Another component AD-PEG-Tf combines the siRNA molecule with the transferrin receptor of the tumor cell surface to target the solid tumors. The majority of pancreatic ductal adenocarcinomas involve mutations in the KRAS oncogene, especially most common in G12D mutation. siG12D LODER provided by Silenseed Ltd is designed to inhibit oncogene KRas G12D mutation specifically. ALN-VSP02 provided by Alnylam Pharmaceuticals and Atu027 provided by Silence Therapeutics AG are both designed to inhibit growth and survival of cancer cells by tumor angiogenesis. ALN-VSP02 is a systemically delivered therapeutic packaged in Tekmira's SNALP delivery formulation and containing two siRNAs designed to target VEGF and kinesin spindle protein (KSP), also known as eglin 5 (Eg5), which disrupts cell division and induces apoptosis. In addition, in vitro studies revealed that Atu027-mediated inhibition of protein kinase N3 function in primary endothelial cells impaired tube formation on extracellular matrix and cell migration (Aleku et al., 2008).
There are five RNAi therapeutics approved by the U.S. FDA to treat ocular diseases, four designed in targeting VEGF and its receptor and one in caspase 2. Bevasiranib provided by Opko Health, Inc. involves in three clinical trials in treating macular edema and degeneration by 2-dT-modified siRNA on 3' end. Similarly, Allergan designed a siRNA targeting on VEGF receptor 1 to treat the same disease. In addition, a synthetic siRNA provided by Quark Pharmaceuticals, QPI-1007, inhibits expression of caspase 2 in retinal ganglion cells to prevent glaucoma, non-arteritic anterior ischemic optic neuropathy (NAION), and other ocular diseases.
There are two trials approved by FDA in treating kidney diseases using the same drug, I5NP, containing siRNA for p53, which arrests cell cycle progression and promotes cellular apoptosis. I5NP is provided by Quark Pharmaceuticals and designed to knockdown p53 to prevent cellular apoptosis of kidney in treating acute renal failure as well as in delayed graft function during kidney transplantation. Pachyonychia congenita is a rare keratin mutant disease, which affects the nails, skin, oral mucosae, larynx, hair and teeth. The majority of pachyonychia congenita involves mutations in the keratin gene, such as K6a, K6b, K16 or K17. A clinical trial using siRNA was applied by Pachyonychia Congenita Project. And, the siRNA was developed and provided by a small company, TransDerm, Inc., to inhibit the expression of the keratin K6a N171K mutation specifically.

4.2 Other approaches

4.2.1 Host protein screening and controlling of viral infection

Large siRNA libraries are constructed to knockdown all proteins known to be encoded by the human and mammalian genomes. Therefore, using siRNA library screening to identify the interacting proteins related to viral infection is a new approach. Several studies were carried out to screen the host factors of viruses, such as HIV, West Nile virus, Dengue virus, hepatitis C virus and influenza (Hirsch, 2010).

Disease	Sponsor	Product	Target gene	Target cell/tissue	Type of RNAi	Status
HIV	City of Hope Medical Center	rHIV7-shI-TAR-CCR5RZ-transduced autologous HPCs	HIV tat and rev	$CD34^+$ Cells	Lentivirus (*in vitro*)	Active, not recruiting
HIV	City of Hope Medical Center	pHIV7-shI-TAR-CCR5RZ treated CD4 cells	HIV tat and rev	T lymphocytes	Lentivirus (*in vitro*)	Phase 0 , terminated
Solid tumors	Calando Pharmaceuticals	CALAA-01	M2 subunit of ribonucleotide reductase	Solid tumors	Nanocomplex, synthetic siRNA	Phase I , recruiting
Pancreatic cancer	Silenseed Ltd	siG12D LODER	KRAS oncogene G12D mutation	Pancreatic ductal adenocarcinoma	Polymeric matrix, synthetic siRNA	Phase I , recruiting
Solid tumors	Alnylam Pharmaceuticals	ALN-VSP02	Vascular endothelial growth factor (VEGF) and kinesin spindle protein (KSP)	Solid tumors, liver	SNALP particle, synthetic siRNA	Phase I , recruiting
Advanced solid tumors	Silence Therapeutics AG	Atu027	Protein kinase N3	Advanced solid tumors	Liposome, 2'-O-methyl modified synthetic siRNA	Phase I , recruiting
Age-related macular degeneration	Allergan	AGN211745	VEGF receptor-1	Macula cells (retina)	Chemically modified siRNA	Phase II , completed
Diabetic macular edema	Opko Health, Inc.	Bevasiranib	VEGF	Retinal vasculature	3'-2 dT-capped synthetic siRNA	Phase II, completed
Age-related macular degeneration	Opko Health, Inc.	Bevasiranib	VEGF	Retinal vasculature	3' 2 dT-capped synthetic siRNA	Phase III, withdrawn
Macular degeneration	Opko Health, Inc.	Bevasiranib	VEGF	Retinal vasculature	3' 2 dT-capped synthetic siRNA	Phase II, completed
Optic neuropathy	Quark Pharmaceuticals	QPI-1007	Caspase 2	Retinal ganglion cells	Synthetic siRNA	Phase I , recruiting

Disease	Sponsor	Product	Target gene	Target cell/tissue	Type of RNAi	Status
Pachyonychia congenita	Pachyonychia Congenita Project (TransDerm, Inc.)	TD101	Keratin K6a N171K mutation	Skin		Phase I , completed
Hyperchole-sterolemia	Tekmira Pharmaceuti-cals Corporation	PRO-040201	ApoB		SNALP particle, synthetic siRNA	Phase I , terminated
Acute renal failure	Quark Pharmaceuti-cals	I5NP	P53	Kidney	Synthetic siRNA	Phase I , completed
Delayed graft function	Quark Pharmaceuti-cals	I5NP	P53	Kidney	Synthetic siRNA	Phase I/II , recruiting

Table 1. RNAi theraputics in clinical trials. (From the U.S. National Library of Medicine, A service of the U.S. National Institute of Health)

Human immunodeficiency virus type 1 (HIV-1) belongs to the family of retroviruses, infects human CD4+ lymphocytes and causes an indolent-type of infection and terminally ended to acquired immunodeficiency syndrome (Alimonti et al., 2003; Guadalupe et al., 2003). Because RNAi provides a strong justification to become a novel but remarkable therapeutic strategy in inhibiting gene expression, including viral mRNAs, many scientists participate in developing new methods using RNAi to treat HIV replication (Berkhout, 2009; Soejitno et al., 2003). In addition to HIV, RNAi is also used in controlling infection of several viruses, such as hepatitis B, hepatitis C, influenza, parainfluenza, CVB3, JEV, HSV2, RSV, PIV, SARS, foot-and-mouth disease and West Nile viruses (Chen et al., 2008; Khaliq et al., 2010; López-Fraga etal., 2008).

4.2.2 Neurodegenerative diseases

Neurodegenerative diseases are characterized by incorrect expression or selective dysfunction of proteins and eventual death of distinct subpopulations of neurons occurred in the central nervous system, such as Alzheimer's, Huntington's and Parkinson's diseases. They are solely caused by the inheritance of genetic mutations and several strategies using RNAi to target the specific mutant genes to treat these diseases in cellular and animal models were developed (Boudreau & Davidson, 2010; Maxwell, 2009). In contrast to these diseases, prion disease is caused by the conversion of a highly conserved prion protein across species, PrPc, into a partially protease-resistant isoform, PrPsc, which aggregates in the brain and is associated with pathogenesis of a neurodegenerative disease (Prusiner, 1991; Prusiner & DeArmond, 1991). However, the function of PrPc is not clear and its ablation represents no deleterious effects. Therefore, RNAi therapeutics should be useful strategies to target and remove normal PrPc to decrease the conversion and aggregation in the adult brain (Verity & Mallucci, 2010).

4.2.3 Immune diseases

As described above, siRNA-based therapeutics have entered clinical trials in treating many diseases. However, it has not been reported that siRNA can be used as an effective alternative to the present medications, such as corticosteroids, for managing allergy in vivo (Suzuki et al., 2009). It has been known that CD40/CD40 ligand (CD40L) interaction enhances Th2 cytokine production. Suzuki and colleagues have developed siRNA-based therapeutics to inhibit CD40 expression and found that decreased CD40 levels attenuated allergy through inhibition of functions of dendritic and B cells and generation of regulatory T cells (Suzuki et al., 2009). Bronchial asthma is a common inflammatory disease associated with allergy and activation of T helper type 2 cells, which secret cytokines to mediate local or systemic inflammation. One of inflammatory factors, interleukin 13 has been identified as a major driver of asthma pathology. Walker et al. used STAT6 siRNA to inhibit its expression and therefore found decreased downstream IL-13 as well as IL-4 and CCL26 protein expression in lung epithelial cells (Walker et al., 2009). The main inflammatory cytokines IL-1 and TNF-α are considered as potential targets for rheumatic diseases therapy. NF-κB is one of the key transcription factors associated with inflammatory pathway. siRNA specific for NF-κB p65 subunit is used in animal models to treat rheumatic diseases. It has been found that NF-κB downstream signaling molecules, such as cyclooxygenase-2, nitric oxide synthase-2, and matrix metalloproteinase-9 (de França et al., 2010; Lianxu et al., 2006).

4.2.4 Cancer gene therapies

Numerous scientists have designed shRNA or siRNAs in various cancer cell and animal models to develop the applications of RNAi in cancer therapeutics. He and colleagues have discussed genes associated with tumor growth and metastasis as well as adjuvant therapies for tumor radiation and chemotherapy (He et al., 2009). In addition to genes discussed by He et al., cyclooxygenase-2 (COX-2) is also a candidate for RNAi suppression, because it involves in tumor angiogenesis. Several in vitro studies have revealed that overexpression of COX-2 inhibits cellular apoptosis and promotes tumor angiogenesis. Therefore, COX-2 may play an important role in developing new vasculature, which involves in tumor growth and metastasis (DuBios et al., 1998; Liu et al., 2001; Tsujii et al., 1998; Wang & DuBois, 2010). Similar to identifying the interacting proteins related to viral infection (Hirsch, 2010), RNAi also paves the way for large scale loss-of-function genetic screens in mammalian cells to understand the cancer biology (Ashworth & Bernards, 2010). It also provides a novel and viable tool help in the identification of targets for treating cancer diseases and of those patients that are respond to a given therapy (Ashworth & Bernards, 2010; Micklem & Lorens, 2007; Nijwening & Beijersbergen, 2010).

5. Conclusion

RNA interference offers great promise for treating various disease states or helping to repair damaged tissue. Especially, initially in vivo studies demonstrated effective tumor suppression in nude mice by chemically synthesized siRNAs. More recently, many researchers have used non-viral or viral vectors for transcription of siRNAs / shRNAs in vitro and in vivo. RNAi technology has quickly been advanced from research discovery to clinical trials as effective gene silencing and therapeutic strategy since its discovery in 1998. Nevertheless, viral siRNA delivery raises several safety and preparation concerns such as immune responses and limited large-scale production. Non-viral siRNA have been developed to enhance transfection efficiency, minimize cytotoxicity and improve the bioactivities of nucleic acids, and then had competent in tackling the barriers in siRNA circulation, permeation into target tissues (ex. eye, central nervous system, muscle, and lung) specific binding to target cells and optimized intracellular trafficking. Recent advances clearly indicate that interdisciplinary approaches using biology, chemistry and engineering play crucial roles in achieving efficient and targeted siRNA delivery in vivo. In certain tissues, it has been demonstrated that a simple injection of naked siRNA will silence gene expression specifically in that tissue. In addition, to achieve local gene silencing in other tissues, a variety of approaches have been pursued to help stabilize the siRNA and to encourage cellular uptake by administration to the site of interest; they include chemical modification of the siRNA or complexation within liposomes or polymers to form nanoparticles. Overall, the field of siRNA delivery has been very focused on the use of nanoparticles.

The application of nanoparticles in medicine is an emerging field of nanobiotechnology (Kim, 2007). As a result of their small size, nanoparticles can penetrate the cell wall and deliver drugs or biomolecules into living systems, usually for a therapeutic purpose. Many different kinds of nanoparticles are known, many have been tested on biosystems, and some approaches have made it into clinical trials (Chen et al., 2010; Strong & West, 2011). Thus, this multifunctional, unique nanoparticulate carrier has the potential to detect diseases, deliver medications, and monitor the ability to change the current scenario of various diseases research and diagnosis in real time. Despite all this, the discovery and characterization of RNAi is not only as a powerful molecular biological tool to suppress the expression of a target gene, but also as an emerging therapeutic strategy to silence disease genes (Harrington, 2001). This work is not intended to give a comprehensive review of the antisense world, but rather to focus on what we know about the mechanism and function of RNAi, and how this molecule can best be applied as a therapy against various diseases.

6. Acknowledgment

We do appreciate the help from the Department of Internal medicine (Kaohsiung Medical University, Taiwan) for kindly providing precious clinical experiences about the application of RNAi.

7. References

Aleku, M., Schulz, P., Keil, O., Santel, A., Schaeper, U., Dieckhoff, B., Janke, O., Endruschat, J., Durieux, B., Röder, N., Löffler, K., Lange, C., Fechtner, M., Möpert, K., Fisch, G., Dames, S., Arnold, W., Jochims, K., Giese, K., Wiedenmann, B., Scholz, A., & Kaufmann, J. (2008). Atu027, a liposomal small interfering RNA formulation targeting protein kinase N3, inhibits cancer progression. *Cancer Research*, 68, 23, 9788-9798. ISSN: 0008-5472.

Andrew, V.O., Jun, Z., & Matthew, D.G. (2005). RNA interference by mixtures of siRNAs prepared using custom oligonucleotide arrays. *Nucleic Acids Research*, 33, 10 e92. ISSN: 1362-4962.

Ashworth, A., & Bernards, R. (2010). Using functional genetics to understand breast cancer biology. *Cold Spring Harbor Perspectives in Biology*, 2, 7, a003327. ISSN: 1943-0264.

Bedi, D., Musacchio, T., Fagbohun, O.A., Gillespie, J.W., Deinnocentes, P., Bird, R.C., Bookbinder, L., Torchilin, V.P., & Petrenko, V.A. (2011). Delivery of siRNA into breast cancer cells via phage fusion protein-targeted liposomes. *Nanomedicine*, (In press). ISSN: 1743-5889.

Berkhout, B. (2009) Toward a durable anti-HIV gene therapy aased on RNA interference. *Annals of the New York Academy of Sciences*, 1175, 3-14. ISSN: 0077-8923.

Bernstein, E., Caudy, A.A., Hammond, S.M., & Hannon, G.J. (2001). Role for a bidentate ribonuclease in the initiation step of RNA interference. *Nature*, 409, 6818, 363–366. ISSN: 0028-0836.

Bisht, S., Bhakta, G., Mitra, S., & Maitra, A. (2005). pDNA loaded calciumphosphate nanoparticles: highly efficient non-viral vector for gene delivery. *International Journal of Pharmaceutics*, 288, 1, 157-168. ISSN: 0378-5173.

Boudreau, R.L., & Davidson, B.L. (2010). RNAi therapeutics for CNS disorders. *Brain Research*, 1338, 112-121. ISSN: 0006-8993.

Brummelkamp, T.R., Bernards, R., & Agami, R. (2002a). Stable suppression of tumorogenicity by virus-mediated RNA interference. *Cancer Cell*, 2, 3, 243-247. ISSN: 1535-6108.

Chen, W., Cormode, D.P., Fayad, Z.A., & Mulder, W.J. (2010). Nanoparticles as magnetic resonance imaging contrast agents for vascular and cardiac diseases. *Nanomedicine and Nanobiotechnology*, (In press). ISSN: 1939-5116.

Chen, Y., Cheng, G., Mahato, R.I. (2008). RNAi for treating hepatitis B viral infection. *Pharmaceutical Research*, 25, 1, 72-86. ISSN 0724-8741.

Choi, Y.S., Lee, J.Y., Suh, J.S., Kwon, Y.M., Lee, S.J. Chung, J.K. Lee, D.S., Yang, V.C., Chung, C.P., & Park, Y.J. (2010). The systemic delivery of siRNAs by a cell penetrating peptide, low molecular weight protamine. *Biomaterials*, 31, 6, 1429-1443. ISSN: 0142-9612.

Chono, S., Li, S.D., Conwell, C.C., & Huang, L. (2008). An efficient and low immunostimulatory nanoparticle formulation for systemic siRNA delivery to the tumor. *Journal of Controlled Release*, 131, 1, 64-69. ISSN: 0168-3659.

Cvetkovic, D., Movsas, B., & Dicker, A.P. (2001). Increased hypoxia correlates with increased expression of the angiogenesis marker vascular endothelial growth factor in human prostate cancer. *Urology*, 57, 4, 821-825. ISSN: 0090-4295.

DuBois, R.N., Abramson, S.B., Crofford, L., Gupta, R.A., Simon, L.S., Van De Putte, L.B., & Lipsky, P.E. (1998). Cyclooxygenase in biology and disease, *FASEB Journal*, 12, 12, 1063-1073. ISSN: 0892-6638.

Dykxhoorn, D.M., & Lieberman, J. (2006). Knocking down disease with siRNAs. *Cell*, 2006, 126, 2, 231-235. ISSN: 0092-8674.

Dykxhoorn, D.M., Palliser, D., & Lieberman, J. (2006). The silent treatment: siRNAs as small molecule drugs. *Gene Therapy*, 13, 6, 541-552. ISSN: 0969-7128.

Elbashir, S.M., Harborth, J., Lendeckel, W., Yalcin, A., Weber, K., & Tuschl, T. (2001a) Duplexes of 21-nucleotide RNAs mediate RNA interference in cultured mammalian cells. *Nature*, 411, 6836, 494-498. ISSN: 0028-0836.

Elbashir, S.M, Lendeckel, W., & Tuschl, T. (2001b). RNA interference is mediated by 21- and 22-nucleotide RNAs. *Genes & Development*, 15, 2, 188-200. ISSN: 0890-9369.

Elbashir, S.M., Martinez, J., Patkaniowska, A., Lendeckel, W., & Tuschl, T. (2001c). Functional anatomy of siRNAs for mediating efficient RNAi in Drosophila melanogaster embryo lysate. The EMBO Journal, 20, 23, 6877-6888. ISSN: 0261-4189.

Felgner, P.L., Gadek, T.R., Holm, M., Roman, R., Chan, H.W., Wenz, M., Northrop, J.P., Ringold, G.M., & Danielsen, M. (1987). Lipofection: a highly efficient, lipid-mediated DNA-transfection procedure. *Proceedings of the National Academy of Sciences of the United States of America*, 84, 21, 7413-7417. ISSN: 0027-8424.

Fire, A., Xu, S., Montgomery, M.K., Kostas, S.A., Driver, S.E., & Mello, C.C. (1998). Potent and specific genetic interference by double-stranded RNA in Caenorhabditis elegans. *Nature* 391, 6669, 806-811. ISSN: 0028-0836.

Fuchs, U., Damm-Welk, C., & Borkhardt, A. (2004). Silencing of disease-related genes by small interfering RNAs. *Current Molecular Medicine*, 4, 5, 507-517. ISSN: 1566-5240.

de Fougerolles, A., Vornlocher, H.P., Maraganore, J., & Lieberman, J. (2007). Interfering with disease: a progress report on siRNA- based therapeutics. *Nature Reviews. Drug Discovery*, 6, 6, 443-453. ISSN: 1474-1776.

de França, N.R., Mesquita Júnior, D., Lima, A.B., Pucci, F.V., Andrade, L.E., & Silva, N.P. (2010). RNA interference: a new alternative for rheumatic diseases therapy. *Revista Brasileira de Reumatologia*, 50, 6, 695-702. ISSN: 0482-5004.

Garnett, M.C. (1999). Gene-delivery systems using cationic polymers. *Critical Reviews in Therapeutic Drug Carrier Systems*, 16, 2, 147-207. ISSN: 0743-4863.

Grimm, D., & Kay, M.A. (2007). Therapeutic application of RNAi: is mRNA targeting finally ready for prime time? *The Journal of Clinical Investigation*, 117, 12, 3633-3641. ISSN: 0021-9738.

Grzelinski, M., Urban-Klein, B., Martens, T., Lamszus, K., Bakowsky, U., Ho¨ bel, S., Czubayko, F., & Aigner, A. (2006). RNA interference-mediated gene silencing of pleiotrophin through polyethylenimine-complexed small interfering RNAs in vivo exerts antitumoral effects in glioblastoma xenografts. *Hum Gene Therapy*, 17, 7, 751-766. ISSN: 1043-0342.

Guadalupe, M., Reay, E., Sankaran, S., Prindiville, T., Flamm, J., McNeil, A., & Dandekar, S. (2003). Severe $CD4^+$ T-cell depletion in gut lymphoid tissue during primary human immunodeficiency virus type 1 infection and substantial delay in restoration following highly active antiretroviral therapy. *Journal of Virology*, 77, 21, 11708-11717. ISSN 0022-538X.

Hammond, S.M., Bernstein, E., Beach, D., & Hannon, G.J. (2000). An RNA-directed nuclease mediates post-transcriptional gene silencing in Drosophila cells. *Nature*, 404, 6775, 293-296. ISSN: 0028-0836.

Hannon, G.J. (2002). RNA interference. *Nature*, 418, 6894, 244-251. ISSN: 0028-0836.

Hannon, G.J., & Rossi, J.J. (2004). Unlocking the potential of the human genome with RNA interference. *Nature*, 431, 7006, 371-378. ISSN: 0028-0836.

Harrington, K.J., Spitzweg, C., Bateman, A.R., Morris, J.C., & Vile, R.G. (2001). Gene therapy for prostate cancer: current status and future prospects. *The Journal of Urology*, 166, 4, 1220-1233. ISSN: 0022-5347.

He, S., Zhang, D., Cheng, F., Gong, F., & Guo, Y. (2009). Applications of RNA interference in cancer therapeutics as a powerful tool for suppressing gene expression. *Molecular Biology Reports*, 36, 8, 2153-2163. ISSN: 0301-4851.

Henschel, A., Buchholz, F., & Habermann, B. (2004). DEQOR: A web-based tool for the design and quality control of siRNA. *Nucleic Acids Research*, 32, 113–20. ISSN: 0305-1048.

Hirsch, A.J. (2010). The use of RNAi-based screens to identify host proteins involved in viral replication. *Future Microbiology*, Vol.5, No.2, pp. 303-311, ISSN 1746-0913.Alimonti, J.B., Ball, T.B., & Fowke, K.R. (2003). Mechanisms of $CD4^+$ T lymphocyte cell death in human immunodeficiency virus infection and AIDS. *Journal of General Virology*, 84, pt7, 1649-1661. ISSN 0022-1317.

Hou, X., Omi, M., Harada, H., Ishii, S., Takahashi, Y., & Nakamura, H. (2001). Conditional knockdown of target gene expression by tetracycline regulated transcription of double strand RNA. *Development, Growth and Differentiation*, 53, 1, 69-75. ISSN: 0012-1592.

Howard, K.A., Paludan, S.R., Behlke, M.A., Besenbacher, F., Deleuran, B., & Kjems, J. (2009). Chitosan/siRNA nanoparticle-mediated TNF-α knockdown in peritoneal macrophages for anti-inflammatory treatment in a murine arthritis model. *Molecular therapy*, 17, 1, 162-168. ISSN: 1525-0016.

Izquierdo, M. (2005). Short interfering RNAs as a tool for cancer gene therapy. *Cancer Gene Therapy*, 12 , 3, 217-227. ISSN: 929- 1903.

Jackson, A.L., Burchard, J., Leake, D., Reynolds, A., Schelter , J., Guo, J., Johnson, J. M., Lim , L., Karpilow, J., Nichols, K., Marshall, W. , Khvorova, A., & Linsley, P.S. (2006). Position-specific chemical modification of siRNAs reduces off-target transcript silencing. *RNA Society*, 12, 7, 1197-1205. ISSN: 1355-8382.

Khaliq, S., Khaliq, S.A., Zahur, M., Ijaz, B., Jahan, S., Ansar, M., Riazuddin, S., Hassan, S. (2010). RNAi as a new therapeutic strategy against HCV. *Biotechnology Advances*, 28, 1, 27-34. ISSN 0734-9750.

Khvorova, A., Reynolds, A., & Jayasena, S.D. (2003). Functional siRNAs and miRNAs exhibit strand bias. *Cell*, 115, 2, 209-216.ISSN: 0092-8674.

Kim, K.Y. (2007). Nanotechnology platforms and physiological challenges for cancer therapeutics. *Nanomedicine*, 3, 2, 103-110. ISSN: 1549-9634.

Kim, S.H., J.H., Lee, S.H., Kim, S.W., & Park, T.G. (2008). Local and systemic delivery of VEGF siRNA using polyelectrolyte complex micelles for effective treatment of cancer. *Journal of Controlled Release*. 2008, 129, 2, 107-116. ISSN: 0168-3659.

Kirchhoff, F. (2008). Silencing HIV-1 in vivo. *Cell*, 134, 4, 566-568. ISSN: 0092-8674.

Klein, T.M., Wolf, E.D., Wu, R., & Sanford, J.C. (1992). High-velocity microprojectiles for delivering nucleic acids into living cells. *Biotechnology*, 24, 384-386. ISSN: 0733-222X.

Lianxu, C., Hongti, J., & Changlong, Y. (2006). NF-κBp65-specific siRNA inhibits expression of genes of COX-2, NOS-2 and MMP-9 in rat IL-1b-induced and TNF-α-induced chondrocytes. *Osteoarthritis and Cartilage*, 14, 4, 367-376. ISSN: 1063-4584.

Liu, C.H., Chang, S.H., Narko, K., Trifan, O.C., Wu, M.T., Smith, E., Haudenschild, C., Lane, T.F., & Hla, T. (2001). Overexpression of cyclooxygenase-2 is sufficient to induce tumorigenesis in transgenic mice. *The Journal of Biological Chemistry*, 276, 21, 18563-18569. ISSN: 0021-9258.

Loo, C., Lowery, A., Halas, N., West, J., & Drezek, R. (2005). Immunotargeted nanoshells for integrated cancer imaging and therapy. *Nano Letters*, 5, 4, 709-711. ISSN: 1530-6984.

López-Fraga, M., Wright, N., & Jiménez, A. (2008). RNA interference-based therapeutics: new strategies to fight infectious disease. *Infectious Disorders Drug Targets*, 8, 4, 262-273. ISSN 1871-5265.

Lorenz, C., Hadwiger, P., John, M., Vornlocher, H.P., & Unverzagt, C. (2004). Steroid and lipid conjugates of siRNAs to enhance cellular uptake and gene silencing in liver cells. *Bioorganic & Medicinal Chemistry Letters*, 14, 19, 4975-4977. ISSN: 0960-894X.

Lu, P.Y., Xie, F.Y., & Woodle, M.C. (2005). Modulation of angiogenesis with siRNA inhibitors for novel therapeutics, *Trends in Molecular Medicine*, 11, 3, 104–113. ISSN: 1471-4914.

Maitra, A. (2005). Calcium phosphate nanoparticles: second-generation nonviral vectors in gene therapy. *Expert Review of Molecular Diagnostics*, 5, 6, 893-905. ISSN: 1473-7159.

Maxwell, M.M. (2009). RNAi applications in therapy development for neurodegenerative disease. *Current Pharmaceutical Design*, 15, 34, 3977-3991. ISSN: 1381-6128.

Micklem, D.R., & Lorens, J.B. (2007). RNAi screening for therapeutic targets in human malignancies. *Current Pharmaceutical Biotechnology*, 8, 6, 337-343. ISSN: 1389-2010.

Minakuchi, Y., Takeshita, F., Kosaka, N., Sasaki, H., Yamamoto, Y., Kouno, M., Honma, K., Nagahara, S., Hanai, K., Sano, A., Kato, T, Terada, M., & Ochiya, T. (2004). Atelocollagen-mediated synthetic small interfering RNA delivery for effective gene silencing in vitro and in vivo. *Nucleic Acids Research*, 32, 13, e109. ISSN: 0305-1048.

Myers, J.W., Jones, J.T., Meyer, T., & Ferrell, J.E. (2003). Recombinant Dicer efficiently converts large dsRNAs into siRNAs suitable for gene silencing. *Nature Biotechnology*, 21, 3, 324–328. ISSN: 1087-0156.

Neumann, E., Schaefer-Ridder, M., Wang, Y., & Hofschneider, P.H. (1982). *The EMBO Journal*, 1, 7, 841- 845. ISSN: 0261-4189.

Nijwening, J.H., & Beijersbergen, R.L. (2010). Using large-scale RNAi screens to identify novel drug targets for cancer. *The Investigational Drugs Journal*, 13, 11, 772-777. ISSN: 1369-7056.

Novarino, G., Fabrizi, C., Tonini, R., Denti, M.A., Malchiodi-Albedi, F., Lauro, G.M., Sacchetti, B., Paradisi, S., Ferroni, A., Curmi, P.M., Breit, S.N., & Mazzanti, M. (2004). Involvement of the intracellular ion channel CLIC1 in microglia-mediated β-amyloid-induced neurotoxicity. *The Journal of Neuroscience*, 24, 23, 5322-5330. ISSN: 0270-6474.

Novina, C., & Sharp, P. (2004). The RNAi revolution. *Nature*. 430, 6996, 161-164. ISSN: 0028-0836.

Olton, D., Li, J., Wilson, M.E., Rogers, T., Close, J., Huang, L., Kumta, P.N., & Sfeir, C. (2007). Nanostructured calcium phosphates (NanoCaPs) for non-viral gene delivery: influence of the synthesis parameters on transfection efficiency. *Biomaterials*, 28, 6, 1267- 1279. ISSN: 0142-9612.

Pille, J.Y., Li, H., Blot, E., Bertrand, J.R., Pritchard, L.L., Opolon, P., Maksimenko, A., Lu, H., Vannier, J.P., Soria, J. Malvy, C., & Soria, C. (2006). Intravenous delivery of anti-RhoA small interfering RNA loaded in nanoparticles of chitosan in mice: safety and efficacy in xenografted aggressive breast cancer. *Human Gene Therapy*, 17, 10, 1019-1026. ISSN: 1043-0342.

Prusiner, S. B. (1991). Molecular biology of prion diseases. *Science*, 252, 5012, 1515-1522. ISSN 0193-4511.

Prusiner, S.B., & DeArmond, S.J. (1991). Molecular biology and pathology of scrapie and the prion diseases of humans. *Brain Pathology*, 1, 4, 297-310. ISSN 1015-6305.

Reynolds, A., Leake, D., Boese, Q., Scaringe, S., Marshall, W.S., & Khvorova, A. (2004). Rational siRNA design for RNA interference. *Nature Biotechnology*, 22, 3, 326-330. ISSN: 1087-0156.

Rhee, J., & Hoff, P.M. (2005). Angiogenesis inhibitors in the treatment of cancer. *Expert Opinion on Pharmacotherapy*, 6, 10, 1701-1711. ISSN: 1465-6566.

Schwarz, D.S., Hutvagner, G., Du, T., Xu, Z., Aronin, N., & Zamore, P.D. (2003). Asymmetry in the assembly of the RNAi enzyme complex. *Cell*, 115, 2, 199-208. ISSN: 0092-8674.

Shim, M.S., & Kwon, Y.J. (2010). Efficient and targeted delivery of siRNA in vivo. *The FEBS Journal*. 2010, 277, 23, 4814-4827. ISSN: 1742-464X.

Sioud, M., & Sorensen, D. (2003). Cationic liposomemediated delivery of siRNAs in adult mice. *Biochemical and Biophysical Research Communications*, 312, 4, 1220-1225. ISSN: 0006-291X.

Soejitno, A., Wihandani, D.M., & Kuswardhani, T. (2009). The therapeutic potential of RNA interference in controlling HIV-1 replication. *Acta Medica Indonesiana*, 41, 4, 215-221. ISSN 0125-9326.

Sokolova, V., & Epple, M. (2008). Inorganic nanoparticles as carriers of nucleic acids into cells. *Angewandte Chemie* (International ed. in English), 47, 8, 1382-1395. ISSN: 1433-7851.

Sorensen, D., Leirdal, M., & Sioud, M. (2003). Gene silencing by systemic delivery of synthetic siRNAs in adult mice. Journal of molecular biology, 327, 4, 761-766. ISSN: 0022-2836.

Strong, L.E., & West, J.L. (2011). Thermally responsive polymer-nanoparticle composites for biomedical applications. Wiley Interdisciplinary reviews. *Nanomedicine and Nanobiotechnology*, (In press). ISSN: 1939-5116.

Suzuki, M., Zheng, X., Zhang, X., Ichim, T.E., Sun, H., Kubo, N., Beduhn, M., Shunnar, A., Garcia, B., & Min, W.P. (2009). Inhibition of allergic responses by CD40 gene silencing. *Allergy*, 64, 3, 387-397. ISSN: 0105-4538.

Suzuki, T, Futaki, S., Niwa, M., Tanaka, S., Ueda, K., & Sugiura, Y. (2002). Possible existence of common internalization mechanisms among arginine-rich peptides. *The Journal of Biological Chemistry*, 277, 4, 2437-2443 ISSN: 0021-9258.

Takei, Y., Katomatsu, K., & Matsuo, S. (2001). Antisense oligodeoxynucleotide targeted to Midkine, a heparin-binding growth factor, suppresses tumorigenicity of mouse rectal carcinoma cells. *Cancer Research*, 61, 23, 8486–8491. ISSN: 0008-5472.

Takei,Y., Kadomatsu, K., Yuzawa, Y., Matsuo, S., & Muramatsu, T. (2004). A small interfering RNA targeting vascular endothelial growth factor as cancer therapeutics. *Cancer Research*, 64, 10, 3365-3370. ISSN: 0008-5472.

Torchilin, V.P., Rammohan, R., Weissig, V., & Levchenko, T.S. (2001). Tat peptide on the surface of liposomes affords their efficient intracellular delivery even at low temperature and in presence of metabolic inhibitors. *Proceedings of the National Academy of Sciences of the United States of America*, 98, 15, 8786-8791. ISSN: 0027-8424.

Tsujii, M., Kawano, S., Tsuji, S., Sawaoka, H., Hori, M., & DuBois, R.N. (1998). Cyclooxygenase regulates angiogenesis induced by colon cancer cells. *Cell*, 93, 5, 705-716. ISSN: 0092-8674.

Uchida, M., Li, X.W., Mertens, P., & Alpar, H.O. (2009). Transfection by particle bombardment: Delivery of plasmid DNA into mammalian cells using gene gun. *Biochimica et biophysica acta*, 1790, 8, 754-764. ISSN: 0006-3002.

Ui-Tei, K., Naito, Y., Takahashi, F., Haraguchi, T., Ohki-Hamazaki, H., Juni, A., Ueda, R., & Saigo, K. (2004). Guidelines for the selection of highly effective siRNA sequences for mammalian and chick RNA interference. *Nucleic Acids Research*, 3, 23, 936-948. ISSN: 0305-1048.

Urban-Klein, B., Werth, S., Abuharbeid, S., Czubayko, F., & Aigner, A. (2005). RNAi-mediated gene-targeting through systemic application of polyethylenimine (PEI)-complexed siRNA in vivo. *Gene Therapy*, 12, 5, 461-466. ISSN: 0969-7128.

Vangasseri, D.P., Han, S.J., & Huang, L. (2005). Lipid–protamine–DNA-mediated antigen delivery. *Current Drug Delivery*, 2, 4, 401- 406. ISSN: 1567-2018.

Vives, E., Brodin, P., & Lebleu, B. (1997). A truncated HIV-1 Tat protein basic domain rapidly translocates through the plasma membrane and accumulates in the cell nucleus. *The Journal of biological chemistry*, 272, 25, 16010-16017. ISSN: 0021- 9258.

Verity, N.C., & Mallucci, G.R. (2010). Rescuing neurons in prion disease. *The Biochemical Journal*, 433, 1, 19-29. ISSN: 0264-6021.

Walker, W., Healey, G.D., & Hopkin, J.M. (2009). RNA interference of STAT6 rapidly attenuates ongoing interleukin-13-mediated events in lung epithelial cells. *Immunology*, 127, 2, 256-266. ISSN: 0019-2805.

Wang, D., & Dubois, R,N. (2010). The role of COX-2 in intestinal inflammation and colorectal cancer. *Oncogene*, 29, 6, 781-788. ISSN: 0950-9232.

Watanabe, K., Harada-Shiba, M., Suzuki, A., Gokuden, R., Kurihara, R., Sugao, Y., Mori,T., Katayama, Y., & Niidome, T. (2009). In vivo siRNA delivery with dendritic poly (l-lysine) for the treatment of hypercholesterolemia. *Molecular BioSystems*, 5, 11, 1306-1310. ISSN: 1742-206X.

Williams, N.S., Gaynor, R.B., Scoggin, S., Verma, U., Gokaslan, T., Simmang, C., Fleming, J., Tavana, D., Frenkel, E., & Becerra, C. (2003). Identification and validation of genes involved in the pathogenesis of colorectal cancer using cDNA microarrays and RNA interference. Clinical Cancer Research, 9, 3, 931-946. ISSN: 1078-0432.

Yang, D., Buchholz, F., Huang, Z., Goga, A., Chen, C.Y., Brodsky, F.M., & Bishop, J.M. (2002). Short RNA duplexes produced by hydrolysis with Escherichia coli RNase III mediate effective RNA interference in mammalian cells. *Proceedings of the National Academy of Sciences of the United States of America*, 99, 15, 9942–9947. ISSN: 0027-8424.

Yang, Y.L., Lin, S. H., Chuang, L. Y., Guh, J. Y., Liao, T. N., Lee, T. C., Chang, W. T., Chang, F. R., Hung, M. Y., Chiang, T. A., & Hung, C. Y. (2007). CD36 is a novel and potential anti-fibrogenic target in albumin-induced renal proximal tubule fibrosis. Journal of Cellular Biochemistry, 101, 3, 735-744. ISSN: 0730-2312.

Yeager, T. (2005). GeneClip U1 Hairpin Cloning Systems for expression of short hairpin RNAs *in vivo*. *Promega Notes*, 89, 21-24.

Yoshida, T., & Nagasawa, T. (2003). epsilon-Poly-L-lysine: microbial production, biodegradation and application potential. Applied microbiology and biotechnology, 62, 1, 21-26. ISSN: 0175-7598.

Yu, J.Y., DeRuiter, S.L., & Turner. D.L. (2002). RNA interference by expression of short interfering RNAs and hairpin RNAs in mammalian cells. *Proceedings of the National Academy of Sciences of the United States of America*, 99, 9, 6047-6052. ISSN: 0027-8424.

Zimmermann, T.S., Lee, A.C., Akinc, A., Bramlage, B., Bumcrot, D., Fedoruk, M.N., Harborth, J., Heyes, J.A., Jeffs, L.B., John, M. Judge, A.D., Lam, K., McClintock, K., Nechev, L.V., Palmer, L.R., Racie, T., Röhl, I., Seiffert, S., Shanmugam, S., Sood, V., Soutschek, J., Toudjarska, I., Wheat, A.J., Yaworski, E., Zedalis, W., Koteliansky, V., Manoharan, M., Vornlocher, H.P., & MacLachlan, I. (2006). RNAi-mediated gene silencing in non-human primates. *Nature*, 441, 7089, 111-114. ISSN: 0028- 0836.

3

Scalable Technology to Produce Pharmaceutical Grade Plasmid DNA for Gene Therapy

Odalys Ruiz Hernández, Miladys Limonta Fernández, Jorge Valdes Hernández, Martha Pupo Peña and Eduardo Martínez Díaz
Center for Genetic Engineering and Biotechnology
Cuba

1. Introduction

The use of gene therapy is a promising process for the prevention, treatment and cure of diseases such as cancer and acquired inmudeficiency syndrome (AIDS); increasing a considerable interest during the last decade (Prather et al., 2003). This process requires considerable amounts of plasmid DNA (pDNA) that should be homogeneous with respect to structural form and DNA sequence (O´Kennedy et al., 2003).

It was shown that naked DNA injected into muscle tissue is expressed in vivo; also the introduction of immunogenic sequences can result in animal vaccination against the encoded peptide (Vogel & Sarver 1995). In general, DNA-based vaccines are considered very safe due, in part, to the lack of genetic integration, and to the absence of specific immune response to the plasmid itself (Robinson, 2000), making its property very attractive. This approach was successfully tested for vaccination against several viral infections such as: West Nile virus vaccine licensed in 2005 by the USDA; in horses; is currently in phase II trial in humans; and the H5N1 influenza DNA vaccine currently undergoing phase I clinical trials (Phue, 2008).

When the concept of a DNA vaccine first popped onto the scene in the early 1990s, it seemed too simple, too easy and too bizarre to be true. Regardless the considerable scientific effort over the past few years, no gene-therapy product has yet reached the market, at the moment. Only several clinical trials have been carried out and thousands of people have received (pDNA) without serious adverse effects (Prazeres et al., 1999). By virtue of the developments made recently in biotechnology and molecular medicine, the speculation of 20 years ago that gene technology would become a powerful tool to cure disease directly, has become reality (Schleef, 1999) and the market of one of these products would exceed US$45 billion.

The trend toward testing DNA vaccines as part of combination trials can be seen in both the large vaccine producers like Merck, Aventis Pasteur and Wyeth as well as in smaller research companies (Powell, 2004). Although the processes of production for many gene-therapy vectors have been developed in pharmaceutical companies, the information of large-scale pDNA production is scarce and usually not available to the scientific community (Xu et al., 2005).

FDA added "Therapeutic plasmid DNA vector" to the list of well-characterized biotechnology product and gene therapy has been moved rapidly from laboratory scale to clinical trials. As a matter of urgency, it is essential to develop new protocols to obtain high-quality plasmids with high yields. The understanding, optimization and validation of steps, from pDNA design and host strain selection to mass-cultivation and purification, are crucial if this novel vaccine technology will become commercially successful (Prather et al., 2003). Innovative methodologies and new engineering tools are needed to expand the window of opportunity for process design. The advantages of the procedure described over existing technology to produce pharmaceutical grade pDNA for gene therapy include a high cell density culture, improved plasmid purity and the elimination of undesirable process additives such as toxic organic extractants and animal derived components or raw materials. By employing this simple, scalable and applicable approach we concluded successfully clinical trial (phase I); and currently is in Phase II using the pIDKE2 plasmid; which is the main component CIGB's candidate vaccine against Hepatitis C virus. The principal topics of this chapter are: Fermentation process including design of high-cell-density culture, Downstream process using tangential flow filtration and chromatography, which are widely accepted methods for pDNA purification and act as orthogonal techniques platform, Scale-up of bioprocess, Quality control of pDNA manufacturing and finally regulatory aspects.

2. Fermentation process to produce plasmid DNA

For the production of large quantities of pDNA an efficient fermentation process needs to be established. The fermentation conditions for optimization of pDNA production in *Escherichia coli (E. coli)* could be fundamental however experimental data are limited. Although the available information is limited in comparison with the extensive recombinant protein production literature, some general rules and methodologies pertaining to the production of pDNA by cultivation of *E. coli* are beginning to emerge (Prather et al., 2003).
A number of recent reports discuss the fermentation strategies used for production of pDNA, but have not addressed the effect of fermentation conditions on the quality of the resulting pDNA. Few studies have been carried out focusing on the quality of plasmid product at the end of the fermentation stage. Because the location of pDNA is intracellular, productivity is proportional to the final cell-density and the specific productivity (amount of pDNA per unit cell mass) too (Yakhchali et al, 2007). Typically, 0.5 - 1 g pDNA per Kg of wet weight biomass is obtained from cultivation media using high copy number plasmid. Therefore the choice of fermentation protocol will be critical in minimizing process contaminants that need to be removed during downstream processing (O´Kennedy et al., 2003).
Generally, these simple processes are based on the growth of *E. coli* in either shake flasks or small laboratory fermentors, usually employing simple media formulation such as Luria Bertani (LB) or Terrific Broth (TB). These processes yield low cell mass, which support modest volumetric plasmid yields that are only sufficient for studies employing limited number of small animals (Prather et al., 2003).
Strategies aimed at increasing plasmid amplification in fermentation include the use of temperature shock, while achievable on a small scale, may be difficult to implement on a large scale. The use of fermentation devices is necessary too, so over the whole propagation of growth at least the following parameters are monitored and documented: temperature, pH, pO2, agitation speed, and the use of some solution like: antifoam, acid, base and in some cases feeding solution.

On the other hand the use of low specific growth rates (μ) is unifying principle in high-quality, high-yield fermentations for pDNA production. Chen et al. 1997 indicated that the pDNA yield is related to the specific growth rate of bacteria during the fermentation. In addition, other authors suggest that the plasmid yields obtained from culture were highest into stationary phase. High specific growth rates are associated with acetate production, plasmid instability and lower percentages of supercoiled plasmid overall (Xu et al., 2005).
The FDA recognizes that open-circle, linear and nicked forms may be fewer effectives therapeutically than supercoiled DNA. Those other forms can be very difficult to separate from the supercoiled plasmid during purification. Therefore, fermentation processes should also be optimized to produce a high percentage of supercoiled plasmid (Carnes, 2005). Large scale *E. coli* fermentation systems for plasmid DNA production have been developed and the success of this process will be dependent on the interactions between the host organism, the recombinant plasmid vector, its copy number, the gene size and the growth environment.

2.1 Host strain

The first consideration in designing an efficient process should be host cell line selection. Host selection requires that the source of the microbial strain must be characterized and free of any adventitious agents, as well as be genotypically and phenotypically well characterized (Prather et al., 2003). Plasmids represent less than 0.5% of the wet biomass and endotoxins and other impurities must be completely removed so the characteristics of the microbial host affect the quality of the purified DNA.
Plasmid production should be in an *E. coli* K12 strain considered non-pathogenic. *E. coli* is usually chosen today as the production host, with its concomitant benefits and drawbacks. The benefits include a high DNA yield and well-established procedures for down-stream processing of the plasmid. However, as a gram-negative bacterium contains highly immunogenic endotoxin or lipopolysaccharides (LPS) in its outer membrane (Glenting, et al, 2005). Popular hosts such as DH5 derivates and XL1 Blue are suitable for plasmid production. Judicious selection of the host strain is also important because this can be minimize the amounts of impurities that needs to be removed by, for example avoiding strains that produce large amounts of carbohydrate such as HB101 (Prazeres et al., 1999). In our experience DH10B have been found to be consistently higher producing pDNA.

2.2 Culture medium

Medium composition and cultivation conditions play an important role by controlling amount of biomass, plasmid copy number and stability. It was reported that the media composition affected cell specific growth rate, and thus influenced in plasmid copy number. Therefore, the effects of medium components on cell growth and plasmid productivity should be evaluated (Xu et al., 2005).
Media composition can dramatically affect yield and consequently the overall cost of production. Media for plasmid production should support high nucleotide pools in cells and supply energy for replication while minimize other cell activity (Carnes, 2005). Through the type and concentration of ingredients used, cultivation medium composition directly dictates the amounts of biomass produced; is therefore likely to influence plasmid volumetric yield (Prather et al., 2003).
Typically, the nutritional requirements are satisfied by either minimal or complex media. The first option contains known quantities of essential nutritional components including

carbon source, nitrogen source and salts and excludes components known to be inhibitory to bacterial growth. Complex media formulations often contain ingredients like yeast extract and peptones that may allow for a higher cell density. Fermentation processes using minimal media are highly reproducible and support higher plasmid copy number (Carnes, 2005). Although standard media can be used for plasmid production, some authors recommend the development of media adapted to the specific plasmid-host system involved in order to increase productivity (Prazeres et al., 1999). Media that supported similar specific growth rates between plasmid-bearing and plasmid-free cells also supported high plasmid stability.

Design of balanced medium is based on bacterial energy requirements and elemental composition (Carnes, 2005). A carbon source provides energy and biomass and is usually the limiting nutrient in *fed-batch* culture. Glucose is the conventional choice as a carbon source because it is inexpensive and very efficiently metabolized. However, high glucose levels have demonstrated to cause undesirable acetate production due to metabolic overflow. The application of glycerol avoids repression of intermediate metabolites and accumulations of inhibitive organic acids to some extent. Therefore, the effect of glycerol addition in culture and feed medium on pDNA production in *E. coli* should be also examined.

On the other hand the selection of nitrogen source and the determination of its concentration are critical to the optimization of plasmid production in recombinant cell fermentation. A nitrogen source and trace metals elements are required for bacterial growth, metabolism and enzymatic reactions. The bacterial requirement for nitrogen can be satisfied by inorganic and organic source. From the development of high density cell culture point of view, organic complex supply of nitrogen from components, such as yeast extract, is essential because it is more effective to support high plasmid yield. Minerals are necessary too for bacterial growth, metabolism and enzymatic reactions. For example it was reported that Magnesium sulphate is often the source of both magnesium and sulphur; and high concentrations are beneficial for the production of homogeneous supercoil plasmid monomers. Therefore, the effects of medium components on cell growth and plasmid productivity should be evaluated to solve the trade-off between higher copy number and reduced specific growth rate (Xu et al., 2005).

2.3 High cell density culture

A further feature of fermentation technology for large scale plasmid production is the performance of high-density culture to obtain large amounts of biomass. *Fed-batch* fermentation provides higher biomass yields than *batch* fermentation because substrate is supplied at such rate, that it is nearly completely consumed; so delivers nutrients over an extended period of time (Carnes, 2005). Both *batch* and *fed-batch* technologies have been successfully employed for plasmid over-production by *E. coli*. *Batch* cultivation, although logistically simple, is severely limited with respect to achieving elevated biomass (Prather et al., 2003).

Nutritional requirements and cellular composition of *E. coli* are well defined. This information that has been reported in literature can be advantageously used in the design of culture media formulation (Table 1) (Carnes, 2005). High cell density (HCD) fermentation requires a balanced medium supplying adequate amounts of nutrients needed for energy, biomass and cell maintenance; and commonly contains carbon and nitrogen sources, various salts and trace metals. HCD process has many inherent advantages, specifically reduces the time required in a fermenter in either a contract manufacturing facility or in captive space.

Element	Dry Weight Percentage
Carbon	50-53
Hydrogen	7
Nitrogen	12-15
Phosphorous	2-3
Sulfur	0.2-1.0
Potassium	1.0-4.5
Sodium	0.5-1.0
Calcium	0.01-1.10
Magnesium	0.1-0.5
Chloride	0.5
Iron	0.02-0.2

Table 1. Elemental component of bacteria.

In *fed-batch* fermentation cells are inoculated into an initial volume of medium that contains all nonlimiting nutrients and an initial concentration of the limiting substrate. These processes start with a *batch* phase, namely phase of biomass build up where the cells grow exponentially (Carnes, 2005) follow by a phase of slow growth, achieved via *fed-batch* technology, where plasmid amplification takes place. Several researches have observed that plasmid copy number increases during both, the late exponential and early stationary phases of growth (Prather et al., 2003). These kinds of cultivations lead to significantly higher biomass yields avoiding the loss of product. The amount of product per cell (or per cell weight) in particular strongly influences the downstream processing scale and therefore, defines another important part of the production costs (Schleef, 1999).

Several feeding strategies have been developed, either automated feedback controlled (e.g., DO-stat, pH-stat, metabolic activity, biomass concentration and substrate concentration) or predetermined (e.g., constant, linear stepwise or exponential feeding). The feeding of nutrients, usually glucose, has been extensively researched and incorporates a range of approaches that span from simple to much elaborated, with each presenting its own advantages and disadvantages. One of the most effective feeding strategies is exponential feeding. This method allows a culture to grow at a predetermined specific rate $< \mu_{max}$ without the need of feedback control. Feeding regimens based on feed rate increase, either simple or following sophisticated algorithms aimed at maintaining a more constant environment thus have been successfully implemented maintaining a desired growth rate (Prather et al., 2003).

However, HCD technique has its draw backs and growth inhibitory by products, such as acetate formed. Acetate formation can be reduced or prevent by altering the fermentation medium or optimization of feeding strategies during *fed-batch* fermentation. According to our literature survey, the effect of acetate on pDNA production in HCD culture has been little investigated (Yakhchali et al, 2007). It has been reported that a minimum acetic acid accumulation and a high plasmid copy number could be obtained when the specific growth rate is about 0.1 h^{-1}.

Using all this approach, we designed a *fed-batch* culture medium according to bacterial element composition to obtain the recombinant host *E. coli* DH10B bearing pIDKE2. This plasmid is the first 650 aa of the Hepatitis C Viral (HCV) polyproteins for DNA immunization expression from the 1b-Cuban isolate genotype (Dueñas et al., 2007). The results show that cell density increased during exponential phase at around 20-21 hrs, to the stationary phase at around 22- 25 hrs, and cell density decreased at 26 hrs. The highest cell mass (29 ± 1.7 g dry cell l^{-1}), plasmid yield (154 ± 2.8 mg pDNA l^{-1}) and specific pDNA yield (0.44 ± 0.02 mg pDNA g^{-1} dry cell weight) were obtained at 24 hours of culture. So we suggest stop the culture in this moment (Ruiz et al, 2009).
The behaviour of *E. coli* (DH10B) in this *fed-batch* fermentation process (red bar in Figure 1) was common because the average of volumetric yield (154± 2.8 mg pDNA l^{-1}) is in the state average of the art (142 mg pDNA l^{-1}). With this culture procedure larger amounts of plasmid pIDKE2 can be obtained in DH10B cells. Several researchers have reported the behaviour of plasmid volumetric yield (mg/L) for different fermentation strategy (Figure 1) (Diogo, 2000, 2001; Durland, 1999; Lahijani, 1996; Shmidt, 2001, 2003; Wang, 2001). As it is shown, plasmid production under non optimized laboratory conditions invariably leads to very low volumetric titters (5-70 mg/L) and DNA production processes that employ simple *batch* cultivation technology yield relatively low biomass and correlatively support low plasmid volumetric yields too (<100 mg/L). However, increasing medium strength, by either adding additional nutrients, employing richer formulation or sophisticated feeding strategy (orange bar), support higher volumetric yield without compromising plasmid quality.

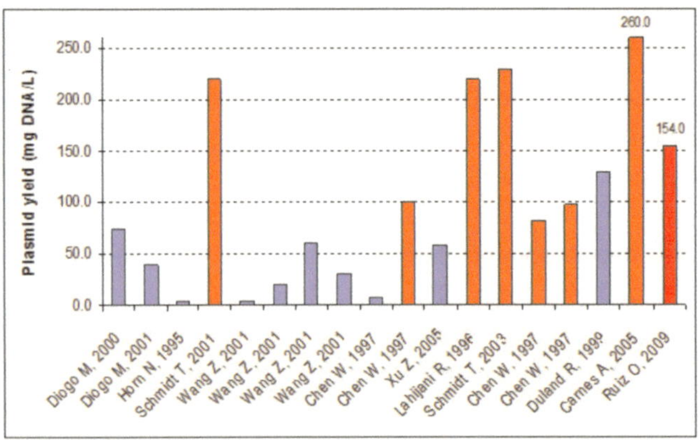

Culture Strategy	Reference
Shake flask 2L (LB medium)	Diogo M, 2000
Batch (TB medium)	Diogo M, 2001
Batch (TBKmedium)	Horn N, 1995
Fed Batch (exponential feeding)	Schmidt T, 2001
Batch (LB medium)	Wang Z, 2001
Batch (LB medium +Glucose)	Wang Z, 2001
Batch (Defined media 1)	Wang Z, 2001
Batch (Defined media 2)	Wang Z, 2001
Fed Batch (manual feeding)	Chen W, 1997
Fed Batch (DO-stat)	Chen W, 1997
Shake flask (Defined media)	Xu Z, 2005
Fed Batch (Temperature shock)	Lahijani R, 1996
Fed Batch (DO-stat)	Schmidt T, 2003
Fed Batch (DO-stat)	Chen W, 1997
Fed Batch (pH-stat)	Chen W, 1997
Batch (Defined media)	Duland R, 1999
Fed Batch (Exponential feeding)	Carnes A, 2005
Fed Batch (Constant feeding)	Ruiz O, 2009

Fig. 1. Plasmid volumetric yields, from several references with different fermentation strategies.

A combination of plasmid and host-strain selection with optimization of fed-batch fermentation can result in yields as high as 260 mg/L (Carnes, 2005). Therefore HCD fermentation techniques for culturing *E. coli* has been developed to improve productivity and to obtain high cell density.

2.4 Scale up

When a molecular biologist thinks of a "large scale" pDNA production, the range of 10-100mg of DNA usually comes to mind. However, at a pharmaceutical production-scale, pDNA requirements may exceed 50g per *batch*. In extreme case, many kilograms of pDNA per year will be needed to fill the ultimate marketing demand for DNA vaccines currently in clinical trials (Prather et al., 2003). The transfer from research scale technology to manufacturing scale requires management of the upscaling process. Such upscaling is not just a simple multiplication of relevant factors, but instead requires highest competence, time investment and incurs cost.

Effective scale-up is essential for successful bioprocessing. Much fermentation processes were successfully scale-up on the basis of a constant volumetric oxygen transfer coefficient (KLa) and power consumption per unit volume (P/V); so they are widely used. However when a particular scale-up strategy is carried out maintaining a specific set of parameters constant, other parameters can not be controlled and may change substantially in unexpected ways (Schleef, 1999).

Current scale-up methods assume that the environment conditions are homogeneously distributed within the large-scale fermentation, as in the small-scale fermentor, however, this is not true. There are so many factors, like hydrodynamics factors, height and geometric configuration of the reactor that would affect the environment of the fluid in the large-scale reactors. The use of traditional empirical methods lead to an increase in mixing and circulation times at large scale. In addition high oxygen demands and high viscosity can cause concentration gradients in oxygen, shear and pH; that can have a significant impact on fermentation yield. Therefore, the choice of scale-up criteria in not an easy task, given the potential sensitive and diverse response of cells to each of the transport phenomena influenced by impeller design, system geometry, scale, fluid properties, and operating parameters.

The primary scale-up criterion of process should be selected based upon the transport property most critical to the performance of the process. If oxygen transfer is the limiting factor, then scale up by equal P/V will be essential. This method is adopted for many authors using larger-scale fermentors, such as these below 1000L capacity (Pollard et al., 2007). Moreover, the suitability of scaled-up methods is usually confirmed by experimental results. Scale-up of plasmid pIDKE2 production from 5L fermentor to 50L pilot scale fermentor was carried out successfully using constant P/V in a *fed batch* process illustrated in epigraph 2.3. Final biomass concentration and specific pDNA yield were increased in comparison with cultures grown on a standard laboratory medium (TB) on *batch* mode as we can see in Figure 2.

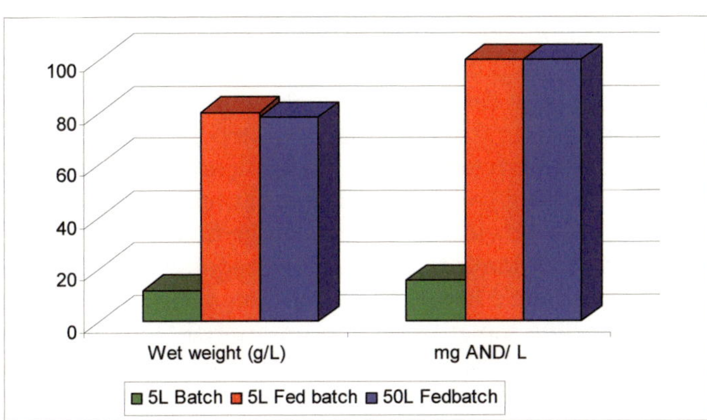

Fig. 2. Effects of culture strategy and scale on pDNA production and cell growth.

The results show that there is no difference in fermentation between small and large bioreactors carried out in *fed-batch* condition. Besides in both cases the cell growth and volumetric plasmid yield were higher than *batch* production (Figure 2). So this fermentation process is very easy to scale up and has been used to provide plasmid yield that are becoming acceptable from a manufacturing viewpoint. The productivity of this process is much higher than the previous works which may be suitable for large scale production of DNA vaccine.

3. Downstream process

Low concentrations of pDNA (0 - 3% dry weight) depending on size and number of plasmid copies in cells of *E. coli* involve an economic challenge in the development of an efficient technology for the production of large quantities of plasmids DNA (pDNA) for therapeutic purposes. The pDNA are macromolecules with hydrodynamic diameter between 150 - 600 nm depending on the molar mass which can be between 3 to 200 MDa; while the chromosomal DNA (cDNA) has a molar mass of 2700 MDa, having similar properties. So, it becomes difficult to separate from pDNA.
There are reports that describe two basic stages: the first one includes the construction and appropriate expression vector, and the choice of host strain, followed by selection and optimization of fermentation conditions. The second one is related with the plasmid isolation and subsequent steps for purification. The purification strategy properly selects and integrates the operation steps; at the beginning carries out cell disruption and after that the clarification and concentration, with the aim to eliminate impurities and cellular debris; simultaneously develop concentration and preparation for further purification of the plasmid. The second step is designed using chromatographic media thus separate pDNA of impurities related to the structure, such as linear and open circular plasmid, chromosomal DNA, RNA, endotoxins and proteins remaining (Limonta et al., 2008).

3.1 Cell disruption by alkaline lysis

The rupture of cells for the release of pDNA is the first and probably the most critical and problematic of all unit operations during the purification processes. The maximum amount of supercoiled plasmid should be obtained to ensure a high performance process. The chemical lysis of the cell was first reported by Birnboim and Doly (Birboim et al., 1979); achieved by breaking the cell wall and membrane with a buffer which contains sodium hydroxide and sodium dodecil sulphate detergent, then begins the release of intracellular products, subsequently is added potassium salt in order to get, as precipitated, cell debris and proteins. The cell disruptions protocols vary taking into account the salt concentration, the sample volume, pH, temperature and time of each step individually.
Several factors may influence the release of plasmid. These include the number of copies of the vector, the host cell, growing conditions and environment. It is valid to note that the duration of this step can affect the yield and purity of the final product. Levy and colleagues (Levy et al., 1999) found that laminar flows were required to break the plasmid and according to their size would take a longer or shorter time the rupture of the cell.
In the alkaline environment the molar mass of cromosomal DNA is denatured, while in a pH range of 12.0 to 12.5 the pDNA double chain remains intact. This pH range is considered appropriate. If the pH of the medium is very low, the cDNA won't be completely denatured, and can cause subsequent purification affectations. On the other hand, high pH levels (higher than 13) cause effects on the structure of pDNA by denaturing irreversibly.

The rupture of the cell occurs as the components are mixed, due to the solubilisation of the cell membrane in alkaline solution containing SDS. This process takes 20 to 40 s to complete, depending on the mixing conditions. Studies have shown that the amount recovered by cells used in the breaking step, depends significantly on the volume of solution used for the treatment of cells (Meacle et al., 2003).

The homogenization of the sample plays an important role, mixing should be accomplished with sufficient intensity to achieve an appropriate level of distribution of chemical reagents. The homogenization is difficult due to changes in the rheological properties of the solution. In the second stage of the rupture process known as neutralization, the pH of the mixture is reduced abruptly broken by the addition of potassium acetate. The change in the physical-chemical conditions of the cDNA causes flocculation and precipitation of a complex of proteins, SDS and other species of high molar mass and RNA. Achieve the optimization of the process of rupture is important for further recovered from pDNA that must be purified in the following stages.

3.2 Plasmid recovery

At the end of the break alkaline forming a precipitate containing cell debris, denatured proteins and nucleic acids, which must be eliminated, using a unit operation in solid-liquid separation, either by centrifugation, filtration or the combination of these operations with the precipitation. The centrifuge with fixed angle rotor operation is commonly used at laboratory scale. However, it is not suitable for large scale production of pDNA. Industrial centrifuges typically operate with a continuous power flow. The centrifugal acceleration of fluid shears and consequently causes the rupture of the material precipitated and the pDNA molecules.

Dead-end filtration is a convenient choice at large-scale operation in the production process of the plasmid. Over 67% of recovered with a purity of 46% of this total was obtained after cutting 99% of the precipitate formed at the end of the break alkaline with filter pore diameter of 5 microns (Prazeres et al., 2004). Another choice at large-scale operation is tangential flow filtration. Once the pellet is separated, the clarified alkaline lysate containing the plasmid can be concentrated removing the impurities. However, neither dead end filtration nor tangential flow filtration remove all the RNA without the uses of critical reagents such as animal-derived compounds (e.g., enzymes), or salts. The use of this unit operation would help to reduce the filtration pressure, in order to avoid precipitate shear and stripping of the chromosomal DNA fragments.

The use of precipitation for the purification of pDNA is reported with the use of natural and chemical precipitants such as calcium chloride salt, after the step of breaking made alkaline to achieve selective precipitation of the cDNA and RNA, obtained as a result, reduction of 50 to 70% of RNA and cDNA, respectively, and the loss of 10% of pDNA. There are also reports of use of other agents which leads to a reduction in volume by concentration and removal of nucleic acids of low molar mass using agents such as isopropanol, polyethylene glycol (PEG) or cetyl trimethylammonium bromide (CTAB) (Lander, 2002; Ribeiro, 2002). Precipitation with ethanol and isopropanol is favourable laboratory scale but not at large scale; it implies a high investment cost. However, the precipitation with the cationic detergent CTAB provides good selectivity and elimination of the cDNA. The use of CTAB and PEG is considered advantageous option for precipitation, but in none of the cases cited by 100% eliminates RNA.

Ultrafiltration and microfiltration are also considered as an option in the first steps of purification. The use of tangential flow ultrafiltration polyethersulfone membrane pore diameter between 100 and 500 kDa, can eliminate 70% of RNA and 90% protein (Butler, 2001). Bussey reported the use of tangential flow ultrafiltration for purification of pDNA (Bussey, 1998). He proposes the use of membranes with a pore diameter between 300-500 kDa, the 500 kDa membranes were used for plasmids ranges between 15-50 kb.

The liquid - liquid extraction is another operation that can be used also for the intermediate step of purification using the aqueous two-phase systems (ATPS). So far they have been reported for the purification of pDNA, two-phase systems formed by PEG and salt polymer K2HPO4 (Ribeiro, 2002), where yields are reported 39, 42 and 100% molar mass PEG 300, 600 or 1000 respectively. The two-phase aqueous systems are easily scaled without a noticeable change in the nature and process efficiency, enabling high yields, a continuous process and reducing operational costs in relation to the costs of other conventional operations. These systems are very useful in the biotechnology industry as K_2HPO_4 salt is very cheap compared to other polymers such as dextran.

Biopharmaceuticals produced from pDNA purity levels required for this component over 90% and is usually achieved by the inclusion in the purification step by the combination of two or three chromatographic processes. The main objective is to separate the pDNA of impurities (in terms of composition and structure). Chromatographic operations described in the literature for the purification of plasmids include properties such as: plasmid size, charge, hydrophobicity, conformation and accessibility to a specific molecular group. Among the most common techniques for obtaining pDNA are: ion exchange chromatography (IEX), the hydrophobic interaction chromatography (HIC), affinity chromatography and exclusion chromatography molecular mass (SEC) (Stadler et al., 2004).

3.3 Purification process development for plasmid DNA gene therapy

Historically, highly purified pDNA recovery is accomplished through the use of cesium chloride / ethidium bromide (CsCL/EtBr) buoyant density gradient separation. This method allows the separation of pDNA by buoyant density into purified bands of different forms: supercoiled plasmid (sc), open circular (oc), linear (l) and multimeric (m).While it yields highly purified plasmid, this approach is not scalable because of personnel safety issues and the hazardous waste considerations associated with the use of cesium chloride and ethidium bromide. In addition the use of ultracentrifugation is also a major impediment to the scale up of this technology.

On the other hand, simple unit operations and the avoidance of critical reagents such as animal-derived compounds (e.g., enzymes), detergents and organic solvents significantly reduce the effort for validation and for precautions regarding patient and operator safety. The employment of these process solutions at large scales requires safety measures such as the design of explosion-proof facilities or use of appropriate protection. It is strictly recommended to spend sufficient time and efforts in upscale-related process development according to GMP. This may end up in a different approach when compared with 'kit' protocols in which convenience and simple robustness play the most important role. Depending on the final application as a therapeutic (single-shot high-dose, or long-term low-dose treatment) or for diagnostics, the specific demands may require individual solutions. Given the complexity of the starting material, certainly any single purification step will not be enough to fulfil the demands of the regulatory authorities. Nevertheless, the aim is to end up with a robust and preferably generic protocol, which is applicable to a variety of plasmids of different sizes (regardless of individual precautions related to stability and sensitivity to shear forces). When developing a multi-step large-scale pDNA Purification process, the design will aim to begin with fast volume reduction. This can be achieved by ultrafiltration or any (chromatographic) capture step, in which recovery (>90%) is more important than maximal capacity.

Currently published processes for pDNA purification include precipitation and extraction of pDNA by organic solvents, ultrafiltration, and predominantly liquid chromatographic techniques which are the most widely used for this purpose. Most of the available processes for pDNA purification are time-consuming and not scalable. Furthermore, due to the application of materials that are not certified for application in humans or due to the application of enzymes of avian or bovine origin and of toxic reagents such as phenol, CsCl, CsBr, etc., these processes do not meet the appropriate guidelines of the regulatory authorities.

Our pDNA purification process is based on alkaline lysis, tangential flow filtration and size exclusion chromatography for extensive removal of RNA as primary downstream steps. Chromatography is considered as the method with highest resolution, therefore being essential for producing pDNA suited for therapeutic applications. It has to be considered that the large pDNA molecules adsorb only at the outer surface of particulate supports. Consequently capacities are usually on the order of hundreds of micrograms of plasmid per millilitre of chromatographic support (Limonta et al., 2010). We used a reverse phase POROS R1 50 matrix which has a dynamic binding capacity between 5 and 1.5 mg pDNA per mL support this matrix is used to purify the pDNA from the remaining impurities, particularly due to its ability to reduce the endotoxin burden to levels below the specifications. Volume reduction of the resulting stream is achieved by tangential flow filtration prior to the final size exclusion chromatography which is used as a polishing step to remove the undesired pDNA isoforms, host proteins and to exchange the buffer for an adequate formulation.

The proposed process reach a 95 % of pDNA, the final genomic DNA content is lower than 5 ng per dose, RNA is not detectable by agarose gel electrophoresis, and protein content is lower than 5 µg per dose and the endotoxin content 0.6 EU per kg body weight. The results demonstrate that process fulfil all regulatory requirements and delivers a pharmaceutical grade pDNA This process does not use or generates significant amounts hazardous materials and no special safety requirements are envisaged. Thus, environmental or safety associated costs are kept to minimum. The reagents used do not pose any special regulatory concern since they are non toxic, non mutagenic and non flammable.

4. Quality control

4.1 Overview

In the US therapeutic gene products are regulated by the FDA Centre for Biologics Evaluation and Research (CBER). In Europe this task is performed by the European Agency for Evaluation of Medical Products (EMEA). The recommendations made by these and others international agencies provide specific quality-control and safety criteria for each therapeutic gene product, reflecting the intended use of the product compliance with Good Laboratory Practice (GLP) and current Good Manufacturing Practice (cGMP). A guiding principle for production of biological products implies to build quality into the product during the process but not to test quality. That is why, it is important to develop appropriated and validated analytical methods for all phases of a GMP process. Quality testings have to be applied since the very beginning to raw material and further established in process and for the purified bulk plasmid. They all must comply with acceptance criteria, regarding identity, purity, potency and safety of the final product.

4.2 MCB and WCB

The Master Cell Bank (MCB) and Working Cell Bank (WCB) are required to ensure each manufacturing run. Quality control methods must be developed to confirm the identity and stability of bacterial host cell and pDNA contained in a MCB and WCB used for the production of pDNA. Cell bank should also be analyzed for cell viability, plasmid copy number, the presence of plasmid-free cells, adventitious agent and viral contaminations. Identity test for pDNA should include analysis of diagnostic restriction enzyme digestion patterns and the full DNA sequence of plasmid. These analyses are typically performed using pDNA isolated from cultures derives from the WCB. Restriction enzyme analysis typically involves digestion of the plasmid with a predefined set of restriction enzymes followed by analysis by an agarose gel electrophoresis analysis and staining with ethidium bromide.

4.3 Control of production process

Likewise for viral vectors the raw materials used in the production process should be characterized. Furthermore, the production process should be controlled by in-process controls. For plasmid vectors these include the control of the amount of plasmid prior to culture harvesting, the amount and form of plasmid after extraction step and the absence of endotoxins in the plasmid pool after extraction step. Specific regulations have been established to provide guidance in the use of vectors in clinical trials for the application and marketing authorization in the production and quality control. Regulatory guidance is given to the environmental protection areas of the patient and not to environmental protein in Europe and in the USA that include: Regulation in Europe, in the Netherlands, in the USA, Good Manufacturing Practice facilities and guidelines that have been established respectively by the Committee for Proprietary Medical Product (CPMP) of the EMEA and CBER of the FDA for the production and control of gene therapeutics and DNA vaccines.

4.3.1 In-process controls

In-process control is required that methods be developed to assay product yield and purity at critical step in the manufacturing process. Bacterial contaminates such as genomic DNA, RNA, protein and endotoxin should be monitored. The amount and purity of plasmid should be controlled prior to culture harvesting and purification steps. The control of the mass of plasmid into the cells prior to culture harvesting is especially important. The monitoring of the pDNA fermentation processes is a key issue in process development, validation and for product approval. Therefore, the reliable analytical methods for the quantification of pDNA from an impure plasmid solution are especially important.

We established a method in which is use the conventional agarose gel electrophoresis for quantification of pDNA pIDKE2. This method consisted in the application of pDNA (pIDKE2) on the range from 113 to 900 ng and defined volumes of the three replicas of the pDNA isolated from 10 mg of bacterial cell pellet by alkaline-treatment procedure assay.

The electronic photograph of the gel is analyzed by image analysis software (software 1D-Manager ver. 2.0) and the plasmid isoform peaks areas for each line were summed (Total Area plasmid). The linear regression between the plasmid mass and the total area plasmid for calibration curve were determined and plasmid mass in each replica was estimated by using the standard calibration curve and taking account the applied volume of the sample. Mean plasmid mass on the sample (between three replicas) was determined with a variation coefficient that should not be superior to 15 %.

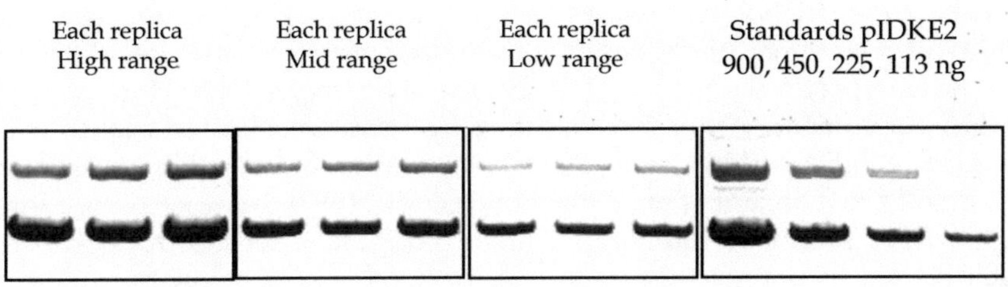

Fig. 3. Electrophoresis agarose gel. Three replicas of sample in the high (lines 1-3), mid (lines 4-6) and low (lines 7-9) range and calibration curve 900, 450, 225 and 113 ng (lines 10-13).

The validation of this method showed that independently of the fact that the applied mass of plasmid is in high, mid and low range, the plasmid mass determinate in the sample were similar (variation coefficient should not be superior to 15 %). A lineal relationship between plasmid amounts versus total plasmid areas was obtained. Three different assays with three replicas of the pDNA standards pIDKE2 calibration curve were run obtaining a determination coefficient (R2) greater than 0.98 ($P \leq 0.01$ in ANOVA regression and $P \geq 0.05$ in ANOVA lack off fit).

Figure 3 shown one assay, this analytical method proved to be specific, linear, precise and accurate in the interval of studied amounts. For the approval of one lot of Wet Biomass, the relation should be more than 0.6 mg of pDNA/gram of Wet Biomass.

4.3.2 Pure bulk plasmid

Quality control testing of pure bulk plasmid must be capable of determining plasmid identity, purity, sterility, potency and safety. Guidelines by the ICH ensure that all tests and analytical protocols should be validated in terms of accuracy, specificity, detection limit, quantification limits, linearity and precision. Guidelines are provided by regulatory agencies for product characterization and in-process controls. Furthermore, analytical methods and product specifications for pDNA are described exhaustively in literature (Horn et al., 1995; Middaugh et al., 1998; Schorr et al., 1995).

In general, identification of a plasmid can be performed by size, sequence or expressed gene of the plasmid. The size can be performed by restriction enzyme mapping. The restriction fragments can be separated by agarose gel electrophoresis, capillary electrophoresis or HPLC. Capillary electrophoretic separation of restriction fragments is superior to gel separation in resolving power, analysis time and quantification (Weiss et al., 1995). The sequence can be performed by sequencing the whole plasmid. Its insert can be performed by automates sequencing method and can be used to check the identity of the plasmid. Chip technology is a promising new technology that allows a confirmation of a sequence of several kilobases. The currently available sequencing methods cannot identify small quantities of a mutated site (<10 %) present in a plasmid preparation (Maschke et al., 1993)

In the final product could be present process-related impurities (genomic DNA, RNA, host proteins and endotoxins) and product-related impurities (open circular (oc), linear DNA isoforms, denatured and multimeric forms) that should be controlled. Contamination of biologics with genomic DNA has always been a mayor Quality Assurance concern due to the possibility of insertional mutagenesis into the recipient genome. Regulatory standards will require level of host cell genomic DNA below 10 µg/mg pDNA (Horn et al., 1995). The host cell DNA contamination can be quantified by Southern blot techniques with a probe specific for host cell gDNA (Levy et al., 2000a), application of the polymerase chain reaction (PCR), real-time PCR (Lahijani et al., 1998; Smith et al., 1999) that assess very low levels of gDNA in the final product. Another technique is agarose-gel electrophoresis, in which gDNA levels should be undetectable. The level of RNA is kept below or undetectable on a 0.8 % agarose gel or by analytical anion-exchange chromatography (Horn et al., 1995). The content of proteins in final plasmid preparations is kept below 10 ng/dose (Sofer & Hagel, 1997); it should be undetectable by bicinchoninic acid (BCA) assay or silver-stained gel.

A specification should exist for the minimum amount of plasmid in the supercoiled form. Regulations may require > 80-90% of the plasmid to be in the supercoiled form. Homogeneity of the plasmid and the different isoforms of pDNA are determined by gel electrophoresis. The proportion of supecoiled and open circular pDNA can be quantified by densitometry scanning of an agarose-gel electrophoresis, capillary electrophoresis or chromatographic techniques.

Denatured supercoiled plasmid runs at the same speed as supercoiled plasmid in agarose gels. This form can be discriminated by HPLC using anion exchange chromatography. The denatured supercoiled plasmid elutes shortly after the main plasmid peak (Schluep et al., 1998). Another method that can be used is the fluorescence-based method SCFluo (Levy et al., 2000b), which is based on the reversible denaturation of sc DNA and the high specificity of the PicoGreen fluorochome for doble-stranded DNA.

It is known that the efficacy of binding of ethidium bromide to supercoiled DNA is different from the efficacy of binding ethidium bromide to closed circular, open circular or lineal DNA (Bauer & Vinograd, 1968). Therefore, it's necessary to determine the relationship between fluorescence and relative band intensity for different configurations of DNA. The linear and open circular material fluoresced with equal intensity and the specific fluorescence of these species is 1.36 ± 0.02 time greater than that supercoiled DNA. A simple and rapid technique to quantify the proportion of supercoiled circular DNA is SCFluo (Levy et al., 2000a), which is a fluorimetric method that is based on the reversible denaturated of scDNA and the high specificity of the PicoGreen fluorochrome for double-stranted DNA.

Endotoxins (lipopolysaccharides) are mayor components of the outer cell wall of gram-negative bacteria and can copurify with the pDNA, which can cause side effects if administered to the recipient. They should be less than 0.1 endotoxin unit (EU)/µg pDNA (Horn et al., 1995) and can be measured by gel-clot assay of aqueous extracts obtained from circulating Limulus polyphemus (horseshoe crab) amoebocytes lysate ('LAL assay'). DNA-concentration (dose) in the product can be measured by spectrophotometer analysis to 260 nm. This value is reliable if the A_{260}/A_{280} ratio will be between 1.75 and 1.85, which means that the DNA product is free from the protein contamination.

Test	Limits	pIDKE2 results
Appearance	Clear, colorless solution	Clear, colorless solution
Identity	5541 pb	5541 pb
Restriction sites	Consistent with Map	Consistent with Map
Biological Activity	> 25 % seroconversion against Co.120 and E2.680	26.6 % vs Co.120 and 33.3 % vs E2.680
Sterility	No growth-14 days in rich media	No growth-14 days in rich media
Endotoxin	≤ 5 EU / kg body weight	0.6 EU/ kg body weight
General Safety	absence of toxic effects	Pass the test
Purity pDNA	≥ 90 %	95 %
RNA	No visualized on 0.8 % Agarose Gel	No visualized on 0.8 % Agarose Gel
pDNA concentration	1.5 - 2.5 mg/mL	1.71 mg/mL
E. coli DNA	≤ 5 ng / dose	≤ 5 ng / dose
Host Protein	≤ 5 µg / dose	1.4 µg / dose
pH	6.7 ± 0.2	6.71

Table 2. Testing results of release purified pIDKE2 compared to specification limits.

In the specific case of the production of pIDKE2 plasmid, analytical methods were followed according to the criteria recommended by the FDA. In table 2 is show a summary of the analytical specifications and final results (Limonta et al., 2008). Limits are according to the specifications of bacterial cell lysates and accepted levels of impurities for the final products described on the Guidance for industry "Considerations for pDNA Vaccines for infectious disease indications."

The results demonstrated that this process meets all regulatory requirements and delivers pharmaceutical grade pDNA. Vaccination with this plasmid (pIDKE2) in HCV chronically-infected individuals was safe, well tolerated and did not impair the ability to respond to non-HCV antigens (Castellanos et al., 2010).

5. Acknowledgments

I would like to thank Pérez, M.; Díaz, M.; Frometa, W.; Martínez, S., for technical support, as well as Márquez, I.; Hernández, S.; Varas, L.; Lugo, V; Bonilla, R. and Fernández, R. for help me with the work.

6. Conclusions

The large-scale plasmid production for gene therapy presents very specific problems as the reproducibility of process. Solutions for these problems and others will undoubtedly have an impact on the economics, efficacy and safety of non-viral approaches to gene therapy. As advances continue in the field of DNA vaccines, factories capable of producing kilograms of pDNA per year must be design.

The choice of a manufacturing route is dictated by the balance between improvements in yield and purity of supercoiled pDNA achieved through the application of new technologies. The Biopharmaceutical industry is a highly regulated sector and to get into a regulatory approval for a new process or product is a major consideration. The recommendations made by some international agencies such as FDA and EMEA provide specific quality-control and safety criteria for each therapeutic gene product. The clinical application of gene therapy and DNA immunization will depend not only on efficacy but also on safety and the ease with which the technology may be adapted for large scale pharmaceutical production.

The advantages of the procedure described over the existing technology to produce pharmaceutical grade pDNA for gene therapy include a high cell density culture, improved plasmid purity and the elimination of undesirable process additives such as toxic organic extractants and animal derived enzymes. By employing this simple, scalable and applicable approach we concluded successfully a phase I clinical trial (Castellanos et al., 2010; Limonta et al., 2010) currently is in Phase II using the pIDKE2 plasmid; which is the principal component of a candidate vaccine against the Hepatitis C virus.

7. References

Bauer, W. & Vinograd, J. (1968). The interaction of closed circular DNA with intercalative dyes. *J. Mol. Biol.* Vol 33, pp. 141–171.

Birboim, H. & Doly, J. (1979). A rapid alkaline extraction procedure for screening recombinant pDNA. *Nucleic acid*, Vol7, pp. 1513-1523.

Bussey, I. (1998). Methods for purifying nucleic acids. International Patent Aplication WO 98/05673.

Butler, E. (2001) Purification of pDNA, US Patent 6,313,285.

Carnes, A. (2005). Fermentation Design for the Manufacture of therapeutic pDNA. *BioProcess International*, pp. 2-7.

Castellanos, Z.; Dorta, Z.; Veliz, G.; Vega, H.; Lorenzo, I.; Ojeda, S.; Dueñas, S.; Alvarez, L.; Martínez, G.; Ferrer, E.; Limonta, M.; Linares, M.; Ruiz, O.; Acevedo, B.; Torres, D.; Márquez, G.; Herrera, L. & Arús E. (2010). Immunization with a DNA vaccine candidate in chronic hepatitis C patients is safe, well tolerated and does not impair immune response induction after anti-hepatitis B vaccination. *J Gene Med.*, Vol12, No. 1, pp.107-116.

Chen, W. (1999). Automated High Yield fermentation of pDNA in Escherichia coli. US Patent 5,955,323. *American Home Products Corporation*, Madison NJ.

Chen, W.; Graham, C. & Ciccarelli, R. (1997). Automated *fed-batch* fermentation with feed-back controls based on dissolved oxygen (DO) and pH for production of DNA vaccines. *J Ind Microbiol Biotechnol*, Vol18, pp.43–48.

Diogo, M.; Queiroz, J.; Monteiro, G.; Martins, S.; Ferreira, G. & Prazeres, D. (2000). Purification of a cystic fibrosis plasmid vector for gene therapy using hydrophobic interaction chromatography. *Biotechnol Bioeng*, Vol68, No. 5, pp.576–83.

Diogo, M.; Ribeiro, S.; Queiroz, J.; Montiero, G.; Tordo, N. & Perrin, P. (2001). Production, purification and analysis of an experimental DNA vaccine against rabies. *J Gene Med*, Vol3, pp.577–584.

Dueñas, S.; Alvarez, L.; Musacchio, A.; Acosta, N.; Falcón, V.; Martínez, G.; Amador, Y.; Guerra, I.; Alvarez, J.; Pérez, A.; Linares, M.; Limonta, M.; Ruiz, O.; Bacardí, D.; Viña, A.; Morales, J.; Torres, D.; Márquez, G.; Marante, J.; de la Rosa, M.; Vega, M.; Aguilar, J.; Soria, Y.; Pichardo, D.; Martínez, E.; Muzio, V.; Vázquez, M.; Acevedo,

B.; Guillén, G.; Cosme, K.; Quintana, M.; López, P. & Herrera, L. (2007). New alternatives for the development of vaccine preparations: contributions to the knowledge on the interaction of recombinant protein viral antigens with nucleic acids. *Biotecnología Aplicada,* Vol24, No. 3-4, pp. 311-314.

Durland, R. & Eastman, E. (1998). Manufacturing and Quality Control of plasmid based gene expression systems. *Adv Drug Deliver,* Vol30, No. 1, pp. 33-48.

Glenting, J. & Wessels, S. (2005). Ensuring safety of DNA vaccines. *Microbial Cell Factories,* Vol 4, No. 26, pp. 1-5.

Horn, N.; Meek, J.; Budahazi, G. & Marquet, M. (1995). Cancer gene therapy using pDNA: purification of DNA for human clinical trials. *Hum Gene Therapy,* Vol6, pp.565–73.

Lahijani, R. (1996). High-Yield production of pBR322- derived plasmids intended for human gene therapy by employing a temperature controllable point mutation. *Hum Gene therapy,* Vol 7, No. 16, pp. 1971-1980.

Lahijani R, Duhon M, Lusby E, Betita H & Marquet M. (1998). Quantization of host cell DNA contaminate in pharmaceutical-grade pDNA using competitive polymerase chain reaction and enzyme-linked immunosorbent assay. *Hum Gene Ther,* Vol9, No.8, pp.1173-1180.

Lander, R. (2002). Fractional precipitation of pDNA from lysate by CTAB. *Biotechnol. Bioeng.,* Vol79, pp. 776-784.

Levy, M.; Ciccolini, S.; Yim, T.; Tsai, N. Titchener, P.; Shamlou, A. & Dunnill, P. (1999). The effects of material properties and fluid flow intensity on pDNA recovering during cell lysis. *Chem. Eng. Sci.,* Vol54, No.14, pp. 3171-3172.

Levy, M.; Collins, J.; Tsai. J.; Shamlou, P.; Ward, J. & Dunnill P. (2000). Removal of contaminant nucleic acids by nitrocellulose filtration during pharmaceutical-grade pDNA processing. *J Biotechnol,* Vol 76, No 2-3, pp. 197-205.

Levy, M.; Lotfian, P.; O'Kennedy, R.; Lo-Yim, M. & Shamlou, P. (2000). Quantitation of supercoiled circular content in pDNA solution using a fluorescence-based method. *Nucleic Acids Res,* Vol 28, No. 12, pp. E57.

Limonta, M.; Márquez, G.; Rey, I..; Pupo, M.; Ruiz, O.; Amador-Cañizares, Y. & Dueñas-Carrera, S. (2008). PDNA Recovery using size-exclusion and perfusion Chromatography. *BioPharmInternational,* Vol21, No 9, pp. 38-47, ISSN 1542-166X.

Limonta, M.; Márquez, G.; Pupo, M. & Ruiz, O. (2010). The Purification of pDNA for clinical trials using membrane chromatography. *Bipharm International.* Vol23, No.2, 46-54, ISSN 1542-166X.

Maschke, H.; Frenz, J.; Belenkii, A.; Karger, B. & Hancock, W. (1993). Ultrasensitive plasmid mapping by high performance capillary electrophoresis. *Electroforesis,* Vol 14, No. 5-6, pp. 509-514.

Meacle, F.; Lander, R.; Shamlou, A. & Titchener, P. (2004). Impact of Engineering flow conditions on pDNA yield and purity in chemical cell lysis operations. *Biotechnology and Bioengineering,* Vol87, No. 3, pp. 293-302.

Middaugh, C.; Evans, R.; Montgomery, D. & Casimiro, D. (1998). Analysis of pDNA from a pharmaceutical perspective. *J Pharm Sci* , Vol87, No. 2, pp. 130-146.

O'Kennedy, R.; Ward, J. & Keshavarz, E. (2003). Effects of fermentation strategy on the characteristic of pDNA production. *Biotecnol. Appl. Biochem,* Vol37, pp. 83-90.

Phue, J.; Jun, S.; Trinh,L.; & Shiloach, J. (2008). Modified *Escherichia coli* B (BL21), a superior producer of pDNA compared with *Escherichia coli* K (DH5α). *Biotechnology and Bioengineering,* Vol 101, No. 4, pp. 831-836.

Pollard, D.; Kirschner, T.; Hunt, G.; Tong. T; Stieber, R. & Salmon, P. (2007). Scale up of a viscous fungal fermentation: Aplication of scale-up criteria with regime analysis and operating boundary conditions. *Biotechnology and Bioengineering*, Vol 96, No. 2, pp. 307-317.

Powell, K. (2004). DNA vaccines-back in the saddle again?. *Nature Biotechnology*, Vol22, No. 7, pp. 799-801.

Prather, K.; Sagar, S.; Murphy, J. & Chartrain, M. (2003). Industrial scale production of pDNA for vaccine and gene therapy: plasmid design, production and purification. *Enzyme and Microbial Technology*, Vol33, pp. 865-883.

Prazeres, D.; Ferreira, G.; Monteiro, G.; Cooney, Ch. & Cabral, J. (1999). Large-scale production of pharmaceutical-grade pDNA for gene therapy. *TIBTECH*, Vol.17, pp. 69-174.

Prazeres, D.; & Ferreira, G. (2004). Design of flowsheets for the recovery and purification of plasmid for gene therapy and DNA vaccination. *Chemical Engineering and Processing*, Vol 43, pp.615-630.

Ribeiro, S. (2002). Isolation of pDNA from cell lysates by aqueous two-phase systems. *Biotechnol. Bioeng.*, Vol78, pp. 376-384.

Robinson, H. (2000). DNA vaccines. *Clin Microbial Newslett*, Vol23, pp. 17-22.

Ruiz, O.; Pérez, M.; Pupo, M.; Limonta, M.; Torres, D.; Martínez, S.; Macias, K.; Diaz, M.; Proenza, Y.; Valdés, J. & Martínez, E. (2009). High cell density culture to produce pDNA for gene therapy in *E. coli*. *Biopharm International*, Vol22, No. 7, pp. 40-45, ISSN 1542-166X.

Schleef, M. (1999). Volume5a: Recombinant Proteins, Monoclonal antibodies and Therapeutic Gene. *Biotechnology*, pp. 445-469. WILEY-VHC, ISBN 3-527-28315-3.

Schluep, T. & Cooney, C. (1998) Purification of plasmid by triplex affinity interaction. *Nucleic Acids Res*, Vol26, No. 19, pp. 4524-4528.

Schmidt, T.; Friehs, K.; Schleef, M.; Voss, C. & Flaschel, E. (2001). In-process analysis of plasmid copy number for fermentation control. *Pacesetter*, Vol5, No. 1, pp.4–6.

Schmidt, T. (2003). Method for the isolation of pDNA. USPatent 6,664,,078 B1. *Qiagen GimbH*, Hilden, DE.

Schorr, J.; Moritz, P.; Seddon, T. & Schleef, M. (1995). Plasmid DNA for human gene therapy and DNA vaccines. Production and quality assurance. *Ann N Y Acad Sci*, Vol 772, pp. 271-273.

Smith, G.; Helf, M.; Nesbet, C.; Betita, H.; Meek, J. & Ferre, F. (1999). Fast and accurate method for quantitating *E. coli* host-cell DNA contamination in pDNA preparations. *Biotechniques*, Vol 23, No. 3, pp. 518-522, 524, 526.

Sofer & Hagel. (1997). Handbook of process chromatography, a guide to optimization, scale-up and validation. (1 ed.) Academic press.

Stadler, J.; Lemmens, R. & Nyhammar, T. (2004). Plasmid DNA purification. *The Journal of Gene Medicine*, Vol6.

Vogel, F. & Sarver, H. (1995). Nucleic acid vaccines. *Clin. Microbiol. Rev.*, Vol8, pp. 406-410.

Wang, Z.; Le, G.; Shi, Y. & Wegrzyn, G. (2001). Medium design for pDNA production based on stoichiometric model. Process. *Biochem*, Vol36, pp.1085–1093.

Weis, G.; Garner, M.; Yarmola, E.; Bocek, P. & Chrambach, A. (1995). A comparison of resolution of DNA fragment between agarose gel and capillary zone electrophoresis in agarose solutions. *Electrophoresis*, Vol16, No. 8, pp. 1345-1353.

Xu, Z.; Shen, W.; Chen, H. & Cen, P. (2005). Effects of medium composition on the production of pDNA vector potentially for human gene therapy. *Journal of Zheijang University SCIENCE*, Vol6B, No. 5, pp. 396-400, ISSN 1009-3095.

Yakhchali, B.; Karami, A.; Aflski, E. & Ahmadi, A. (2007). PDNA production for genetic inmunization in *Fed-batch* fermentation with feed back controls based on dissolved oxygen (DO) ahd pH. *Journal of Sciences*, Vol 18, No. 2, pp. 129-133, ISSN 1016-1104.

4

Small Interfering RNAs: Heralding a New Era in Gene Therapy

Maro Bujak[1], Ivana Ratkaj[2], Mirela Baus Loncar[1],
Radan Spaventi[3] and Sandra Kraljevic Pavelic[2]
[1]*Rudjer Boskovic Institute, Division of Molecular Medicine, Laboratory for Systems Biomedicine, Zagreb,*
[2]*Department of Biotechnology, University of Rijeka, Rijeka,*
[3]*Galapagos Research Centre, Zagreb,*
Croatia

1. Introduction

Last decades have witnessed a tremendous expansion in knowledge and availability of the genome sequence, which was of great importance for advancements in the field of gene therapy. This led to improved strategies based on use of nucleic acids with sequences complementary to specific target genes in treatment of many diseases. Especially, advancements have been achieved in discovery and use of diverse RNA molecules other than messenger RNAs (mRNAs), transfer RNAs (tRNAs), or ribosomal RNAs (rRNAs). Such RNA molecules, known as non-coding RNAs (ncRNAs), serve diverse biological roles some of which are still elusive (Gesteland 2006). Generally, the ncRNA molecule is functional even when it does not encode for a protein. Recent evidence provided by many projects including the Encode project (The Encyclopedia Of DNA Elements) suggests that larger part of the genomes of mammals and other complex organisms is transcribed into ncRNAs. These ncRNAs are transcribed from both exon and intron DNA regions, and include small interfering RNAs (siRNAs), micro RNAs (miRNAs) and small nucleolar RNAs (snoRNAs), while many of such molecules remain yet to be discovered. A vast amount of evidence demonstrates that ncRNAs play essential roles in cellular physiology. Some biological processes known to be regulated by ncRNAs include transcriptional regulation of genes, gene silencing, messenger RNA stability and translation, development, proliferation, haematopoiesis, apoptosis, protein translocation and chromosome replication (Bühler 2007, Mattick 2006, Lee 1993).

There is no doubt that RNA regulatory networks are critical for determining our most complex traits, and they play an important role in disease pathogenesis as well. The specific disease phenotypes might indeed result from deficiency of one or more specific ncRNA instead from protein structural defects, as is usually expected. A challenge for the future might thus be to map the whole cells/organisms complement of ncRNAs and to understand their biological role. Up to now, the use of ncRNAs as a research tool has greatly improved gene therapy approaches for various diseases (Gallaso 2010), but also substantially improved drug discovery and target validation. In this book chapter, we will therefore focus on the use of a particular approach, namely RNAi for improved gene silencing for both, therapeutic approaches and identification of new therapeutic targets.

2. RNA interference

RNA interference (RNAi) is an evolutionary conserved cellular defence mechanism that protects plants and vertebrates from viruses and transposable genetic elements, but is also involved in direct development and gene expression in general (Lecellier 2004,Vastenhouw 2004, Meister 2004). Two types of ncRNA molecules - micro RNA (miRNA) and small interfering RNA (siRNA) are involved in the RNAi mechanism through binding to mRNA molecules. Through this process, either increase or decrease of mRNA activity or repression of translation occurs (Hannon 2002). Small interfering RNAs are 20-25 nucleotides long double-stranded RNA molecules, that play a variety of biological roles. The most notable one is its involvement in the RNAi pathway, where it interferes with the expression of a specific gene (Devi 2006, Elbashir 2001a). siRNA may also be involved in RNAi-related pathways, such as shaping the chromatin structure. Similarly, miRNAs are short non-coding, 19-22 nucleotides long, functional RNA molecules that play important regulatory roles by sequence-specific base pairing on the 3' untranslated region (3'-UTR) of target messenger mRNAs, promoting mRNA degradation or inhibiting translation (Bartel 2004). RNAi is thus a post-transcriptional gene silencing mechanism employed to silence an endogenous gene, e.g. by the introduction of a homologous dsRNA. The selective and rapid degradation of the transcript ensured in the RNAi pathways makes it a valuable laboratory technique in biotechnology and medicine for controlled silencing of genes. For that purpose, synthetic dsRNA are usually introduced into cells to suppress expression of specific genes of interest (Elbashir 2002).

The RNAi pathway is initiated by the Dicer enzyme, which cleaves long double-stranded RNA (dsRNA) molecules (500-1000 nucleotides) into short siRNA fragments of ~20 nucleotides or pre-miRNAs into mature miRNA (Figure 1) (Elbashir 2001b). While miRNAs have incomplete base pairing to a target and inhibit the translation of many different mRNAs with similar sequences, siRNAs have perfect complementarity and induce mRNA cleavage only in a single, specific target (Pillai 2007). Interestingly, about one-third of human protein-coding genes are controlled by miRNAs (Du 2005), while siRNAs participate in chromosome dynamics and formation of heterochromatin (Mattick 2005). Exogenous siRNAs may be derived from experimentally introduced double-stranded RNAs (dsRNAs) or viral RNAs (Fire 1998). Endogenous siRNA (endo-siRNA) precursors are derived from repetitive sequences ,transposons, sense–antisense pairs or long stem-loop structures (Babiarz 2008; Watanabe 2008). RNAi interference can be exerted through naturally occurring antisense transcripts (NATs) that are complementary to other RNA transcripts (Osato 2007). They are involved in alternative splicing, genomic imprinting, and X-chromosome inactivation as well (Zhang 2004). Based on the locus of their transcription, NATs can be divided into two groups, namely cis-NATs and trans-NATs. Cis-NATs are transcribed from the same genomic locus as their target, but from the opposite DNA strand, therefore forming a perfect match with their targets (Wang 2005). So far, five orientations have been identified, among which the so-called 'head to head' orientation where both transcripts align their 5' ends is considered to be the most common (Lavorgna 2004). On the other hand, trans-NATs are transcribed on different genome locations and are complementary to multiple transcripts resulting, however, in a number of mismatches

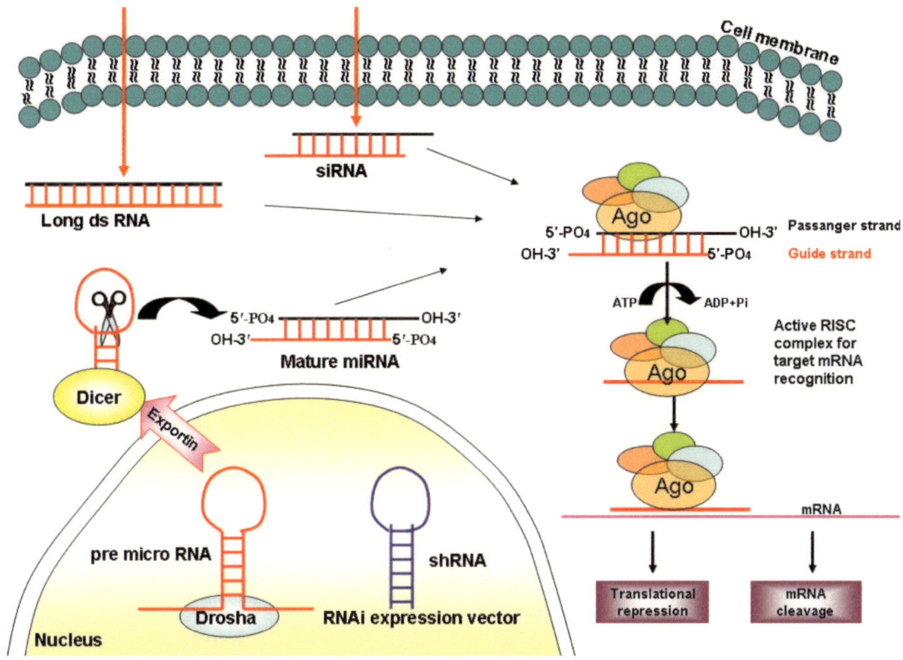

Fig. 1. Pre-micro RNA and shRNA are expressed in the nucleus, exported to the cytoplasm and processed into a mature form by the 'Dicer' enzyme. It is possible to exogenously introduce synthetic RNAi constructs directly into the cytoplasm and to specifically silence the target gene. Long double-stranded RNA (dsRNA) and hairpin structures are cut into smaller strands, namely interfering siRNA by Dicer, leaving ~2nt overhangs at the 3′ end and phosphate group at the 5′ end. The guided strand is incorporated into the RNA-induced silencing complex (RISC), while the passenger strand is discarded. Active RISC complex uses the guide strand to cleave complementary target, which causes mRNA degradation and translational repression. The same RISC complex may carry out several cleavage cycles. Long primary transcripts of miRNA genes (pri-miRNA) are cleaved by Drosha to produce a stem-loop structured precursor, pre-microRNA (pre-miRNA). Subsequently, it leaves the nucleus through the nuclear pores and enters the cytoplasm, where is being processed by Dicer. Mature ds miRNA is loaded onto the RISC. Only one strand is successfully incorporated into the RISC, while the other is eliminated. Interaction between miRNA and target RNA is characterized by imperfect base pairing. Namely, the guide miRNA strands usually form bulge structures due to mismatches with its target sequence. Consequently, there is no perfect complementarity between base pairs. In this way, miRNA together with the RISC induce repression of protein translation (Jackson 2003; Bartel 2004).

(Carmichael 2003). miRNAs are typical representatives of trans-NATs involved in transcriptional silencing, translation repression, deadenylation and heterochromatin formation. miRNA genes are found in introns of non-coding or coding genes and in exons of non-coding genes.

Both miRNAs and siRNAs molecules have two strands, one named the 'passenger strand' and the other called the 'guide strand'. The passenger strand is the one to be degraded, while the guide strand further incorporates into the RNA-induced silencing complex (RISC)

(Lee 2004) in an ATP-independent process performed directly by the protein components of the RISC (Leucschner 2006; Gregory 2005). This complex contains the Argonautes (Ago) proteins that cleave the passenger strand and liberate the guide strand from the siRNA duplex (Liu 2004; Meister 2004). Activated RISC is then capable of cleaving target mRNAs. The guide strand recognizes homologous sequence of the target mRNA. When mRNA is associated with the guide strand (template) in the RISC complex, it is cleaved by the Ago proteins (Matranga 2005, Leuschner 2006). In this process, template siRNA remains intact and serves for subsequent cycles of mRNA cleavage. The mRNAs cleaved by the RISC are degraded by cellular exonucleases. In this way, the translation of mRNA is ceased (Hall 2005).

The third group of interfering RNA molecules is comprised of Piwi-interacting RNAs (piRNAs) that are processed from single-stranded RNA precursors transcribed from intergenic repetitive elements, transposons or large piRNA clusters. They are associated with the Piwi subfamily proteins, and therefore do not depend upon Dicer. piRNAs are highly abundant in germ cells and at least some of them are involved in transposon silencing through heterochromatin formation or RNA destabilization (Vagin 2006). The precise mechanisms and the functions of most piRNAs are still unknown.

2. Barriers to RNAi-based therapies

Various RNAi therapy approaches *in vivo* are hampered by unwanted side effects such as induction of immune response and toxicity, including the activation of Toll-like receptors (TLRs), type I interferon responses and competition with the endogenous RNAi pathway components (Marques 2005). Several reports have shown that chemical modifications of siRNA can attenuate immune reaction by abrogating interferon (IFN) and cytokine induction (Judge 2005, Sioud 2005, 2006). Family of Toll-like receptor proteins (TLRs) are known to be involved in the recognition of pathogen molecules such as viral dsRNAs, and are central to the activation of immune cell response. TLRs recognise siRNAs in a sequence-dependent manner in the endosome prior to the siRNAs cytoplasm internalization. In particular, the so-called 'off-target' effects of siRNAs are widely recognized as an issue associated with the use of siRNAs (Jackson 2003). Off-target effect is undesired down-regulation of non-targeted transcripts, either by miRNAs or siRNAs. This phenomenon mainly occurs due to lack of complementarity between siRNAs and target mRNAs. RNAi machinery tolerates single mutations located in the centre of siRNA molecules without losing the gene silencing ability. In this manner, some siRNAs have the ability to silence other genes besides complementary target genes. These problems may, however, be partially overcome by the use of computer algorithms in combination with the experimental validation procedures that ensure optimized siRNA sequences complementary to the target mRNA inducing minimal immune responses.

Additionally, silencing 'off-target' genes other than interferon-induced pathway represents nowadays the major problem in designing effective siRNA approaches, which impedes the clinical usage of RNAi (Jackson 2003, Persengiev 2004, Birmingham 2006). Indeed, cross-hybridization of interfering RNA molecules may partially match the sequence of non-target genes and consequently knockdown these genes. miRNAs require only a small match at the 5' end of the anti-sense strand as to induce such "off-target" effect while similarly, the insertion of the sense siRNA strand into the RISC complex instead of the anti-sense strand should significantly contribute to unwanted gene silencing as well (Jackson 2003). Finally, "off-target" effects may occur due to the seed-sequence-dependent binding, where "off-targeted" genes contain matches between the seed region of siRNA and their sequences in the 3'UTR (Jackson 2006a). Increase of the RNAi specificity has, however, been achieved by minimizing sense strand incorporation into activated RISC and selective thermodynamic stabilization of the sense strand 5' ends by incorporation of locked nucleic acids (LNA) (Schwarz 2003, Elmen 2005).

Though the siRNA macromolecules have strong negative anionic charge deriving from the phosphates on their surface that enables spontaneous passage across the negatively charged cell membrane, a variety of biological barriers should be overcome for *in vivo* delivery. These barriers include filtration, phagocytosis and degradation in the bloodstream, passage across the vascular endothelial barrier, diffusion through the extracellular matrix, uptake into the cell, escape from the endosome and unpackage and release of siRNA to the RNA interference (RNAi) machinery (Whitehead 2009).

For example, naked siRNAs are relatively unstable in blood and serum in its native form, though more stable in comparison to single-stranded RNAs (Whitehead 2009). What happens to siRNAs when entering blood is rapid degradation by ribonucleases, a rapid renal excretion and non-specific uptake by the reticuloendothelial system. According to studies in rats that received naked siRNA intravenously, a rather short half-life of 6 min and a clearance of 17.6 mL/min was documented (Soutschek 2004). Poor pharmacokinetic properties of siRNA arise from endogenous RNAses degradation and rapid elimination by kidney filtration due to small molecular masses (~7 kDa) (Soutschek 2004).

Recently, even a novel elimination pathway for siRNAs *in vivo* has been identified, where liver-enriched siRNA is secreted into the gallbladder and then excreted into the intestine (Huang 2011). After their delivery into the bloodstream, siRNAs are subjected to rapid clearance from blood through liver accumulation and renal filtration, but up until now, it has been believed that the siRNAs elimination could be carried out only by the renal system.

Unpredictable biological stability and cellular uptake of siRNAs may be partially surmounted by chemically modifying the siRNA structure including backbone, base and sugar modifications without affecting gene silencing.

If however, administered siRNAs survive in the plasma, they encounter a problem of extravagation through the tight vascular endothelial junctions (Juliano 2009). Interestingly, transport of macromolecules across tumour endothelium was found to be more efficient than transport across normal endothelium that was leaky and had discontinuous vascular structures with poor lymphatic drainage (Jang 2003). Additionally, siRNA diffuses through the extracellular matrix, a dense network of collagen and carbohydrates surrounding a cell (Zamečnik 2003), and it finally reaches its last destination - the cytoplasm of the target cell. Here, siRNAs incorporate into RNAi machinery and encounter target mRNAs. At this point, endosomes represent a natural barrier to internalisation and subsequent degradation of siRNAs (Boussif 1995, Oliveira 2007). However, the use of acid-responsive delivery carriers may improve escape of siRNA from endosomes, as the endosome environment is naturally mildly acidic. In addition, fusogenic peptides that undergo acid-triggered conformational changes may also accelerate endosomal escape of nucleic acids, and are liberated from carriers in the last stage of delivery (Medina-Kauwe 2005, Cho 2003).

3. Chemical modifications

Delivery of siRNAs in their unmodified form has several advantages over chemically modified forms ensuring maximal efficiency (maximized RNAi per siRNA molecule) and avoiding potentially inefficient and time/labour-consuming modification process.

Nevertheless, the use of chemical modifications was found to reduce cleavage of RNA duplexes by nucleases, scale down the activation of innate immune response, lower the incidence of off-target effects, and improve pharmacodynamics (Behlke 2008). For example, phosphorothioate (PS) linkage is one of the simplest modifications of the siRNA backbone. Studies showed that toxicity and loss of silencing activity could pose a hurdle when phosphorothioate-modified siRNAs are employed (Manoharan 2004, Mahato 2005). A better alternative to backbone modification is the boranophosphonate linkage, which is more effective at silencing than phosphorothioate siRNAs, and is 10 times more nuclease resistant in comparison with unmodified siRNAs. Furthermore, boranophosphate siRNAs are more potent than unmodified siRNAs, and act through the standard RNAi pathway (Hall 2004).

Another chemical modification of interest is ribose ring-like modification of RNA at 2′-position of the ribose ring. These modifications include 2′-O-methyl (2′-OMe), 2′ deoxy-2′-fluoro modifications and locked nucleic acid. They increase siRNA stability against endonucleases and reduce immune response activation (Chiu 2003). In addition, 2′-OMe modifications at specific positions within the siRNA region reduce the number of off-target transcripts and the magnitude of their regulation without significantly affecting silencing of the intended targets (Jackson 2006b). Interestingly, 2′-OMe modifications reduce the hybridisation free energy that compensates for somewhat weaker base pairing (Inoue 1987, Lesnik 1993). It was proved that 2′-OMe modifications greatly prolonged siRNA half-live in the plasma (Chiu and Rana 2003), but a number of siRNAs currently used in clinics had been designed prior to findings on 2′-OMe modification benefits to siRNA application *in vivo*. Further on, ribose modification or locked nucleic acid (LNA) also protracts the functional half-life of siRNA *in vivo* by two different mechanisms: 1) enhancing the protection of RNA from degradation by enzymes, and 2) stabilizing the siRNA duplex structure indispensable for silencing activity (Elmen 2005). Such modified RNA nucleotide is modified *via* a methylene bridge connecting the 2′ oxygen with the 4′ carbon of the ribose ring (Bondensgaard 2000, Braasch 2001), which produces a locked ribose conformation known to increase the hybridization properties of oligonucleotides (Kaur 2006). LNA is highly compatible with the siRNA intracellular machinery and preserves the molecule integrity (Braasch 2003, Elmen 2005). There is, however, a possibility that production of non-natural molecules might occur upon degradation of chemically modified siRNAs, as these RNAs may produce unsafe metabolites or trigger unwanted effects.

4. siRNA delivery systems

Obstacles to efficient delivery of siRNA *in vivo* might be overcome by diverse approaches aimed at increasing cellular uptake, protecting from enzymatic degradation, bypassing the immune recognition and improving the pharmacokinetics properties. These delivery systems, namely bioconjugation, complex formation with lipids and polymers, viral vectors, encapsulation into lipid particles and non-pathogenic bacteria vector are designed to specifically localize siRNA in desired tissue, which minimizes side effects and decreases the concentrations of siRNA required for efficient gene scilencing *in vivo*.

4.1 Bioconjugation

Conjugation of siRNAs with lipids and polymers increases thermodynamic stability, protects siRNAs′ strands from nucleases and improves the biodistribution and pharmacokinetic profiles of siRNAs along with their targeting to specific cell types (Cheng 2006, Lorenz 2004, Soutschek 2004, Wolfrum 2007, DiFiglia 2007, Mahat 1999; Schepers 2005). Therefore, conjugation of siRNA with lipids either enhances the uptake *via* receptor-mediated endocytosis, or increases penetration across the cell membrane, as demonstrated by the studies where cholesterol-conjugated siRNAs were effectively delivered to cells in cell culture, liver and other organs (Cheng 2006). Indeed, cholesterol conjugation increases hydrophobicity and cellular association of nucleic acids (Lorenz 2004), and conjugation of cholesterol with anti-ApoB siRNAs efficiently lowers the level of ApoB mRNA in the mice liver and jejunum leading to decline in the blood cholesterol level (Soutschek 2004). Similar approach was successfully applied to deliver siRNAs in murine vaginal mucosal tissue for prevention and inhibition of potentially lethal herpes simplex type 2 infections. It seems that cholesterol-siRNA conjugates incorporate into circulating lipoprotein particles, and are efficiently internalized by hepatocytes *via* a receptor-mediated process. Pre-binding of cholesterol-siRNA conjugates to lipoparticles dramatically improves silencing efficiency in mice and distribution of lipoparticle cholesterol-siRNA conjugate in various tissues (Wolfrum 2007). Intrastriatal injection of cholesterol-siRNA conjugates silenced mutant huntingtin gene in a transgenic mouse model for Huntington's disease, attenuating neuronal pathology as well as delaying the abnormal behavioural phenotype (DiFiglia 2007).

Furthermore, siRNAs may be conjugated to peptides termed protein transduction domains (PTDs). The latter have the ability to translocate across the cell membrane and therefore to efficiently deliver siRNAs into cells. PTDs consist of short amino acid sequences with stretches that have positively charged amino acids arginine and lysine, which facilitate their translocation through the plasma membrane. Such amphipathic molecules interact with negatively charged head groups of the plasma membrane *via* their positive amino acid residues. siRNA is finally released in the cytoplasm upon reduction of the disulfide bond. The uptake of peptides-siRNA conjugates is rapid, effective and occurs without the need for specific receptors, which provides an important role for these conjugates in siRNAs delivery into all kinds of mammalian cells *in vivo* (Mahat 1999, Schepers 2005).

4.2 Complex formation with lipids and polymers

Bioconjugation substantially improves delivery of siRNA, but still fails to ensure reversible binding of siRNAs for controlled release of siRNAs into target cells, protection of siRNAs from nuclease degradation and serum binding during transit through the circulation, escape from endosomal compartment, biocompatibility as to escape hosts immune response, and resistance to liver and kidney rapid clearance.

Cationic polymers interact with siRNAs spontaneously and self-assemble in a process induced upon electrostatic interactions that results in formation of nanoparticles known as polyplexes. The efficiency of siRNA polyplexes to silence genes of interest depends on several factors such as capability to bind cellular membranes, cellular uptake rate and escape from endosomes.

Several cationic polymers have been widely investigated as siRNA carriers *in vitro* and *in vivo* (Mahato 1997), and their design has been optimized in the cell cultures (Friend 1996, Xu 1996).

Cationic polymers spontaneously form complexes with nucleic acids due to electrostatic interactions between positively charged amine groups of the polycations and negatively charged phosphate groups of the nucleic acids. These interactions enhance the uptake of cationic polymers by cells and increase transfection efficiency (Han 2000). Among cationic polymers employed for gene delivery, polyethylenimine (PEI) is one of the most common ones in siRNA delivery *in vitro* and *in vivo*. PEIs of various molecular weights, degrees of branching and other modifications have been largely used for transfection of siRNAs in different cell lines and live animals. For instance, siRNA targeted towards the HER2 growth receptor was delivered intraperitoneally to subcutaneous tumours as siRNA/PEI complex, and significantly reduced tumour growth. Moreover, pain receptors for N-methyl-D-aspartate were effectively knocked down in rats by specific PEI/siRNA delivered intrathecally (Tan 2005). PEIs should thus play an important role for non-viral siRNA delivery *in vivo*, if toxicity and limited biodegradability issues are appropriately addressed.

On the other hand, cationic lipids are constructed by protonable polyamines linked to dialkyl or cholesterol anchors, and represent one of the most widely used strategies for *in vivo* delivery of siRNA (Whitehead 2009). Physicochemical properties of lipid/nucleic acid complexes (nanoparticles) are influenced by the relative proportions of each component, structure of the cationic lipids head group, co-lipid molar and charge ratio, particle size of complexes, and liposome size (Mahato 1998, Spagnou 2004). Electrostatic interactions between siRNA and cationic liposomes may provoke relatively uncontrolled interaction processes giving rise either to the excessive size of the formed lipid/siRNA complex and its poor stability, or to incomplete encapsulation of siRNA molecules posing a risk of their potential enzymatic or physical degradation prior to delivery into the cells (Spagnou 2004, Keller 2005).

Still, cationic lipids complexed with siRNAs of interest were successfully used in nonhuman primates (Akinc 2008, Frank-Kamenetsky 2008), and are currently being evaluated in several clinical trials.

Still, some shortcomings of using the lipid-siRNA biocunjugates remain. Major obstacles refer to the plasma stability for intravenous applications (Mahato 1998,1999, Keller 2005), where they interact with serum proteins, lipoproteins, heparin and glycosaminoglycans in the extracellular matrix precipitating the aggregation or release of nucleic acids from the complexes before reaching the target cell. Cationic lipids activate the complement system resulting in rapid clearance by macrophages (Mahato 1997).

However, polyethylene glycol (PEG) coating of liposomal carriers (Lia 2005) substantially lowers their interaction with serum proteins and with the proteins of the complement system thus improving the complexes circulation time. It is now widely accepted that PEGylation-aided stabilization of the lipid/nucleic acid complexes leads to the reduction in macrophage clearance.

Cationic lipids represent a convenient and flexible method for siRNA delivery. Indeed, various approaches to designing cationic lipid structure and liposome composition have been successfully developed in combination with diverse reliable methods for their preparation. This ensures increased *in vivo* efficiency tailored for different models and diseases.

Recently, a promising siRNA delivery carrier, namely stable nucleic acid lipid particles - SNALPs, has been described (Zimmermann 2006). SNALPs consist of a lipid bilayer containing a mixture of cationic and fusogenic lipids that enable cellular uptake and endosomal release of siRNAs. These particles are additionally coated with the polyethylene glycol-lipid (PEGylated lipid) conjugate that provides neutral hydrophilic exterior and stabilizes the particle during formulation. The silencing effect of SNALP-conjugated siRNAs is more potent (>100-fold) than that of systemic administration of cholesterol-conjugated siRNAs targeted against ApoB in mice. Another study confirming higher potency of SNALP-conjugated siRNAs was performed in mice (Morrissey 2005). Chemically modified siRNAs against hepatitis B virus (HBV) were conjugated with SNALPs and administered intravenously into mice carrying replicating HBV. The results confirmed improved efficacy and longer half-life of siRNA encapsulated in SNALPs in the plasma and liver compared to unformulated siRNA (Morrissey 2005).

Another newly described delivery vehicle for siRNAs is the liposome-siRNA-peptide complex (LSPCs) that showed a potential in therapy of neurodegenerative disorders (Pulford 2010). For that purpose, intravenous injections were used for transvascular delivery of siRNA complexed with LSPCs across the blood-brain barrier to the brain. The LSPCs complex consisted of a modified peptide from the rabies virus glycoprotein that acts as a ligand for acetylcholine receptors (AchR), a small peptide that links siRNA with modified peptide and liposomal nanoparticle. This complex effectively delivered siRNA to neuronal cells expressing AchR in brain. Furthermore, LSPCs' liposomes increased the stability of siRNA/peptide complex in serum during vascular transport. This approach proved promising in the treatment of prion diseases as well. For example, LSPCs coupled with the prion protein (PrP) siRNA were shown to significantly suppress cellular prion protein PrP^{C} expression and to eliminate misfolded protease-resistant isoform of the cellular prion protein PrP^{RES} in the AchR-expressing cells *in vitro* (Pulford 2010). Similarly, LSPCs injected intravenously in mice efficiently bypassed serum degradation and the PrP siRNAs were delivered to AchR- and PrP^{C}- expressing neurons in brain. Still, these promising results need to be proved for the future human siRNA therapy and possible beneficialy effects in case of prion disease, neurodegenerative disorders such as Alzheimer's disease or viral encephalitis.

At last, it is worth to mention that it has become possible recently to quantitatively estimate the disassembling ratio of nanoparticles complexes with nucleic acids in complex biological media such as serum (Buyers 2009). The measurement is performed by the use of fluorescence fluctuation spectroscopy (FES) that quantifies nanomolar concentrations of released siRNA. First measurements showed that the gene silencing efficacy of siRNA polyplexes in the serum depends on the serum concentrations. These findings will aid in the development of siRNAs polyplexes and other nanoparticle nucleic acid as delivery systems.

4.3 Viral and non-pathogenic bacterial vectors

It is well-known that siRNA-mediated gene silencing is usually transient in cell culture and lasts for only a couple of days. Such short-term knockdown is not sufficient for studying phenotypic effects that require longer duration of knockdown of the target protein. Moreover, transient transfection of siRNA varies in efficiency between different cell types, but the key to resolving this problem is stable expression of RNAi effector molecules from plasmids or viral vectors (Amarzguioui 2005). There are several viral vectors used therein: double-stranded adeno-associated viruses (AAV), lentiviral vectors and adenoviruses (Brummelkamp 2002a, Zufferey 1998, Andersson 2005, Yoo 2007). However, the most commonly used approach involves RNA polymerase III-mediated transcription of short hairpin structures (shRNA) with a stem of 19–29 bp and a short loop of 4–10 nt. Besides, siRNAs may be introduced by viral vectors and transcribed from separate expression units, from either the same or two separate plasmids. Finally, the effector molecules may be expressed as a chimera of siRNA and miRNA (Figure 2).

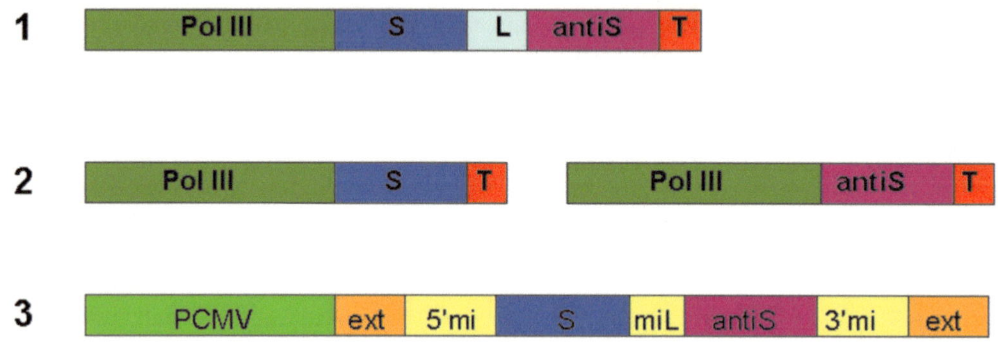

Fig. 2. Construction of expression cassettes for 1) shRNA and 2) siRNA 3) miRNA. PIII: pol III promoter, PCMV: pol II promoter S: siRNA sense strand, antiS: siRNA antisense strand, L: loop, T: terminator, 5′mi: 5′ pri-miRNA sequence, 3′mi: 3′ pri-miRNA, ext: extraneous transcript sequences. Correct excision of the siRNA from the heterologous transcript is directed by 50mi and 30mi sequences.

AAV vectors are the safest and thus most promising viral gene delivery vehicles known to date (Grimm 2003). The wild-type AAV viruses are non-pathogenic in humans, persistently infect a large variety of dividing and non-dividing cells, and do not integrate into chromosomes. Despite these advantages, their clinical application is restricted due to their potential in some mutagenic and/or oncogenic transformations and host immune responses, and high production costs.

Non-pathogenic bacteria may also be used as delivery vectors. For example, transkingdom RNAi (*tk*RNAi) uses non-pathogenic bacteria to produce and deliver therapeutic short hairpin RNA (shRNA) encoding plasmid DNA into target cells for precise gene silencing (Krühn 2009). Plasmid or TRIP vector contains shRNA of interest and is controlled by bacteriophage T7 promoter. TRIP vector also contains the *Inv* locus from *Yersinia pseudotuberculosis* that encodes invasin, which helps bacteria to enter into β-1 integrin-positive mammalian cells. Listeriolysin O, an additional product of TRIP vector coded by the HlyA gene, makes it possible for shRNA to escape from entry vesicles. TRIP vectors are introduced into competent non-pathogenic *Escherichia coli* strains BL21(DE3). This technique showed very good results in silencing catenin-β1 in human colon cancer cells *in vitro* as well as *in vivo* (Xiang 2006). It is also suitable for targeting the multidrug resistance (MDR)-mediating drug extrusion pump ABCB1 (MDR/P-gp) in multidrug resistant cancer cells, but it is not yet as good as conventional siRNA (Nieth 2003, Stein 2008) and virally delivered shRNAs (Kaszubiak 2007). With additional ongoing improvements, *tk*RNAi may become a powerful tool for delivery of RNAi effectors for the reversal of cancer MDR in future.

5. Targeted siRNA

Considerable effort has been invested in targeted siRNA delivery *in vivo*. For that purpose, important requirements must be fulfilled including stability, prolonged circulation in the body, high accessibility to target tissues, specific binding to target cells, active endocytosis in the cell and siRNA activity in the target cells. Only then, one can expect maximized delivery and optimal concentration in the target tissue. Targeted siRNA design may also prevent non-specific siRNA distribution. Ligands that recognize cell-specific receptors expressed by the target cells can be conjugated to polymers and cationic lipids in order to promote specific cellular uptake *via* receptor-mediated endocytosis (Dubey 2004, Lu 2005). Folate receptor is one of the most popular target molecules in cancer-specific gene and drug delivery (Gosselin 2002). Folic acid is essential for rapid cell growth, thus many cancer cells over-express folate receptors. They have binding sites for FA and monoclonal antibodies. FA is convenient for conjugation with liposomal and polymeric siRNA carriers with or without the polyethylene glycol spacer. In the study presented by Kim et al. (Kim 2006), FA-conjugated polyethylenimine enhanced gene silencing *via* receptor-mediated endocytosis. Another group of receptors that are potential targets for efficient siRNA delivery are integrins and transferrin. The arginine-glycine-aspartic acid (RGD) motif has been used for target delivery of drugs and genes because of its ability to bind to integrins expressed on the activated endothelial cells found in tumour vasculature (Schiffelers 2004, Kim 2004). In addition, cyclodexstrin-based polycation delivery system can be used to target metastatic tumours (Hu-Lieskovan 2005). Aptamers can be used for site-specific delivery of siRNA, as they possess high affinity and specificity for their target. Prostate-specific membrane antigen (PSMA)-specific aptamers can be internalized into PSMA expressing-like prostate cancer cells (Hicke 2000, Pestourie 2005). Antigen-conjugated siRNA carriers are an alternative (Park 2002, Mamot 2005). HER-2 siRNA-carrying liposomes decorated with transferrin receptor-specific antibody fragments silenced the HER-2 gene in xenograft tumours in mice, significantly inhibiting tumour growth (Pirollo 2007).

6. Local and systemic delivery

The administration of siRNA can be local or systemic depending on the types of target tissues and cells. siRNA can be directly applied to some organs like eye or skin, as well as muscle *via* local delivery. Systemic siRNA delivery is the only way for metastatic and haematological cancer cells. Local delivery has several advantages, such as low effective doses, simple formulation, low risk of inducing systemic side effects and facilitated site-specific delivery (Dykxhoorn 2003). Local injections of siRNA into the eye were used in initial clinical trials for age-related macular degeneration (Oh 2009). Moreover, intranasal siRNA administration for pulmonary delivery and direct injection into the central nervous system were also tested in clinical trials (Howard 2006, Bitko 2005, Zhang 2004). Systemic delivery by intravenous (i.v.), intraperitoneal (i.p.) or oral administration is convenient for target sites that are not readily accessible. This especially refers to metastatic tumours. Thus, for example, Yano et al. (Yano 2004) showed that human bcl-2 oncogene targeting siRNA complexed with cationic liposomes injected i.v. inhibited tumour growth in a mouse liver metastasis model.. Another research carried out by Morrissey et al. (Morrissey 2005) revealed efficient and persistent antiviral activity after injection of siRNA encapsulated in lipid vesicle into the hepatitis B virus mouse model. Moreover, in systemic delivery, siRNA must maintain active form in circulation and be able to reach target tissues after passing through multiple barrier organs.

siRNA technology is a promising application of naturally occurring processes in the human body. There is evidence that mature miRNAs, mRNA and signal peptides are loaded into exosomes (Thery 2002), small membrane-bound particles derived from the endocytic compartment that are secreted and act as intercellular mediators of biological information

(Graner 2009). Barr virus (EBV)-infected cells secrete exosomes containing EBV-miRNA that are transferred to uninfected neighbouring cells (T-cells) in the peripheral blood of patients helping to spread the virus (Rechavi 2009). Cancer cells can affect function of immune system *via* exosomes by inhibiting functions of T cells and natural killer cells (Zhang 2011), thus avoiding immunosurveillance. The fact that mast cells-derived exosomes can carry mRNAs for more that 1300 genes and more than 100 miRNAs (Zhang 2011) clearly demonstrates the potential of this intercellular genetic exchange mechanism as a target in treatment of various diseases. Knowledge of this process will be highly beneficial in terms of siRNA therapy application.

7. RNAi as a research tool

Knocking down the genes of interest by using siRNAs has turned out to be an important laboratory tool for large-scale RNAi screens, especially in the field of medical research. There are several methods for siRNA generation. Direct chemical synthesis is an obvious choice for creating siRNA library, but this could be a rather expensive option for most researchers, so that the only large-scale synthetic siRNA library was made for Novartis by Qiagen and Dhamarcon. Vector-based approach has lower cost enabling not only high transfection efficiency and delivery of siRNA expression cassettes but also the selection of transfected cells. The basic idea is to use pol III promoters followed by DNA coding for shRNA that structurally resembles miRNA (Brummelkamp 2002, Miyagishi and Taira 2002, Sui 2002, Xia 2002, Yu 2002). It is possible as well to use dual Pol III promoters (Chen 2005, Zheng 2004) or even two tandem Pol III promoters (Lee 2002), which is less popular method due to its more laborious construction. Some other promoters like T7 and CMV can be used for constructing siRNA vectors (Xia 2002, Holle 2004). Bacteriophage T7 promoter is not functional in mammalian cells. CMV promoter, on the other hand, is RNA polymerase II promoter, which is stronger promoter than Pol III resulting in more transcribes from the same vector that are capped at the 5′-end and tailed at the 3′-end with a long poly (A) sequence. These modifications are well-tolerated, indicating that such approach might be used for *in vivo* research purposes. If lentivirus and retrovirus are used, it is possible to make stable knockdown cells as a consequence of genome integration. So far, three large-scale siRNA libraries have been constructed, two for academic research (Paddison 2004, Berns 2004, Michiels 2002) and one for industrial sector by Galapagos, with more libraries covering a whole mammalian genome on the horizon. siRNA libraries are usually designed to explore and study target genes central to important biological pathways, which is important for development of novel therapeutic options. Because disease pathogenesis is driven by the alteration in multiple genes and/or pathways, it is expected that modulation of gene activity by siRNA might produce a therapeutic benefit. Thus, Galapagos library targeted over 4,900 human druggable transcripts like G-protein-coupled receptors, ion channels and nuclear hormone receptors. Bernards and colleagues constructed human RNAi library (the 'NKi library') covering 7,914 human genes (Michiels 2002). Genes implicated in cancer and other diseases, as well as genes coding for major cellular pathways like cell cycle, transcription regulation, stress signalling, proteolysis and metabolism are included in the library. However, a rather robust method in the laboratory environment turned out to pose quite a lot of technical challenges when used for treatment *in vivo*. For example, siRNAs are large molecules (~13kDa) with phosphodiester backbone bearing strong negative anionic charge that hampers diffusion through the anionic cell membrane surface. Until nowadays, numerous delivery strategies have been developed to circumvent this problem, some of them being successfully employed for introduction of siRNAs into cells *in vitro* and *in vivo*. These systems are based on the use of diverse compounds or materials and viruses complexed to siRNAs, *e.g.*. chitosan-based siRNA nanoparticle delivery (Howard 2006), adenovirus-mediated siRNA delivery (Uchida 2004), antibody-mediated delivery of siRNAs *via* cell-surface receptors (Song 2005), or bioconjugation (Cheng 2006). Improved siRNA delivery (Whitehead 2009) resulted in efficient silencing of disease-associated genes, including allelic variants in tissue culture and animal models (De Paula 2007) that fostered interest in developing RNAi-based reagents for clinical applications, *e.g.*. cancer treatment, viral infections, autoimmune diseases and neurodegenerative diseases. However, blood stability, targeted delivery, poor intracellular uptake and non-specific immune stimulation are major bottlenecks in modern approaches to delivery of RNAi reagents in clinics. On the other hand, low siRNA production costs (Hall 2005) in comparison to antibodies and other therapeutic proteins make them appealing novel drugs. siRNAs possess favourable pharmacokinetic properties, can be delivered to a wide range of organs, and are increasingly considered as a basis for development of next generation targeted drugs.

Diverse RNAs may be also useful to mimic or antagonize miRNAs that are central to regulation of oncogenic or tumor suppressor pathways (Chen 2005). For example, Nohata et al. (Nohata 2011) observed that restoration of *miR-1* in cancer cells inhibits cell proliferation, invasion and migration, supporting the hypothesis that *miR-1* functions as a tumour suppressor in head and neck squamous cell carcinoma (HNSCC). Furthermore, transgelin 2 (TAGLN2), a potential oncogene, is directly regulated by *miR-1*. Silencing of *TAGLN2* significantly inhibited cell proliferation and invasion in HNSCC cells (Nohata 2011).

Recent clinical trials using siRNAs to cure age-related macular degeneration (Bevasiranib by Opko Health, Inc., Miami, USA; phase III) and respiratory syncytial virus infection (ALN-RSV01 by Alnylan, Cambridge, USA; phase II) have proved the therapeutic potential of RNAi pathways. In other studies with siRNA employed for treatment of disease *in vivo*, multiple non-specific effects were also observed. One of them occurs due to delivery of siRNA into target cells by lipid-mediated transfection, resulting in combined transfection and siRNA-specific effects (Fedorov 2005). Furthermore, common non-specific effect is the interferon-induced response (Sledz, 2003). For example, in patients with blinding choroidal neovascularisation receiving intravenous injections of siRNA, targeting vascular endothelial growth factor to block angiogenesis induced strong immune system response (Kleinman 2008). These common issues might be adequately addressed by careful optimization of concentration, delivery method and siRNA design. Nonetheless, proof of concept for RNAi-mediated specific gene silencing efficacy in humans was recently reported in a clinical trial of melanoma (Davis 2010). Nanoparticle-mediated siRNA delivery was employed for treatment of melanoma patients. Intracellular localized nanoparticles were detected in all tumour biopsies obtained upon treatment in amounts that correlated with dose levels of administered nanoparticles. Furthermore, a reduction of specific messenger RNA - M2 subunit of ribonucleotide reductase (RRM2) and the protein (RRM2) levels were observed as well (Davis 2010).

In conclusion, implementation of siRNA in clinical applications for treatment of disease through RNAi will be beneficial for such disorders that exert the symptoms *via* dominant-negative or gain-of-function mechanism. Here, we clearly foresee the challenge of inducing endogenous degradation of mutant RNAs while leaving wild-type transcripts unaffected.

8. Acknowledgments

This work was supported by the Foundation of Croatian Academy of Sciences and Arts and the Croatian Ministry of Science, Education and Sports (grants number 335-0982464-2393 and 335-0000000-3532).

9. References

Akinc A., *et al.* 2008. A combinatorial library of lipid-like materials for delivery of RNAi therapeutics. *Nat. Biotechnol.* 26: 561–569

Amarzguioui M., Rossi J.J., Kim D. 2005. Approaches for chemically synthesized siRNA and vector-mediated RNAi. *FEBS Letters* 579: 5974–5981.

Andersson M.G., et al. 2005. Suppression of RNA interference by adenovirus virus-associated RNA. *J. Virol.* 79: 9556–9565

Babiarz J.E., Ruby J.G., Wang Y., Bartel D.P. & Blelloch R. 2008. Mouse ES cells express endogenous shRNAs, siRNAs, and other Microprocessor-independent, Dicer-dependent small RNAs. *Genes Dev.* 22: 2773–2785

Bartel D.P. 2004. MicroRNAs: Genomics, biogenesis, mechanism, and function. *Cell* 116: 281–297

Behlke M.A. 2008. Chemical modification of siRNAs for in vivo use. *Oligonucleotides* 18: 305-320

Berns K., Hijmans E.M., Mullenders J. et al. 2004. A large-scale RNAi screen in human cells identifies new components of the p53 pathway. *Nature* 428: 431-437

Birmingham A., Anderson E.M., Reynolds A., Ilsley-Tyree D., Leake D., Fedorov Y., Baskerville S., Maksimova E., Robinson K., et al. 2006. 3' UTR seed matches, but not overall identity, are associated with RNAi off-targets. *Nat. Methods.* 3: 199-204

Bitko V., Musiyenko A., Shulyayeva O. & Barik S. 2005. Inhibition of respiratory viruses by nasally administered siRNA. *Nat Med* 11: 50–55

Bondensgaard K., Petersen M., Singh S.K., Rajwanshi V.K., Kumar R., Wengel J. and Jacobsen J.P. 2000. Structural studies of LNA: RNA duplexes by NMR: Conformations and implications for RNase H activity. *Chemistry* (Easton) 6: 2687–2695.

Boussif O., Lezoualc'h F., Zanta M.A., Mergny M.D., Scherman D., Demeneix B. & Behr J-P. 1995. A versatile vector for gene and oligonucleotide transfer into cells in culture and in vivo: polyethylenimine. *Proc Natl Acad Sci* USA 92: 7297–7301

Braasch D.A. and Corey D.R. 2001. Locked nucleic acid (LNA): Fine-tuning the recognition of DNA and RNA. *Chem. Biol.* 8: 1–7

Braasch D.A., Jensen S., Liu Y., Kaur K., Arar K., White M.A. and Corey D.R. 2003. RNA interference in mammalian cells by chemically-modified RNA. *Biochemistry* 42: 7967–7975

Brummelkamp T.R., Bernards R. & Agami R. 2002a. Stable suppression of tumorigenicity by virus-mediated RNA interference. *Cancer Cell* 2: 243–247

Brummelkamp T.R., Bernards R., Agami R. 2002b. A system for stable expression of short interfering RNAs in mammalian cells. *Science* 296: 550-553

Buyens K., Meyer M., Wagner E., Demeester J., De Smedt S.C., Sanders N.N. 2009. Monitoring the disassembly of siRNA polyplexes in serum is crucial for predicting their biological efficacy. *Journal of Controlled Release* 141: 38-41

Bühler M., Moazed D. 2007. Transcription and RNAi in heterochromatic gene silencing. *Nature structural & molecular biology* 14: 1041-1048

Carmichael G.G. 2003. "Antisense starts making more sense". *Nat Biotechnol* 21: 371–372.

Chen C.Z. 2005a. MicroRNAs as Oncogenes and Tumor Suppressors. *New Eng. J. Med.* 353: 1768-1771

Chen M., Zhang L., Zhang H.Y. et al. 2005b. A Universal Plasmid Library Encoding All Permutations of siRNA. *Proc Natl Acad Sci* USA 120: 2356-2361

Cheng K., Ye Z., Guntaka R.V. and Mahato R.I. 2006. Enhanced hepatic uptake and bioactivity of type a1(I) collagen gene promoter-specific triplex-forming oligonucleotides after conjugation with cholesterol. *J. Pharmacol. Exp. Ther.* 317: 797–805

Chiu Y.L. and Rana T.M. 2002. RNAi in human cells: Basic structural and functional features of small interfering RNA. *Mol. Cell* 10: 549–561

Chiu Y.L. and Rana T.M. 2003. siRNA function in RNAi: A chemical modification analysis. *RNA* 9: 1034–1048

Cho Y.W., Kim J-D. & Park K. 2003. Polycation gene delivery systems: escape from endosomes to cytosol. *J Pharm Pharmacol* 55: 721–734.

Davis M.E., Zuckerman J.E., Choi C.H.J., Seligson D., Tolcher A., Alabi C.A., Yen Y. Heidel J.D. & Ribas A. 2010. Evidence of RNAi in humans from systemically administered siRNA via targeted nanoparticles. *Nature* Vol 464: 1067-1070

De Paula D., Vito M., Bentley R.L.B. and Mahato R.I. 2007. Hydrophobization and bioconjugation for enhanced siRNA delivery and targeting. *RNA* 13: 431–456.

Devi G.R. 2006. siRNA-based approaches in cancer therapy. *Cancer Gene Therapy* 13: 819–829

DiFiglia M., Sena-Esteves M., Chase K., Sapp E., Pfister E., Sass M., Yoder J., Reeves P., Pandey R.K., Rajeev K.G. et al. 2007. Therapeutic silencing of mutant huntingtin with siRNA attenuates striatal and cortical neuropathology and behavioral deficits. *Proc Natl Acad Sci* USA 104: 17204–17209.

Donze O. and Picard D. 2002. RNA interference in mammalian cells using siRNAs synthesized with T7 RNA polymerase. *Nucleic Acids Res.* 30: e46

Du T. and Zamore P.D. 2005. microPrimer: the biogenesis and function of microRNA. *Development* 132: 4645–4652

Dubey P.K., Mishra V., Jain S., Mahor S. & Vyas S.P. 2004. Liposomes modified with cyclic RGD peptide for tumor targeting. *J Drug Target* 12: 257–264

Dykxhoorn D.M., Novina C.D., and Sharp P.A. 2003. Killing the messenger: Short RNAs that silence gene expression. *Nat. Rev. Mol. Cell Biol.* 4: 457–467.

Dykxhoorn DM, Palliser D. & Lieberman J. 2006. The silent treatment: siRNAs as small molecule drugs. *Gene Ther* 13: 541–552

Elbashir S.M., Harborth J., Lendeckel W., Yalcin A., Weber K., and Tuschl T. 2001a. Duplexes of 21-nucleotide RNAs mediate RNA interference in cultured mammalian cells. *Nature* 411: 494–498

Elbashir S.M., Lendeckel W., and Tuschl T. 2001b. RNA interference is mediated by 21- and 22-nucleotide RNAs. *Genes & Dev.* 15: 188–200

Elbashir S.M., Harborth J., Weber K. and Tuschl T. 2002. Analysis of gene function in somatic mammalian cells using small interfering RNAs. *Methods* 26: 199–213

Elmen J., Thonberg H., Ljungberg K., Frieden M., Westergaard M., Xu Y., Wahren B., Liang Z., Orum H., Koch T., et al. 2005. Locked nucleic acid (LNA) mediated improvements in siRNA, stability and functionality. *Nucleic Acids Res*. 33: 439–447

ENCODE Project Consortium. 2007. Identification and analysis of functional elements in 1% ofthe human genome by the ENCODE pilot project.Nature. 14;447(7146):799-816

Fedorov Y. et al. 2005. "Different delivery methods-different expression profiles." *Nat Methods* 2: 241

Fire A. *et al.* 1998 Potent and specific genetic interference by double-stranded RNA in *Caenorhabditis elegans*. *Nature* 391: 806–811

Frank-Kamenetsky M. *et al.* 2008. Therapeutic RNAi targeting PCSK9 acutely lowers plasma cholesterol in rodents and LDL cholesterol in nonhuman primates. *Proc. Natl. Acad. Sci. USA* 105: 11915–11920

Friend D.S., Papahadjopoulos D., Debs R.J. 1996. Endocytosis and intracellular processing accompanying transfection mediated by cationic liposomes. *Biochim Biophys Acta*. 1278: 41–50.

Gesteland R.F., Cech T.R. and Atkins J.F. (eds) 2006. The RNA World, 3rd edn. Cold Spring Harbor Laboratory Press

Gosselin M.A. & Lee R.J. 2002. Folate receptortargeted liposomes as vectors for therapeutic agents. *Biotechnol Annu Rev* 8: 103–131

Graner M.W., Alzate O., Dechkovskaia A.M., Keene J.D., Sampson J.H., Mitchell D.A., et al. 2009. Proteomic and immunologic analyses of brain tumor exosomes. FASEB J. 23:1541–57

Gregory R., Chendrimada T., Cooch N., Shiekhattar R. 2005. "Human RISC couples microRNA biogenesis and posttranscriptional gene silencing". *Cell* 123: 631–40

Grimm D. and Kay M.A. 2003. From virus evolution to vector revolution: use of naturally occurring serotypes of adeno-associated virus (AAV) as novel vectors for human gene therapy. *Curr. Gene Ther*. 3:281–304

Hall A.H., Wan J., Shaughnessy E.E., Ramsay Shaw B., and Alexander K.A. 2004. RNA interference using boranophosphate siRNAs: Structure–activity relationships. *Nucleic Acids Res*. 32:5991–6000

Hall T.M. Structure and function of argonaute proteins. 2005. *Structure*. 13:1403-1408

Han S., Mahato R.I., Sung Y.K., and Kim S.W. 2000. Development of biomaterials for gene therapy. *Mol. Ther*. 2: 302–317

Hannon G.J. 2002. RNA interference. *Nature* 418: 244–251

Hicke B.J. and Stephens A.W. 2000. Escort aptamers: A delivery service for diagnosis and therapy. *J. Clin. Invest*. 106:923–928.

Holen T., Amarzguioui M., Wiiger M.T., Babaie E. and Prydz H.2002. Positional effects of short interfering RNAs targeting the human coagulation trigger Tissue Factor. *Nucleic Acids Res*. 30:1757–1766

Holle L., Hicks L., Song W., Holle E., Wagner T., Yu X. 2004. Bcl-2 targeting siRNA expressed by a T7 vector system inhibits human tumor cell growth in vitro. *Int J Oncol*, 24: 615-621

Howard K.A., Rahbek U.L., Liu X., Damgaard C.K., Glud S.Z., Andersen M.O., Hovgaard M.B., Schmitz A., Nyengaard J.R., Besenbacher F. et al. 2006 RNA interference *in vitro* and *in vivo* using a chitosan/siRNA nanoparticle system. *Mol Ther* 14: 476–484

Hu-Lieskovan S., Heidel J.D., Bartlett D.W., Davis M.E. and Triche T.J. 2005. Sequence-specific knockdown of EWS-FLI1 by targeted, nonviral delivery of small interfering RNA inhibits tumor growth in a murine model of metastatic Ewing's sarcoma. *Cancer Res.* 65: 8984–8992

Huang Y., Hong J., Zheng S., Ding Y., Guo S., Zhang H., Zhang X., Du Q., Lisng Z., 2011. Elimination pathways of systemically delivered siRNA. *Molecular Therapy* 19: 381-385

Inoue H., Hayase Y., Imura A., Iwai S., Miura. K., and Ohtsuka E. 1987. Synthesis and hybridization studies on two complementary nona(29-O-methyl)ribonucleotides. *Nucleic Acids Res.* 15: 6131–6148

Jackson A.L., Burchard J., Schelter J., Chau B.N., Cleary M., Lim L., 2006a. Widespread siRNA "off-target" transcript silencing mediated by seed region sequence complementarity. *RNA.* 12:1179-87.

Jackson A.L., Bartz S.R., Schelter J., Kobayashi S.V., Burchard J., Mao M., Li B., Cavet G., and Linsley P.S. 2003. Expression profiling reveals off-target gene regulation by RNAi. *Nat. Biotechnol.* 21: 635–637.

Jackson A.L., Burchard J., Leake D., Reynolds A., Schelter J.,Guo J., Johnson J.M., Lim L., Karpilow J., Nichols K. et al. 2006b. Position-specific chemical modification of siRNAs reduces"off-target" transcript silencing. *RNA* 12: 1197–1205

Jang S.H., Wientjes M.G., Lu D. & Au J.L.-S. 2003 Drug delivery and transport to solid tumors. *Pharm Res* 20: 1337-1350

Judge A.D., Sood V., Shaw J.R., Fang D., McClintock K. and MacLachlan I. 2005. Sequence-dependent stimulation of the mammalian innate immune response by synthetic siRNA. *Nat.Biotechnol.* 23: 457–462

Juliano R., Bauman J., Kang H. and Ming X., 2009. Biological barriers to therapy with with with antisense and siRNA oligonucleotides. *Mol Pharm* 6: 686-695.

Kaszubiak A., Holm P.S., Lage H.. 2007. Overcoming the classical multidrug resistance phenotype by adenoviral delivery of anti-MDR1 short hairpin RNAs and ribozymes. *Int J Oncol;* 31:419-30

Kaur H., Arora., Wengel J., Maiti S.,. 2006. "Thermodynamic, Counterion, and Hydration Effects for the Incorporation of Locked Nucleic Acid Nucleotides into DNA Duplexes". *Biochemistry* 45: 7347–55

Keller M. 2005. Lipidic carriers of RNA/DNA oligonucleotides and polynucleotides: What a difference a formulation makes! *J. Control. Release* 103: 537–540

Kim B., Tang Q., Biswas P.S., Xu J., Schiffelers R.M., Xie F.Y., Ansari A.M., Scaria P.V., Woodle M.C., Lu P. et al. 2004. Inhibition of ocular angiogenesis by siRNA targeting vascular endothelial growth factor pathway genes: therapeutic strategy for herpetic stromal keratitis. *Am J Pathol 165*: 2177–2185

Kim D.H., Behlke M.A., Rose S.D., Chang M.S., Choi. S., and Rossi, J.J. 2005. Synthetic dsRNA Dicer substrates enhance RNAi potency and efficacy. *Nat. Biotechnol.* 23: 222–226

Kim S.H. Mok H. Jeong J.H. Kim S.W. & Park T.G. 2006. Comparative evaluation of the target-specific GFP gene scilencing efficiencies for antisense ODN, synthetic siRNA, and siRNA plasmid complexed with PEI-PEG-FOL conjugate. Bioconjug Chem 17: 241-244

Kleinman M.E., Yamada K., Takeda A., Chandrasekaran V., Nozaki M., Baffi J. Z., Albuquerque R.J.C., Yamasaki S., Itaya M., Pan Y., Appukuttan B., Gibbs D., Yang Z., Karikó K., Ambati B.K., Wilgus T.A., DiPietro L.A., Sakurai E., Zhang K., Smith J.R., Taylor E.W. & Ambati J. 2008. Sequence- and target-independent angiogenesis suppression by siRNA via TLR3 *Nature* 452:591-597

Krühn A., Wang A., Fruehauf J.H., Lage H. 2009. Delivery of short hairpin RNAs by transkingdom RNA interference modulates the classical ABCBI-mediated multidrug-resistant phenotype of cancer cells. *Cell Cycle* 8: 3349-3354

Lavorgna G., Dahary D., Lehner B., Sorek R., Sanderson C.M., Casari G. 2004. "In search of antisense". *Trends Biochem Sci.* 29 : 88–94

Lee R.C., Feinbaum R.L. & Ambros V. 1993. The *C. elegans* heterochronic gene *lin-4* encodes small RNAs with antisense complementarity to *lin-14*. *Cell* 75: 843–854

Lee N.S., Dohjima T., Bauer G. et al. 2002. Expression of small interfering RNAs targeted against HIV-1 rev transcripts in human cells. *Nat Biotechnol* 20: 500-505

Lecellier C.H., Voinnet O. 2004. RNA silencing: no mercy for viruses? Immunol Rev 198: 285–303

Lee Y.S., Nakahara K., Pham J.W., Ki K., He Z., Sontheimer E.J. and Carthew R.W. 2004. Distinct roles for Drosophila Dicer-1 and Dicer-2 in the siRNA/miRNA silencing pathways. *Cell* 117: 69–81.

Lesnik, E.A., Guinosso, C.J., Kawasaki, A.M., Sasmor, H., Zounes, M., Cummins, L.L., Ecker, D.J., Cook, P.D., and Freier, S.M. 1993. Oligodeoxynucleotides containing 29-O-modified adenosine: Synthesis and effects on stability of DNA:RNA duplexes. *Biochemistry* 32: 7832–7838

Leuschner P.J., Ameres S.L., Kueng S., and Martinez J. 2006. Cleavage of the siRNA passenger strand during RISC assembly in human cells. *EMBO Rep.* 7: 314–320

Lia S-D., Chono S. & Huang L. 2005 Efficient gene silencing in metastatic tumor by siRNA formulated in surface-modified nanoparticles. *J Control Release* 126: 77–84

Liu J., Carmell M.A., Rivas F.V., Marsden C.G., Thomson J.M., Song J.J., Hammond S.M., Joshua-Tor L. and Hannon G.J. 2004. Argonaute2 is the catalytic engine of mammalian RNAi. *Science* 305: 1437–1441

Lorenz C., Hadwiger P., John M., Vornlocher H.P., and Unverzagt C. 2004. Steroid and lipid conjugates of siRNAs to enhance cellular uptake and gene silencing in liver cells. *Bioorg. Med. Chem. Lett.* 14: 4975–4977

Lu P.Y., Xie F.Y. & Woodle M.C. 2005 Modulation of angiogenesis with siRNA inhibitors for novel therapeutics. *Trends Mol Med* 11: 104–113

Mahat R.I., Monera O.D., Smith L.C., and Rolland A. 1999. Peptide-based gene delivery. *Curr. Opin. Mol. Ther.* 1: 226–243

Mahato R.I., Rolland A., and Tomlinson E. 1997. Cationic lipidbased gene delivery systems: Pharmaceutical perspectives. *Pharm. Res.* 14: 853–859

Mahato R.I., Cheng K., and Guntaka R.V. 2005. Modulation of gene expression by antisense and antigene oligodeoxynucleotides and small interfering RNA. *Expert Opin. Drug Deliv.* 2: 3–28

Mahato R.I., Anwer K., Tagliaferri F., Meaney C., Leonard P., Wadhwa M.S., Logan M., French M., and Rolland A. 1998. Biodistribution and gene expression of lipid/plasmid complexes after systemic administration. *Hum. Gene Ther.* 9: 2083–2099

Mahato R.I., Smith L.C., and Rolland A. 1999. Pharmaceutical perspectives of nonviral gene therapy. *Adv. Genet.* 41: 95–156

Mamot C., Drummond D.C., Noble C.O., Kallab V., Guo Z., Hong K., Kirpotin D.B. & Park J.W. 2005. Epidermal growth factor receptor-targeted immunoliposomessignificantly enhance the efficacy of multiple anticancer drugs in vivo. *Cancer Res* 65: 11631–11638

Manoharan M. 2004. RNA interference and chemically modified small interfering RNAs. *Curr. Opin. Chem. Biol.* 8: 570–579

Marques J.T. and Williams B.R. 2005. Activation of the mammalian immune system by siRNAs. *Nat. Biotechnol.* 23: 1399–1405

Matranga C., Tomari Y., Shin C., Bartel D.P., and Zamore P.D. 2005. Passenger-strand cleavage facilitates assembly of siRNA into Ago2-containing RNAi enzyme complexes. *Cell* 123: 607–620

Mattick J.S., and Makunin I.V. 2006. Non-coding RNA *Human Molecular Genetics* 15: 17-29

Mattick J.S. and Makunin I.V. 2005 Small regulatory RNAs in mammals. *Hum. Mol. Genet.* 14: 121–132

Medina-Kauwe L.K., Xie J. & Hamm-Alvarez S. 2005 Intracellular trafficking of nonviral vectors. *Gene Ther* 12: 1734–1751

Meister G. and Tuschl T. 2004. Mechanisms of gene silencing by double-stranded RNA. *Nature* 431: 343–349

Michiels F., van Es H., van Rompaey L. et al. 2002. Arrayed adenoviralexpression libraries for functional screening. *Nat Biotechnol* 20: 1154-1157

Miyagishi M., Taira K. 2002. U6 promoter-driven siRNAs withfour uridine 3' overhangs efficiently suppress targeted gene expressionin mammalian cells. *Nat Biotechnol* 20: 497-500

Milligan J.F. and Uhlenbeck O.C. 1989. Synthesis of small RNAsusing T7 RNA polymerase. *Methods Enzymol.* 180: 51–62

Morrissey D.V., Lockridge J.A., Shaw L., Blanchard K., Jensen K., Breen W., Hartsough K., Machemer L., Radka S., Jadhav V. et al. 2005. Potent and persistent in vivo anti-HBV activity of chemically modified siRNAs. *Nat Biotechnol* 23: 1002–100

Myers J.W., Jones J.T., Meyer T., and Ferrell Jr. J.E. 2003. Recombinant Dicer efficiently converts large dsRNAs into siRNAs suitable for gene silencing. *Nat. Biotechnol.* 21: 324–328

Nieth C., Priebsch A., Stege A., Lage H.. 2003. Modulation of the classical multidrug resistance (MDR) phenotype by RNA interference (RNAi). *FEBS Lett.* 545:144-50.

Nohata N., Sone Y., Hanazawa T., Fuse M., Kikkawa N., Yoshino H., Chiyomaru T., Kawakami K., Enokida H., Nakagawa M., Shozu M., Okamoto Y. and Seki N. 2011. miR-1 as a tumor suppressive microRNA targeting TAGLN2 in head and neck squamous cell carcinoma. *Oncotarget* 2: 29 - 58

Oh Y-K. & Park T.G. 2009 siRNA delivery systems for cancer treatment. *Adv Drug Deliver Rev* 61: 850–862

Oliveira S., Van Rooy I., Kranenburg O., Storm G. & Schiffelers R.M. 2007 Fusogenic peptides enhance endosomal escape improving siRNA-induced silencing of oncogenes. *Int J Pharm* 331: 211–214.

Osato N., Suzuki Y., Ikeo K., Gojobori T. 2007. "Transcriptional interferences in cis-natural antisense transcripts of humans and mice". *Genetics* 176: 1299–306

Paddison P.J., Caudy A.A., Bernstein E., Hannon G.J., and Conklin D.S. 2002. Short hairpin RNAs (shRNAs) induce sequence-specific silencing in mammalian cells. *Genes & Dev.* 16: 948–958.

Paddison P.J., Silva J.M., Conklin D.S. et al. 2004. A resource forlarge-scale RNA-interference-based screens in mammals. *Nature* 428: 427-431

Park J.W., Hong K., Kirpotin D.B., Colbern G., Shalaby R., Baselga J., Shao Y., Nielsen U.B., Marks J.D., Moore D., Papahadjopoulos D., Benz C.C. 2002. Anti-HER2 immunoliposomes: enhanced efficacy attributable to targeted delivery. *Clin Cancer Res.* 8(4): 1172-81

Persengiev S.P., Zhu X., Green M.R. 2004. Nonspecific, concentration dependent stimulation and repression of mammalian gene expression by small interfering RNAs (siRNAs). *RNA* 10:12-18

Pestourie C., Tavitian B., and Duconge F. 2005. Aptamers against extracellular targets for in vivo applications. *Biochimie* 87: 921–930

Pillai R.S., Bhattacharyya S.N., Filipowicz W. 2007. "Repression of protein synthesis by miRNAs: how many mechanisms?". *Trends Cell Biol* 17: 118–26

Pirollo K.F., Rait A., Zhou Q., Hwang S.H., Dagata J.A., Zon G., Hogrefe R.I., Palchik G. & Chang E.H. 2007 Materializing the potential of small interfering RNA via a tumor-targeting nanodelivery system. *Cancer Res* 67: 2938–2943

Pulford B., Reim N., Bell A., Veatch J., Forster G., bender H., Meyerett C., Hafeman S., Michel B., Johnson T., Wyckoff A.C., Miele G., Julius C., Kranich J., Schenkel A., Dow S., Zabel M.D. 2010. Liposome-siRNA-Peptide Complexes Cross the Blood-Brain Barrier and Significantly Decrease PrPc on Neuronal Cells and PrPres in Infected Cell Cultures *Plos ONE* 5: e11085

Rechavi O., Erlich Y., Amram H., Flomenblit L., Karginov F.V., Goldstein I., et al. 2009. Cell contact-dependent acquisition of cellular and viral nonautonomously encoded small RNAs. *Genes Dev* 23:1971-9

Reynolds A., Leake D., Boese Q., Scaringe S., Marshall W.S., and Khvorova A. 2004. Rational siRNA design for RNA interference. *Nat. Biotechnol.* 22: 326–330

Schepers U. 2005. RNA interference in practice: Principles, basics, and methods for gene silencing in C. elegans, Drosophila, and mammals. Wiley-VCH, NewYork.

Schiffelers R.M., Ansari A., Xu J., Zhou Q., Tang Q.,Storm G., Molema G., Lu P.Y., Scaria P.V. & Woodle M.C. 2004 Cancer siRNA therapy by tumor selectivedelivery with ligand-targeted sterically stabilized nanoparticle. *Nucleic Acids Res* 32: e149.

Schwarz D.S., Hutvagner G., Du T., Xu Z., Aronin N., Zamore P.D. 2003 Asymmetry in the assembly of the RNAi enzyme complex. *Cell.* 115:199-208

Sioud M. 2004. Therapeutic siRNAs. *Trends Pharmacol. Sci.* 25: 22–28

Sioud M. 2005. Induction of inflammatory cytokines and interferon responses by double-stranded and single-stranded siRNAs is sequence-dependent and requires endosomal localization. *J. Mol. Biol. 348*: 1079–1090

Sioud M. 2006. Single-stranded small interfering RNA are more immunostimulatory than their double-stranded counterparts: Acentral role for 29-hydroxyl uridines in immune responses. *Eur. J.Immunol.* 36: 1222–1230

Sledz C. et al. 2003 Activation of the interferon system by short-interfering RNAs. *Nat Cell Biol* 5: 834-9

Song et al.2005 Antibody mediated *in vivo* delivery of small interfering RNAs via cell-surface receptors. *Nature Biotechnology* 23: 709 - 717

Soutschek J., Akinc A., Bramlage B., Charisse K., Constien R., Donoghue M., Elbashir S., Geick A., Hadwiger P., Harborth J., et al. 2004. Therapeutic silencing of an endogenous gene by systemic administration of modified siRNAs. *Nature* 432: 173–178

Spagnou S., Miller A.D., and Keller M. 2004. Lipidic carriers of siRNA: Differences in the formulation, cellular uptake, and delivery with plasmid DNA. *Biochemistry* 43: 13348–13356.

Stein U., Walther W., Stege A., Kaszubiak A., Fichtner I., Lage H. 2008. Complete in vivo reversal of the multidrug resistance phenotype by jet-injection of anti-MDR1 short hairpin RNA-encoding plasmid DNA. *Mol Ther.* 16:178-86

Sui G., Soohoo C., Affar el B et al. 2002. A DNA vector-based RNAi technology to suppress gene expression in mammalian cells. *Proc Natl Acad Sci* USA, 16: 5515-5520

Tan P-H., Yang L-C., Shih H-C., Lan K-C. & Cheng J-T. 2005. Gene knockdown with intrathecal siRNA of NMDA receptor NR2B subunit reduces formalin-induced nociception in the rat. *Gene Ther* 12: 59–66

Taylor D.D., Gercel-Taylor C. 2005. Tumour-derived exosomes and their role in cancer-associated T-cell signalling defects. *Br J Cancer* 92: 305–11

Thery C., Zitvogel L., Amigorena S. 2002 Exosomes: composition, biogenesisand function. *Nat Rev Immunol* 2: 569–79

Uchida et al. 2004. Adenovirus-Mediated Transfer of siRNA against Survivin Induced Apoptosis and Attenuated Tumor Cell Growth *in Vitro* and *in Vivo*. *Molecular Therapy* 10, 162–171

Vagin V. V. *et al.* 2006. A distinct small RNA pathway silences selfish genetic elements in the germline. *Science* 313: 320–324

Valadi H., Ekstrom K., Bossios A., Sjostrand M., Lee J.J., Lotvall J.O., 2007. Exosome-mediated transfer of mRNAs and microRNAs is a novel mechanism of genetic exchange between cells. *Nat Cell Biol* 9: 654-9

Zámečník J., Vargová L., Homola A., Kodet R & Syková E. 2003. Extracellular matrix glycoproteins and diffusion barriers in human astrocytic tumours. *Neuropathol Appl Neurobiol* 30: 338–350

Zhang H.-G., and Grizzle W. E. 2011. Exosomes and cancer: A newly described pathway of immune suppression. *Clin Cancer Res* 17: 959-64

Zhang X., Shan P., Jiang D., Noble P, Abraham N., Kappas A. & Lee P 2004. Small interfering RNAtargeting hemeoxygenase-1 enhances ischemia-reperfusion-induced lung apoptosis. *J Biol Chem* 279: 10677–10684

Zhang Y., Liu X.S., Liu Q.R., Wei L. 2006. "Genome-wide in silico identification and analysis of cis natural antisense transcripts (cis-NATs) in ten species". *Nucleic Acids Research* 34: 3465–75

Zheng L., Liu J., Batalov S., Zhou D., Orth A., Ding S., Schultz P.G. 2004. An approach to genomewide screens of expressed small interfering RNAs in mammalian cells. *Proc Natl Acad Sci* USA 101: 135-40

Zimmermann T.S., Lee A.C., Akinc A., Bramlage B., Bumcrot D., Fedoruk M.N., Harborth J., Heyes J.A., Jeff L.B., John M. et al. 2006. RNAi-mediated gene silencing in non-human primates. *Nature* 441: 111–114

Zufferey R., Dull T., Mandel R.J., Bukovsky A., Quiroz D., et al. 1998. Self-inactivating lentivirus vector for safe and efficient in vivo gene delivery.*J. Virol.* 72:9873–9880

Wang X.J., Gaasterland T., Chua N.H. 2005. "Genome-wide prediction and identification of cis-natural antisense transcripts in Arabidopsis thaliana". *Genome Biol* 6: 30

Watanabe T. *et al.* 2008. Endogenous siRNAs from naturally formed dsRNAs regulate transcripts in mouse oocytes. *Nature* 453: 539–543

Whitehead K.A., Langer R., and Anderson D.G. 2009. Knocking down barriers: advances in siRNA delivery. *Nat Drug Discov* 8: 129-138

Wolfrum C., Shi S., Jayaprakash K.N., Jayaraman M., Wang G., Pandey R.K., Rajeev K.G., Nakayama T., Charrise K., Ndungo E.M. et al. 2007. Mechanisms and optimization of in vivo delivery of lipophilic siRNAs. Nat Biotechnol 25:1149–1157

Xia H., Mao Q., Paulson H.L., Davidson B.L. 2002. siRNAmediated gene silencing in vitro and in vivo. *Nat Biotechnol* 20: 1006-1010.

Xiang S., Fruehauf J., Li C.J. 2006. Short hairpin RNAexpressing bacteria elicit RNA interference in mammals. *Nat Biotechnol* 24: 697-702

Xu Y., Szoka F.C. Jr. 1996. Mechanism of DNA release from cationic liposome/DNA complexes used in cell transfection. *Biochemistry* 35: 5616–5623

Yang D., Buchholz F., Huang Z., Goga A., Chen C.Y., Brodsky F.M., and Bishop J.M. 2002. Short RNA duplexes produced by hydrolysis with Escherichia coli RNase III mediateeffective RNA interference in mammalian cells. *Proc. Natl. Acad.Sci.* 99: 9942–9947

Yano J., Hirabayashi K., Nakagawa S-I., Yamaguchi T., Nogawa M., Kashimori I., Naito H., Kitagawa H., Ishiyama K., Ohgi T. et al. 2004. Antitumor activity of smallinterfering RNA/ cationic liposome complex in mouse models of cancer. *Clin Cancer Res* 10: 7721–7726

Yoo J.Y., et al. 2007. VEGF-specific short hairpin RNA-expressing oncolytic adenovirus elicits potent inhibition of angiogenesis and tumor growth. *Mol.Ther.* 15:295–302

Yu J.Y., DeRuiter S.L., Turner D.L. 2002. RNA interference by expression of short-interfering RNAs and hairpin RNAs in mammalian cells. *Proc Natl Acad Sci* USA 99, 6047-6052

5

MicroRNAs in Disease and Health: Diagnostic and Therapeutic Potentials

Mohammad Reza Noori-Daloii[1] and Azim Nejatizadeh[2]
[1]*Department of Medical Genetics, Faculty of Medicine, Tehran University of Medical Sciences;*
[2]*Research Center for Molecular Medicine, Faculty of Medicine, Hormozgan University of Medical Sciences, Iran*

1. Introduction

In the past decade, relevance and application of genomics and proteomics technologies in early detection of diseases have verified that numerous categories of diseases could be diagnosed at early stage which would be helpful in initiation of treatment. As a result of human genome studies, a shift has occurred from mRNAs to noncoding RNAs as a main regulator of human genome. The sequence analyses of genomes in eukaryotes indicated that simple unicellular organisms, invertebrates and mammals have approximately 25%, 80% and 98%, respectively, of their genomes composed of noncoding DNA regions [1]. In higher eukaryotic organisms, approximately, the entire genome is transcribed as consisting of rRNA, tRNA, introns, 5' and 3' untranslated regions, and microRNAs. It also has been proposed that mammalian miRNAs are originated from transposons and repeats [2,3]. Moreover, it is showed that miRNAs could be developed from pseudogenes [4]. Exisisting analyses of the human genome reflects that the protein coding genes are low as 23500, indicating that a large segment of human genome consists of non-coding protein genes. Open reading Frames comprise less than 2%, repetitive sequences around 46% and non-coding parts of protein-coding genes (introns, 5' and 3'-UTRs) around 25-27% of 3.2 billion bases in the human genome [5,6]. As the human genome and its functions are being explored, the roles of non-coding RNAs are becoming more evident in specific cellular functions. Members of non-coding RNAs include microRNAs and small nucleolar RNAs which are believed to have well preserved functions in various species. MiRNAs are functional molecules that have recently emerged as important regulators of gene expression at the posttranscriptional and translational levels. Endogenous miRNAs are involved in a variety of physiological and pathological processes in human. Target mRNA specification is defined by sequence complementarity between the seed sequence and the target mRNA. The technological advances and applications of functional RNA molecules for medicine provide important insights into molecular mechanisms affecting human health and disease and could eventually lead to the discovery of diagnostic biomarkers and the development of novel gene therapies [7].

In this chapter, we first address the synthesis, mechanisms of action and functions of miRNAs. Then, we focus on recent advances and technologies in miRNA. Next, we discuss the clinical applications of miRNA. At last, we review current knowledge of the roles of miRNAs in various diseases and determine the advantages and potential challenges of microRNA-based approaches compared to conventional drug-based therapies.

2. MiRNA biology and function

Micro ribonucleic acids (miRNAs) are a large class of endogenously expressed single stranded, evolutionarily conserved small non-coding RNAs, typically 17-25 ribonucleotides in length that are found in many plants, animals and DNA viruses regulating gene expression in a sequence-dependent manner [8]. MiRNA has revealed the great potential regulating roles in various aspects of biological and pathological processes. They were first discovered in worms in 1993, *Caenorhabditis elegans, lin-4,* capable of modulating the protein expression of *lin-14* opened up a new role for small RNAs in regulating gene expression [9]. While more than 3,000 miRNAs have now been identified in animals, plants and viruses, the human genome has been estimated to code up to 1000 miRNAs that are expected to regulate a third of all genes. A plethora of predicted mRNA targets, it is believed that these small RNAs have an enormous regulatory potentials [10,11]. In mammals, miRNAs derive from a large primary transcript, referred to as a pri-miR, transcribed by RNApolymerase II/III in nucleus. The pri-miR, which is likely hundreds to thousands of nucleotides long, experiences nuclear cleavage by a ribonuclease III called Drosha and the double-stranded DNA binding protein DGCR8/Pasha to generate a hairpin shaped ~70-nucleotide pre-miRNA. Then, pre-miRNA is transported to the cytoplasm by the nuclear export factor exportin 5, and undergoes another processing where they serve as substrates of RNase Dicer and its cofactors (PACT and TRBP) to generate ~22 nt miRNA duplexes. RNA duplex is unwound into a mature single-stranded miRNA, and loaded into RNA-induced silencing complex (RISC). Although most miRNAs in plants hybridize to target mRNAs with perfect complementarity, in animals the 5' proximal "seed" region (nucleotides 2 to 8) appears to be the primary determinant of the pairing specificity of the miRNA to the 3' untranslated region (3'-UTR) of a target mRNA. MiRNA then binds to complementary sites in the 3'-untranslated region (3'-UTR) of target mRNA and regulate its expression either by causing degradation of mRNA or repression of their translation, depending on the degree of complementarity between the miRNA and its target [12-17]. Alternatively, pre-miRNAs are derived directly from size-matched introns. These are referred to as 'mitrons' skip the Drosha–DGCR8 processing step and are spliced out of their host genes. These lariats are debranched, refolded into the stem-loop structure of typical pre-miRNAs, and then enter the canonical pathway [18]. Of note, Drosha, DGCR8, and Dicer are the well-established regulators of miRNA processing. Defects in the miRNA biogenesis machinery could be intimately related to various diseases including cancer.

3. MiRNA-mediated gene regulation

The expression of miRNAs is vibrant depending on tissue types, metabolic status and disease condition. A potent trait of miRNA-based regulation is the capability of individual miRNAs to regulate multiple functionally related mRNAs, which itself regulates multiple metabolic genes [19,20]. Approximately half of all known miRNA genes are grouped in the genome and transcribed as polycistronic primary transcripts with the remainder expressed as individual transcripts from intergenic or intronic site. Regardless of genomic organization, miRNAs function in a distinct yet cooperative manner to regulate cellular processes by coordinately targeting related proteins [21,22]. Furthermore, miRNAs often go to families of narrowly related or the same sequences. As of their homology in the seed sequence, the associated miRNAs are able to target the same mRNAs, which increases the effectiveness of repression. The number of validated mature human miRNA approaches over 1 thousand, with individual miRNAs capable to repress multiple genes. Of note, miRNAs have emerged as important regulators of every biological process involved with differentiation, cellular proliferation, tissue development and cell-type specific function and homeostasis. As a consequence, dysregulation of miRNAs have been implicated with impairment of regulatory networks. In fact, a multiple number of pathologies are associated with altered miRNAs expression [23]. It is becoming progressively more evident that the aberrant expression of miRNAs is causally related to a diversity of disease states. Stress-induced upregulation of miRNAs be able to result in the downregulation of a set of targeted mRNAs, whereas downregulation of miRNAs can lead to upregulation of target mRNAs. At last, it is the pattern of miRNA-induced gene expression that contributes to the consequential disease phenotype [24]. It was shown that diverse forms of stress alleviate mRNAs from miRNA repression by releasing mRNAs from P-bodies (cytoplasmic bodies containing mRNA degradation enzymes) and promotes their entry into polysomes, thereby enhancing translation of the preexisting mRNA [25]. Both changes in expression and function in response to stress increase their influence under conditions of disease states. The apparent roles of miRNAs in disease have led to an increasing interest in miRNA regulation as a therapeutic and diagnostic approach [26]. The role of miRNAs-mediated regulation in viral infection is becoming more evident. The outcome of miRNA repression is not well understood. Some reports showed that miRNA regulation led to translational inhibition, without affecting mRNA levels. Although there are accumulating reports that mRNA degradation is a consequence of miRNA regulation, it is unclear whether it is a consequence of translational repression or a separate pathway of miRNA regulation [27-30].

4. MiRNAs expression profile analysis

Investigating and implementing efficient tools for detection, quantification, and functional analysis of miRNAs is essential to explore the role of miRNAs signatures in health and disease process. Various studies exploited high throughput methods to analyze global miRNA expression in clinical samples. As a common platform, Oligonucleotide miRNA microarray analysis has been extensively used as high-throughput method for the evaluation of global expression levels in a large number of samples [31,32]. An original miRNA microarray platform by means of locked nucleic acid–modified capture probes has also been emerged. This procedure allows miRNAs with single nucleotide differences to be discriminated. Furthermore, MiRAGE, a form of serial analysis of gene expression to evaluate miRNA levels, and RAKE an RNA primed, array-based, Klenow enzyme high-throughput assay, have also been built up to find out miRNA expression profiles [33,34]. Of note, the above-mentioned techniques were mainly developed to determine the cancer-specific expression levels, however, the use of high-throughput arrays for investigating miRNA expression in non-neoplastic diseases is beginning to emerge. A number of miRNAs are up regulated in the brains of demised Alzheimer's patients, implicating impairment of miRNA expression in neurodegenerative disorders [35]. A microarray-based approach has also been used to profile miRNA expression in response to environmental stresses such as hypoxia. A method to weigh miRNA expression is the bead-based flow cytometric approach. Individual polystyrene beads coupled to miRNA complementary probes are marked with fluorescent tags. After hybridization with size-fractionated RNAs and streptavidin-phycoerythrin staining, the beads are analyzed using a flow-cytometer to measure bead color and phycoerythrin, demonstrating miRNA characteristics and loads respectively. The technique provides great specificity for intimately related miRNAs because hybridization happens in solution. [36]. Quantitative real-time polymerase chain reaction (qRT-PCR) have also been widely used to miRNA research due to its cost-effectiveness, high throughput and higher detection [37]. Up to now, the most successful approach in terms of specificity and sensitivity is a two-step approach via looped miRNA-specific reverse transcription primers and TaqMan probes. Multiplex PCR approaches for miRNAs have also been reported [38]. All of these technologies facilitating miRNAs expression profiling are essential for validation of microarray data. The high throughput capability of array-based platforms make them an attractive option for miRNA studies compared with lower throughput techniques such as Northern blotting and cloning. High-throughput analysis of miRNA expression in various diseases only demonstrates that some miRNAs are over expressed while others are markedly reduced in other tissues. These are exclusively correlative data. In other words, high throughput platforms to gauge miRNA expression provide only correlative evidence that atypical miRNA processing. These techniques only convey us modest about the underlying miRNA expression problem. Besides, the threshold of differential miRNA expression required so as to impact biological processes is unknown for most disease-associated miRNAs. Of importance, the development of methods to manipulate miRNA expression has made possible examinaions into the cellular processes involved by differentially expressed miRNAs. 2-O-Methyl antisense single-strand oligonucleotides and locked nucleic acid–modified oligonucleotides have been developed as miRNA inhibitors, making the suppression of endogenous miRNA activity and its downstream effect on mRNA expression achievable [39-42]. The effect of target miRNA knockdown on cell morphology and function can be determined using standard assays for processes such as cell proliferation, migration, invasion, and angiogenesis. Cell-based assays that examine the role of miRNA in human disease are also recently emerged. Numerous studies in cancer cell lines, using either antisense inhibition or over expression of individual miRNAs, show a direct functional link between aberrant miRNA expression and an individual tumor [43-46]. It is well-known that cancer-based cell assays are suitable for biochemical experimentation. MiRNA mimicry, a complementary method to inhibition, newly used in vitro to identify cellular processes and phenotypic changes associated with specific miRNAs transfected into cell lines; which will be explained at the last section. Disruption in miRNA expression is not the only change that can modify the regulation of target mRNAs. Mutations in the 3′ UTR of the candidate disease genes that disrupt miRNA binding sites can also affect diseases through reduced or total loss of miRNA-mediated regulation.

5. Biological functions of miRNAs

While the "seed" region is most important for miRNA–mRNA interactions, applying this principle only leads to prediction of many miRNA targets that cannot be validated in vivo, raising the possibility that further imperative rules manage miRNA–mRNA interaction. A prevailing aspect of all targets is that miRNAs usually target UTR sites that do not have a complex secondary structure and are located in accessible regions of the RNA. Since this model was proposed, several additional targets have been characterized *in vivo*, and approximately all are consistent with the proposed accessibility criteria [47,48]. MiRNAs are regulators of gene expression that control many biological processes in growth, development, differentiation, and metabolism. Their expression levels, small size, and mode of action pose unique challenges in studies elucidating the function of miRNAs. New technologies for identification, expression profiling and target gene validation will make easy the study of their involvement to biological processes and disease. Such information will be crucial to utilize the upcoming knowledge of miRNAs for the development of new human therapeutics. It is remarkable to think about whether individual miRNAs function separately on specific targets or if they can also function in a combinatorial manner. For instance, the effects of single miRNAs can be found in the regulation of lin-28 mRNA by *lin-4*, the first known miRNA, discovered in 1993 and was shown to have significant functions in developmental timing of stage-specific cell lineages [49]. By contrast, many miRNA clusters inhabit in related introns of paralogous genes. These polycistronic miRNAs could be classified into the similar miRNA family based on sequence similarity in the miRNA 50 region, implying that they might cooperatively control frequent sets of targets or molecular events. Besides to coordinately regulating a single mRNA, several members of a miRNA family can control sequential events [50]. Given the ability of miRNAs to regulate multiple genes, it will be interesting to examine whether they function through many of the same paradigms as transcription factors, such as combinatorial regulation and regulation of whole genetic programs. Genetic studies in *Caenorhabditis elegans, Drosophila melanogaster* have identified important functions of specific miRNAs in the coordination of cell proliferation and death during development, stress resistance, fat metabolism and brain morphogenesis [51,52]. For the past few years, one primary focus of the investigators studying mammalian miRNAs was to recognize and catalog the complete miRNA list and its expression pattern using cloning, bioinformatics and gene expression approaches. With these efforts nearing conclusion in the near future, the focus is shifting to the clarification of miRNA function. Several technological advances including bioinformatic prediction algorithms, reporter assays, in situ hybridizations, overexpression and silencing technologies, were developed to infer miRNA function. Here, we review the basic knowledge on miRNAs functions, especially highlighting recently discovered miRNA functions. The recent progress of miRNA involvements in organs development will be discussed.

5.1 Pivotal functions of miRNAs in development and or differentiation

Examining mice lacking the essential miRNA-processing enzyme Dicer is essential to investigate the role of miRNAs in development. Targeted deletion of Dicer in mice causes embryonic lethality before embryonic day (E) 7.5. Dicer-deficient embryonic stem (ES) cells are defective in differentiation both in vitro and in vivo, and do not form the three germ layers normally located in embryoid bodies derived from ES cells, suggesting an essential role for miRNAs in development [53]. In fact, without *lin-4*, *C. elegans* is unable to make the transition from the first to the second larval stage due to a differentiation defect, which is caused by a failure to posttranscriptionally repress the *lin-14* gene, which is the target gene of *lin-4* [54]. Similarly, without *let-7*, a failure of larval-to-adult transition was observed [55]. Therefore, miRNA function might be essential for 'fine tuning' developmental incidents during the defined events of organogenesis. MiR-1–1 and miR-1–2 are rich in the developing heart. Enrichment of miR-1–1 is primarily observed in the atrial precursors before becoming omnipresent in the heart, whereas a miR-1–2 enhancer is particular for the ventricles in the developing heart; therefore, miR-1–1 and miR-1–2 might have chamber-specific effects in vivo [56]. MiR-1 in flies regulates the Notch signaling pathway by directly targeting mRNA of the Notch ligand, Delta, demonstrating that miR-1 functions to persuade differentiated cardiac cells from an equivalency group of progenitor cells [57,58]. MiRNAs regulate key events during neurogenesis in various species. In mammals, miR-134 is particularly expressed in the rat dendritic spine in hippocampal neurons. It binds to 3' UTR of Limk1 and represses local LimK1 translation, which results in inhibition of dendriticspine growth. Stimuli such as brain-derived neurotrophic factor can mitigate this suppression. This finding revealed that miRNAs can be key regulators of neuronal structure and plasticity [59]. MiRNAs control key events during neurogenesis. In zebrafish, maternal zygotic Dicer mutant embryos have severe defects in the development of the neurocoel and the neural tube. These developmental defects are saved by members of the miR-430 family, indicating that the latter are the major miRNAs involved in the neurogenic defects [60]. MiRNAs can also be important regulators of neuronal structure and plasticity in mammals [61]. A discrete set of miRNAs is exclusively expressed in pluripotent embryonic stem cells but not in differentiated embryoid bodies, suggesting a role in stem cell self-renewal [62]. Understanding how miRNAs are processed and how they are integrated into the complex regulatory networks that direct the developmental, homeostatic and physiological processes of organisms are extremely crucial.

5.2 Cell proliferation and apoptosis

MiRNAs have been shown to regulate main genes for cancer progression that coordinately manages cell proliferation and apoptosis. MiRNAs regulate pathways controlled by genes such as p53, MYC and RAS. Moreover, miR17-92 cluster was shown to be competent to operate as a functional switch between cell proliferation and apoptosis. The fly miRNA, Bantam, was originally characterized from a fly P-ELEMENT screen for genes that promote cell proliferation and suppress apoptosis during tissue growth [63]. Its sequence complementarity with the 3' UTR and its functional antagonism of the pro-apoptotic *hid* gene were the first clues for the translational repression of *hid* by *Bantam* [63, 64]. In addition, fly *miR-14* was recognized through a *P-element* screen for inhibitors of apoptotic cell death. Deficiency in miR-14 enhances cell death that is induced by the cell death activator, *Reaper*, and results in defective stress responses and fat metabolism. Loss of *miR-14* also leads to an elevated level of Drice, an apoptotic effector caspase, indicating a direct or indirect repression of Drice by *miR-14* [65].

5.3 Contribution to maintain tissue identity

Yu et al. conducted a genome-wide analysis of the expression profiles of miRNA targets in human, *mouse* and *Drosophila*. They found that the expression levels of miRNA targets are significantly lower in all mouse mature tissues and *Drosophila* later life stages than in the embryos. These results point out that miRNAs may play roles in determining the timing of tissue differentiation during the larva period of *Drosophila* development and maintaining the tissue identity during adulthood [66].

5.4 As regulators for noise filtering and buffering

Eukaryotic cells are noisy milieus in which transcription often happens in a bursting manner, causing the number of mRNAs per cell to swing significantly [67]. In positive regulatory loops, noise or stochastic fluctuations of gene transcripts and protein molecules leads to randomly switching cell phenotypes in yeast, while a negative regulator adding in the positive regulatory loops often helps in reducing such noise in biological systems and making a strong result for cell development. Because miRNAs can adjust target protein levels more rapidly at the posttranscriptional level, they may significantly shorten the response delay and, in turn, provide more effective noise buffering. The miRNA *miR-17* might play a role in preventing noise-driven transition from apoptosis to cell proliferation. It is possible that miRNAs serve to buffer stochastically fluctuating expression of genes in positive regulatory loop. MiRNAs provide a common mechanism in buffering gene expression noise by frequently regulating positive regulatory loops [68,69].

Up to date, miRNAs have been shown to be involved in a range of cellular processes primarily developmental and metabolic processes including: cell proliferation, cell differentiation, developmental timing, fat metabolism, apoptosis, insulin secretion, stem cell maintenance, neuronal patterning, and haematopoietic lineage differentiation. Table 1 lists a number of the main important miRNAs that are associated with defined biological processes and some of the target genes through which they exert their regulatory function.

6. MiRNAs- associated disease mechanisms

MiRNAs- Associated Disease Mechanisms are quietly abundant so as because of time and place limitations, it is impossible to discuss in detail the all respective involved mechanisms. We then describe the essentials and needful accordingly. The high sequence conservation of many miRNAs among faintly related organisms suggests strong evolutionary pressure and involvement in main physiological processes by miRNAs. In fact, miRNA deficiencies or excesses are correlated with a range of clinically imperative diseases including myocardial infarction, virus infection, Alzheimer's disease, metabolic diseases, cancers, and many others [70-73]. Calin and colleagues found that a region containing miR-15 and miR-16 at chromosome 13q14 was commonly deleted in the majority of chronic lymphocytic leukemia cases [74]. It is quite clear that many miRNAs are associated with primary human tumors, and more than 50% of human miRNAs genes are located at genomic regions implicated in cancers, such as common breakpoint regions and fragile sites [75,76]. Discovery of the role of miRNAs in various pathological processes has shed light to the possible applications of miRNA in molecular diagnostics and prognostics, particularly for cancer. It is obvious that miRNAs in deleted or amplified regions in cancer samples contain altered expression levels. The impaired expression of various miRNAs throughout oncogenesis may advance or impede the tumor formation by modulating the expression of critical genes involved in cancer cell proliferation or survival. Though the vast majority of associations between miRNAs and human disease are coupled with tumorigenesis, there is accumulating evidence that miRNAs most probably are involved in multiple diseases. An investigation has added indirect support that miRNA changes are causal, rather than consequential, of cellular transformation [77]. One of them is fragile X mental retardation (FXMR) caused by absence or mutation of the fragile X mental retardation protein. Experimental results from *Drosophila melanogaster* indicate that FXMR may be a part of *RISC* [78]. The syndrome most often results from trinucleotide expansion of the CGG repeat in the 5′ UTR of the *FMR1*

microRNA	Target gene (s)	Biological Functions
Mammalian		
miR-1	HAND, HDAC4	Cardiomyocyte /skeletal muscle differentiation and proliferation
miR-10a	HOXA1	Megakaryocytopoiesis
miR-27b	CYP1B1	Regulation drug metabolising enzymes
miR-32	Retrovirus PFV-1	Antiviral defence
miR-103	Multiple targets of cell cycle	Cell cycle progression
miR-132	P250GAP	Neuronal morphogenesis
miR-143	ERK5	Adipocyte differentiation
miR-155	AT1R	Angiotensin II related processes
miR-221	c-KIT	Erythropoiesis
miR-196a	HOXB8	Developmental patterning
miR-132	TRAF6	Regulation innate immune response
miR-133	nPTB, SRF	Myoblast/skeletal muscle differentiation and proliferation
miR-134	LIMK1	Regulation of dendritic spine development
miR-375	MTPN	Regulation of insulin secretion
miR-130a	MAFB	Megakaryocytopoiesis
miR-15a	BCL2	Regulation of granulopoiesis
miR-146a-b	IRAK1	Regulation macrophage inflammatory response
Caenorhabditis elegans		
let-7	lin-41, hbl-1	Regulation of developmental transition between the last larval stage (L4) and the adult stage
lin-4	lin-14, lin-28	Regulation of developmental transition between the first two larval stages, L1 and L2
Drosophila melanogaster		
Bantam	hid	Promotion of cell proliferation and suppression of apoptosis
miR-14	Unknown	Suppression of apoptosis and regulation of fat metabolism
Mus musculus		
miR-181	Unknown	Promotion of haematopoietic differentiation towards the B-cell lineage
miR-196	Hoxb8	Unknown
Zea mays		
miR-166	rld1	Regulation of leaf morphogenesis

Abbreviations: HAND2, hand transcription factor; HDAC4, histone deacetylase 4; CYP1B1, cytochrome P450 1B1; PFV1, primate foamy virus type 1; P50GAP (RICS), Rho GTPase-activating protein; ERK5, extracellular signal regulated kinase 5; AT1 R, angiotensin II type 1 receptor; c-KIT, stem cell factor receptor; HOXB8, homeobox B8; TRAF6, TNF receptor-associated factor 6;nPTB, neuronal polypyrimidine tract-binding protein;SRF, serum response factor; LIMK1, Lim domain containing protein kinase 1; MTPN, myotrophin; Hoxb8, homeobox B8; rld1, rolled leaf1; MAFB, v-maf musculoaponeurotic fibrosarcoma oncogene homologue B; BCL2, B-cell lymphoma 2; IRAK1, IL-1 receptor associated kinase;

Table 1. MicroRNAs associated with experimentally defined functions and targets.

gene, causing hypermethylation and defeat of FMR1 expression [79]. Biochemical studies using recombinant FMRP and FXR1P suggest that FMR1P, FXR1P, and FXR2P proteins perform as acceptor molecules for Dicer-processed miRNAs and help direct gathering of miRNA [80]. The dAGO1 is indispensable for miRNA-directed gene silencing in Drosophila, showing a functional interaction with dFMR1, strengthens the dispute that failing in miRNA-mediated translation repression during neural development could result into fragile X syndrome [81,82]. It has been shown that expression of many miRNAs is altered in heart disease and that various types of heart disease are associated with discrete alterations in miRNA expression [83]. Such changes intimately look like the miRNA expression patterns observed in fetal cardiac tissue, indicating a novel mode of regulation for the transcriptional changes in cardiac failure. Numerous miRNAs were found to be dysregulated in two mouse models of cardiac hypertrophy. MiR-9 and miR-128a were overexpressed in the brains of Alzheimer's patients and 16 miRNAs were differentially expressed in the brains of schizophrenics. A mutation in the 3' UTR of the SLITRK1 gene that is associated with Tourette's syndrome led to enhanced repression by miR-189 [84-87]. Several hundreds of miRNAs were identified in human but currently, only a couple of specific targets have been experimentally validated. As predicted by bioinformatical analysis, a single miRNA can potentially target different mRNAs.

MiRNA regulation has also been implicated in virus-induced diseases. In fact, cellular miRNA expression may confer host immunity against viral infections; whereas viruses may have evolved to utilize miRNA machinery for their replication. It was observed that production of miRNAs by RNA viruses or cytoplasmic DNA viruses is unlikely, due to the compartmentalization of miRNA processing in the nucleus, as well as the fact that Drosha processing of miRNAs from RNA viruses would result in cleavage of the viral genome [88]. Increasing evidence suggests that viruses interact with the miRNA machinery [89]. Host miRNAs can also be used for viral replication as well as antiviral defense. The small size of miRNA precursors makes them also potentially ideal for use by oncogenic viruses as inhibitors of host cell defense pathways. For example, Human Papilloma Virus 16 (HPV16), is associated with cervical cancer, incorporates into miRNA genes at a rate 3 times higher than to the rest of the genome [90]. In fact, Cellular microRNAs have regulatory functions and direct antiviral consequences. A cellular microRNA effectively restricts the accumulation of the retrovirus primate foamy virus type 1 (PFV-1) in human cells. Viral Tas protein suppresses microRNA-directed functions in mammalian cells and displays cross-kingdom antisilencing activities [91]. Epstein-Barr virus (EBV) is a large DNA virus that preferentially infects human B cells and expresses a number of microRNA genes. The small RNA profile of cells infected by EBV was recorded and discovered that EBV miRNAs originated from five different double-stranded RNA precursors clustered in two regions of the EBV genome. Epstein-Barr virus use RNA silencing as a method for gene regulation of host and viral genes in a non-immunogenic manner [92]. Nearly and likely more, 11 viruses have been shown to encode their own miRNAs. These viral miRNAs stand for potential antiviral targets and might also serve as diagnostic markers for viral infection or stage of infection. Viruses use miRNAs in various ways, such as to inhibit viral or host transcripts or to recruit host miRNAs for viral replication.

7. MiRNAs and cancer

The aberrant expression of miRNA in cancers and the fact that approximately half of miRNA genes are localized in cancer-associated genomic regions or in fragile sites indicates the potential role of miRNAs as oncogenes or tumor suppressor genes in human carcinogenesis. MiRNA acts as oncomiRNA or tumor suppressors to affect the tumorigenesis if their target mRNAs were encoded by tumor suppressor genes or ontogenesis. MiRNAs still mainly intact in conventionally collected, formalin-fixed and paraffin-embedded tissues and even a modest number of miRNAs are adequate to discriminate human tumors according to the developmental lineage and differentiation state of the tumors [93-95]. The first association between miRNAs and cancer was identified by Croce and colleagues when the miR-15a-16-1cluster was implicated as a putative tumor suppressor gene mapping to chr 13q14, a small genomic region frequently deleted or translocated in chronic lymphocytic leukemia [96]. Since the predicted number of miRNAs in the human genome is as many as 1000. Regulation mediated by these genes has possibly a great impact on gene expression because, based on computional predictions, a single miRNA can target dozens of genes. Each cancer tissue has a particular miRNA signature and miRNA based cancer sorting is a very effective and potential tool. A subset of cancer-related miRNAs are persistently involved in a variety of cancers so that the miR-17-92, miR-106b-25 and miR-221-222 clusters, miR-155, let-7, miR-34a, miR-200 and others were revealed to play key roles in a variety of oncogenic processes [97,98]. Other miRNAs are expressed only in tumors of a limited tissue type and may be the most precise approach of defining not only the cell of origin, though the state of differentiation of a tumor. Moreover, miRNA signatures specify tumor subtypes and can help envisage prognosis and reaction to therapy. It is likely that numerous further essential oncomir-regulated targets/pathways with additional oncomirs will persist to be described in this fast-moving field [99,100]. To initiate and maintain a tumor, cancer cells must obtain the ability to proliferate autonomously, elude apoptosis and self-renew. To expand progress and metastasize, solid tumors also require stimulating angiogenesis, attacking normal tissue boundaries and becoming motile. Cancer-related miRNAs are implicated in each of these steps. For example, miR-15a-16 expression is downregulated in nearly all cases of CLL and prostate cancer; while miR-25/92 are upregulated in the majority human cancers. MiR-34a, which is transactivated by p53, one of the main tumor suppressor genes recurrently inactivated in human tumors, operates as a tumor suppressor miRNA by inducing cell cycle arrest and apoptosis in breast and lung cancer cells. This miRNA inhibits the expression of cyclin D1 and the cyclin-dependent kinase CDK6, which force cell cycle progression from G1 to S phase, as well as SIRT1, suppresses p53 transcriptional activity and the expression of its targets p21 and PUMA [101-103]. MiRNAs also play a main role in regulating cancer cell self-renewal. A self-renewing pool of immature cancer cells within a tumor, are thought to serve as a self-renewing reserve to generate new cancer cells. These cells are also relatively resistant to chemotherapy and radiotherapy and likely play a major role in tumor recurrence after therapy. The let-7 family of miRNAs, which is not expressed in CSC (or other types of normal stem cells), acts as a master regulator of self-renewal in breast CSC. Processing of the let-7 primary transcripts to the mature miRNA is inhibited at several steps by lin28, which is only expressed in stem cells [104-106]. Invasion of contiguous tissue and metastasis by epithelial cancer cells is another key step in tumor progression and is thought to involve a process termed epithelial mesenchymal transition. Epithelial cancer cells at the periphery of the tumor employ in a complex crosstalk with stromal cells leading to a global re-programming of gene expression with loss of epithelial traits and acquisition of mesenchymal properties, including invasion and motility [107]. Tumor-associated miRNAs along with validated target genes are presented in Table 2.

miRNAs	Cancer	Expression	Targets
miR-21	Breast, Colon, Lung, Pancreas, Brain, Liver	Up	CDK6, PDCD4, FAS, IL6R TPM1, CDKN1A, SOCS5
miR-25/92	Leukemia, Lung, Stomach, Colon, Prostate, Thyroid	Up	CDKN1C, BCL2L11
miR-142	Aggressive B cell leukemia	Up	Translocated c-MYC gene
miR-155	Chronic lymphocytic leukemia	Up	BIC RNA
miR-186	Chronic lymphocytic leukemia	Up	IgVh gene
miR-221	Thyroid, Stomach, Pancreas, Prostate, Melanoma	Up	CDK1B, CDKN1C, KIT
Let-7	Breast, Lung	Down	LIN28, HMGA2, kRAS, NF2
miR-335	Breast	Down	SOX4, MERTK
miR-372/3	Breast, Testicular germ cells	Down	LATS2, CD44, CD24
miR-15/16	Chronic lymphocytic leukemia	Down	BCL2, PDCD4, JUN, MCL1,RAB21, PRIM1
miR-17/20/93/106	Lung, Stomach, Colon, Pancreas, Prostate, Leukemia, Thyroid	Up	E2F1, CDKN1A, RUNX1, NCOA3

Table 2. Tumor-associated miRNAs along with validated target genes.

Overall, it is proposed that miRNAs may regulate tumorigenesis through a overabundance of possible oncogenic mechanisms. Genomic deletion or epigenetic silencing of a miRNA that normally represses expression of one or more oncogenes might lead to increased oncogenic expression. Alternatively, amplification, overexpression, or loss of epigenetic silencing of a gene encoding an miRNA that targets one or more tumor suppressor genes could inhibit the activity of an anti-oncogenic pathway [108]. Besides, mutations affecting the sequence of the mature miRNA or target mRNA could modify binding of the miRNA to its related targets leading to alterations in the balance of critical growth regulatory proteins [109]. The onco-microRNA expression profiling of human malignancies has also identified several diagnostic and prognostic cancer signatures. Furthermore, some miRNAs are downregulated in cancer, such as let-7 and miR-34a. The widespread differential expression of miRNA genes between malignant and normal cells is a complex phenomenon and may engage multiple mechanisms, including miRNA transcriptional control by tumour suppressor genes, oncogenes, epigenetic mechanisms and genomic abnormalities [109,110].

Moreover, germ-line and somatic mutations in miRNAs or polymorphisms in the mRNAs targeted by miRNAs may also participate to cancer predisposition and progression. It has been suggested that alterations in miRNA genes play a serious role in the pathophysiology of many human cancers [111].

7.1 MiRNAs and esophageal carcinoma

MiRNA plays role as oncomiRNA or tumor suppressors to influence the tumorigenesis if their target mRNAs were encoded by tumor suppressor genes or ontogenesis. Aberrant miRNA expression has been identified and confirmed in esophageal carcinoma. MiRNAs expression profiling differs markedly between esophageal squamous cell carcinoma and esophageal adenocarcima, indicates that these two main forms of esophageal carcinoma have distinct etiologic and pathologic characteristics. The miRNAs which are highly expressed in tumor can work as tumor promoter by targeting and inhibiting diverse tumor suppressor genes that itself were involved in carcinogenesis of esophagus [112-114]. Apart from identifying different cancer-related miRNAs, efforts were made to recognize their target genes, messenger RNAs and receptors, which will result into their contribution in cancer treatment. For example, one of the putatively identified targets of miR-21 is PTEN [115]. A decrease in functional PTEN causes constitutive activation of downstream components of the PI3K/AKT pathway, leading to tumor progression and metastasis. Thus, down-regulation of PTEN by miR-21 may contribute to transformation and increased tumor cell survival [116]. Epigenetic silencing of tumor suppressor genes is an additional mechanism of cancer development. In fact, the expression of tumor suppressor being able to get altered in epigenetic silencing mechanism via expression of miRNA. It was found that miR-127, located in a CpG island, identified in hematological cancers and deleted by loss of heterozygosity in solid tumors [117]. Further investigation is required for improved thoughtful their role in carcinogenesis of esophageal carcinoma and for better application in the future.

7.2 MiRNAs and breast cancer

MiR-10b, miR-125b and *miR-145*, are down-regulated and *miR-21, miR-155*, get up-regulated in breast cancer. *MiR-125b* gene is located at chromosome 11q23-24, one of the regions most frequently deleted in breast, ovarian, and lung tumors [118, 119]. *MiR-145* was progressively down-regulated from normal breast tissue to cancer with high proliferation index. The expression of various *let-7* miRNAs was down-regulated in breast cancer samples with either lymph node metastasis or higher proliferation index [120]. It was found that upregulation of *miR-10b* commences breast cancer invasion and metastasis [121]. The justification for using miRNAs as potential therapeutic targets is underlined by the fact that miRNA overexpression in cancer cells has a pathogenic effect.

7.3 MiRNAs and lung cancer

let-7 expression is recurrently reduced in lung cancers and associated with decreased post operative survival [122, 123]. It was shown that *miR-155* was over-expression, while *miR-17-92* cluster was over-expressed [124]. An *in vitro* experiment has revealed that overexpression of *let-7* results in the inhibition of lung cancer cell growth. Furthermore, Dicer protein expression is reduced in a fraction of lung cancers with a prognostic impact on the survival of surgically treated patients [125].

7.4 MiRNAs and hematological malignancies

It was shown that two miRNA genes located at 13q14.3 within a 30-kb region of minimal loss in. Both of these genes, miR-15a and miR-16-1, are down-regulated in more than 60% of CLL cases. Cluster miR-15b, miR-16-2, along with a different promoter, was found on chromosome 3q25–26.169. These miRNAs are less intensively expressed in normal cells; however, they may play a role in cases of 13q14 deletions [126,127]. It was also found that down-regulation of miR-16-1 and miR-15a expression correlates with allelic loss at 13q14, could be essential for clinical classification of CLL. Patients with a normal karyotype or deletion of 13q14 as the sole genetic abnormality have a better prognosis than those with a complex karyotype [128,129]. Indeed, the miRNA expression profile is associated with progression in CLL and be able to serve as a potential prognostic marker. As the investigation on lymphoma showed an elevation in the amount of miR-155/ BIC RNA happening in lymphomas derived from B cells, therefore *miR-155* possibly will play a role in the pathogenesis of B cell lymphomas [130]. *MiR-142* located at a spot of rearrangement linked to human leukemia that causes an aggressive B cell leukemia due to up-regulation of a translocated c-MYC gene. Moreover, it was revealed that miR-142 expression is higher in B-lymphoid and myeloid lineages compared to other hematopoetic tissues [131, 132].

7.5 MiRNAs and brain tumors

Microarray studies of glioma tissue have demonstrated a number of miRNAs implicated in glioma formation and propagation. MiR-7, -10b, -15b, -21, -26a, -124, -128, -137, -181a, -181b, -221, -451, play a role in human glioma. The majority of miRNAs are underexpressed in proliferating glioma cells with the important exception of miR-10b, -21, and -221 [133]. MicroRNAs regulate oncogenes implicated in brain tumor formation. Interestingly, microRNAs may also dictate the invasiveness and aggressiveness of tumors. MicroRNAs are significant regulators of cellular proliferation and differentiation so that it was found that miR-124 and miR-137 are downregulated [134]. On the other hand, microRNAs have been shown to work as tumor suppressors where downregulation of miR-181a and miR-181b involved in glioma formation was reported suggesting a tumor suppressor role for miRNAs [135]. Evidence for a role of miRNA in brain tumorigenesis recently emerged via the involvement of miRNA in medulloblastoma by demonstrating that miR- 124 modulates cell-cycle regulation in medulloblastoma cells. They showed that miR-124 expression is significantly decreased in medulloblastoma [136]. Therefore, strong evidence raising that miRNAs are integrally involved in brain tumor development and progression was proven. The discovery of the role miRNAs in brain tumors has also revealed a new category of therapeutic targets.

7.6 MiRNAs and cardiovascular diseases

MiRNAs are fundamental for heart development and regulating the expression of genes which play a part in cardiac function including the conductance of electrical signals, heart muscle contraction, and heart growth and morphogenesis. The most abundant miRNAs in heart are miR-1, let-7, miR-133, miR-126-3p, miR-143, miR-30c, and miR-22 [136]. It was found that loss-of-function of miR-1 prevented heart arrhythmia, whereas miR-1 overexpression led to heart arrhythmia in normal and infarcted hearts. The same also showed that both gain- and loss-of function of miR-1 affect conductivity through affecting potassium channels [137]. MiR-1, miR-133 and miR-208 are considered muscle specific, being primarily expressed in cardiac and skeletal muscles and also the intronic miRNAs including miR-208a, miR-208b, and miR-499 control muscle performance [138-140].

MiRNA expression profiles in a given tissue are dependent on the disease state. In order to adjust to the workload and impaired cardiac function, the heart may react by undergoing large cardiac remodeling known as cardiac hypertrophy. Invstigators established an association between miRNAs and hypertrophy by demonstrating that stress regulated miRNAs could activate both positive and negative persuade on the hypertrophic growth response [141,142]. Investigation on three various types of failing hearts showed that around 50% of miRNA were differentially expressed in at least one disease group, while seven miRNAs revealed similar regulation in all three disease states [143]. Another study revealed that a large fraction of miRNAs were either up- or down regulated in the same direction in fetal and failing heart compared with normal heart [144]. Changes in miRNA expression profiles in experimental models may also provide further insights into our understanding of heart failure. Arrhythmias arise due to heart disease or mutation in ion channel genes, however, miRNAs, such as miR-1 and miR-133 have been implicated to function in cardiac conduction system. The involvement of miR-1 in cardiac conductance was further confirmed by over expression studies in normal and infarcted rat hearts so as upregulation of miR-1 in individuals with coronary heart disease [145,146].

Myocardial vascularization subsequent MI needs signaling by angiogenic growth factors, such as vascular endothelial growth factor and fibroblast growth factor. MiR-126 is an endothelial cell–specific miRNA that plays an critical role in neoangiogenesis following MI and in maintenance of vascular integrity. The actions of miR-126 reflect its potentiation of mitogen-activated protein kinase signaling downstream of VEGF and FGF. Spred-1, an intracellular inhibitor of the Ras/mitogen-activated protein kinase pathway, serves as a key target for repression by miR-126. These findings suggest that strategies to raise miR-126 expression in the ischemic myocardium could enhance cardiac repair [147,148]. For the first time, it was showed that aberrant expression of miRNAs in the vascular walls after carotid artery balloon angioplasty in rats. This team identified p27 (Kip1) and p57 (Kip2) as potential targets for these miRNAs in these cells. Further by knocking down miR-221 and miR-222 in rat carotid arteries, they revealed therapeutic potential for these miRNAs in suppressing cell proliferation in vivo and neointimal lesion formation after angioplasty [149, 150].

The role of miRNAs in regulating endothelial cells in response to hypoxia was also studied [151]. They observed miR-210 upregulation in human endothelial cells in response to hypoxia affecting cell survival, migration, and differentiation. MiR-210 overexpression in normoxic endothelial cells stimulated angiogenesis whereas the opposite was observed with miR-210 blockade. Furthermore, a Dicer knockdown approach was used to examine the implication of miRNA in regulating the redox state and angiogenic response of human microvascular endothelial cells. The reduced miRNA levels induced expression of the transcription factor HBP1 that negatively regulates expression of p47phox of the NADPH oxidase complex. This study provides the first evidence that redox signaling in cells is subjected to regulation by miRNA [152].

Taken together, it seems clear that miRNAs have a central role in regulating gene expression in the heart. These studies indicate that miRNAs are important during heart development and adult cardiac physiology, and modulate a diverse spectrum of cardiovascular functions in vivo. Furthermore, these studies also have implications for understanding complex pathways, e.g., interactions between miRNAs, cell signaling and transcription factors, involved in heart diseases and can lead to potential opportunities in manipulating miRNAs as therapeutic targets.

8. Diagnostic and prognostic value of miRNA: as novel promising biomarkers

Make use of blood biomarkers was proved to be a reasonable means for early detection of some diseases. Since abnormal miRNA expression seems to characterize many diseases, increasing evidence indicates that the specific miRNA expression can be applied not only for diagnosis but also for classification of different tumors. The distinctive expression profile of miRNAs in different types and at different stages of cancer, and in other diseases, suggest that miRNA can be exploited as novel biomarkers for disease diagnostics and might present a new strategy for miRNA gene therapy. At the same time, risk stratification and prognosis assessment have become a major concern in the era of personalised medicine. Although, gene expression profiling has reached a plateau in this regard, recent miRNA studies illustrate great promise whereas aberrant miRNA profiling and or abnormal miRNA levels in tissues or in plasma can perform as a robust predictor of overall survival and disease outcome in various disorders. Because numerous miRNAs are expressed in a tissue-specific manner and their levels in different organs vary in association with disease states, these small molecules represent an attractive new class of highly specific biomarkers [153-157]. Some reports have previously illustrated the potential of these small RNA molecules as biomarkers in cancerous patients [158]. Moreover, serum of patients with autoimmune disorders exhibits increased amounts of certain miRNAs. Another study showed that miR-155 and miR-146a are raised in samples from patients with rheumatoid arthritis [159]. One report revealed that the miRNA profile in the serum of type 2 diabetic patients is considerably different from those of healthy
individuals and includes three miRNAs that were not associated with other disorders [160-162]. Recent evidence revealed that profile of miRNAs expression correlated with clinicopathological attributes and disease consequence. Because abundant studies demonstrated that miRNAs are implicated in cancer development and metastasis, miRNAs have great cancer diagnostic and prognostic potentials. Several miRNAs was showed to be associated with prognostic factors and disease progression in chronic lymphocytic leukemia [163]. Furthermore, high expression of miR-155 and low expression of let-7a-2 were associated with poor prognosis in human lung cancer [164]. For instance, a number of studies demonstrated that MicroRNA profiling acts as a tool to understand prognosis, and manage therapy response and resistance in breast cancer [165-167]. They revealed that expression level of miR-210 in early initiation of the disease was associated negatively with overall survival, suggesting that miR-210 could be free prognostic factor for breast cancer. MiRNA microarray profiling in breast cancer was also shown a positive correlation with epidemiological and pathological features of the disease so that miR-21 was associated with pathological features including advanced tumor stage, lymph node metastasis, and poor survival [168]. Taken together, in cancerous conditions, microRNAs expression profiling is certainly considered widely as a novel prognostic and diagnostic tool in clinical setting compared to mRNA; because, firstly that miRNAs stability in paraffin-embedded tissues is higher and remain primarily intact in plasma/serum compared with mRNA, due to lack of endogenous RNase activity. Secondly, a small number of miRNAs likely is adequate to distinguish cancers from normal [169,170]. These findings suggest that miRNA profiling is far more informative than usual mRNA profiling. Furthermore, predictive miRNA

expression signatures may be identified within tumor groups that predict the rate of progression risk, survival or existence of metastases. Lastly, miRNAs could be a target or tool for cancer prevention or therapeutic intervention. Hence, with mounting facts concerning miRNAs associated with molecular signatures and clinicopathological characteristics of various disorders, it is deemed that miRNAs may verify useful as diagnostic and prognostic means in the future.

9. MiRNA–based therapeutics

MiRNAs have great potential to be developed as a novel class of therapeutic targets. The exclusive biogenesis and mechanism of miRNA action allocate it to be free from the problems including off-target effects and drawbacks of siRNA which greatly hamper therapeutic use of siRNA. The benefit on specificity and toxicity, and the striking feature of multiple targeting potential, miRNA will also become an excellent tool for gene intervention. It is well known that miRNA levels are either upregulated or downregulated in various diseases. Therefore, miRNAs need to be finely modulated so as to either knockdown pathogenic or aberrantly expressed miRNAs or induce expression of optimistic miRNAs to threshold levels. There are several approaches to attain these *in vivo* and *in vitro*. In cancer therapy, reasonable approaches for therapy would comprise achieving "gain" or "loss" of miRNA roles in the cancer cells. Because many miRNAs have been identified to impart tumor suppressive effects, restoring their expression could produce therapeutic effects. It was found that ectopic overexpression of let-7 tumor suppressor miRNA inhibited the growth of lung, liver and pancreatic cancer cells. Moreover, systemic administration of miR-26a using adeno-associated virus in an animal model of hepatocellular carcinoma inhibited tumor progression. These findings demonstrated an important target miRNA with tumor suppressive activity and signified that adenoviral vector-based delivery might be a clinically viable approach [171,172]. Besides, synthetic miRNA mimics have also been introduced to re-establish miRNA function within the tumor. In case of oncogenic miRNAs, a number of approaches have been designed and tested to attain their downregulation [173]. For oncogenic miRNAs, multiple approaches have been designed and tested to achieve their downregulation. These approaches include the use of anti-miRNA oligonucleotides (AMOs), small molecule inhibitors, miRNA sponges and miRNA masking. Of note, downregulation of miRNAs could be approached via its biogenesis. In a one investigation, several small organic molecules were screened to block miR-21 function and azobenzene was identified as an efficient inhibitor of miR-21 expression [174]. An additional approach is the application of synthetic mRNA consisting multiple pairing sites for endogenous miRNA [175]. These synthetic mRNAs, known as miRNA sponges, act by sucking up the target miRNAs and blocking their regulatory function in the cell [176].

Taken together, to date, two strategies have been introduced to exploit miRNAs as a novel and effective therapeutic tool. These include inhibition strategy and replacement strategy. Antisense inhibition of mature miRNA is one the inhibition strategies. Antisense miRNA Oligonucleotides (ASOs) are currently the most easily approachable technology for inhibiting miRNAs therapeutically. Anti-miRNA ASOs (AMOs) have been used by many groups to inhibit miRNA activity in cell culture. A group of investigators demonstrated that oligonucleotides carrying 2'sugar modifications (including 2'- (2'-F) and locked nucleic acid (LNA) plus phosphorothioate backbone modification, most probably works as successful inhibitors of miRNAs in cell culture [177–180]. It seems that there are other factors vital for effective miRNA targeting, which will be imperative to appreciate to develop the most compelling AMOs for therapeutics. The most likely AMO binding site is the RISC-loaded miRNA, and there is indirect proof to support that. How this results in degradation is not clear, it may engage accelerated turnover of the miRNA complex [181]. Further approaches for modulating or improving oligonucleotide distribution *in vivo* include liposomal formulation and conjugation chemistry. Some progress has been made in liposomal delivery of ASOs [182,183]. However, route of administration, toxicity, and the cost made limited employing of oligonucleotide/liposome complex in practice. These limitations are needed to be addressed effectively in order to develop from a laboratory implement to a commercially practical therapeutic and clinical setting [184,185]. An alternative approach to targeting miRNAs therapeutically is by inhibiting its processing. This could be achieved by inhibiting Drosha, Dicer, or other miRNA pathway components, which could access by small molecule drugs. The anticipated pleiotropic effects of this approach may be challenging. On the other hand, an oligonucleotide complementary to an individual pri-miRNA designed to interrupt the hairpin structure could prevent Drosha recognition or processing [186,187]. It could also be potential to target pri-miRNAs with ASOs that function by an RNase H mechanism. One team showed inhibition of a pre-miRNA hairpin in the cytoplasm with a siRNA targeted to the loop region, requiring much higher doses of siRNA than a typical mRNA target [188]. The next effective approach is replacement strategy. One approach to achieve this is through the introduction of a double-stranded miRNA mimetic, corresponding to the endogenous Dicer product and analogous in structure to a siRNA. This approach will likely face all the same impediments that siRNA therapeutics currently encounter, mainly the trouble of systemic delivery to tissues. Nucleotide modifications to improve stability to nuclease degradation and avoid quick renal clearance of the dsRNA from the blood were widely investigated, and a general understanding of what kinds of modifications are beneficial [189- 191]. The current progress in therapeutic delivery of siRNA indicates that augmentation of miRNA function with dsRNA mimetics will ultimately be promising.

A substitute strategy for therapeutic miRNA replacement is a gene therapy approach. This involves expression of a short hairpin RNA (shRNA) from a polymerase II or III promoter, in a DNA or viral vector that is subsequently processed by Dicer prior to loading into RISC. Benefits to this approach are the potential for more persistent silencing compared to double-stranded siRNA or miRNA mimetics, plus the simplicity of expressing several miRNAs from one transcript. Modified adenovirus or adeno-associated virus (AAV) vectors also were effective for gene delivery to the liver and the brain. They are restricted by the immune response to the adenovirus, and still limited in the tissues so as they can competently infect [192,193].

Recently, further therapeutic potentials for miRNAs clinical applications over stem cells signatures have been emerged. Particularly, in majority of malignant tumors, heterogeneous population of cells exist so as a proportion of which have been assigned the related stem cells. These cells are involved in tumorigenesis owing to their capability to self-renew and proliferation. At the same time, the ability of miRNAs to control many target genes gets them smart candidates for regulating stem cell self-renewal. Compelling evidence supports that specific miRNAs are differentially expressed in stem cells. It was showed that miRNAs are required to enable stem cells to overcome the G1-S checkpoint and achieve self-renewal. The exploitation of such miRNAs would smooth the progress of the regulation of the stem cells motivating tumorigenesis. An extra stem cell/miRNA therapeutic possibility is the use of mesenchymal stem cells as promising tumor-targeted vectors for miRNA therapeutics. Of note, the advantages and challenges of miRNA-based therapeutics compared with conservative and routine treatments are needed taken into account comprehensively [194-198]. The advantages involve regulation of many components of the same pathway/cellular via miRNA, stable and durable, and effective in vivo regulation of the miRNA. In contrast, the potential challenges include delivery of the miRNA modulator, off-target effects of unintended targets of a miRNA, toxicity of the miRNA modulator. It is important to keep in mind that a single miRNA can comprise both favorable and pathogenic effects. Besides, siRNA/miRNA specific delivery to target cell populations using approaches of nanobiotechnology is just beginning and looks promising. In a word, with the development in miRNA field, these small molecules are invaluable means for various areas of basic and applied research and, more importantly, for therapeutic intervention [199, 200].

10. References

[1] Szymanski M, Barciszewska MZ, Erdamann VA, Barciszewski J. A new frontier for molecular medicine: Noncoding RNAs. Biochimica et Biophys Acta 2005;1756:65-75.

[2] Sevignani C, Calin GA, Siracusa LD, Croce CM. Mammalian micro RNAs: a small world for fine-tuning gene expression. Mamm Genome 2006;17:189-202.

[3] Lim LP, Lau NC, Garrett-Engele P, Grimson A, Schelter JM, Castle J, et al. Microarray analysis shows that some microRNAs down-regulate large numbers of target mRNAs. Nature 2005;433:769-773.

[4] Devor EJ. Primate microRNAs miR-220 and miR-492 lie within processed pseudogenes. J Hered 2006;97:186-190.

[5] Venter JC, Adams MD, Myers EW, Li PW, Mural RJ, Sutton GG, et al. The sequence of the human genome. Science 2001;291:1304-1351.

[6] Lander ES, Linton LM, Birren B, Nusbaun C, Zody MC, Baldwin J, et al. Initial sequencing and analysis of the human genome. Nature 2001;409:860-921.

[7] Mattick JS, Makunin IV. Small regulatory RNAs in mammals. Hum Mol Genet 2005;14:121-132.

[8] Bartel, D. P. MicroRNAs: Genomics, biogenesis, mechanism, and function. Cell 2004;116:281–297.

[9] Lee RC, Feinbaum RL, Ambros V: The C. elegans heterochronic gene lin-4 encodes small RNAs with antisense complementarity to lin-14. Cell 1993;75:843–854.

[10] Berezikov E, Guryev V, van de Belt J, Wienholds E, Plasterk RH, Cuppen E. Phylogenetic shadowing and computational identification of human microRNA genes. Cell 2005;120:21–24.

[11] Bartel DP. MicroRNAs: genomics, biogenesis, mechanism and function. Cell 2004;116:281-97.

[12] Denli AM, Tops BB, Plasterk RH, Ketting RF, Hannon GJ. Processing of primary microRNAs by the Microprocessor complex. Nature 2004;432:231–235.

[13] Gregory RI, Yan KP, Amuthan G, Chendrimada T, Doratotaj B, Cooch N, Shiekhattar R. The microprocessor complex mediates the genesis of microRNAs. Nature 2004;432:235–240.

[14] Lee Y, Ahn C, Han J, Choi H, Kim J, Yim J, et al. The nuclear RNase III Drosha initiates microRNA processing. Nature 2003;425:415– 419.

[15] Pillai RS, Bhattacharyya SN, Filipowicz W. Repression of protein synthesis by miRNAs: how many mechanisms? Trends Cell Biol 2007;17:118–126.

[16] Valencia-Sanchez MA, Liu J, Hannon GJ, Parker R. Control of translation and mRNA degradation by miRNAs and siRNAs. Genes Dev 2006;20:515–524.

[17] Standart N, Jackson RJ. MicroRNAs repress translation of m7Gpppcapped target mRNAs in vitro by inhibiting initiation and promoting deadenylation. Genes Dev 2007;21:1975–1982.

[18] Ruby JG, Jan CH, Bartel DP. Intronic microRNA precursors that bypass Drosha processing. Nature 2007;448:83–86

[19] Esau C, Davis S, Murray SF, Yu XX, Pandey SK, Pear M, et al. miR-122 regulation of lipid metabolism revealed by in vivo antisense targeting. Cell Metab 2006;3:87–98.

[20] Krutzfeldt J, Rajewsky N, Braich R, Rajeev KG, Tuschl T, Manoharan M, et al. Silencing of microRNAs in vivo with 'antagomirs'. Nature 2005;438:685–689.

[21] Mourelatos Z, Dostie J, Paushkin S, Sharma A, Charroux B, Abel L, Rappsilber J, Mann M, Dreyfuss G. miRNPs: a novel class of ribonucleoproteins containing numerous microRNAs. Genes Dev. 2002;16:720–728.

[22] Stefani G, Slack FJ. Small non-coding RNAs in animal development. Nat Rev Mol Cell Biol 2008;9:219 -230.

[23] Chang TC. Mendell JT: microRNAs in vertebrae physiology and human disease. Annu Rev Genomics Hum Genet 2007;8:21-239.

[24] Mann DL. MicroRNAs and the failing heart. N Engl J Med. 2007;356:2644–2645.

[25] Bhattacharyya SN, Habermacher R, Martine U, Closs EI, Filipowicz W. Relief of microRNA-mediated translational repression in human cells subjected to stress. Cell 2006;125:1111–1124.

[26] Couzin J. MicroRNAs make big impression in disease after disease. Science 2008; 319:1782–1784.

[27] Pillai RS, Battacharyya SN, Artus CG, Zoller T, Cougot N, Basuyk E. Inhibition of translational initiation by Let-7 microRNA in human cells. Science 2005;309:1573–1576.

[28] Petersen CP, Bordeleau ME, Pelletier J, Sharp PA. Short RNAs repress translation after initiation in mammalian cells. Mol. Cell 2006;21:533–542.

[29] Humphreys DT, Westman BJ, Martin DI, Preiss T., MicroRNAs control translation initiation by inhibiting eukaryotic initiation factor 4E/cap and poly (A) tail function. Proc. Natl. Acad. Sci. U. S. A. 2005;102:16961–16966.

[30] Jing Q, Haung S, Guth S, Zarubin T, Motoyama A, Chen J. Involvement of microRNA in AU rich element-mediated mRNA instability. Cell;2005:623–634.

[31] Kim VN, Nam JW. Genomics of microRNA. Trends Genet 2006;22:165-173

[32] Liu CG, Calin GA, Meloon B, Gamliel N, Sevignani C, Ferracin M, et al. An oligonucleotide microchip for genome-wide microRNA profiling in human and mouse tissues. Proc Natl Acad Sci USA 2004;101:9740-9744

[33] Castoldi M, Schmidt S, Benes V, et al. A sensitive array for microRNA expression profiling (miChip) based on locked nucleic acids (LNA). RNA 2006;12: 913-20.

[34] Nelson PT, Baldwin DA, Scearce LM, Oberholtzer JC, Tobias JW and Mourelatos Z. Microarray-based, high-throughput gene expression profiling of microRNAs. Nat Methods 2004;1:155–161

[35] Lukiw, WJ. Micro-RNA speciation in fetal, adult and Alzheimer's disease hippocampus. Neuroreport 2007;18:297–300.
[36] LuJ, Getz G,Miska EA, et al. MicroRNA expression profiles classify human cancers. Nature 2005;435: 834-8.
[37] Chen C, Ridzon DA, Broomer AJ, Zhou Z, Lee DH, Nguyen JT, et al. Real-time quantification of microRNAs by stem-loop RT-PCR. Nucleic Acids Res 2005;33:e179
[38] Lao K, Xu NL,YeungV, Chen C, Livak KJ, Straus NA. Multiplexing R T-PCR for the detection of multiple miRNA species in small samples. Biochem Biophys Res Commun 2006;343:859.
[39] Hutvagner G, Simard MJ, Mello CC, Zamore PD. Sequence-specific inhibition of small RNA function. PLoSBiol 2004;2:E98.
[40] Meister G, Landthaler M, Dorsett Y,Tuschl T. Sequence-specific inhibition of microRNA and siRNA-induced RNA silencing. RNA 2004;10:544-50.
[41] Boutla A, Delidakis C, Tabler M. Developmental defects by antisense-mediated inactivation of micro RNAs 2 and 13 in Drosophila and the identification of putative target genes. Nucleic Acids Res 2003;31:4973-80.
[42] Orom UA, Kauppinen S, Lund AH. LNA-modified oligonucleotides mediate specific inhibition of micro-RNA function. Gene 2006;372:137-41.
[43] Matsubara H, Takeuchi T, Nishikawa E, Yanagisawa K, Hayashita Y, Ebi H, et al. Apoptosis induction by antisense oligonucleotides against miR-17-5p and miR-20a in lung cancers overexpressing miR-17-92. Oncogene (epub ahead of print).
[44] O'Donnell KA, Wentzel EA, Zeller KI, Dang CV and Mendell JT. c-Myc-regulated microRNAs modulate E2F1 expression. Nature 2005;435:839–843.
[45] Hayashita Y, Osada H, Tatematsu Y, Yamada H, Yanagisawa K, Tomida S et al. A polycistronic microRNA cluster, miR-17-92, is overexpressed in human lung cancers and enhances cell proliferation. Cancer Res 2005;65:9628–9632.
[46] Cimmino A, Calin GA, Fabbri M, Iorio MV, Ferracin M, Shimizu M et al. miR-15 and miR-16 induce apoptosis by targeting BCL2. Proc Natl Acad Sci USA 2005;2102:13944–13949.
[47] Zhao Y. et al. Serum response factor regulates a muscle-specific microRNA that targets Hand during during cardiogenesis. Nature 2005;436: 214–220
[48] Didiano D. and Hobert O. Perfect seed pairing is not a generally reliable predictor for miRNA-target interactions. Nat. Struct. Mol. Biol.2006;13: 849–851
[49] Moss EG et al. The cold shock domain protein LIN-28 controls developmental timing in C. elegans and is regulated by the lin-4 RNA.Cell 1997;88:637–646
[50] Wightman B, Ha I & Ruvkun G. Posttranscriptional regulation of the heterochronic gene lin-14 by lin-4 mediates temporal pattern formation in C. elegans. Cell 1993;75:855–862.
[51] Brennecke J, Hipfner DR, Stark A, Russell RB & Cohen SM. bantam encodes a developmentally regulated microRNA that controls cell proliferation and regulates the proapoptotic gene hid in Drosophila. Cell 2003;113:25–36.
[52] Xu P, Vernooy SY, Guo M. & Hay BA. The Drosophila microRNA Mir-14 suppresses cell death and is required for normal fat metabolism. Curr. Biol. 2003:13:790–795.
[53] Bernstein E. et al. Dicer is essential for mouse development. Nat. Genet 2003;35:215–217
[54] Lee RC, Feinbaum RL, Ambros V.The C. elegans heterochronic gene lin-4 encodes small RNAs with antisense complementarity to lin-14. Cell 1993;75:843–854

[55] Reinhart BJ, Slack FJ, Basson M et al. The 21-nucleotide let-7 RNA regulates developmental timing in Caenorhabditis elegans. Nature 2000;403:901–906
[56] Zhao, Y. et al. (2005) Serum response factor regulates a muscle-specific microRNA that targets Hand2 during cardiogenesis. Nature 2005;36:214–220
[57] Kwon C. et al. MicroRNA1 influences cardiac differentiation in Drosophila and regulates Notch signaling. Proc. Natl. Acad. Sci. U. S.A. 2005;102:18986–18991.
[58] Artavanis-Tsakonas S. et al. Notch signaling: cell fate control and signal integration in development. Science 1999;284:770–776
[59] Schratt GM. et al. A brain-specific microRNA regulates dendritic spine development. Nature 2006;439: 283–289
[60] Giraldez AJ. et al. MicroRNAs regulate brain morphogenesis in zebrafish. Science 2005:308;833–838
[61] Schratt GM. et al. A brain-specific microRNA regulates dendritic spine development. Nature 2006;439: 283–289
[62] Houbaviy HB. et al. Embryonic stem cell-specific MicroRNAs. Dev. Cell 2005;5:351–358.
[63] Hipfner DR, Weigmann K. & Cohen SM. The Bantam gene regulates Drosophila growth. Genetics 2002;161:1527–1537.
[64] Brennecke J, Hipfner DR, Stark A, Russell RB. & Cohen SM. Bantam encodes a developmentally regulated microRNA that controls cell proliferation and regulates the proapoptotic gene hid in Drosophila. Cell 2003;113:25–36.
[65] Xu P, Vernooy SY, Guo M& Hay BA. The Drosophila microRNA mir-14 suppresses cell death and is required for normal fat metabolism. Curr. Biol. 2003;13:790–795.
[66] Yu Z, Jian Z, Shen SH et al. Global analysis of microRNA target gene expression reveals that miRNA targets are lower expressed in mature mouse and Drosophila tissues than in the embryos. Nucleic Acids Res 2007;35:152–164.
[67] Blake WJ, Balazsi G, Kohanski MA et al. Phenotypic consequences of promoter-mediated transcriptional noise. Mol Cell 2006;24:853–865.
[68] Brandman O, Ferrell JE Jr, Li R, et al. Interlinked fast and slow positive feedback loops drive reliable cell decisions. Science 2005:310:496–498
[69] Ferrell JE. Self-perpetuating states in signal transduction: positive feedback, double-negative feedback and bistability. Curr Opin Cell Biol 2002;14:140–148.
[70] Wiemer EA. The role of microRNAs in cancer: no small matter. Eur. J. Cancer. 2007; 43:1529-1544.
[71] Sullivan CS, Grundhoff AT, Tevethia S, Pipas JM, Ganem D. SV40-encoded microRNAs regulate viral gene expression and reduce susceptibility to cytotoxic T cells. Nature 2005;35:682-686.
[72] Krutzfeldt, J.; Stoffel, M. MicroRNAs: a new class of regulatory genes affecting metabolism. Cell. Metab. 2006;4:9-12.
[73] Nelson PT, Keller JN. RNA in brain disease: no longer just "the messenger in the middle". J. europathol. Exp. Neurol. 2007;66:461-468
[74] Calin GA, Dumitru CD, Shimizu M, Bichi R, Zupo S, Noch E, et al. Frequent deletions and down-regulation of micro- RNA genes miR15 and miR16 at 13q14 in chronic lymphocytic leukemia. Proc. Natl. Acad. Sci. USA 2002;99:15524-15529.
[75] Calin GA, Liu CG, Sevignani C, Ferracin M, Felli N, Dumitru CD et al. MicroRNA profiling reveals distinct signatures in B cell chronic lymphocytic leukemias. Proc. Natl. Acad. Sci. USA 2004;101:11755-11760.

[76] He H, Jazdzewski K, Li W, Liyanarachchi S, Nagy R, Volinia S, et al. The role of microRNA genes in papillary thyroid carcinoma. Proc. Natl. Acad. Sci. USA 2005;102:19075-19080.

[77] Kumar MS, Lu J, Mercer KL, GolubTR, Jacks T. Impaired microRNA processing enhances cellular transformation and tumorigenesis. Nat. Genet. 2007;39:673-677.

[78] Ishizuka A, Siomi M C, Siomi H. A Drosophila fragile X protein interacts with components of RNAi and ribosomal proteins. Genes Dev. 2002;16:2497–508

[79] Jin P, Alisch RS and Warren, ST. RNA and microRNAs in fragile X mental retardation. Nat Cell Biol 2004;6:1048–1053.

[80] Plante I, Davidovic L, Ouellet DL, Gobeil LA, Tremblay S, Khandjian EW et al. Dicer-derived microRNAs are utilized by the fragile X mental retardation protein for assembly on target RNAs. J Biomed Biotechnol 2006: 64347.

[81] Jin P, Zarnescu DC, Ceman S, Nakamoto M, Mowrey J, Jongens TA et al. Biochemical and genetic interaction between the fragile X mental retardation protein and the microRNA pathway. Nat Neurosci 2004;7:113–117

[82] Okamura K, Ishizuka A, Siomi H and Siomi MC. Distinct roles for Argonaute proteins in small RNA-directed RNA cleavage pathways. Genes Dev 2004;18:1655–1666.

[83] Ikeda S, Kong S W, Lu J, Bisping E, Zhang H, Allen PD et al. Altered microRNA expression in human heart disease. Physiol. Genomics 2007;31:367-373.

[84] Van Rooij E, Sutterland LB, Liu N, Williams AH, Mcanally J, Gerard RD, et al. A signature pattern of stress-responsive micro-RNAs that can evoke cardiac hypertrophy and heart failure. Proc Natl. Acad. Sci. U.S.A. 2006;103:18255–18260

[85] Lukiw WJ. Micro-RNA speciation in fetal, adult and Alzheimer's disease hippocampus. Neuroreport 2007;18:297–300.

[86] Perkins DO, Jeffries CD, Jarskog LF, Thomson JM, Woods K, Newman MA, et al. MicroRNA expression in the prefrontal cortex of individuals with schizophrenia and schizoaffective disorder. Genome Biol. 2007;8:R27.

[87] Abelson JF, Kwan KY, O'roak BJ, Beak DY, Stillman AA, Morgan TM, et al. Sequence variants in SLITRK1 are associated with Tourette's syndrome. Science 2005;310:317–320.

[88] B.R. Cullen, Viruses and microRNAs, Nat. Genet. 2006;38 S25–S30.

[89] Sullivan CS, Grundhoff A, Tevethia S, Treisman R, Pipas JM, Ganem D. Expression and function of microRNAs in viruses great and small. Cold Spring Harb. Symp.Quant. Biol. 2006;71:351–356.

[90] Calin GA, Sevignani C, Dumitru CD, Hyslop T, Noch E, Yendamuri S, et al. Human microRNA genes are frequently located at fragile sites and genomic regions involved in cancers. Proc Natl Acad Sci U S A. 2004;101:2999–3004.

[91] Lecellier CH, Dunoyer P, Arar K, Lehmann C, J, Eyquem S, Himber C, Saib A, Voinnet O. A cellular microRNA mediates antiviral defense in human cells. Science 2005;308:557–60

[92] Pfeffer S, Zavolan M, Grüsser FA, Chien M, Russo JJ, Ju J, et al. Identification of Virus-Encoded MicroRNAs. Science 2004; 304:734–6.

[93] Lu J, Getz G, Miska EA, Alvarez-Saavedra E, Lamb J, Peck D . MicroRNA expression profiles classify human cancers. Nature 2005; 435: 834-838

[94] Calin GA, Sevignani C, Dumitru CD, Hyslop T, Noch E, Yendamuri S, et al. Human microRNA genes are frequently located at fragile sites and genomic regions involved in cancers. Proc Natl Acad Sci USA 2004; 101: 2999-3004

[95] Esquela-Kerscher A, Slack FJ. Oncomirs - microRNAs with a role in cancer. Nat Rev Cancer 2006; 6: 259-269

[96] Calin GA, Dumitru CD, Shimizu M, Bichi R, Zupo S, Noch E, et al. Frequent deletions and downregulation of micro-RNA genes miR15 and miR16 at 13q14 in chronic lymphocytic leukemia. Proc Natl Acad Sci USA 2002; 99:15524-9.

[97] Lu J, Getz G, Miska EA, Alvarez-Saavedra E, Lamb J, Peck D, et al. MicroRNA expression profiles classify human cancers. Nature 2005;435:834-8.

[98] Volinia S, Calin GA, Liu CG, Ambs S, Cimmino A, Petrocca F, et al. A microRNA expression signature of human solid tumors defines cancer gene targets. Proc Natl Acad Sci USA 2006;103:2257-61.

[99] Shell S, Park SM, Radjabi AR, Schickel R, Kistner EO, Jewell DA, et al. Let-7 expression defines two differentiation stages of cancer. Proc Natl Acad Sci USA 2007; 104:11400-5.

[100] Iorio MV, Visone R, Di Leva G, Donati V, Petrocca F, Casalini P, et al. MicroRNA signatures in human ovarian cancer. Cancer Res 2007; 67:8699-707.

[101] Chang TC, Wentzel EA, Kent OA, Ramachandran K, Mullendore M, Lee KH, et al. Transactivation of miR-34a by p53 broadly influences gene expression and promotes apoptosis. Mol Cell 2007; 26:745-52.

[102] Sun F, Fu H, Liu Q, Tie Y, Zhu J, Xing R, et al. Downregulation of CCND1 and CDK6 by miR-34a induces cell cycle arrest. FEBS Lett 2008; 582:1564-8.

[103] Yamakuchi M, Ferlito M, Lowenstein CJ. miR-34a repression of SIRT1 regulates apoptosis. Proc Natl Acad Sci USA 2008; 105:13421-6.

[104] O'Brien CS, Farnie G, Howell SJ, Clarke RB. Are stem-like cells responsible for resistance to therapy in breast cancer? Breast Dis 2008; 29:83-9.

[105] Yu F, Yao H, Zhu P, Zhang X, Pan Q, Gong C, et al. let-7 regulates self renewal and tumorigenicity of breast cancer cells. Cell 2007; 131:1109-23.

[106] Ibarra I, Erlich Y, Muthuswamy SK, Sachidanandam R, Hannon GJ. A role for microRNAs in maintenance of mouse mammary epithelial progenitor cells. Genes Dev 2007; 21:3238-43

[107] Korpal M, Lee ES, Hu G, Kang Y. The miR-200 family inhibits epithelial-mesenchymal transition and cancer cell migration by direct targeting of E-cadherin transcriptional repressors ZEB1 and ZEB2. J Biol Chem 2008; 283:14910-4.

[108] Ventura A, Jacks T. MicroRNAs and cancer: short RNAs go a long way. Cell. 2009;136:586–591.

[109] Garzon R, Calin GA, Croce CM. MicroRNAs in Cancer. Annu Rev Med. 2009;60:167–179.

[110] Cho WC. OncomiRs: the discovery and progress of microRNAs in cancers. Mol Cancer. 2007;6:60.

[111] Calin GA, Croce CM. MicroRNA signatures in human cancers. Nat Rev Cancer. 2006;6:857–866.

[112] Si ML, Zhu S, Wu H, Lu Z, Wu F, Mo YY. miR-21-mediated tumor growth. Oncogene 2007; 26: 2799- 2803

[113] Meng F, Henson R, Lang M, Wehbe H, Maheshwari S, Mendell JT, et al. Involvement of human micro-RNA in growth and response to chemotherapy in human cholangiocarcinoma cell lines. Gastroenterology 2006; 130: 2113-2129
[114] Luthra R, Singh RR, Luthra MG, Li YX, Hannah C, Romans AM, et al. MicroRNA-196a targets annexin A1: a microRNA-mediated mechanism of annexin A1 downregulation in cancers. Oncogene 2008; 27: 6667-6678.
[115] Zhu S, Wu H, Wu F, Nie D, Sheng S, Mo YY. MicroRNA-21 targets tumor suppressor genes in invasion and metastasis. Cell Res 2008; 18: 350-359.
[116] Sansal I, Sellers WR. The biology and clinical relevance of the PTEN tumor suppressor pathway. J Clin Oncol 2004; 22:2954-2963.
[117] Calin GA, Sevignani C, Dumitru CD, Hyslop T, Noch E, Yendamuri S, Shimizu M, Rattan S, Bullrich F, Negrini M, Croce CM. Human microRNA genes are frequently located at fragile sites and genomic regions involved in cancers Proc Natl Acad Sci USA 2004; 101: 2999-3004
[118] Negrini M, Rasio D, Hampton GM, Sabbioni S, Rattan S, Carter SL, Rosenberg AL, Schwartz GF, Shiloh Y, Cavenee WK. Definition and refinement of chromosome 11 regions of loss of heterozygosity in breast cancer: identification of a new region at 11q23.3. Cancer Res. 1995; 55:3003–7.
[119] Rasio D, Negrini M, Manenti G, Dragani TA, Croce CM. Loss of heterozygosity at chromosome 11q in lung adenocarcinoma: identification of three independent regions. Cancer Res. 1995;55:3988–91.
[120] Iorio MV, Ferracin M, Liu CG, Veronese A, Spizzo R, Sabbioni S, et al. MicroRNA gene expression deregulation in human breast cancer. Cancer Res. 2005; 65:7065–70.
[121] Ma L, Teruya-Feldstein J, Weinberg RA: Tumour invasion and metastasis initiated by microRNA-10b in breast cancer. Nature 2007, 449:682-688.
[122] Fu SW, Chen L, Man YG. miRNA Biomarkers in Breast Cancer Detection and Management. J Cancer. 2011;24:116-22.
[123] Takamizawa J, Konishi H, Yanagisawa K, Tomida S, Osada H, Endoh H, et al. Reduced expression of the let-7 microRNAs in human lung cancers in association with shortened postoperative survival. Cancer Res. 2004; 64:3753–6.
[124] Yanaihara N, Caplen N, Bowman E, Seike M, Kumamoto K, Yi M, et al. Unique microRNA molecular profiles in lung cancer diagnosis and prognosis. Cancer Cell. 2006; 9:189–98.
[125] Karube Y, Tanaka H, Osada H, Tomida S, Tatematsu Y, Yanagisawa K, et al. Reduced expression of Dicer associated with poor prognosis in lung cancer patients.Cancer Sci. 2005; 96:111–5.
[126] Calin GA, Dumitru CD, Shimizu M, Bichi R, Zupo S, Noch E, et al. Frequent deletions and down-regulationof microRNA genes miR15 and miR16 at 13q14 in chronic lymphocytic leukemia. Proc Natl Acad Sci U S A. 2002; 99:15524–9.
[127] Lagos-Quintana M, Rauhut R, Yalcin A, Meyer J, Lendeckel W, Tuschl T. Identification of tissue-specific microRNAs from mouse. Curr Biol. 2002; 12:735–9.
[128] Calin GA, Liu CG, Sevignani C, Ferracin M, Felli N, Dumitru CD, et al. MicroRNA profiling reveals distinct signatures in B cell chronic lymphocytic leukemias. Proc Natl Acad Sci U S A. 2004; 101: 11755–60.

[129] Juliusson G, Oscier DG, Fitchett M, Ross FM, Stockdill G, Mackie MJ, et al. Prognostic subgroups in B-cell chronic lymphocytic leukemia defined by specific chromosomal abnormalities. N Engl J Med. 1990; 323:720–4.
[130] Eis PS, Tam W, Sun L, Chadburn A, Li Z, Gomez MF, Lund E, Dahlberg JE. Accumulation of miR-155 and BIC RNA in human B cell lymphomas. Proc Natl Acad Sci U S A. 2005; 102: 3627–32
[131] Gauwerky CE, Huebner K, Isobe M, Nowell PC, Croce CM.Activation of MYC in a masked t(8;17) translocation results in an aggressive B-cell leukemia. Proc Natl Acad Sci U S A. 1989;86:8867–71.
[132] Chen C, Z, Li L, Lodish HF, Bartel DP. MicroRNAs modulate hematopoietic lineage differentiation. Science 2004; 303:83–6.
[133] Silber J, Lim DA, Petritsch C, Persson AI, Maunakea AK, Yu M, et al: miR-124 and miR-137 inhibit proliferation of glioblastoma multiforme cells and induce differentiation of brain tumor stem cells. BMC Med 2008;6:14.
[134] Shi L, Cheng Z, Zhang J, Li R, Zhao P, Fu Z, et al: hsa-mir-181a and hsa-mir-181b function as tumor suppressors in human glioma cells. Brain Res 2008;1236:185–193.
[135] Pierson J, Hostager B, Fan R, Vibhakar R: Regulation of cyclin dependent kinase 6 by microRNA 124 in medulloblastoma. J Neurooncol 2008;90:1–7.
[136] Lagos-Quintana, M., Rauhut, R., Yalcin, A., Meyer, J., Lendeckel W., & Tuschl, T. (2002). Identification of tissue-specific micro-RNAs from mouse. Current Biology, 12, 735–739
[137] Yang B, Lin H, Xiao J, et al. The muscle-specific microRNA miR-1 regulates cardiac arrhythmogenic potential by targeting GJA1 and KCNJ2. Nat Med 2007;13:486–491
[138] van Rooij E, Quiat D, Johnson B A, Sutherland LB, Qi X.,Richardson JA, et al. Family of microRNAs encoded by myosin genes governs myosin expression and muscle performance. Developments in Cell2009;17: 662–673
[139] van Rooij E, Sutherland LB, Qi X, Richardson JA, Hill J,& Olson EN. Control of stress-dependent cardiac growth and gene expression by a microRNA. Science 2007;316:575–579.
[140] Zhao Y, Ransom JF, Li A, Vedantham V, von Drehle M., Muth AN, et al. Dysregulation of cardiogenesis, cardiac conduction, and cell cycle in mice lacking miRNA-1-2.Cell 2007;129: 303–317
[141] Care A, Catalucci D, Felicetti F, Bonci D, Addario A, Gallo P, et al. MicroRNA-133 controls cardiac hypertrophy. Nature Medicine2007;13: 613–618.
[142] van Rooij E, Sutherland LB, Q X, Richardson JA, Hill J,& Olson E N. Control of stress-dependent cardiac growth and gene expression by a microRNA. Science 2007;316:575–579.
[143] Ikeda S, Kong SW, Lu J, Bisping E, Zhang H, Allen PD, et al. Altered microRNA expression in human heart disease. Physiological Genomics 2007;31:367–373.
[144] Naga Prasad SV, Duan ZH, Gupta MK, Surampudi VS, Volinia S, Calin GA, et al. Unique microRNA profile in end-stage heart failure indicates alterations in specific cardiovascular signaling networks. Journal of Biological Chemistry2009;284: 27487–27499
[145] Luo X, Lin H, Pan Z, Xiao J, Zhang Y, Lu Y, et al. Down-regulation of miR-1/miR-133 contributes to reexpression of pacemaker channel genes HCN2 and HCN4 in hypertrophic heart. Journal of Biological Chemistry 2008; 283: 20045–20052

[146] Yang B, Lin H, Xiao J, Lu Y, Luo X, Li B, The muscle-specific microRNA miR-1 regulates cardiac arrhythmogenic potential by targeting GJA1 and KCNJ2. Nature Medicine 2008;13: 486–491.

[147] Wang S, Aurora A, Johnson B, Qi X, McAnally J, Hill J, et al. An endothelial-specific microRNA governs vascular integrity and angiogenesis. Dev Cell. 2008;15:261–271.

[148] Fish JE, Santoro MM, Morton SU, Yu S, Yeh RF, Wythe JD, et al. miR-126 regulates angiogenic signaling and vascular integrity. Dev Cell. 2008;15:272–284

[149] Ji R, Cheng Y, Yue J, Yang J, Liu X, Chen H, et al. MicroRNA expression signature and antisense-mediated depletion reveal an essential role of microRNA in vascular neointimal lesion formation. Circulation Research 2007;100:1579–1588

[150] Liu X, Cheng Y, Zhang S, Lin Y, Yang J, & Zhang C. A necessary role of miR-221 and miR-222 in vascular smooth muscle cell proliferation and neointimal hyperplasia.Circulation Research 2009;104: 476–487

[151] Fasanaro P, D'Alessandra Y, Di Stefano V, Melchionna R, Roman S, Pompilio G, et al. MicroRNA-210 modulates endothelial cell response to hypoxia and inhibits the receptor tyrosine kinase ligand Ephrin-A3. Journal of Biological Chemistry 2008;283:15878–15883.

[152] Shilo S, Roy S, Khanna S, & Sen CK. Evidence for the involvement of miRNA in redox regulated angiogenic response of human microvascular endothelial cells. Arteriosclerosis, Thrombosis, and Vascular Biology 2008; 28:471–477.

[153] Lu J, Getz G, Miska EA, et al. MicroRNA expressionprofiles classify human cancers. Nature 2005; 435:834–838.

[154] Volinia S, Calin GA, Liu CG et al. A microRNA expression signature of human solid tumors defines cancer gene targets. Proc Natl Acad Sci USA 2006; 103:2257–2261.

[155] Santarelli L, Strafella E, Staffolani S, Amati M, Emanuelli M, Sartini D, et al. Association of MiR-126 with Soluble Mesothelin-Related Peptides, a Marker for Malignant Mesothelioma. PLoS One. 2011; 1:e18232

[156] Schmitz KJ, Helwig J, Bertram S, Sheu SY, Suttorp AC, Seggewiß J, et al. Differential expression of microRNA-675, microRNA-139-3p and microRNA-335 in benign and malignant adrenocortical tumours. J Clin Pathol. 2011; 6:1-7

[157] Lee SK, Calin GA. Non-coding RNAs and cancer: new paradigms in oncology. Discov Med. 2011 ;11:245-54

[158] Chen X, Ba Y,Ma L et al. Characterization of microRNAs in serum: a novel class of biomarkers for diagnosis of cancer and other diseases. Cell Res 2008; 18: 997–1006.

[159] Duroux-Richard I, orgensen C, Apparailly F. miRNAs and rheumatoid arthritis - promising novel biomarkers. Swiss Med Wkly 2011. 2011;141:w13175

[160] Stanczyk J, Pedrioli DM, Brentano F et al. Altered expression of MicroRNA in synovial fibroblasts and synovial tissue in rheumatoid arthritis. Arthritis Rheum 2008; 58: 1001–1009.

[161] Brase JC, Wuttig D, Kuner R, Sültmann H. Serum microRNAs as non-invasive biomarkers for cancer. Molecular Cancer 2010;9:306-405

[162] G. A. Calin, M. Ferracin, A. Cimmino, et al., "A microRNA signature associated with prognosis and progression in chronic lymphocytic leukemia," The New England Journal of Medicine 2005;17: 1793–1801, 2005.

[163] N. Yanaihara, N. Caplen, E. Bowman, et al., "Unique microRNA molecular profiles in lung cancer diagnosis and prognosis," Cancer Cell 2006;9: 189–198.

[164] N Yanaihara N, Caplen E. Bowman et al., "Unique microRNA molecular profiles in lung cancer diagnosis and prognosis," Cancer Cell 2006;9:189–198..
[165] M. V. Iorio, P. Casalini, E. Tagliabue, S. Menard, and C. M. Croce, "MicroRNA profiling as a tool to understand prognosis, therapy response and resistance in breast cancer," European Journal of Cancer 2008;4: 2753–2759.
[166] A.J Lowery, N Miller, RE McNeill, and M. Kerin, "MicroRNAs as prognostic indicators and therapeutic targets:potential effect on breast cancer management," Clinical Cancer Research, vol. 14, no. 2, pp. 360–365, 2008.
[167] C Camps, F M Buffa S, Colell, et al. "Hsa-miR-210 is induced by hypoxia and is an independent prognostic factor in breast cancer,". Clinical Cancer Research 2008:108:.1340–1348
[168] L.-X. Yan, X.-F. Huang, Q. Shao, et al., "MicroRNA miR-21 overexpression in human breast cancer is associated with advanced clinical stage, lymph node metastasis and patient poor prognosis," RNA 2008;2348–2360.
[169] Mitchell PS, Parkin RK, Kroh EM, et al., "Circulating microRNAs as stable blood-based markers for cancer detection," Proceedings of the National Academy of Sciences of the United States of America 2008;105:10513–10518.
[170] B. Hasemeier, M. Christgen, H. Kreipe, and U. Lehmann, "Reliable microRNA profiling in routinely processed formalin-fixed paraffin-embedded breast cancer specimens using fluorescence labelled bead technology," BMC Biotechnology 2008; 8.
[171] Takamizawa J, Konishi H, Yanagisawa K, et al. Reduced expression of the let-7 microRNAs in human lung cancers in association with shortened postoperative survival. Cancer Res 2004;64:3753-6.
[172] Johnson SM, Grosshans H, Shingara J, et al. RAS is regulated by the let-7 microRNA family. Cell 2005;120:635-47.
[173] Kota J, Chivukula RR, O'Donnell KA, et al. Therapeutic microRNA delivery suppresses tumorigenesis in a murine liver cancer model. Cell 2009;137:1005-17.
[174] Tsuda N, Ishiyama S, Li Y, et al. Synthetic microRNA designed to target glioma-associated antigen 1 transcription factor inhibits division and induces late apoptosis in pancreatic tumor cells. Clin Cancer Res 2006;12:6557-64.
[175] Gumireddy K, Young DD, Xiong X, et al. Small-molecule inhibitors of microrna miR-21 function. Angew Chem Int Ed Engl 2008;47:7482-4.
[176] Ebert MS, Neilson JR, Sharp PA. MicroRNA sponges: competitive inhibitors of small RNAs in mammalian cells. Nat Methods 2007;4:721-6
[177] Meister G, Landthaler M, Dorsett Y, Tuschl T., Sequence-specific inhibition of microRNA- and siRNA-induced RNA silencing, RNA 2004;10:544–550.
[178] Hutvagner G, Simard MJ, Mello CC, Zamore PD., Sequence-specific inhibition of small RNA function, PLoS Biol. 2 (4) (2004) E98.
[179] Davis S, Lollo B, Freier S, Esav C., Improved targeting of miRNAwith antisense oligonucleotides, Nucleic Acids Res. 2006;34:2294–2304.
[180] Orom UA, Kauppinen S, Lund AH., LNA-modified oligonucleotides mediate specific inhibition of microRNAfunction, Gene 2006;372:137–141.
[181] Dass CR. Liposome-mediated delivery of oligodeoxynucleotides in vivo. Drug Deliv 2002;9:169–180.

[182] Dritschilo A, Huang CH, Rudin CM, Marshall J,Collins B, Dul JL, et al. Phase I study of liposome-encapsulated c-raf antisense oligodeoxyribonucleotide infusion in combination with radiation therapy in patients with advanced malignancies, Clin. Cancer Res. 2006;12:1251–1259.

[183] Yi R, Qin Y, Macara IG, Cullen BR. Exportin-5 mediates the nuclear export of pre-microRNAs and short hairpin RNAs. Genes Dev. 2003;17:3011–3016.

[184] Lund E, Guttinger S, Calado A, Dahlberg JE, Kutay U. Nuclear export of microRNA precursors, Science 2004;303:95–98.

[185] Lee YS, Kim HK, Chung S, Kim KS, Dutta A. Depletion of human micro-RNA miR-125b reveals that it is critical for the proliferation of differentiated cells but not for the down-regulation of putative targets during differentiation, J. Biol. Chem. 2005;280:16635–16641.

[186] Y.S. Lee, H.K. Kim, S. Chung, K.S. Kim, A. Dutta, Depletion of human micro-RNA miR-125b reveals that it is critical for the proliferation of differentiated cells but not for the down-regulation of putative targets during differentiation, J. Biol. Chem. 2005;280:16635–16641.

[187] Chiu YL, Rana TM. siRNA function in RNAi: a chemical modification analysis. RNA 2003;9:1034–1048.

[188] Czauderna F, Fechtner M, Dames S, Aygun H, Klippel A, Pronk GJ, et al. Structural variations and stabilising modifications of synthetic siRNAs in mammalian cells. Nucleic Acids Res. 2003;31:2705–2716.

[189] B.A. Kraynack, B.F. Baker, Small interfering RNAs containing full 2′-Omethylribonucleotide-modified sense strands display Argonaute2/ eIF2C2-dependent activity. RNA 2006;12:163–176.

[190] H. Xia, Q. Mao, H.L. Paulson, B.L. Davidson, siRNA-mediated gene silencing in vitro and in vivo, Nat. Biotechnol. 2002;20:1006–1010.

[191] Buchschacher Jr GL, Wong-Staal F. Development of lentiviral vectors for gene therapy for human diseases, Blood 2000;95:2499–2504

[192] Clarke MF, Dick JE, Dirks PB, et al. Cancer stem cellsMperspectives on current status and future directions:AACRWorkshop on Cancer Stem Cells. Cancer Res 2006;66:9339^44.

[193] Suh MR, Lee Y, Kim JY, et al. Human embryonic stem cells express a unique set of microRNAs. Dev Biol 2004;270:488-98.

[194] Bernstein E, Kim SY, Carmell MA, et al. Dicer is essential for mouse development. Nat Genet 2003; 35:215-7.

[195] Kanellopoulou C, Muljo SA, KungA L, et al. Dicerdeficient mouse embryonic stem cells are defective in differentiation and centromeric silencing. Genes Dev 2005;19:489-501.

[196] Hatfield SD, Shcherbata HR, Fischer KA, Nakahara K, Carthew RW, Ruohola-Baker H. Stem cell division is regulated by the microRNA pathway. Nature 2005;435:974-8.

[197] Dwyer RM, Potter SM, Harrington KA, et al.Monocyte chemotactic protein-1 (MCP-1) secreted by primary breast tumours stimulates migration of mesenchymal stem cells (MSCs). Clin Cancer Res 2007;13:5020-7.

[198] Seto, AG. The road toward microRNA therapeutics. Int J Cell Biol 2010;4:32-39

[199] Brian D. Brown1 & Luigi Naldini. Exploiting and antagonizing microRNA regulation for therapeutic and experimental applications. Nature Reviews Genetics 10, 578-585.

[200] Metias SM1, Lianidou E, Yousef GM. MicroRNAs in clinical oncology: at the crossroads between promises and problems. J Clin Pathol 2009;62:771-776

6

Gene Therapy Strategies Incorporating Large Transgenes

Jennifer Johnston, Christopher B. Doering and H. Trent Spencer
Emory University
U.S.A

1. Introduction

The application of nucleic acid therapeutics sometimes requires the transfer of relatively large transgenes. For example, treatment of diseases such as hemophilia A, sickle cell disease, muscular dystrophy, or cystic fibrosis requires the transfer of coding sequences or complex regulatory elements, which can exceed 4.5 kilobases (kb). In general, transgenes are inserted into expression cassettes that can then be incorporated into either viral or nonviral vectors. The vector chosen depends not only on the therapeutic application but also on the size of the expression cassette. The size of the expression cassette depends on the size of the transgene and the requirement of specific regulatory elements necessary for appropriate transgene expression (for example, internal promoters, enhancers, insulators and other regulatory elements). Larger expression cassettes complicate gene therapy applications using viral vectors by (1) limiting the types of vectors available due to encapsidation limitations, (2) increasing the complexity of the transferred nucleic acid sequence, which, for example, can inadvertently introduce splice donor and acceptor sites, and (3) reducing the titer of viral vector that can be produced. Due to these hurdles, gene therapy strategies utilizing large expression cassettes are limited in vector design. One avenue of decreasing the size of transgenes is to genetically engineer minimal complementary DNA (cDNA) cassettes by eliminating regions that encode for non-functional aspects of the encoded protein. For example, the cDNA of human dystrophin, the missing functional gene in Duchenne's Muscular Dystrophy, is approximately 11 kb. Due to its large size, a truncated functional version termed, mini-dystrophin, is utilized, thereby reducing the transgene size to 6 kb. A similar strategy has also been evaluated for the cDNA encoding factor VIII (FVIII), mutations of which cause hemophilia A. The transgene size has been reduced by eliminating an entire domain, thus reducing the transgene size by >2.5 kb. A second strategy that has been evaluated involves dividing a larger transgene into smaller sub-transgenes that can then be incorporated into separate vectors to be delivered simultaneously. Nonviral gene-delivery systems, on the other hand, are not as constrained by the size of the expression cassette. Despite this advantage, nonviral vectors are currently not widely used because of inefficient gene transfer. However, rapid progress is being made with transposons circumventing limited transfer by capitalizing on their ability to integrate within the genome. For example, the *Sleeping Beauty* transposon has been used to insert a number of large expression cassettes into the human genome, including the 6.5 kb β-globin expression cassette for the treatment of sickle cell disease. Therefore, these vectors hold much promise for gene therapy applications with large expression cassettes.

The gene therapy field has a reasonable level of understanding regarding how to transfer and manage some of the larger therapeutic payloads, and excellent progress has been achieved for some diseases. The transfer of the cDNA sequence encoding FVIII incorporates many of the strategies used to transfer large transgene sequences. Therefore, this chapter will focus on the methods developed to transfer the FVIII transgene. But the strategies described in this chapter can be, and have been, used to transfer similarly large nucleic acid sequences. For example, as shown in Figure I, several parameters have been manipulated to achieve safe gene transfer and high level expression. This chapter will describe (1) the various gene transfer platforms, such as viral and nonviral gene transfer systems that are available and their likely applications to the transfer of large sequences, (2) various methods and techniques for modifying large transgene sequences for greater expression, and (3) the introduction of various accessory sequences, such as internal promoters in viral vectors and the WPRE sequence, both of which may aid in RNA expression and export from the nucleus. Because the transfer of the FVIII cDNA sequence has incorporated many of these parameters, it is an excellent model for developing strategies requiring the transfer of large nucleic acid sequences.

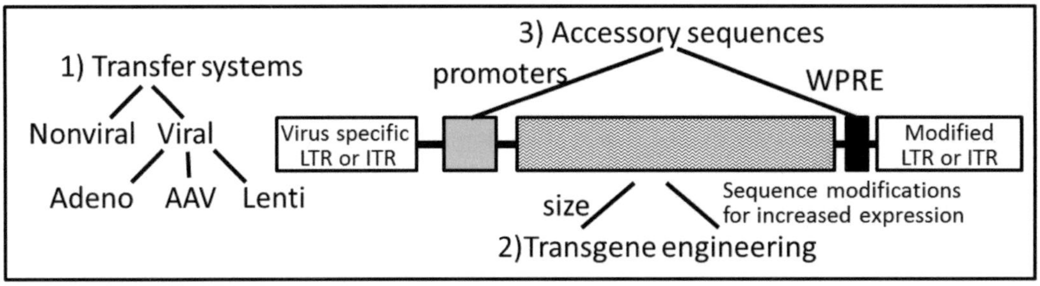

Fig. I. Schematic of a gene therapy expression cassette.

The various parameters noted above can potentially be modified in order to achieve efficient gene transfer and expression of large nucleic acid sequences.

2. Hemophilia A as a disease model for the transfer of large transgenes

Hemophilia A is an X-linked bleeding disorder attributed to the loss of a functionally secreted FVIII protein. Approximately 1 in every 5,000 males have hemophilia A, equating to approximately 400,000 people across the globe (Doering and Spencer, 2009). The current treatment consists of repetitive prophylactic administration of recombinant or plasma concentrated FVIII as a means of protein replacement. However, this treatment doesn't alleviate all the symptoms. Chronic joint pain can be experienced regardless of receiving optimal care. In addition, plasma concentrated FVIII historically has resulted in the transmission of blood borne pathogens (HIV, Hepatitis, etc.) to hemophilia patients and has thus, for the most part, been replaced with the administration of recombinant FVIII. Unfortunately, the recombinant form of FVIII is not available to a significant percentage (approximately 75%) of the individuals affected by the disease (Doering and Spencer, 2009). This is mainly due to the expense of treating hemophilia A, which on average can be $250,000 for recombinant FVIII product per year. Recombinant FVIII is costly because it is difficult to make resulting in periodic product shortages. It also has a low half-life in the circulation requiring repetitive multi-weekly administration to achieve prophylaxis. Further complicating the current therapy, some individuals who receive this treatment develop an immunogenic response in the form of neutralizing antibodies against the administered FVIII. These inhibitors make managing a bleeding episode in these individuals extremely complicated. Therefore, new therapeutic approaches are being developed to treat hemophilia A.

A monogenic disorder, such as hemophilia A, is a prime candidate for gene therapy for a number of reasons. First, the gene responsible for hemophilia A has been isolated and well characterized, which has led to useful preclinical mouse (Bi et al., 1995) and dog models (Kingdon & Hassell, 1981) as well as a newly described sheep model (Porada et al., 2010). Second, the delivery of FVIII is not restricted to certain cell types. In fact, any tissue with exposure to the vasculature is an appropriate cellular target in that FVIII only needs to be secreted into the bloodstream for effectiveness. This makes a gene therapy approach relatively straightforward and achievable. Third, the therapeutic window is large. Only a moderate increase in FVIII (2-5% of normal equating to 2-5ng/ml) is required to be therapeutically effective while levels as high as 150% of normal have not been associated with adverse effects such as thrombosis (VandenDriessche et al., 2001). As a result, a number of viral and nonviral delivery strategies have been postulated.

2.1 Previous clinical trials

Three clinical trials to date have been conducted. Each utilized the human cDNA FVIII sequence, but all three differed in the manner whereby the nucleic acid sequence was incorporated into the patients' cells. The first trial by Roth et al. (2001) admitted six subjects with severe hemophilia A. Dermal fibroblasts were biopsied from each patient from the upper arm, expanded in tissue culture dishes in a laboratory incubator and electroporated (exposed to a voltage shock in order to perturb the cell membrane layer), resulting in the incorporation of the cDNA sequence into the fibroblast cells. After culturing, stably modified clones were selected and implanted into the omentum of each patient. Transient FVIII expression was observed within three of the patients for up to 6 months, with one patient expressing 4 percent of the normal amount of FVIII twelve weeks after implanting the genetically modified cells. However, the levels of FVIII diminished to less than 0.5% of normal a year later. The second trial included eleven subjects (Powell et al., 2003). Four doses (2.8×10^7, 9.2×10^7, 2.2×10^8, and 4.4×10^8 TU/kg) of a retroviral vector based on the Moloney murine leukemia virus (MoMLV) were administered via peripheral vein injection over three consecutive days. No adverse effects were observed throughout the 53 week study. Yet once again only a transient expression of FVIII was achieved. Eight of the patients demonstrated greater than 1% of normal FVIII levels on two or more occasions yet these levels were not sustained throughout the study and could be associated with the administration of exogenous recombinant FVIII. The final trial was performed by GenStar Therapeutics. One patient was injected intravenously with an adenovirus, which contained the full-length human FVIII cDNA. The patient acquired an immune reaction to the virus and the trial was abruptly closed (Berlfein, 2003).

2.2 The FVIII transgene

The three clinical trials for hemophilia A used the human FVIII cDNA sequence instead of the wild-type FVIII gene sequence. This is due to the large size of the wild-type FVIII gene.

In its entirety, the F8 gene is approximately 180 kilobases (kb) long and is comprised of 26 exons. It is transcribed into a 9010 base pair (bp) transcript with a short 5′ untranslated region (150bp) and a large 3′ untranslated region (1806bp), and a 7056 bp open reading frame the encodes the FVIII protein. The open reading frame of the FVIII transcript is translated into a protein containing a short 19 amino acid signal peptide, which is necessary for cellular excretion, and the 2332 amino acid protein with a distinct domain structure denoted A1-A2-B-A3-C1-C2. The B domain, comprising a total of 907 amino acids, is not found within the functional protein. Instead it contains sequence motifs recognized by both intracellular and extracellular proteases (Bowen, 2002). For example, FVIII is cleaved intracellularly after Golgi processing at two separate arginine residues within the B domain yielding a FVIII heterodimer composed of a heavy chain (A1 and A2 domains, as well as a shortened B domain) and a light chain (A3, C1 and C2 domains) held together by a calcium ion bridge. Further cleavage occurs extracellularly in which thrombin cleavage releases the remainder of the B domain resulting in FVIII activation (Lenting et al., 1998).
Large transgenes, such as the FVIII transgene, complicate gene therapy applications using viral vectors by (1) limiting the types of vectors available due to encapsidation limitations (see Table I) and (2) reducing the titer of viral vector that can be produced (Kumar et al., 2001; Radcliffe et al., 2008; Yacoub et al., 2007). The different human cDNA transgene lengths chosen for the clinical trials are a reflection of these limitations. The GenStar Therapeutics trial, unlike the other two trials, utilized an adenovirus which has fewer encapsidation constraints than other viral vectors available for gene transfer. As a result, it was the only trial to utilize the full-length cDNA 7kb sequence. The Powell clinical trial, on the other hand utilized a retrovirus. Although retroviruses have the capability of encapsulating 7kb of exogenous DNA, incorporating a 7kb transgene into a retrovirus results in diminished viral titer making it difficult to achieve a high enough number of viral particles to be effective. Reducing the size of the insert, however, can increase viral titer (Yacoub et al., 2007). For this reason, many groups are using viral vectors and have reduced the size of the cDNA to approximately 4.5 kb. This can be accomplished by removing sequence that encodes the B domain, which has been found to be dispensable for the coagulation activity of FVIII (Toole et al., 1986).

	Adenovirus	Adeno-associated virus	Lentivirus	Transposons
Insert Size	45kb	4.0kb	7kb	10kb
Chromosomal Integration	No	* No	Yes	Yes
Route of gene delivery	Ex vivo and in vivo	Ex vivo and in vivo	Ex vivo	Ex vivo and in vivo
Titer	10^{11}	10^{12}	10^{8}	N/A
Host immunological response	Extensive	Moderate	Few	None
Pre-existing immunity	Yes	Yes	Unlikely	No
Safety concerns	Inflammatory Response, Toxicity	Inflammatory Response, Toxicity	Risk of Insertional Mutagenesis	Risk of Insertional Mutagenesis

* A low frequency (up to 10%) of wild-type adeno-associated vectors has been found to integrate within chromosome 19 (Kotin et al., 1990).

Table I. Properties of major gene transfer methods used in gene therapy.

As demonstrated above, the complications associated with the large FVIII transgene has led researchers to find innovative ways to apply gene therapy techniques to the transfer of the FVIII transgene. The following sections will discuss the methods that have been proposed for the pre-clinical testing of gene transfer technologies for FVIII. These methods will be outlined in reference to which vector is being used, since each vector is accompanied with its own set of limitations (Table 1). Both viral and nonviral vectors will be discussed, highlighting the strategies utilized to overcome the limitations experienced due to the use of a large transgene.

3. Viral vectors

Within the field of gene therapy, many viral vectors have been considered for the modification of cells, including both nonintegrating and integrating vectors. Nonintegrating vectors, such as the adenoviral and adeno-associated viral vectors, persist within cells extrachromosomally. As nonintegrating viruses, there is the risk that the vector genome will be lost, particularly if the modified cell divides. Yet, adenoviral vectors and adeno-associated viral vectors are appealing in that they efficiently transduce both dividing and non-dividing cells. If non-dividing cells are targeted then it is possible that long term expression can be achieved with these vectors. This quality allows these vectors to be able to target the most likely primary endogenous producers of FVIII, the terminally differentiated non-dividing hepatocytes.

Since adenoviral vectors are not constrained by insert size, they were among the first to be used as therapeutic gene transfer vectors within clinical trials. However as mentioned previously in reference to the GenStar FVIII clinical trial, systemic administration of adenoviral vectors resulted in acute toxicity (as evidenced by elevation of liver enzymes) as a result of the induction of pro-inflammatory cytokines and chemokines directed against the viral capsid proteins (Aruda, 2006; Brunetti-Pierri et al., 2004; Schnell et al., 2001; Muruve, et al., 1999; Yang et al., 1994). This toxicity can be circumvented if adenoviral vectors are administered neonatally, capitalizing on the immaturity of the immune system during early development. Therefore, adenoviral vectors are now being considered for use within neonates to induce FVIII tolerance. This was recently achieved within hemophilia A mice after intravenous injection of 5×10^{12} vector particles/kg administered at three days of age (Hu et al., 2011). FVIII levels peaked at ~650% of normal on day six, but declined with animal growth as a result of episomal vector loss. Therefore, the single administration of adenoviral vectors within neonates was not able to achieve sustained therapeutic levels of FVIII. However, tolerance to the transgene and viral capsid proteins was achieved as noted by the lack of adverse effects after subsequent vector administration (Hu, 2011). It is worthwhile to note that this therapy could also be beneficial, in the absence of subsequent vector administration, to prevent the development of inhibitors to FVIII which currently complicates protein replacement therapy. In the context of gene therapy for hemophilia A, adenoviral vectors are only being considered for the induction of FVIII tolerance within neonates due to the extensive inflammatory response observed after presentation of the vector to the systemic circulation. This is unfortunate since the vector can withstand the large size of the FVIII transgene as well as any number of regulatory elements used within the field for expression enhancement or safety. Adeno-associated viral vectors, on the other hand, are being extensively evaluated for use within gene therapy.

3.1 Gene transfer of FVIII with adeno-associated viral vectors

The adeno-associated viruses are relatively small viruses, composed of a linear single-stranded DNA genome of approximately 4.6 kb. As of 2009, twelve different serotypes have been isolated from both human and non-human primates (a number which is expected to increase), all of which vary in transduction efficiency and tissue tropism (Youjin and Jun, 2009). Serotype 2 (AAV-2) was the first adeno-associated virus to be sequenced and cloned, and was therefore the first serotype to be used within gene transfer studies (Hermonat and Muzyczka, 1984; Laughlin et al., 1983; Samulski et al, 1982). Wild-type AAV-2 was found to encode two large open reading frames, composed of the replication (Rep78, Rep68, Rep52, and Rep40) and capsid genes (VP1, VP2, and VP3). To accommodate transgenes, these genes were removed leaving behind the inverted terminal repeats required for replication and packaging into a viron (Youjin and Jun, 2009). AAV-2 and other AAV serotypes have the ability to efficiently transduce both non-dividing and dividing cells (Hallek et al., 1998). This quality makes modifying hepatocytes *in vivo* possible, making them a potentially ideal vector for FVIII delivery. In this aspect, hepatocytes have been modified by a number of adeno-associated viral serotypes. For example, AAV-2, after intraportal administration, transferred a canine B domain deleted version of FVIII to liver cells, which resulted in partial phenotypic correction of hemophilia A mice. Although FVIII activity initially peaked to 8% of normal, expression was not sustained, declining to 2% nine months after injection (Sarkar et al., 2003). These findings, although confirmed independently by Jiang et al. (2003), are contradictory to similar preclinical and clinical studies for hemophilia B in which therapeutically effective levels of FIX are sustained over time (Manno et al., 2005 and Schuettrumpt et al., 2005). This is because FIX is a significantly smaller transgene than FVIII with a cDNA of 2.8 kb. This smaller sequence allows for the inclusion of larger regulatory elements (such as liver specific promoters and enhancers) within the adeno-associated viral vector that are not able to be incorporated after the inclusion of the FVIII cDNA sequence. Within the Jiang (2003) and Sarkar (2003) reports, a minipromoter was all that could be incorporated into the AAV-2 vector to promote FVIII expression. Therefore, it was concluded that regulatory elements, that were unable to be included in the AAV-2 vector (due to insert size restraints associated with adeno-associated viral vectors), were required to enhance FVIII expression. A follow up study evaluated additional adeno-associated viral serotypes (AAV-5, AAV-7, and AAV-8) to determine if other serotypes were more efficient at transducing hepatocytes than AAV-2. For the inefficient transfer of large transgenes, it was hypothesized that by increasing hepatocyte transduction, limited expression could be overcome without the inclusion of regulatory expression-enhacement elements. They found that AAV-8 was superior to other serotypes regardless of route of administration (intraportally or intravenously) producing near normal physiological levels of FVIII (0.58 $\pm$ 0.2 IU/mL) six months post administration at a vector dose of 1 x 10^{11} vector copies / mouse (Sarkar et al., 2004). A similar comparison was performed by Jiang et al. (2006), comparing four serotypes (AAV-2, AAV-5, AAV-6, and AAV-8), within both mice and dogs. Within mice, transduction efficiency was found to be least with AAV-5 and greatest with AAV-8. However for dogs, no substantial difference was observed among the serotypes. Remarkably though, FVIII expression was sustained in some dogs (2 to 5% of normal) for up to three years, resulting in decreased occurrences of spontaneous bleeds (Jiang et al., 2006). This was a significant contribution to the field being the first multiyear report of therapeutic efficacy and safety within dogs. Albeit, high vector doses of 6 x 10^{12} and 2.7 x 10^{13} vector genomes/kilogram were required to yield these subtherapeutic levels of FVIII.

Despite the phenotypic improvements noted above, the inclusion of regulatory elements to the vector for enhancing the expression of FVIII would have been the simplest way to address the limited hepatocyte transduction that was seen with AAV-2. Yet since adeno-associated viral vectors are restricted in their genetic carrying capacity, other avenues had to be evaluated to overcome this limitation. Some reports show packaging of genomes greater than 5kb within adeno-associated vectors (Alloca et al., 2008 and Grieger and Samulski, 2005). For example, it is reported that an AAV-8 viral vector was produced containing the B domain deleted human FVIII transgene as well as a full length promoter and enhancer, totaling 5.75 kb (Lu, 2008). However, extensive examination within this report as well as by Wu (2010) clearly showed that inserts ranging from 4.7 kb to 8.7 kb result in heterogenous virons of varying genome lengths, typically containing truncations at the 5′ end. Thus, increasing the size of the adeno-associated vector genome leads to the formation of defective viral particles encapsulating incomplete transgene sequences (Dong et al., 1996).

For these reasons, several groups are attempting to overcome the packaging limitation with the use of two different vectors, one for the heavy chain and one for the light chain of FVIII. This strategy resulted from the demonstration of secretable biologically active FVIII following co-transfection within Chinese hamster ovary cells of two plasmids separating the heavy and light chains (Burke et al, 1986 and Yonemura et al., 1993). Within these cells the two polypeptide chains were able to reconstitute a functional FVIII heterodimer that was secreted into the cellular media. Although this strategy may be unique to hemophilia A gene therapy applications due to the structural properties of the protein, similar strategies could be implemented in other large transgenes. This strategy was first performed in C57BL/6 mice by intraportal administration (Burton et al., 1999). These mice were chosen since this strain does not elicit an immune response to the FVIII transgene, allowing expression to be measured without any contraindications. As a result, greater than physiological levels of FVIII were produced. These results were then extended into the hemophilia A mouse model where therapeutic levels of FVIII were achieved in a dose-dependent manner. High levels of transduction were noted with twelve percent of hepatocytes being modified with both vectors. Complicating the issue, a chain imbalance was noted with a 25 to 100 fold excess of light chain. This was found to be due to inefficient translational or posttranslational processing that could not be circumvented by changing the administration ratio of heavy to light chain vectors (Scallan et al., 2003). When extended to the hemophilia A dog model, only partial phenotypic correction was achieved, irrespective of adeno-associated serotype used. Although only modest levels of FVIII were observed in the dogs (ranging from 1 to 8% of normal), these levels were found to be sustained for at least two years (Sarkar et al., 2006).

Another strategy used to overcome the inability of adeno-associated vectors to deliver large genes is trans-splicing. Trans-splicing attempts to repair the truncated FVIII mRNA *in vivo* by delivering the remaining downstream pre-mRNA. Within this strategy, a pre-trans-splicing molecule is delivered by an adeno-associated vector in which complementary mRNA sequences are located at the 5′ end of the molecule designed to be spliced with the preexisting truncated FVIII mRNA due to a strong splice site at the 3′ end. In this way, a shortened version of the transgene can be delivered *in vivo* to restore the disease phenotype. This method was performed in hemophilia A mice (Chao et al., 2003). Hemophilia A mice were created by inserting a neomycin resistance gene into the sixteenth exon of FVIII (Bi et al., 1995). As a result truncated FVIII mRNA is still expressed within these mice. By delivering a pre-trans-splicing molecule containing complementary sequence to intron 15, a functional FVIII pre-mRNA was spliced together *in vivo* resulting in phenotypic correction within eight of the ten injected mice.

Despite these efforts the fact remains that nonintegrating adeno-associated viral vectors are unable to stably transduce cells. Therefore, many groups are focusing on the use of integrating viral vectors such as gamma-retroviral and lentiviral vectors. Lentiviral vectors, such as HIV and SIV, have been analyzed for their use within gene therapy since 1996 in which Naldini and colleagues revealed the ability of these vectors to overcome the need for cell division during transduction. Being able to transduce both dividing and non-dividing cells gives lentiviral vectors the same advantage as adeno-associated viral vectors. For this reason, lentiviral vectors are likely to make up a second generation of therapeutic vectors to be tested in clinical trials.

3.2 Gene transfer of FVIII with lentiviral vectors

Stable integration of a transgene can be achieved with integrating viruses, such as gamma-retroviral and lentiviral vectors. However, genomic integration of a viral vector has concerned the gene therapy community because of the possibility of cellular transformation due to integration of the transgene near an oncogene. This process has been termed insertional mutagenesis, and can cause misregulation of oncogene expression, which could subsequently lead to malignancy. Historically, insertional mutagenesis has been debatable due to the lack of data confirming its occurrence. However, recent data has confirmed the possibility of insertional mutagenesis due to retroviruses. First, retroviruses have been found to insert into the genome near promoters of transcriptionally active genes, setting the stage for the disrupted regulation of downstream genes (Wu et al., 2003). Second, direct proof of insertional mutagenesis has been documented in human gene therapy clinical trials for the treatment of severe combined immune deficiency syndrome that used gamma-based retroviruses (Hacein-Bey-Abina et al., 2003). In the initial clinical trials, of the 20 treated children, 5 have developed a T-cell leukemia-like disorder. The cause of the leukemia has been found to be due to integration of the gamma-retrovirus upstream of the oncogene, LMO2. Integration at this site disrupted the regulation of the oncongene increasing the expression of LMO2. The confirmation of insertional mutagenesis with gamma-retroviral vectors halted their use for clinical development for hemophilia. However, no direct evidence for insertional mutagenesis has been documented for recombinant lentiviral-based retroviruses. Instead, lentiviral vectors have been promising vectors for the delivery of the FVIII transgene because, like adeno-associated viral vectors, they are able to transduce both dividing and non-dividing cells, (Naldini et al., 1996) but unlike adeno-associated viral vectors are not as constrained by the size of the transgene. For these reasons, lentiviral vectors are ideal for gene therapy applications aimed for the treatment of hemophilia A.

The first lentiviral vectors contained all of the viral genes except for the envelope gene (Naldini et al., 1996). Since then numerous safety measures have been taken to ensure the safety of the virus in the unlikely event of generating a replication competent lentivirus. Second generation HIV-based vectors removed 5 of the 9 viral genes, eliminating accessory genes (Quinonez & Sutton 2002). As an added precaution second generation lentiviral vectors have been designed as replication incompetent self-inactivating (SIN) vectors. This has been accomplished by removing 133 bps from the 3′ long terminal repeat (LTR). LTRs flank viral DNA at both the 3′ and 5′ ends and are involved in the integration process (for further discussion refer to Sinn et al., 2005). During the process of integration, the 3′LTR is copied and becomes the 5′LTR in the integrated sequence, which inactivates the integrated

5′LTR. Further safety measures resulted in the third generation lentiviral vectors, in which 2 more viral genes (the tat and the rev genes) were eliminated. To date these third generation lentiviral vectors have been used for gene therapy applications without any adverse complications (Cartier et al., 2010).

Lentiviral vectors have a carrying capacity of approximately 7kb exogenous DNA. Although still constrained by encapsidation limitations, lentiviruses can be used to shuttle a number of transgenes that are restricted within the adeno-associated viral vector. However, as the insert size increases the viral particles produced (as measured by viral titer) can decrease (Yacoub et al., 2007). This phenomenon has been observed by several laboratories that use the 4.5 kb B domain deleted FVIII transgene. Because of this limitation, focus has been on reducing the insert size within the lentiviral vector. One component of the viral vector, which can be considered to be removed for this purpose, is the woodchuck post-transcriptional regulatory (WPRE) sequence (~ 600bp).

Zufferey et al. (1999) incorporated a WPRE sequence at the 3′ end of the transgene and demonstrated a 2- to 5- fold increase in expression. The enhancement in expression appears to be due to increased export of unspliced mRNA (Zuffery et al., 1999). Viral vectors used for the purpose of gene therapy utilize cDNA sequences, which are not spliced due to vector size constraints and therefore experience limited export of the mRNA. This limited export of unspliced transgene mRNA compounds the low level expression obstacle experienced historically. Thus, the inclusion of either splice donor and acceptor sites or a WPRE sequence appears to be ideal. As a result, the WPRE has routinely been incorporated into viral vectors. However, a recent report showed that the function of WPRE as a transgene expression enhancer may not be as advantageous as previously determined. The enhancement of transgene expression due to a WPRE sequence was found to be dependent on the promoter and cell line used. In general, the WPRE sequence enhances transgene expression, but in some instances no increase and even a decrease in transgene expression is observed. It was concluded that the function of the WPRE is more complex than originally assumed and should be evaluated in conjunction with every transgene (Klein et al., 2006). For this reason, the WPRE was evaluated in the context of an optimized high-expressing FVIII transgene and found to be negligible in regards to transgene expression as assessed by both transcript number and FVIII activity (Johnston et al., 2010). The effects were also negligible in regards to viral transduction. For these reasons, the WPRE can be considered for removal from some lentiviral backbones in order to reduce the insert size.

To further overcome issues of FVIII expression several bioengineered FVIII constructs have been proposed, many of which target the efficient transport of FVIII from the endoplasmic reticulum to the golgi (Dorner et al., 1987). For example, removal of the B domain, besides shortening transgene length, was also found to be beneficial by increasing mRNA production 20-fold (Meulien et al., 1988). However, efficient secretion of FVIII requires N-linked glycosyl residues found within the B domain. Therefore, retaining these sites within a truncated B domain may be a preferred shortened FVIII construct (Miao et al., 2004). In addition to the above engineering schemes, amino acid substitutions within the A1 domain were incorporated in order to diminish binding to an ER resident protein chaperone, which resulted in enhanced FVIII production (Marquette et al., 1995 and Swaroop et al., 1997). A B domain deleted porcine FVIII transgene was also evaluated revealing a 10 - 14 fold increase in expression compared to a human FVIII transgene (Doering et al., 2002). Its subsequent transfer within hemophilia A mice resulted in high-level FVIII expression that could be sustained even after low-toxicity pretransplantation conditioning (Ide et al., 2007). Together, these studies demonstrated the ability of a high-expressing porcine FVIII construct to function *in vivo*. A comparison of these transgenes revealed the superiority of the porcine B-domain-deleted FVIII with a 36 to 225-fold increase in FVIII expression (Dooriss et al., 2009). These findings suggested that the current low-level expression obstacle could be eliminated if the sequences that are responsible for the enhanced secretion of porcine FVIII were identified. To accomplish this, human/porcine FVIII chimeras were constructed that revealed sequences within the A1 and A3 domains to be responsible for enhanced secretion of porcine FVIII (Gangadharan et al., 2006). The result was a hybrid human/porcine construct comprising ~ 90% human FVIII, designated HPFVIII, which has been shown to maintain the high-expression characteristics of the porcine sequence. This optimized HPFVIII transgene has recently been used to treat hemophilia A mice, which resulted in therapeutic levels of FVIII being observed after modifying hematopoietic stem cells (HSC) *ex vivo* with lentiviral vector (Doering et al., 2009). A codon optimized FVIII cDNA also has been reported and shown to enhance expression after *in vivo* administration to neonatal hemophilia A mice (Ward et al., 2011).

Reduction in transgene titers due to issues associated with transgene size can be overcome by targeting various cell populations *ex vivo* then expanding the genetically modified cells. Therefore, despite diminished titer production, preclinical progress has been made with lentiviral vectors encoding the 4.5kb B domain deleted FVIII transgene. And, by targeting specific cells, viral transduction can be optimized and enhanced, which further overcomes the reduction in titer due to transgene size. In addition, *ex vivo* modification of cells is considered safer than the *in vivo* delivery of recombinant virus since it eliminates the possible transmission to germline cells, as well as avoiding any systemic toxicity that can result due to direct presentation of the vector particle (Van Damme et al., 2004). *Ex vivo* modification also eliminates the issue of modifying antigen-presenting cells, possibly eliminating the development of an immune response to the transgene.

Ex vivo gene therapy for hemophilia A has been analyzed within a broad range of cell types (Viiala et al., 2009). Cellular alternatives considered include embryonic stem (ES) cells, bone marrow derived mesenchymal cells, blood outgrowth endothelial cells (BOECs), and HSCs (as discussed previously). Stem cells are a reasonable alternative in that they have unlimited replicative potential and contain the ability to differentiate into a wide range of cells. However, the initial use of stem cells within the field of gene therapy resulted in low expression levels. This was thought to either be due to gene inactivation as a result of extensive differentiation (McIvor, 1987) or an inability to effectively transduce stem cells. Regardless, promising results were published utilizing an inducible system for FVIII within ES cells. However, both ethical and safety concerns have inhibited the continuation of these studies (Kasuda et al., 2008). This is due to the controversy surrounding the generation of ES cells from human embryos, as well as the formation of teratomas which arose from undifferentiated ES cells used for insulin production (Fujikawa et al., 2005). Fortunately, induced pluripotent stem cells (iPS) appear to be comparable to ES cells and have thus been considered to treat monogenic disorders in order to alleviate the ethical concerns surrounding stem cell usage. iPS cells are derived from adult somatic cells which have been reprogrammed to have stem cell characteristics. Significant progress has been made utilizing iPS cell-based therapy for murine hemophilia A (Xu et al., 2009). However, these methods are fairly new and still do not address the potential formation of teratomas. Therefore, many obstacles need to be addressed before this therapy can reach the clinics (for further discussion refer to Liras, 2011). Another cell type, bone marrow derived mesenchymal cells, initially yielded therapeutic levels of FVIII from transduced human mesenchymal cells within immunodeficient mice. Yet FVIII plasma levels deteriorated gradually in spite of the persistence of gene modified cells, suggesting transcriptional repression within this cell type (Van Damme et al., 2004). Human BOECs can be isolated from the peripheral blood of healthy donors and were considered as FVIII gene transfer targets because they express von Willebrand factor (vWF). vWF binds with high affinity to FVIII in the circulation and protects FVIII from degradation and uptake by antigen presenting cells (possibly eliminating the development of an immune response to the transgene) (Dasgupta et al., 2007). Therefore, it was hypothesized that modifying these cells to also express FVIII would result in the secretion of FVIII complexed to vWF, which would result in an increased half-life of FVIII, secreted at sites of injury. After transduction, BOECs expressed high levels of FVIII measured at 1.6 pmol/million cells/24hrs, which lasted for over thirty days in culture. FVIII was found to be stored within the same vesicles as VWF within the BOECs but was not found to be released upon agonist stimulation, unlike vWF. Instead, FVIII appeared to be released in a constitutive manner (van den Biggelaar et al., 2009). When BOECs were implanted into immunocompetent hemophilic mice, FVIII levels were within the therapeutic range for a total of 27 weeks. Afterwards, the levels declined to baseline due to loss of the implanted BOECs (Matsui, et al., 2007). Although a benefit for FVIII secretion with vWF was not directly tested, the proof of concept was shown for the expression of FVIII from BOECs. Another cell target, which has been considered, is skeletal muscle cells. Skeletal muscles cells are an ideal target for *in vivo* gene transfer in that skeletal muscle cells are terminally differentiated and provide a consistent source of FVIII persisting throughout the lifetime of an individual. For these reasons, Jeon et al. (2010) injected 10^7 lentiviral particles intramuscularly into the thigh of rats and found plasma FVIII levels to increase slightly above that of control mice for up to 4 weeks before deteriorating. Despite the need for follow up studies in order to achieve therapeutic levels of FVIII with this strategy, the results suggested that the *in vivo* administration of a lentivirus targeted at skeletal muscle cells may be an effective strategy for the treatment of hemophilia A. Most *in vivo* strategies, however, are aimed at targeting hepatocytes, the endogenous producer of FVIII. Lentivirus is administered via either the portal vein or intravenously. Unfortunately this strategy in the case of FVIII (a protein with extensive immunogenicity properties), results in the presentation of anti-FVIII antibodies due to the possible transduction of antigen presenting cells. To overcome this, a miRNA sequence was incorporated downstream of the WPRE sequence which would prevent expression within hematopoietic cells (including cells which make up the immune system). This method was found to be very effective in eliminating a FIX immune response (Brown et al., 2007), but alone was unable to do so with FVIII. Instead the FVIII-miRNA lentivirus had to be pseudotyped with the baculovirus envelope glycoprotein GP64, which has been shown to restrict transduction away from hematopoietic stem cells (Schauber et al., 2004). Combined, the miRNA incorporation and the GP64 pseudotyping were able to restrict FVIII expression to the liver, eliminating the presence of inhibitors, while resulting in about 9% of normal levels of FVIII (0.1U/mL), which was sustained in mice for a total of 60 weeks (Matsui, 2010). This study was significant in that it modified the current *in vivo* lentiviral gene transfer of FVIII making it safer by restricting expression within the liver.

In contrast to focusing on transferring the missing or malfunctioning gene, constructs that encode proteins that can bypass the missing protein can be used to overcome the difficulties associated with the size of the transgene. In the case of hemophilia A, a smaller gene such as FVII can be used to bypass the need for FVIII. FVII is an extrinsic pathway coagulation factor that along with thromboplastin initiates the blood coagulation proteolytic cleavage cascade and has been shown in a recombinant form to be an alternative treatment for hemophilia A (Jurlander et al., 2001). For these reasons, Ohmori et al. (2008) transduced HSCs *ex vivo* with a simian immunodeficiency virus (SIV)-based lentiviral vector encoding an activated form of FVII expressed from a platelet specific promoter (the GPIbα promoter). As a result, FVII was found to localize to the cell surface following platelet activation within transplanted FVIII-deficient mice. Due to species-specific interactions, the murine TF was unable to interact with the human form of FVII resulting in unimproved hemophilia conditions within the FVIII-deficient mice. However, when a murine FVII was incorporated into the SIV-based lentiviral vector, the clot time and rate of clot formation were significantly reduced, decreasing the mortality rate after tail clipping (Ohmori et al., 2008). In addition, FVII was recently incorporated into an adeno-associated vector (AAV-8) being able to overcome the encapsidation limitations of the vector due to the shorter size of FVII. Yet it was shown that within hemophilic dogs, large doses of vector were required to be efficacious (Margaritis et al., 2009). Therefore, a bioengineered FVII variant with enhanced intrinsic activity was recently utilized in order to reduce the dose of *in vivo* administered vector. However, adverse thrombotic effects were observed in treated mice, which limits enthusiasm for this therapy. (Margaritis et al., 2011).

4. Nonviral vectors

Unlike viral vectors, nonviral vectors themselves do not risk evoking an immunological response, are less expensive to produce, and are less limited by the size of the transgene. As a result, naked DNA gene transfer was among the first methods to be utilized in a clinical trial for hemophilia A (Roth et al., 2001). However, this strategy results in transient gene expression because of limited uptake by target cells and further limited integration into the genome of these cells (a process that unless further manipulated occurs only randomly through nonhomologous recombination) (Essner et al., 2005). This issue can be overcome by promoting stable integration into the cell's genome with the use of a transposable element. Transposable elements, although mostly inactive, are found to be littered throughout the human genome (Deininger and Batzer, 2002). In an active form, transposable elements (transposons) have the ability to jump from one location in the genome to another by a "cut-and paste" method through the enzyme transposase, which is encoded within the element. In order for a transposon to be utilized as a gene transfer vehicle, two components must be delivered to the target cell, (1) the transgene flanked by inverted repeat/direct repeat elements that are recognized for integration, and (2) a transposase which can be encoded within the same plasmid or within a second plasmid. These plasmids can be taken up into cells after being complexed to a cationic polymer such as polyethylenimine (PEI).

Although transposons can carry an expansive amount of DNA, transposons are still somewhat limited by insert size. Integration efficiency has been shown to decrease with the size of the transgene (Essner et al., 2005). This is due to both the difficulties in delivering plasmids containing larger inserts as well as the limitations of the transposase. For example, the transposase enzyme associated with the *Sleeping Beauty* transposon, the most notable nonviral gene-delivery system currently used, is only able to transpose up to 10kb.

4.1 Gene transfer of FVIII with a transposon

Transposons have been utilized as a nonviral vector for gene therapy of hemophilia A by a number of groups. The *Sleeping Beauty* transposon system was engineered from an inactive

Tc1-like transposable element found within fish (Ivics et al., 1997). It has since been used to insert a number of large expression cassettes into the human genome, including the 6.5 kb α-globin expression cassette for the treatment of sickle cell disease (Zhu et. al, 2007). For hemophilia A, the *Sleeping Beauty* transposon/transposase system was utilized by Liu et al. (2006) to express the human B domain deleted FVIII cDNA within endothelial cells. FVIII levels remained at ~12% of normal after intravenous plasmid injection through the temporal vein of neonatal hemophilia A mice. However, the presence of inhibitors to FVIII resulted in only partial phenotypic correction (Liu et al., 2006). In order to circumvent the presence of inhibitors, the Largaespada group tolerized neonatal, one day old, hemophilia A mice to FVIII with a facial vein injection of 0.1U/g of recombinant human FVIII. Eight to twelve weeks later, two high pressure tail vein injections of a *Sleeping Beauty* transposon were administered. As a result, 16% of normal FVIII levels were seen within these mice at eighty-four days after plasmid injection, which was found to be sustained for 6 months. No inhibitors were detected and an improvement in clotting function was noted (Ohlfest et al., 2005).

The high-pressure method of delivery is accomplished by injecting a high volume into the systemic circulation (termed hydrodynamic injections). Within the mouse, this results in DNA uptake followed by expression within the liver. Designed to overcome the difficulties of delivering DNA to the nucleus of a cell, high-volume high-pressure injection is not yet applicable for people (Essner et al., 2005). Therefore, other methods of transposon delivery are being explored. One method that is being studied is the cell specific delivery of a transposon by encapsulation within a nanocapsule. A recent report by Kren et al. (2009) utilized a novel dispersion atomization technique to encapsulate the *Sleeping Beauty* transposon system. The engineered nanocapsule was targeted to liver sinusoidal endothelial cells (LSECs) by coating the capsule with an endogenous ligand for the hyaluronan receptor found on LSECs. Inside the nanocapsule a single plasmid was encapsulated containing both a cis-acting transposase as well as the B domain deleted canine FVIII transgene. Eight-week old hemophilia A mice were injected with 25μg of nanocapsule via tail vein injection. FVIII levels were measurable for a total of 11 months.

The size limitations of transposons have recently been expanded. Recently, a number of improvements have been made resulting in a hyperactive transposase, which appears to be able to improve transpositional efficiency to transgenes greater than 10kb (Zayed et al., 2004). These improvements will be useful for the transfer of large transgenes and expression cassettes within gene therapy.

5. Conclusion

Gene delivery systems are available for the routine delivery of nucleic acid sequences below approximately 3 kb. As the transgene size increases beyond this, the complexity of transferring the larger sequences increases as well. Many systems have been tested for transferring large transgene sequences and some have shown reasonable promise. In general, viral vectors efficiently transfer these larger sequences, but several hurdles hamper gene transfer, namely: (1) limitations in the size of genetic material that can be packaged in a viral vector, (2) the inadvertent introduction of splice donor and acceptor sites, and (3) reduction of viral titer. Therefore, although efficient gene transfer systems are available, and clinical trials have confirmed the usefulness of some systems, there is still a need for improved gene transfer systems for large payloads. Even though optimal systems are not available, several strategies can be used to transfer large nucleic acid sequences. These strategies revolve around manipulating the various components of the expression cassette, specifically (1) introducing the sequence into multiple viral or nonviral gene transfer system to determine the best for the specific transgene (2) modifying the transgene sequence, for example by deleting coding sequences that may not be important to the function of the expressed protein, and (3) removing various accessory sequences that may not be necessary, or incorporating accessory sequences with optimal expression properties, such as stronger promoter elements. The transfer of FVIII is an excellent example of how some of these limitations were overcome. The transgene that encodes FVIII is very large (7kb). Within the context of expressing FVIII for the treatment of hemophilia A, both viral and nonviral vectors have been tested. Viral vectors were first used to provide proof-of-principle that hemophilia A could be treated by gene therapy (VandenDriessche et al., 1999). However, the efficiency of FVIII gene transfer has hampered the progress of developing a gene therapy treatment for hemophilia A. Since then, the FVIII transgene has been truncated from 7kb to 4.5kb by removing the B domain, a non-functional region of the protein. A number of groups have focused on shortening FVIII even further by dividing FVIII into two smaller sub-transgenes, one encoding the heavy chain and another encoding the light chain. Besides focusing on the FVIII transgene itself, other components of the expression cassette have also been evaluated, such as removal of the WPRE sequence and testing of various promoters. Despite these innovative methods, viral vector design is limited, prohibiting the addition of other regulatory or safety sequences. Nonviral vector systems, on the other hand, are not as constrained by the size of the expression cassette. However, these vectors have been historically associated with inefficient and unstable gene transfer. The *Sleeping Beauty* transposon may be able to circumvent this disadvantage by stably integrating the transgene into the target cell's genome. Overall, tremendous progress has been made to overcome the limitations associated with large expression cassettes. We now have a reasonable level of understanding, within the gene therapy field, of the limitations of the various gene transfer systems. The ability to transfer larger and more complex genetic expression cassettes will allow for more sophisticated approaches for targeting and treating diseases that currently are not being addressed because of transfer limitations.

6. References

Allocca, M., Doria, M., Petrillo, M, Colella, P., Garcia-Hoyos, M., Gibbs, D., Kim, S.R., Maguire, A., Rex, T.S., Di Vicino, U., Cutillo, L., Sparrow, J.R., Williams, D.S., Bennett, J., and Auricchio, A. (2008) Serotype-dependent packaging of large genes in adeno-associated viral vectors results in effective gene delivery in mice. *Journal of Clinical Investigation*, Vol. 118, No. 5, (May), pp. 1955-1964, ISSN 0021-9738

Aruda, VR. (2006) Toward gene therapy for hemophilia A with novel adenoviral vectors: success and limitations in canine models. *Journal of Thrombosis and Haemostasis*, Vol. 4, No. 6, (June), pp. 1215-1217, ISSN 1538-7933

Berlfein, J. (2003) Clinical trial update. *Hemaware*, Vol. 8, No. 5, (September), pp. 52-53

Bi, L., Lawler, A.M., Antonarakis, S.E., High, K.A., Gearhart, J.D., and Kazazian, H.H. (1995) Targeted disruption of the mouse factor VIII gene produces a model of haemophilia A. *Nature Genetics*, Vol. 10, No. 1, (May), pp. 119-121, ISSN 1061-4036

Brown, B.D., and Cantore, A., Annoni, A., Sergi, L.S., Lombardo, A., Della Valle, P., D'Angelo, A., and Naldini, L. (2007) A microRNA-regulated lentiviral vector mediates stable correction of hemophilia B mice. *Blood*, Vol. 110, No. 13, (December), pp. 4144-4152, ISSN 0006-4971

Brunetti-Pierri, N., Palmer, D.J., Beaudet, A.L., Carey, K.D., Finegold, M., and Ng, P. (2004) Acute toxicity after high-dose systemic injection of helper-dependent adenoviral vectors into nonhuman primates. *Human Gene Therapy*, Vol. 15, No. 1, (January), pp. 35-46, ISSN 1043-0342

Burke, R.L., Pachl, C., Quiroga, M., Rosenberg, S., Haigwood, N., Nordfang, O., and Ezban, M. (1986) The functional domains of coagulation factor VIII:C. *Journal of Biological Chemistry*, Vol. 261, No. 27, (September), pp. 12574-8, ISSN 0021-9258

Burton, M., Nakai, H., Colosi, P., Cunningham, J., Mitchell, R., and Couto, L. (1999) Coexpression of factor VIII heavy and light chain adeno-associated viral vectors produces biologically active protein. *Proceedings of the National Academy of Sciences*, Vol. 96, No. 22, (October), pp. 12725-12730, ISSN 0027-8424

Bowen, D.J. (2002) Haemophilia A and haemophilia B: molecular insights. *Molecular Pathology*, Vol. 55, No. 1, (February), pp. 1-18, ISSN 1472-4154

Cartier, N., Hacein-Bey-Abina, S., Von Kalle, C., Bougnères, P., Fischer, A., Cavazzana-Calvo, M., and Aubourg, P. (2010) Gene therapy of x-linked adrenoleukodystrophy using hematopoietic stem cells and a lentiviral vector. *Bull Acad Natl Med*, Vol. 194, No. 2, (February), pp. 255-64, ISSN 0001-4079

Chao, H., Mansfield, S.G., Bartel, R.C., hiriyanna, S., Mitchell, L.G., Garcia-Blanco, M.A., and Walsh, C.E. (2003) Phenotype correction of hemophilia A mice by spliceosome-mediated RNA trans-splicing. *Nature Medicine*, Vol. 9, No. 8, (August), pp. 1015-1019, ISSN 1078-8956

Dasgupta, S., Repesse, Y., Bayry, J., Navarrete, A.M., Wootla, B., Delignat, S., Irinopoulou, T., Kamaté, C., Saint-Remy, J.M., Jacquemin, M., Lenting, P.J., Borel-Derlon, A., Kaveri, S.V., and Lacroix-Desmazes, S. (2007) VWF protects FVIII fron endocytosis by dendritic cells and subsequent presentation to immune effectors. *Blood*, Vol. 109, No.2 , (January), pp. 610-612, ISSN 0006-4971

Deininger, P. and Batzer, M. (2002) Mammalian Retroelements. *Genome Research*, Vol. 12, No. 10, (October), pp. 1455-1465, ISSN 1088-9051

Doering, C., Parker, E., Healey, J., Craddock, H., Barrow, R., and Lollar, P. (2002) Expression and characterization of recombinant murine FVIII. *Journal of Thrombosis and Haemostasis*, Vol. 88, No. 3, (September), pp. 450-458, ISSN 1538-7933

Doering, C. and Spencer, T. (2009) Advancements in gene-transfer based therapy for hemophilia A. *Expert Review of Hematology*, Vol. 2, No. 6, (December), pp. 673-683, ISSN 1747-4086.

Doering, C., Denning, G., Doriss, K., Gangadharan, B., Johnston, J., Kerstann, K., McCarty, D., and Spencer, T. (2009) Directed Engineering of a High-expression chimeric transgene as a strategy for gene therapy of hemophilia A. *Molecular Therapy*, Vol. 17, No. 7, (July), pp. 1145-1154, ISSN 1525-0016

Dong, J.Y., Fan, P.D., and Frizzell, R.A. (1996) Quantitative analysis of the packaging capacity of recombinant adeno-associated virus. *Human Gene Therapy*, Vol. 7, No. 17, (November), pp. 2101-2112, ISSN 1043-0342

Dooriss, K.L., Denning, G., Gangadharan, B., Javazon, E.H., McCarty, D., Spencer, H.T., and Doering C.B. (2008) Comparison of factor VIII transgenes bioengineered for improved expression in gene therapy of hemophilia A. *Human Gene Therapy*, Vol. 20, No. 5, (May), pp. 465-478, ISSN 1043-0342

Dorner, A.J., Bole, D.G., and Kaufman, R.J. (1987) The relationship of N-linked glycosylation and heavy chain-binding protein association with the secretion of glycoproteins. *Journal of Cell Biology*, Vol. 105, No. 6, (December), pp. 2665-2674, ISSN 0021-9525

Essner, J.J., McIvor, R. S., and Hackett, P.B. (2005) Awakening gene therapy with *Sleeping Beauty* transposons. *Current Opinion in Pharmacology*, Vol. 5, No. 5, (October), pp.513-519, ISSN 1471- 4892

Gangadharan, B., Parker, E., Ide, L., Spencer, T., and Doering, C. (2006) High level expression of porcine FVIII from genetically modified bone marrow-derived stem cells. *Blood*, Vol. 107, No. 10, (May) pp. 3859-3864, ISSN 0006-4971

Grieger, J.C., and Samulski, R.J. (2005) Packaging capacity of adeno-associated virus serotypes: impact of larger genomes on infectivity and postentry steps. *Journal of Virology*, Vol. 79, No. 15, (August), pp. 9933-9944, ISSN 1098-5514

Hacein-Bey-Abina, S., von Kalle, C., Schmidt, M., Le Deist, F., Wulffraat, N., McIntyre, E., Radford, I., Villeval, J.L., Fraser, C.C., Cavazzana-Calvo, M., and Fischer, A. (2003) A serious adverse event after successful gene therapy for X-linked severe combined immunodeficiency. *New England Journal of Medicine*, Vol. 348, No. 3, (January), pp. 255-256, ISSN 0028-4793

Hallek, M., Girod, A., Braun-Falco, M., Wendtner, C.M., Bogedain, C., and Hörer, M. (1998) Recombinant adeno-associated virus vectors. *IDrugs*, Vol. 1, No. 5, (September), pp. 561-573, ISSN 1369-7056

Hermonat, P.L., and Muzyczka, N. (1984) Use of adeno-associated virus as a mammalian DNA cloning vector: transduction of neomycin resistance into mammalian tissue cultured cells. *Proceedings of the National Academy of Sciences*, Vol. 81, No. 20, (October), pp. 6466-6470, ISSN 0027-8424

Hu, C., Clea, R., Suzuki, M., Lee, B., and Lipshutz, G.S. (2011) Neonatal helper-dependent adenoviral vector gene therapy mediates correction of hemophilia A and tolerance to human factor VIII. *Proceedings of the National Academy of Sciences*, Vol. 108, No. 5, (Feruary), pp. 2082-2087, ISSN 0027-8424

Ide, L., Gangadharan, B., Chiang, K., Doering, C., and Spencer, T. (2007) Hematopoietic stem-cell gene therapy of hemophilia A incorporating a porcine FVIII transgene and nonmyeloablative conditioning regimens. *Blood*, Vol. 110, No. 8, (October), pp. 2855-2863, ISSN 0006-4971

Ivics, Z., Hackett, P.B., Plasterk, R.H., and Izsvak, Z. (1997) Molecular reconstruction of *Sleeping Beauty*, a Tc1-like transposon from fish, and its transposition in human cells. *Cell*, Vol. 91, No. 4, (November), pp. 501-510, ISSN 0092-8674

Jeon, H., Oh, T.K., Kim, O.H., and Kim, S.T. (2010) Delivery of Factor VIII gene into skeletal muscle cells using lentiviral vector. *Yonsei Medical Journal*, Vol. 51, No. 1, (January), pp. 52-57, 0513-5796

Jiang, H., Lillicrap, D., Patarroyo-White, S., Liu, T., Qian, X., Scallan, C.D., Powell, S., Keller, T., McMurray, M., Labelle, A., Nagy, D., Vargas, J.A., Zhou, S., Couto, L.B., and

Pierce GF. (2006) Multiyear therapeutic benefit of AAV serotypes 2, 6, and 8 delivering factor VIII to hemophilia A mice and dogs. *Blood*, Vol. 108, No. 1, (July), pp. 107-115, ISSN 0006-4971

Johnston, J.M., Moot, R., Doering, C., and H. Trent Spencer. (2010) Generation of an optimized lentiviral vector encoding a high-expression fVIII transgene for gene therapy of hemophilia A. Proceedings of the 13th Annual American Society of Gene and Cell Therapy Meeting, ABST#230, Washington D.C., May, 2010

Jurlander, B., Thim, L., Klausen, NK., Persson, E., Kjalke, M., Rexen, P., Jørgensen, T.B., Østergaard, P.B., Erhardtsen, E., and Bjørn, S.E. (2001) Recombinant activated factor VII (rFVIIa): characterization, manufacturing, and clinical development. *Seminars in Thrombosis and Hemostasis*, Vol. 27, No. 4, (August) pp. 373-384, ISSN 0094-6176

Kasuda, S., Kubo, A., Sakurai, Y., Irion, S., Ohashi, K., Tatsumi, K., Nakajima, Y., Saito, Y., Hatake, K., Pipe, S., Shima, M., and Yoshioka, A. (2008) Establishment of embryonic stem cells secreting human factor VIII for cell-based treatment of hemophilia A. *Journal of Thrombosis and Haemostasis*, Vol. 6, No. 8, (August), pp. 1352-1359, ISSN 1538-7933

Kingdon, H.S. and Hassell, T.M. (1981) Hemophilic dog model for evaluating therapeutic effectiveness of plasma protein fraction. *Blood*, Vol. 58, No. 5, (November), pp. 868-872, ISSN 0006-4971

Klein, R., Ruttkowski, B., Knapp, E., Salmons, B., Gunzburg, W, and Hohenadl, C. (2006) WPRE-mediated enhancement of gene expression is promoter and cell line specific. *Gene*, Vol. 372, (May), pp. 153-161, ISSN 0378-1119

Kotin, R.M., Siniscalco, M., Samulski, R.J., Zhu, X.D., Hunter, L., Laughlin, C.A., McLaughlin, S., Muzyczka, N., Rocchi, M., and Berns, K.I. (1990) Site-specific integration by adeno-associated virus. *Proceedings of the National Academy of Sciences*, Vol. 87, No. 6, (March), pp. 2211-5, ISSN 0027-8424

Kren, B., Unger, G., Sjeklocha, L., Trossen, A., Korman, V., Diethelm-Okita, B., Reding, M., and Steer, C. (2009) Nanocapsule-delivered *Sleeping Beauty* mediates therapeutic Factor VIII expression in liver sinusoidal endothelial cells of hemophilia A mice. *Journal of Clinical Investigation*, Vol. 119, No. 7, (July), pp. 2086-2098, ISSN 00219738

Kumar, M., Keller, B., Makalou, N., and Sutton, R.E (2001) Systemic determination of the packaging limit of lentiviral vectors. *Human Gene Therapy*, Vol. 12, No. 15, (October), pp. 1893-905, ISSN 1043-0342

Laughlin, C.A., Tratschin, J.D., Coon, H., and Carter, B.J. (1983) Cloning of infectious adeno-associated virus genomes in bacterial plasmids. *Gene*. Vol. 23, No. 1, (July), pp. 65-73, ISSN 0378-1119

Lenging, P.J., van Mourik, J.A., and Mertens, K. (1998) The life cycle of coagulation factor VIII in view of its structure and function. *Blood*, Vol. 92, No. 11, (December), pp. 3983-3996, ISSN 0006-4971

Liras, A. (2011) Induced human pluripotent stem cells and advanced therapies. Future perspectives for the treatment of haemophilia? *Thrombosis Research*, Vol. 10, (March), pp. 1-6, ISSN 0049-3848

Liu, L., Mah, C., and Fletcher, B. (2006) Sustained FVIII expression and phenotypic correction of hemophilia A in neonatal mice using an endothelial-targeted *Sleeping Beauty* transposon. *Molecular Therapy*, Vol. 13, No. 5, (May), pp. 1006-1015, ISSN 1525-0016

Lu, H., Chen, L., Wang, J., Huack, B., Sarkar, R., Zhou, S., Xu, R., Ding, Q., Wang, X., Wang, H., and Xiao, W. (2008) Complete correction of hemophilia A with adeno-associated viral vectors containing a full-size expression cassette. *Human Gene Therapy*, Vol. 19, No. 6, (June), pp. 648-654, ISSN 1043-0342

Manno, C.S., Pierce, G.F., Arruda, V.R., Glader, B., Ragni, M., Rasko, J.J., Ozelo, M.C., Hoots, K., Blatt, P., Konkle, B., Dake, M., Kaye, R., Razavi, M., Zajko, A., Zehnder, J., Rustagi, P.K., Nakai, H., Chew, A., Leonard, D., Wright, J.F., Lessard, R.R., Sommer, J.M., Tigges, M., Sabatino, D., Luk, A., Jiang, H., Mingozzi, F., Couto, L., Ertl, H.C., High, K.A., and Kay, M.A. (2005) Successful transduction of liver in hemophilia by AAV-Factor IX and limitations imposed by the host immune response. *Nature Medicine*, Vol. 12, No. 3, (March), pp. 342-347, ISSN 1078-8956

Margaritis, P., Roy, E., Aljamali, M.N., Downey, H.D, Giger, U., Zhou, S., Merricks, E., Dillow, A., Ezban, M., Nichols, T.C., and High, K.A. (2009) Successful treatment of canine hemophilia by continuous expression of canine FVIIa. *Blood*, Vol. 113, No. 16, (April), pp. 3682-3689, ISSN 0006-4971

Margaritis, P., Roy, E., Faella, A., Downey, H.D., Ivanciu, L., Pavani, G., Zhou, S., Bunte, R.M., and High, K.A. (2011) Catalytic domain modification and viral gene delivery of activated Factor VII confers hemostasis at reduced expression levels and vector doses in vivo. *Blood*, Vol. 118, No. 4, (February), pp. 1-22, ISSN 0006-4971

Marquette, K.A., Pittman, D.D., and Kaufman, R.J. (1995) A 110-amino acid region within the A1-domain of coauglation factor VIII inhibits secretion from mammalian cells. *Journal of Biological Chemistry*, Vol. 270, No. 17, (April), pp. 10297-10303, ISSN 0021-9258

Matsui, H., Masaru, S., Brown, B., Labelle, A., Hegadorn, C., Andrews, C., Hebbel, R., Galipeau, J., Hough, C., and Lillicrap, D. (2007) *Ex vivo* gene therapy for hemophilia A that enhances safe delivery and sustained *in vivo* factor VIII expression from lentivirally engineered endothelial progenitors. *Stem Cells*, Vol. 25, No. 10, (October), pp. 2660-2669, ISSN 1066- 5099

Matsui, H., Hegadorn, C., Ozelo, M., Burnett, E., Tuttle, A., Labelle, A., McCRay, P.B., Naldini, L., Brown, B., Hough, C., and Lillicrap, D. (2011) A microRNA-regulated and GP64-pseudotyped lentiviral vector mediates stable expression of FVIII in a murine model of hemophilia A. *Molecular Therapy*, Vol 1., (February), pp. 1-8, ISSN 1525-0016

McIvor, R.S., Johnson, M.J., Miller, A.D., Pitts, S., Williams, S.R., Valerio, D., Martin, D.W., and Verma, I.M. (1987) Human purine nucleoside phosphorylase and adenosine deaminase: gene transfer into cultured cells and murine hematopoietic stem cells by using recombinant amphotropic retroviruses. *Molecular and Cellular Biology*, Vol. 7, No. 2, (February), pp. 838-846, ISSN 1098-5549

Meulien, P., Faure, T., Mischler, F., Harrer, H., Ulrich, P., Bouderbala, B., Dott, K., Sainte Marie, M., Mazurier, C., Wiesel, M.L., van de Pol, H., Cazenave, J.P., Courtney, M., and Pavirani, A. (1988) A new recombinant procoagulant protein derived from the cDNA encoding human factor VIII. *Protein Engineering*, Vol. 2, No. 4, (October), pp. 301-306, ISSN 0269-2139

Miao, H.Z., Sirachainan, N., Palmer, L., Kucab, P., Cunningham, M.A., Kaufman, R.J., and Pipe, S.W. (2004) Bioengineering of coagulation factor VIII for improved secretion. *Blood*, Vol. 103, No. 9, (May), pp. 3412-3419, ISSN 0006-4971

Muruve, D.A., Barnes, M.J., Stillman, I.E., and Libermann, T.A. (1999) Adenoviral gene therapy leads to rapid induction of multiple chemokines and acute neutrophil-dependent hepatic injury *in vivo*. *Human Gene Therapy*, Vol. 10, No. 6, (April), pp. 965-976, ISSN 1043-0342

Naldini, L., Blömer, U., Gallay, P., Ory, D., Mulligan, R., Gage, F.H., Verma, I.M., and Trono D. (1996) *In vivo* gene delivery and stable transduction of non-dividing cells by a lentiviral vector. *Science*, Vol. 272, No. 5259, (April), pp. 263-267, ISSN 0036-8075

Ohlfest, J.R., Frandsen, J.L., Fritz, S., Lobitz, P.D., Perkinson, S.G., Clark, K.J., Nelsestuen, G., Key, N.S., McIvor, R.S., Hacket, P.B., and Largaespada, D.A. (2005) Phenotypic correction and long-term expression of factor VIII in hemophilic mice by immunotolerization and nonviral gene transfer using the *Sleeping Beauty* transposon system. *Blood*, Vol. 105, No. 7, (April), pp. 2691-2698, ISSN 0006-4971

Ohmori, T., Ishiwata, A., Kashiwakura, Y., Madoiwa, S., Mitomo, K., Suzuki, H., Hasegawa, M., Mimuro, J., and Sakata, Y. (2008) Phenotypic correction of Hemophilia A by ectopic expression of activated factor VII in platelets. *Molecular Therapy*, Vol. 16, No.8, (August), pp. 1359-1365, ISSN 1525-0016

Porada, C.D., Sanada, C., Long, C.R., Wood, J.A., Desai, J., Frederick, N., Millsap, L., Bormann, C., Menges, S.L., Hanna, C., Flores-Foxworth, G., Shin, T., Westhusin, M.E., Liu, W., Glimp, H., Zanjani, E.D., Lozier, J.N., Pliska, V., Stranzinger, G., Joerg, H., Kraemer, D.C., and Almeida-Porada, G. (2010) Clinical and molecular characterization of a re-established line of sheep exhibiting hemophilia A. *Journal of Thrombosis and Haemostasis*, Vol. 8, No. 2, (Feruary), pp. 276-85, ISSN 1538-7933

Powell, J.S., Ragni, M.V., White, G.C., Lusher, J.h, Hillman-Wiseman, C., Cole, V., Jolly, D., Ramanathan-Girish, S., Roehl, H., Lu, B, and Hurst, D. (2003) Phase 1 trial of FVIII gene transfer for severe hemophilia A using a retroviral construct administered by peripheral intravenous infusion. *Blood*, Vol. 102, No. 6, (September), pp. 2038–45, ISSN 0006-4971

Quinonez, R. and Sutton, R. (2002) Lentiviral vectors for gene delivery into cells. *DNA and Cell Biology*, Vol. 21, No. 12, (December), pp. 937-951, ISSN 1044-5498

Radcliffe, P., Sion, C.J.M., Wilkes, E.J., Custard, E.J., Beard, G.L., Kingsman, S.M., and Mitrophanous, K.A. (2008) Analysis of factor VIII mediated suppression of lentiviral vector titres. *Gene Therapy*, Vol. 15, No. 4, (February), pp. 289-297, ISSN 0969-7128

Roth, D.A., Tawa, N.E., O'Brien, J.M., Treco, D.A., and Selden, R.F. (2001) Nonviral transfer of the gene encoding coagulation factor VIII in patients with severe hemophilia. *New England Journal of Medicine*, Vol. 344, No. 23, (June), pp. 1735–42, ISSN 0028-4793

Sarkar, R., Xiao, W., and Kazazian, H.H. (2003) A single adeno-associated virus (AAV) murine factor VVIII. *Journal of Thrombosis and Haemostasis*, Vol. 1, No. 2, (February), pp. 220-226, ISSN 1538-7933

Sarkar, R., Tetreault, R., Gao, G., Wang, L., Bell, P., Chandler, R., Wilson, J.M., and Kazazian, H.H. Jr. (2004) Total correction of hemophilia A mice with canine FVIII using an AAV 8 serotype. *Blood*, Vol. 103, No. 4, (February), pp. 1253-1260, ISSN 0006-4971

Sarkar, R., Mucci, M., Addya, S., Tetreault, R., Bellinger, D., Nichols, T., and Kazazian, H. (2006) Long-term efficacy of adeno-associated virus serotypes 8 and 9 in hemophili A dogs and mice. *Human Gene Therapy*, Vol. 17, No. 4, (April), pp. 427-439, ISSN 1043-0342

Samulski, R.J., Berns, K.I., Tan, M., and Muzyczka, N. (1982) Cloning of adeno-associated virus into pBR322: rescue of intact virus from the recombinant plasmid in human cells. *Proceedings of the National Academy of Sciences*, Vol. 79, No. 6, (March), pp. 2077-2081, ISSN 0027-8424

Scallan, C.D., Liu, T., Parker, A.E., Patarroyo-White, S.L., Chen, H., Jiang, H., Vargas, J., Nagy, D., Powell, S.K., Wright, J.F., Sarkar, R., Kazazian, H.H., McClelland, A., and Couto, L.B. (2003) Phenotypic correction of a mouse model of hemophilia A using AAV2 vectors encoding the heavy and light chains of FVIII. *Blood*, Vol. 102, No. 12, (December), pp. 3919-3926, ISSN 0006-4971

Schauber, C.A., Tuerk, M.J., Pacheco, C.D., Escarpe, P.A., and Veres, G. (2004) Lentiviral vectors pseudotyped with baculovirus gp64 efficiently transduce mouse cells *in vivo* and show tropism restriction against hematopoietic cell types *in vitro*. *Gene Therapy*, Vol. 11, No., 3, (February), pp. 266-275, ISSN 0969-7128

Schnell, M.A., Zhang, Y., Tazelaar, J., Gao, G.P., Yu, Q.C., Qian, R., Chen, S.J., Varnavski, A.N., LeClair, C., Raper, S.E., and Wilson, J.M. (2001) Activation of innate immunity in nonhuman primates following intraportal administration of adenoviral vectors. *Molecular Therapy*, Vol. 5, No. 1, (May), pp. 708-22, ISSN 1525-0016

Schuettrumpf, J., Herzog, R.W., Schlachterman, A., Kaufhold, A., Stafford, D.W., and Arruda, V.R. (2005) Factor IX variants improve gene therapy efficacy for hemophilia B. *Blood*, Vol. 105, No. 6, (March), pp.2316-2323, ISSN 0006-4971

Sinn, P.L., Sauter, S.L., and McCray, P.B. (2005) Gene therapy progress and prospects: Development of improved lentiviral and retroviral vectors - design, biosafety, and production. *Gene Therapy*, Vol. 12, No. 14, (July), pp. 1089-1098, ISSN 0969-7128

Toole, J.J., Pittman, D.D., Orr, E.C., Murtha, P., Wasley, L., and Kaufman, R.J. (1986) A large region (approximately equal to 95 kDa) of human factor VIII is dispensable for in vitro procoagulant activity. *Proceedings of the National Academy of Sciences*, Vol. 83, No. 16, (August), pp. 5939-42, ISSN 0027-8424

Van Damme, A., Chuah, M., Collen, D., and VandenDriessche, T. (2004) Onco-retroviral and lentiviral vector-based gene therapy for hemophilia: Preclinical Studies. *Seminars in Thrombosis and Hemostasis*, Vol. 30, No. 2, (April), pp. 185-195, ISSN 0094-6176

Van den Biggelaar, M., Bouwens, E., Kootstr,a N., Hebbel, R., Voorberg, J., and Mertens, K. (2009) Storage and regulated secretion of factor VIII in blood outgrowth endothelial cells. *Haematologica*, Vol. 94, No. 5, (May), pp. 670-678, ISSN 0390-6078

VandenDriessche, T., Vanslembrouck, V., Goovaerts, I., Zwinnen, H., Vanderhaeghen, M.L., Collen, D., and Chuah, M.K. (1999) Long-term expression of human coagulation factor VIII and correction of hemophilia A after *in vivo* retroviral gene transfer in factor VIII-deficient mice. *Proceedings of the National Academy of Sciences*, Vol. 96, No. 18, (August), pp. 10379-84, ISSN 0027-8424

VandenDriessche T, Vanslembrouck V, Goovaerts I, VandenDriessche, T., Collen, D., and Chuah, M.K. (2001) Viral vector-mediated gene therapy for hemophilia. *Current Gene Therapy*, Vol. 1, No. 3, (September), pp. 301-315, ISSN 1566-5232

Viiala, N., Larsen, S., and Rasko, J. (2009) Gene Therapy for Hemophilia: Clinical Trials and Technical Tribulations. *Seminars in Thrombosis and Hemostasis*, Vol. 35, No. 1, (February), pp. 81-92, ISSN 0094-6176

Ward, N.J., Buckley, S.M., Waddington, S.N., VandenDriessche, T., Chuah, M.K.L., Nathwani, A.C., McIntosh, J., Tuddenham, E.G.D., Kinnon, C., Thrasher, A.J., and McVey, J. (2011) Codon optimization of human factor VIII cDNAs leads to high-level expression. *Blood*, Vol. 117, No. 3, (January), pp. 798-807, ISSN 0006-4971

Wu, X., Li, Y., Crise, B., and Burgess, S.M. (2003) Transcription start regions in the human genome are favored targets for MLV integration. *Science*, Vol. 300, No. 5626, (June), pp. 1749-1751, ISSN 0036-8075

Wu, Z., Yang, H., and Colosi, P. (2010) Effect of genome size on AAV vector packaging. *Molecular Therapy*, Vol. 18, No. 1, (January), pp. 80-86, ISSN 1525-0016

Xu, D., Alipio, Z., Fink, L., Adcock, D., Yang, J., Ward, D., and Ma, Y. (2009) Phenotypic correction of murine hemophilia A using an iPS cell-based therapy. *Proceedings of the National Academy of Sciences*, Vol. 106, No. 3, (January), pp. 808-813, ISSN 0027-8424

Yacoub, N., Romanowska, M., Haritonova, N., and Foerster, J. (2007) Optimized production and concentration of lentiviral vectors containing large inserts. *Journal of Gene Medicine*, Vol. 9, No. 7, (July), pp. 579-584, ISSN 1521-2254

Yang, Y., Nunes, F.A., Berencsi, K., Furth, E.E., Gönczöl, E., and Wilson, J.M. (1994) Cellular immunity to viral antigens limits E1-deleted adenoviruses for gene therapy. *Proceedings of the National Academy of Sciences*, Vol. 91, No. 10, (May), pp. 4407-4411, ISSN 0027-8424

Yant, S., Meuse, L., Chiu, W., Ivics, Z., Isvak, Z., and Kay, M. (2000) Somatic integration and long-term transgene expression in normal and haemophilic mice using a DNA transposon system. *Nature Genetics*, Vol. 25, No. 1, (May) pp. 35-41, ISSN 1061-4036

Yonemura, H., Sugawara, K., Nakashima, K., Nakahara, Y., Hamamoto, T., Mimaki, I., Yokomizo, K., Tajima, Y., Masuda, K., Imaizumi, A., Funatsu, A., and Miyazaki, J. (1993) Efficient production of recombinant human factor VIII by co-expression of the heavy and light chains. *Protein Engineering*, Vol. 6, No. 6, (August), pp. 669-74, ISSN 0269-2139

Youjin, S., and Jun, Y. (2009) The treatment of hemophilia A: from protein replacement to AAV-mediated gene therapy. *Biotechnology Letters*, Vol. 31, No. 3, (March), pp. 321-328, ISSN 0141-5492

Zayed, H., Izsvák, Z., Walisko, O., and Ivics, Z. (2004) Development of hyperactive *Sleeping Beauty* transposon vectors by mutational analysis. *Molecular Therapy*, Vol. 9, No. 2, (February), pp. 292-304, ISSN 1525-0016

Zhu, J., Kren, B.T., Park, C.W., Bilgim, R., Wong, P.Y., and Steer, C.J. (2007) Erythroid-specific expression of beta-globin by the *Sleeping Beauty* transposon for Sickle cell disease. *Biochemistry*, Vol. 46, No. 23, (June), pp. 6844-58, ISSN 1507-1521

Zufferey, R., Donello, J.E., Trono, D., and Hope, T.J. (1999) Woodchuck hepatitis virus posttranscriptional regulatory element enhances expression of transgenes delivered by retroviral vectors. *Journal of Virology*, Vol. 73, No. 4, (April), pp. 2886-2892, ISSN 1098-5514

Part 2

Evaluation of Gene Therapy

7

Recent Advances and Improvements in the Biosafety of Gene Therapy

Jaichandran Sivalingam[1,2] and Oi Lian Kon[1,2]
[1]*Division of Medical Sciences, Laboratory of Applied Human Genetics, Humphrey Oei Institute of Cancer Research, National Cancer Centre,*
[2]*Department of Biochemistry, Yong Loo Lin School of Medicine, National University of Singapore, Singapore*

1. Introduction

1.1 Overview of gene therapy

Progress in understanding the cellular and molecular bases of human health and disease in recent decades has spawned research in the fields of regenerative medicine and gene therapy. These novel approaches to medical treatments offer new possibilities of mitigating, and even curing, a plethora of medical conditions ranging from rare inherited monogenic disorders, metabolic diseases, infections and even complex disorders such as cancer.

In a simplified form, gene therapy can be defined as any procedure aimed at genetically altering or modifying cells or tissues with exogenous genetic materials that encompasses RNA, DNA and even oligonucleotides. These molecules may be directly delivered, *in vivo* into patients, often with the goal of targeting particular tissues (or organs). Alternatively, patients' cells may be isolated, expanded and modified *ex vivo* before reimplantation into the same subject (figure 1).

Whilst gene therapy appears to be a relatively new concept in the field of biomedicine, the original conceptualization of treating diseases by genetic engineering dates back as early as the 1940s. Avery, MacLeod and McCarthy pioneered the notion and demonstrated that genes could be transferred within nucleic acids (Avery et al., 1944). Early visionary investigators such as Tatum (Tatum, 1966) envisioned " that viruses will be effectively used for man's benefit, in theoretical studies in somatic-cell genetics and possibly in genetic therapy..." And at the end of that same decade, the earliest experimentation of gene delivery in humans was carried out controversially by Rogers and colleagues, who explored the idea of using Shope papilloma virus to treat three patients with arginase deficiency (Wolff & Lederberg, 1994). The decades that followed witnessed tremendous advances in recombinant DNA technology and enabled the first approved human gene therapy clinical trial in 1990 for treating infants with adenosine deaminase deficiency (Blaese et al., 1995). By the turn of the millennium, almost 4000 patients had received gene therapy from more than 500 clinical trials worldwide (Scollay, 2001), albeit with varying and limited successes. Nonetheless, these trials were helpful in highlighting several aspects of gene therapy that demanded improvements and refinements to achieve meaningful therapeutic efficacy and patient safety.

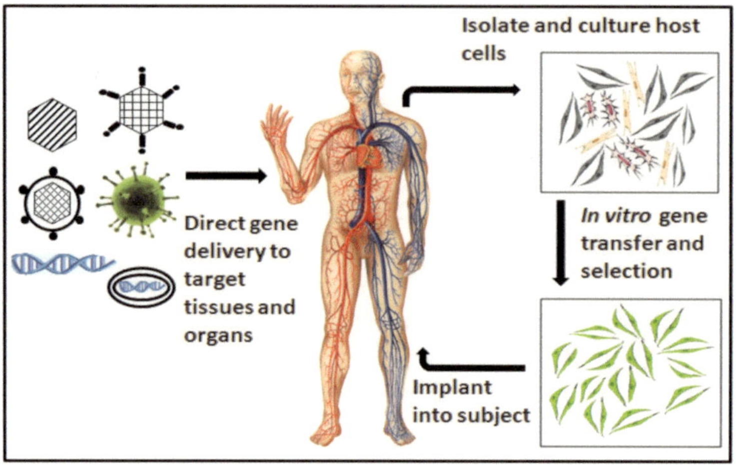

Fig. 1. Gene-based therapy. Left: *In vivo* administration of vector to modify cells in target organs or tissues directly. Right: *Ex vivo* modification of primary somatic cells that are reimplanted into the same subject (autologous cell therapy). Viral or non-viral vectors may be used to deliver transgenes.

Gene delivery can be achieved using either viral vectors or non-viral vectors. The latter may be episomally maintained or integrated into the host genome. To date, five main classes of viral vectors have been tested for clinical applications. These include retroviruses (RV), adenoviruses, adeno-associated viruses (AAV), lentiviruses and herpes simplex viruses (HSV) (Walther & Stein, 2000). Non-viral vectors most often utilize plasmid DNA which can be delivered into cells or tissues by physical methods such as electroporation, gene-gun bombardment, sonoporation, hydrodynamic injection or by chemical methods that utilize calcium phosphate, polymeric carriers, cell-penetrating peptides, cationic and anionic lipids (Niidome & Huang, 2002).

Gene therapy was initially conceptualized as ideal treatment for monogenic disorders such as adenosine deaminase, alpha-1-antitrypsin, ornithine transcarbamoylase and clotting factor (factors VIII and IX) deficiencies. These were considered ideal candidates as reconstitution of the missing protein in each case should alleviate or abolish the disease phenotype. The spectrum of gene therapy applications has now broadened considerably to every area of molecular medicine to include restoration of cellular and metabolic functions in various diseases, immuno-reconstitution of tumor cells in cancer immunotherapy, targeted cancer cell ablation in suicide gene therapy, treatment of infectious diseases, genetic manipulation, reprogramming of cancer and stem cell fate, reversing degenerative vascular and brain disorders, to name just a few.

Although gene therapy is conceptually appealing, the high hopes of translating such treatments into standard clinical practice has yet to be fulfilled, in part as initial enthusiasm from a few clinical successes have been marred by adverse, and even fatal, iatrogenic complications in a limited number of treated patients. Reactions to these sentinel events reiterate the need to understand and evaluate the genotoxic risks for any given gene therapy approach and for pertinent biosafety improvements to be incorporated into current treatment modalities. This chapter reviews current improvements to gene therapy with a focus on biosafety and highlights the essential advances and developments that could garner greater clinical acceptance for gene therapy applications.

1.2 Gene therapy clinical trials- successes and adverse outcomes

As of 2010, the Wiley Journal of Gene Medicine clinical trials database reported a total of 1644 gene therapy clinical trials, the majority (64.5%) of which were directed at cancer and related diseases (last accessed on 7th February 2011) (figure 2) . Given the greater depth of understanding of molecular virology, the broad tropism of viral vectors and their superior efficiencies of gene transfer, transgene delivery *via* viral vectors has been the favoured and most feasible option (67 % of all trials).

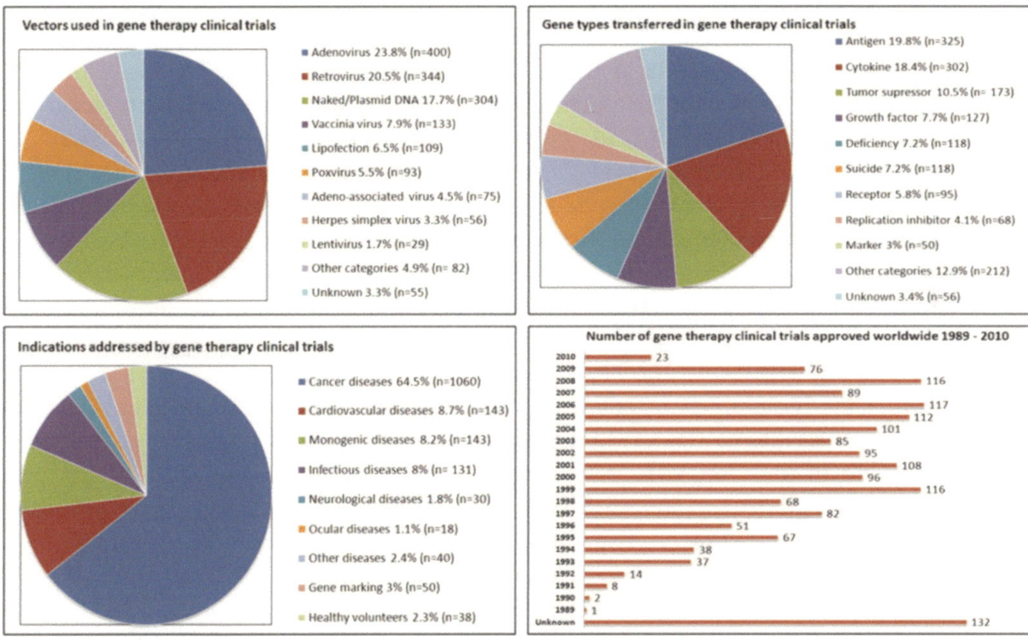

Fig. 2. Characteristics of clinical gene therapy trials. Categorisation of gene therapy trials according to indications, vectors used, gene types transferred and annual number of approved trials. (*Images reproduced from Journal of Gene Medicine clinical trials database (http://www.wiley.com/legacy/wileychi/genmed/clinical/)).*

Despite the impressive number of gene therapy trials, it is worth noting that only a small number of these trials reported clinically meaningful and long term outcomes. The first clinical success was for the treatment of X-linked severe combined immunodeficiency (SCID-X1) (Cavazzana-Calvo et al., 2000), a disease characterised by immature development of the immune system due to mutations in the interleukin-2 receptor common gamma chain gene (*IL2Rγ*). Nine of ten treated patients achieved long term immune reconstitution following implantation with gene modified hematopoietic stem cells and marked clinical improvement (Hacein-Bey-Abina et al., 2003). More success stories echoed from similar clinical trials in London, U.K., of the same disorder (Gaspar et al., 2004). In the years that followed, long term therapeutic efficacy was also reported in clinical trials for another form of SCID disorder due to adenosine deaminase deficiency (SCID-ADA) (Aiuti et al., 2009). In 2006, gene therapy scored more successes when impressive results were reported in two patients treated for X-linked chronic granulomatous disease (CGD) (Ott et al., 2006), caused by inactivating mutations of gp91phox (*CYBB*) gene and characterised by neutrophil dysfunction and recurrent serious infections. More recent and notable clinical success has been reported for gene therapy of Wiskott-Aldrich syndrome (Boztug et al., 2010), X-linked adrenoleukodystrophy (Cartier et al., 2009), Leber's congenital amaurosis and Parkinson's disease.

Although these impressive clinical outcomes provided incontrovertible proof-of-principle, it soon became evident that treatment benefits could occur in tandem with significant adverse effects when serious iatrogenic complications were reported in a small number of patients. The first gene therapy death was reported in 1999 from an ornithine transcarbamoylase trial conducted at the University of Pennsylvania. This was ascribed to a massive immune response to the adenoviral vector used in that trial (Raper et al., 2003). Gene therapy suffered the heaviest blows in the years 2003 to 2006, and attracted close scrutiny by regulatory authorities and the medical fraternity when five successfully treated SCID-X1 patients (from two different clinical trials) developed T-cell lymphoblastic leukemia, three to six years after treatment with autologous bone marrow-derived CD34+ hematopoietic cells transduced with a murine leukaemia virus (MLV) gammaretroviral vector to express the *IL2Rγ* gene (Howe et al., 2008; Hacein-Bey-Abina et al., 2008). Random integration of the MLV gamma retroviral vector that had strong enhancer elements in the long terminal repeat (LTR) regions resulted in the insertional activation of LIM domain only-2 (*LMO2*) proto-oncogene. This mutagenic event likely promoted clonal proliferation of T cells that culminated in acute lymphoblastic leukaemia. In a different trial in 2007, Targeted Genetics Corporation was forced to halt its gene therapy trial for rheumatoid arthritis involving intra-articular injection of an adenoviral vector expressing *tgAAC94*, following the death of a patient. In this case however, investigations by the US Food and Drug Administration (FDA) exonerated gene therapy as the direct cause of death (Frank et al., 2009), although there was evidence of vector-induced immune response; and the trials have since recommenced. The inherent risks of insertional mutagenesis by viral vectors surfaced again in another clinical trial in the year 2006 for treatment of CGD. Two adult CGD patients infused with granulocyte colony-stimulating factor (*G-CSF*)-mobilized peripheral blood CD34+ cells transduced with MLV gammaretroviral vector expressing $gp91^{phox}$ had markedly improved neutrophil functions and resistance to life threatening infections. Regrettably, both subjects later developed myelodysplasia and one subject died from this complication (Stein et al., 2010). Myelodysplasia probably developed from random integration of the gammaretroviral vector that activated the expression of a proto-oncogene, *MDS-EVI1*) (Stein et al., 2010). As of this writing, the most recent case of adverse gene therapy outcome, brought to light by the American Society of Gene and Cell therapy (http://www.asgct.org/media/news-releases/?c=505) affected one of ten Wiskott-Aldrich syndrome patients treated at the Hannover Medical School using a gammaretroviral vector similar to that used in the SCID-X1 trials. This patient was reported to have developed leukaemia. A comprehensive clinical evaluation of this adverse event is yet to be disclosed.

In summary, there is clear evidence that gene therapy can be clinically effective. Moreover, it offers the only treatment for certain serious life threatening diseases that are currently untreatable or poorly treated. An important issue that must be addressed if gene therapy is to mature from experimental treatment to standard of care is that of biosafety. The occurrence of serious iatrogenic outcomes, albeit uncommon, has brought into sharp focus the inherent risks of genetic modifications.

2. Biosafety considerations of gene therapy

2.1 Genotoxicity potential of gene therapy

The potential for genotoxicity in gene therapy is not unexpected. Initial studies investigating the integration site preferences of different viral vectors such as human immunodeficiency virus, avian sarcoma-leukosis virus and MLV gammaretrovirus, drew attention to the potential for insertional mutagenesis arising from random or quasi-random genomic integrations, aggravated by the marked propensity of these vectors to target transcription start sites and active genes (Mitchell et al., 2004). Even before reports of adverse events surfaced in clinical trials, a 2002 retroviral gene marking study in murine bone marrow cells already reported a high frequency of vector-induced hematopoietic disorders, including leukemia, caused in part by insertional activation of an oncogene (Li, Z. et al., 2002). Different strategies are being actively explored to reduce the genotoxic potential of current viral vectors. The main focus areas are to devise methods for: (a) appropriate tissue targeting of systemically delivered vectors, (b) disabling the capacity for generating replication competent viruses; (c) mitigating immune responses to vectors and/or transgene products; (d) avoiding germ-line modifications; (e) preventing unintended vector dissemination; and (f) directing the integration of transgenes into genomic safe harbors.

2.2 Insertional mutagenesis

Insertional mutagenesis refers to the induction of deleterious mutations to genes, promoters, enhancers or other regulatory elements that alter gene expression as a consequence of exogenous vector integration into the genome. Although a major concern of integrating vectors, even non-integrating vectors have a low but finite possibility of random genomic integration (Wang, Z. et al., 2004).

Prior to cases of gene therapy induced oncogenesis in recent clinical trials, the risk of malignant transformation from integrating vectors was considered theoretically plausible but unlikely to occur in practice. With hindsight, treatment-induced malignancies could have been predicted on the basis that as many as 1% of genes encoded in the genome are implicated in one or more forms of cancer (Futreal et al., 2004). Although oncogenesis is a process that requires multiple genetic hits, random integration of vectors into multiple genomic sites could sufficiently generate the right "cocktail" of aberrations in different oncogenes and/or tumor suppressor genes (Hanahan & Weinberg, 2000), Moreover, as the formerly regarded gene deserts are now known to be richly populated with different classes of non-protein-coding RNAs with key roles in cellular maintenance and cancer development (Farazi et al., 2011), evaluation of genotoxic risk of integration events requires extra caution.

Viral vectors do not integrate randomly but have a propensity for transcriptionally active units and transcription start sites in mammalian cells (Mitchell et al., 2004). Such studies have been instrumental in developing integration maps or profiles of the different viruses, highlighting their potential risks based on their propensity to integrate near transcription start sites, into active transcriptional units, close to oncogenes or tumor suppressor genes. Even disruptive integrations into other genes such as those necessary for cell survival or metabolism may be deleterious. Thus, insertional mutagenesis is a real risk that needs to be seriously addressed rather than being dismissed as inconsequential as was the attitude prior to reports of adverse gene therapy clinical outcomes.

Much has been learned about the molecular pathogenesis of oncogenesis associated with integrating viral vectors. MLV gammaretroviral vectors have a predilection for integrating close to transcription start sites (Mitchell et al., 2004) and to perturb their expression possibly due to the strong enhancer effect inherent in the LTRs (Modlich et al., 2006). However, this effect alone may not be sufficient for complete oncogenic evolution as a clinical trial for SCID-ADA in ten patients treated with a similar MLV retroviral vector reported no untoward outcomes (median duration of follow-up of 4 years) (Aiuti et al., 2009). This has led to the speculation that other factors such as the nature of the expressed transgene (*IL2Rγ versus ADA*), the underlying disease, the cell types selected for transgenic modification and other patient-specific intrinsic factors could be necessary accessory factors to oncogenesis.

In contrast to retroviral vectors, no overt adverse events have been reported thus far from the use of other viral vectors such as lentiviral, adenoviral, HSV or AAV vectors. Some studies even suggest that lentiviral vectors pose significantly lower risks of insertional oncogenesis compared to retroviral vectors due to differences in their integration preferences (Montini et al., 2006). Generally, non-integrating vectors such as adenoviruses, recombinant AAV and HSV which are predominantly maintained as episomes are not considered to be mutagenic given their minute possibility of inducing rare random integrations in the genome. On the other hand, AAV which can integrate into the AAVS1 locus in the presence of viral proteins Rep68 or Rep78 (Smith, 2008), must be considered as having intermediate risks.

2.3 Tools for evaluating potential for genotoxicity

The reality of vector-induced oncogenesis need not be a fatal impediment to the goal of clinical gene therapy. Tools are now available to interrogate transgenically-modified cells *ex vivo* for undesirable genomic alterations and to evaluate tumorigenic potential. The ability to perform comprehensive biosafety assessments *ex vivo* before *in vivo* treatment could be a feasible approach to exploit the benefits of gene replacement while minimizing treatment risks to a clinically acceptable level.

A first step to genotoxicity analysis of any given modality would be to review databases for adverse outcomes encountered in past or ongoing clinical trials which can be accessed at several websites e.g. Wiley clinical trials database (http:// www.wiley.com/ legacy/ wileychi/genmed/clinical/), the US National Institutes of Health ClinicalTrials.gov (http://www.genetherapynet.com/clinicaltrialsgov.html) and Clinigene (http:// www.clinigene.eu/search-published-human-gene-therapy-clinical-trials-database/).

This section focuses on the biosafety assessment of *ex vivo* gene modified cells, with an emphasis on key features to monitor and molecular biology tools that aid the evaluation. The importance of bioinformatic tools in biosafety evaluation cannot be overemphasized. This section will also highlight useful programs, internet resources and databases.

2.4 Mapping genome integration sites

It is imperative to document integration events in gene modified cells, and prudent to do so even for episomal vectors that have a low probability of random integration (Stephen et al., 2008; Wang, Z. et al., 2004). Integration events are detailed with reference to their physical distance relative to promoter sites, transcription start sites, exons or introns, oncogenes, tumor suppressor genes, non-protein coding genes, CpG islands, repetitive elements and transcription factor and micro-RNA binding sites. Such integration profiles aid genotoxicity risk evaluation when comparing across vector types, modified cell types and the nature of transgenes.

Integration events within cells can be experimentally retrieved and identified by plasmid rescue, ligation mediated PCR (LM-PCR) (Laufs et al., 2003), inverse PCR (Silver & Keerikatte, 1989) or linear amplification mediated PCR (LAM-PCR)(Schmidt, M. et al., 2007). Sequence data can be analyzed for vector-flanking sequences by programs such as IntegrationSeq (Giordano et al., 2007) which may then be queried using programs such as NCBI-BLAST (http://blast.ncbi.nlm.nih.gov/) or UCSC-BLAT (http:// www. genome.ucsc.edu/) to identify their genomic positions (figure 3). In recent years, several programs have been developed to automate the process of genome mapping. IntegrationMap (Giordano et al., 2007), SeqMap (Peters et al., 2008) and QuickMap (Appelt et al., 2009) are examples of web-based programs that are useful for annotating genome mapping information such as proximity to genes, neighbouring gene identity, exon/intron localization, distance from transcription start sites, repeat element localization and Gene Ontology functions. QuickMap (http://www.gtsg.org), most recently developed, provides a more comprehensive evaluation which includes information about proximity to oncogenes, pseudogenes, CpG islands, fragile sites, transcription factor and micro-RNA binding sites. Identity of potential cancer genes can be derived from lists compiled from the human cancer gene census (Futreal et al., 2004) or the retroviral tagged cancer gene database, RTCGD (http://rtcgd.abcc.ncifcrf.gov, mouse cancer genes). Another useful database with a comprehensive compilation of known oncogenes and tumor suppressor genes (Wang, G.P. et al., 2008) can be accessed at the following website (http:// microb230.med.upenn.edu/ protocols/cancergenes.html) hosted by the University of Pennsylvania School of Medicine.

Another useful aspect of genomic profiling of integration sites is its application for the long-term monitoring of the clonality of *in vivo* implanted gene modified cells (Wang, G.P. et al., 2010). Integration profiles of gene modified cells determined pre-implantation can be periodically monitored post-implantation to detect the emergence of dominant clones. Deviation from a polyclonal pattern of growth could imply selection of a dominant clone of cells by virtue of a growth advantage or a greatly increased proliferation rate. This ought to alert close scrutiny for the likelihood of insertional oncogenesis. Gerrits et al. have recently demonstrated the use of tagged vectors with variable barcode signatures to track different clones *in vivo* (Gerrits et al., 2010). Such innovative techniques could be applied to enhance monitoring the clonality of implanted cells *in vivo* and increase the sensitivity of detecting potential oncogenic alterations.

2.5 Characterizing the modified genome

There are relevant concerns that integrating and non-integrating vectors can potentially alter the genomic architecture of cells. Copy number gains and deletions have been observed in transformed cancer cell-lines and to a lesser extent on cells treated with gene therapy vectors (Stephen et al., 2008). Recent advances to the array based technology have made it possible to study amplifications or deletions to the genome at very high resolutions with probes that span the genome on average at 2.5 kb intervals (Hester et al., 2009). As with most array based techniques, copy number analysis relies on a relatively homogeneous population of cells as events in a minor population of polyclonal cells may be masked or under-represented in the analysis that would otherwise highlight the effects that are observed in the dominant population of cells.

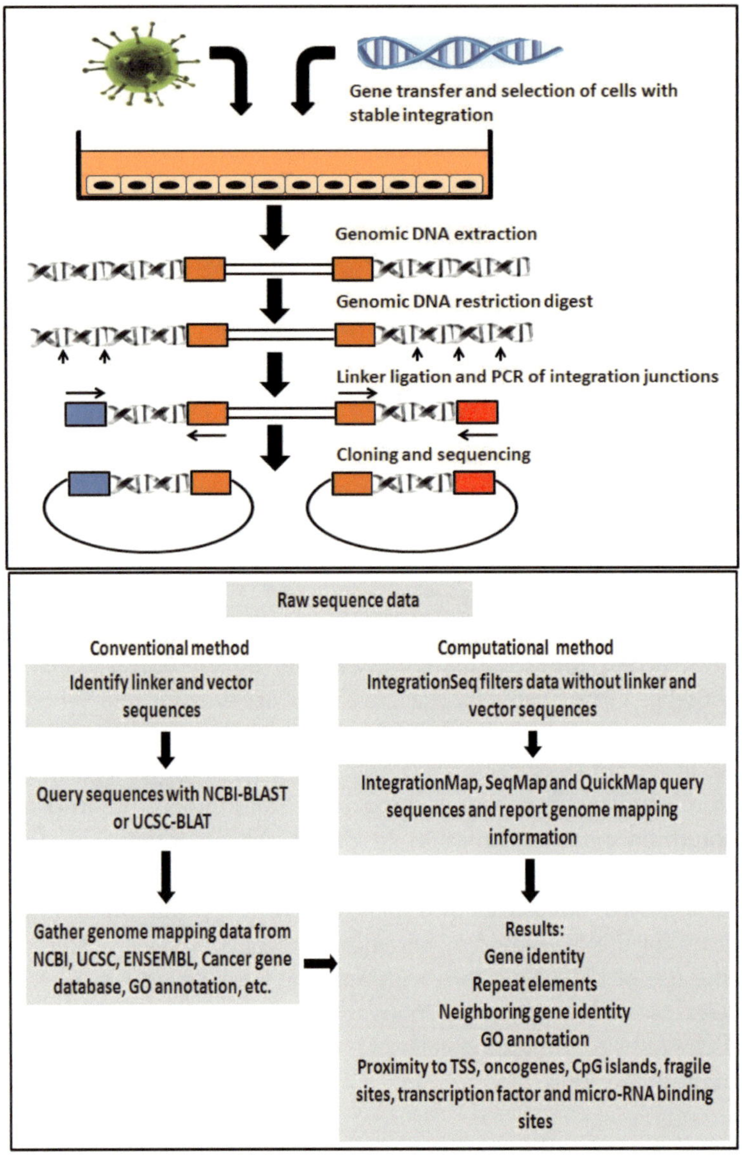

Fig. 3. Experimental recovery of integration events and computational analysis of integration site distribution in mammalian cell genomes. Top: Integration events in cells may be retrieved by digesting genomic DNA (with restriction enzymes that do not cleave within the vector sequences). Appropriate adapters are ligated to restriction fragments to serve as priming sites for PCR amplification of integration junctions which can then be cloned and sequenced. *(Adapted from Ciuffi et al., 2009.)* Bottom: Vector flanking raw sequence data may be selected with programs such as IntegrationSeq and queried using UCSC-BLAT or NCBI-BLAST to retrieve relevant genomic information. Computational programs such as IntegrationMap, SeqMap and QuickMap automate the process of genome mapping and provide the necessary genomic information required for biosafety assessment. *(Adapted from Peters et al., 2008.)*

Another serious genomic alteration that can be mediated by gene therapy vectors is chromosomal aneuploidy and/or gross structural abnormalities such as deletions and translocations, which are common hallmarks of transformed cells. Several studies have reported unexpected but rare cytogenetic abnormalities in cells treated with AAV (Miller, D.G. et al., 2005), retroviral vectors (Modlich, 2005) and non-viral vectors such as phiC31 phage integrase-mediated plasmid integration (Liu, J. et al., 2006). The inciting causes of such cytogenetic abnormalities are unclear, namely whether from direct effects of vector integration and repair or from recombination events secondary to vector integration.

Gross chromosomal rearrangements in gene modified cells can be evaluated by spectral karyotyping or multi-color FISH. However, karyotyping requires that a sufficient number of metaphases should be examined if rare rearrangements are not to be missed. Array based comparative genomic hybridization detects copy number abnormalities (deletions or amplifications) at high resolution, provided a fairly homogeneous cell population is analyzed. However, even high resolution copy number analysis could not be expected to detect aberrations in a rare subpopulation of cells. Genome sequencing to identify vector integration junctions can potentially identify translocations at high (nucleotide level) resolution provided junctional fragments can be confidently identified. However, this method (currently performed at relatively high cost) generates large datasets that require specialized bioinformatic analysis and awareness of technical artifacts (Koboldt et al, 2010). In conclusion, effective cytogenetic analysis should combine sequencing techniques (for integration site retrieval), multicolor karyotyping, whole genome copy number and possibly deep genome sequencing analysis as a complementary suite of techniques to completely characterize the chromosomes of gene modified cells.

2.6 Transcriptome and epigenome analysis

A necessary complement to genome analyses is to determine effects of gene transfer (however accomplished, but especially if the transgene is known to have integrated) on the transcriptome of gene modified cells. In this regard, it is worth noting that vector insertions are often accompanied by deletions of genomic regions (Miller, D.G. et al., 2002) that may in turn alter the epigenetic status of the cell if key histone proteins or histone modifying enzymes are affected. Thus it may also be relevant to determine effects of gene transfer on the epigenome.

Comparing the global transcriptomes of naïve and vector treated cells may help to identify genes whose expression are perturbed by vector treatment. Many technical platforms based on hybridization to gene-specific oligonucleotide probes are now available for genome-wide transcriptome analysis and, being unbiased, are the method of choice. Such data, in practice, reveals significantly altered gene expression mainly in the dominant cell population, though not necessarily in minor subpopulations. Ideally the transcriptome of a homogeneous or, preferably, clonal population of cells with a single known vector integration is more informative. The presence of multiple integration sites in a clonal population confounds attempts to distinguish effects attributable to any particular integration. Likewise, the study of a heterogeneous cell population would mask the transcriptional features of a minor subpopulation within a mixed culture. Therefore, microarray studies would yield useful information only when a sufficient number of clonal populations from different integration sites are characterized. Given that viral vectors mediate integrations into multiple sites, such clonal studies would be highly impractical. Clonal studies are especially important when integrations have been identified close to oncogenes. Transcriptome analysis aims not only to identify individual genes with significantly altered expression but should also map individual aberrations to molecular pathways. There is a plethora of non-proprietary microarray analysis and bioinformatic software tools for data evaluation and analysis. For example, useful tools are hosted by groups such as the Gene Ontology (http://www.geneontology.org/GO.tools.microarray.shtml), Genomics and Bioinformatics Group from NIH (http://discover.nci.nih.gov/tools.jsp) and DAVID (http://david.abcc.ncifcrf.gov/home.jsp).

Epigenetic changes refer to the changes in the acetylation, methylation, sumoylation and phosphorylation patterns of histone proteins, which in turn may affect the dynamic chromatin architecture and determine the active or repressed status of genes. It also encompasses changes in CpG methylation status of DNA near promoter regions which may influence gene expression. Transgene integrations may directly attenuate gene expression, have a negative or positive effect on genes based on copy number aberrations of the genome or affect histone modifying enzymes which in turn may affect the epigenetic and gene expression status of cells. Global epigenetic status of cells are presently studied using a combination of global transcriptome analysis, cytosine methylation pattern, nucleosome positioning assay and chromatin immunoprecipitation (ChIP) based assays to determine transcription factor binding sites (Fazzari & Greally, 2010). The on-going human epigenome project (http://www.epigenome.org/) that aims to document the DNA methylation patterns of all human genes is likely to provide invaluable insights into the role of epigenetics in human diseases. However, the study of epigenetics is currently hampered by a lack of simple, high quality and high-throughput techniques. Technical advances should deepen knowledge of this important domain of human genetics.

2.7 *In vitro* and *in vivo* tumorigenicity studies

Transformed cells acquire altered phenotypes that can be detected under *in vitro* conditions to distinguish them from untransformed cells. Anchorage independent growth, loss of contact inhibition, resistance to apoptosis, increased proliferation rate and extended cell passaging are common characteristics of transformed cells.

Simple *in vitro* assays demonstrate the anchorage independent growth and increased proliferation rates of cells. The soft agar colony formation assay involves enumerating colonies (clonal propagation of cells) formed from individual cells in the absence of substrate adhesion. Anchorage independent cells typically form colonies while normal cells do not as they rely on surface attachment for proliferation. Assays that quantify incorporation of bromo-deoxyuridine (BrdU), reduction of tetrazolium compounds (e.g. 3-(4,5-Dimethylthiazol-2-yl)-2,5-diphenyltetrazolium bromide) and colony formation are direct or indirect measures of cellular proliferation rates. Modlich and colleagues (Modlich et al., 2009) recently introduced another assay, termed the *in vitro* immortalization assay, which tests tumorigenic potential of virally transduced murine hematopoietic stem cells (HSCs) based on their replating capacity, thus obviating the need to use animal models.

Most *in vitro* biosafety assays seek to evaluate deviations from normal cellular characteristics. A more realistic evaluation of tumorigenicity would be to determine the potential to induce tumors *in vivo.* Two main models are used to evaluate the tumorigenic potential either of *ex vivo* modified cells or systemically delivered viral vectors. In the first model, gene modified human cells are implanted into immunocompromised mice that are known to support the engraftment of xenogeneic cells. It is helpful to know that different strains of immunocompromised mice have different capacities to mount immune responses depending on which components of the immune system are still functional. Mouse strains that are most severely immunocompromised can be expected to have high sensitivity as tumorigenic hosts because low numbers of implanted cells will give rise to visible tumors. Such sensitive models are useful for the detection of rare populations of oncogenic cells in a heterogeneous population of otherwise untransformed cells. The absence of tumor formation should not immediately exonerate cells of their tumorigenic potential. It is essential to establish from immunohistology of the implantation sites or in the case of HSCs implantation, immunocytometric blood analysis that the implanted cells have indeed engrafted *in vivo* in animals that fail to form tumors. The second model is useful to evaluate the genotoxic potential of HSCs transduced with different gene therapy vectors. It is based on the transduction and transplantation of HSCs derived from a tumor-prone mouse model that lacks the tumor suppressor, cyclin dependent kinase inhibitor 2A (*cdkn2a*) gene (Montini et al., 2009). This assay thus evaluates tumorigenic risk in an already tumor-prone cell line and was used to compare the oncogenic potential of retroviral and lentiviral vectors, and to assess the benefits of introducing self-inactivating (SIN) long terminal repeats (LTR) in these vectors. However, a caveat is that due to the intrinsic oncogenic potential of the cdkn2-/- HSCs, the effects of subtle but relevant insertional mutagenic events may be masked or misinterpreted. Besides murine models, long-term studies can also be performed in pre-clinical animals such dogs and non-human primates (Kim, Y.J. et al., 2009) where the clonality of implanted cells can be dynamically monitored by documenting integration profiles of recovered cells to ascertain if dominant clones with clone-specific integration patterns have emerged.

3. Recent developments in biosafety enhancement of gene therapy

Comprehensive molecular studies of adverse outcomes of gene therapy trials have advanced our understanding of mechanisms that likely caused clinical complications. This has, in turn, spurred the development of safer vectors. In parallel, more sensitive experimental techniques for biosafety evaluations enable higher confidence in pre-clinical assessments of biosafety before treatments are implemented in clinical trials. This section reviews recent developments that enhance biosafety of gene therapy.

3.1 Improvements to viral vectors

Gene transfer *via* viral vectors remains the most prevalent choice in clinical trials of gene therapy. Knowledge of genotoxic risks that are inherent in viral life cycles and their biology have guided modifications aimed at improving the biosafety of viral vectors. The basic approaches are summarised in figure 4. They include the use of viral vectors that do not integrate or that do so with a more random and less selective integration spectrum, the inclusion of self-inactivating LTR elements and chromatin insulators to reduce neighborhood effects of integrated vectors on gene expression and the use of cell- or tissue-specific promoters for physiological and tissue-specific gene expression.

3.1.1 Replication defective vectors

Apart from certain oncolytic cancer gene therapies that use conditionally replicating viruses, most clinical applications rely on replication-incompetent viral vectors as virus replication *in*

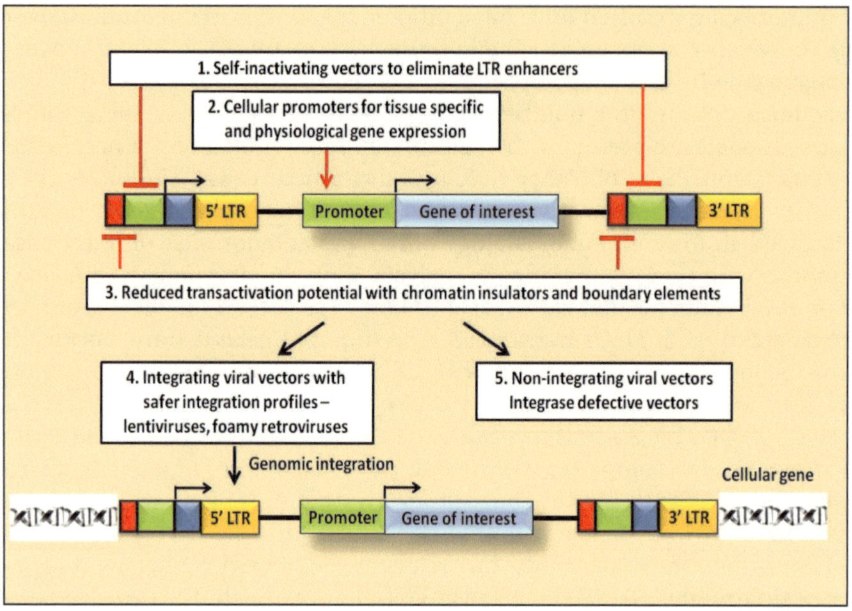

Fig. 4. Strategies to improve biosafety of integrating viral vectors. Integrating viral vectors have been shown to mediate transactivation of genes close to integration sites. This risk can be reduced by using self-inactivating vectors devoid of strong LTR enhancers, cellular promoters, incorporating chromatin insulators and other boundary elements and lastly by the selective use of viral vectors with intrinsically safer integration profiles. *(Adapted from Kohn and Candotti, 2009.)*

vivo could pose a serious health and mutagenic hazard to patients. Replication-defective vectors are generally designed to lack viral genes necessary for their replication and packaging and therefore need to be produced in helper cell lines which provide the necessary components (gag/pol, env and rev, as is the case for HIV-lentivirus) for their packaging *in trans*. Unintended homologous recombination between the replication-defective vector and packaging constructs or endogenous viral sequences in the human genome may potentially cause reversion to a replication-competent virus. Such a risk has been greatly mitigated through improved packaging constructs or packaging cell lines that have little or no homology to the vector that encodes the therapeutic gene to greatly minimise the likelihood of recombination.

Other avenues of improvements have been in the methods used to rigorously screen vector batches for contamination with replication competent viruses. Assays that detect recombination between gene transfer vector and helper vectors based on their known structures are available for detecting replication competent-AAV (Tenenbaum et al., 2003), replication competent adenovirus (Chuah et al., 2003) and replication competent retrovirus (Sinn et al., 2005). However, the development of accurate assays for RCL (replication competent lentivirus) detection has been more challenging due to the difficulty of predicting their genomic organizations. Nevertheless, recent assay developments such as the product-enhanced reverse transcriptase (PERT) assays (Sinn et al., 2005) and combination of p24 ELISA and psi-gag PCR (Cornetta et al., 2010) ought to increase the sensitivity and accuracy of screening for RCL contamination in clinical grades of viral stocks.

In summary, improvements to packaging cell-lines or helper constructs have minimized the risk of reversion to replication competency while improved screening methods should help prevent the unintentional clinical administration of viral vectors contaminated with replication competent viruses.

3.1.2 Self-inactivating vectors

Retroviral and lentiviral vectors have intrinsic promoter and enhancer activities in their LTR regions which have been implicated in the aberrant activation of neighboring genes. This potential to activate oncogenes, combined with other concurrent factors is the basis for insertional oncogenesis. Several studies have shown that the risks of insertional gene activation can be drastically reduced by deleting the strong internal promoter/enhancer elements in the U3 regions of the LTR of retroviral and lentiviral vectors. The concept of self-inactivating (SIN) vector requires the replacement of the U3 regions of the 5′ LTR with a heterologous promoter (such as CMV) and partial deletion of the U3 enhancer elements in the 3′LTR. The process of viral vector integration involves copying of the 3′LTR (now devoid of enhancer elements) to the 5′LTR and deletion of the 5′LTR-CMV promoter. The final result is a transcriptionally inert 5′LTR incapable of transactivating genes (Schäfer-Korting et al., 2010). Neoplastic transformation rates of bone marrow derived murine HSCs transduced with lentiviral and retroviral vectors with and without SIN elements have been compared (Montini et al., 2009; Modlich et al., 2009; Bosticardo et al., 2009). These studies demonstrated significantly reduced but not complete abrogation of oncogenicity (Bosticardo et al., 2009) of vectors bearing the SIN elements. These studies also highlighted that even with SIN vectors, insertional mutagenesis was still possible from internal enhancer/promoter elements and the choice of the internal promoter may reduce overt genotoxicity. Thus, although the development of SIN vectors has been an important step in improving biosafety, further refinements such as the use of cellular promoters devoid of enhancer elements and with decreased potential to induce activation of neighboring genes are necessary.

3.1.3 Chromatin insulators and cellular promoters

SIN vectors depend on an internal promoter to drive transgene expression. However, enhancer effects of the internal promoter in transactivating neighboring oncogenes has been a possible mechanism for neoplastic transformation associated with SIN vectors (Bosticardo et al., 2009; Modlich et al., 2009). The internal promoter of choice should ideally drive a high level of transgene expression without affecting the transcriptional status of neighboring genes. Thus, the use of moderately active internal promoters such as the phosphoglycerate kinase (PGK), elongation factor-1α (EF1α) or WAS promoter has been recommended to reduce the likelihood of neighborhood effects causing inadvertent gene activation (Zychlinski et al., 2008). The potential of vector-encoded promoters to transactivate host genes may be evaluated using *in vitro* assays (Weber & Cannon, 2007).

Another potential biosafety feature that has been explored is the inclusion of chromatin insulators to shield neighboring genes from the effects of vector-borne enhancers (Nienhuis et al., 2006). Insulator elements serve as barriers that separate transcriptionally active genomic regions (euchromatin) from heterochromatin and also prevent long-range interactions between enhancer/ regulatory elements and neighboring promoters, thereby reducing the risk of unintended transactivation of proximate genes. Insulator elements are typically cloned into the 3′ LTRs from where they are copied into the 5′LTRs following genomic integration, thus flanking and isolating the transgene cassette. Zychlinski et al. reported moderately positive results with reduced transformation of murine HSCs when a 250 basepair (bp) core element of chicken hypersensitive site 4 (cHS4) insulator was incorporated into the viral vector (Zychlinski et al., 2008). More encouraging results of reduced transactivation were reported of a 77 bp element consisting of the β-globin 5′ HS4 insulator and a homologous region from human T-cell receptor BEAD-1 insulator (Ramezani et al., 2008). However, insulators may function in a tissue-specific manner or may be effective only against certain promoters/enhancers. Thus more work is needed to screen different insulator elements and test them in different cell types and with different promoter/enhancer configurations. Incorporation of strong polyadenylation signals in LTRs of vector is another option that has been explored to ensure the proper transcriptional termination of transgenes and to minimise the risk of internal promoters transcribing downstream coding sequences (Nienhuis et al., 2006). However, this carries the potential risk of premature transcript termination and transcriptional inactivation of neighbouring genes. Although the biosafety afforded by improved transcriptional termination is largely speculative, Schambach et al. did report encouraging results of improved transcriptional termination using upstream sequence elements in lentiviral and gammaretroviral SIN vectors (Schambach et al., 2007). Further evaluations in *in vitro* and *in vivo* models are necessary to determine if tightly regulated transcriptional termination translates to a reduced risk of insertional oncogenesis.

In summary, stringent selection of cellular promoters devoid of enhancer elements, inclusion of chromatin insulators and improved transcriptional termination should significantly enhance the biosafety of current SIN vectors.

3.1.4 Integrase defective vectors

Risks of insertional mutagenesis can be better managed if the frequency of genomic integration is reduced or if episomally maintained vectors are utilized. Virally encoded integrases bind to attachment regions (att) in the LTRs and mediate genomic integration of retro- and lentiviruses. Recent years have seen the developments of integrase defective vectors (IDV) which are generated either by mutating the viral integrase genes or att regions of the LTR (Sarkis et al., 2008). These altered vectors combine the efficient transduction capability of viruses with the higher biosafety of non-integrating vectors, although IDVs are not completely devoid of integration potential. Integrase defective retro- and lentiviral vectors have been developed, with the latter being more prevalent in use as lentiviral transduction is not limited to mitotic cells.

Integrase defective lentiviral vectors (IDLV) have been generated *via* mutations to integrase proteins at their catalytic domains, LTR-interacting N-terminal domains or non-specific DNA-binding C-terminal domains. Of these, the D64V and D116N mutations in the integrase catalytic domains have been more widely studied and reported to reduce residual integrase activity by 100- to 1000-fold compared with wild-type vectors (Apolonia et al., 2007) but with uncompromised transgene expression *in vivo* and about 2- to 10-fold decrease in expression *in vitro* (Apolonia et al., 2007). IDLV transduced cells can maintain stable transgene expression in the non-dividing state and may find useful applications in gene transfer to post-mitotic cells such as in muscle, liver and retina. They may also be useful in immuno gene therapy applications such as DNA vaccination where only transient expression of the transgene is required. Another application being explored is the use of IDLV as an episomal gene delivery technique for expressing site-specific integration factors such as zinc finger nucleases (ZFNs) (Lombardo et al., 2007), transposons (Vink et al., 2009) and recombinases (Moldt et al., 2008). Lastly, IDLV may be developed as a safer alternative to non-integrating viral vectors such as AAV which are known to integrate quasi-randomly into the genome at low frequencies (Smith, 2008).

3.1.5 Novel and hybrid viral vectors

Ideal gene therapy vectors should be capable of accommodating large inserts and of efficient gene transfer in a broad range of cell types, while maintaining stable transgene expression with negligible genotoxicity. Much effort has been directed to designing and combining the positive traits of different viral vectors in a bid to refine therapeutic gene delivery.

As mentioned in the preceding section, IDVs combine the traits of broad tropism and efficient transduction of wild-type viruses with improved biosafety of episomal vectors. IDLV combined with Sleeping Beauty transposon/transposase, ZFNs and FLP/FRT recombinases are hybrid vectors tailored to integrate transgenes in a site-specific manner as directed by the transgene expressed proteins. Such a design also ensures that integrations are altered from the quasi-random pattern of the wild-type lentivirus to those directed by the coding proteins. Another example of a chimeric lentiviral vector with altered integration specificity was described by Gijsbers et al. (Gijsbers et al., 2010) who demonstrated retargeted integration specificity when artificial chromatin tethers were fused to a lentiviral-integrase interacting protein called lens epithelium-derived growth factor/p75 (LEDGF/p75). By replacing the DNA/chromatin interacting domain of LEDGF/p75 with heterochromatin 1β (*CBX1*), lentiviral integrations were retargeted to genomic loci bound by *CBX1*. This study also raises possibilities of designing both viral and non-viral vectors with LEDGF/p75 fusion proteins targeting safer genomic sites.

Hybrid HSV/AAV vectors have been constructed in an attempt to combine the large insert cloning capacity of non-integrating HSV vectors (up to 150 kb) with the site-specific integration property of AAV vectors into a genomic hotspot, the AAVS1 locus, and to a certain extent, randomly (De Oliveira & Fraefel, 2010). Other HSV-based hybrid vectors include the episomally maintained HSV/EBV and randomly integrating HSV/RV vectors.

Given the propensity of MLV gammaretroviral vectors to mediate insertional mutagenesis, vectors with safer integration profiles are being developed and investigated actively. For instance, the non-pathogenic foamy spumaretrovirus has shown promise in treating canine leukocyte deficiency without any reported adverse outcomes for up to 2 years (Bauer et al., 2008). These vectors also had a more favourable integration profile i.e. decreased frequency of integrating near oncogenes. While novel hybrid vectors appear promising, continued long-term efficacy and biosafety studies are necessary before they can be serious candidates for clinical gene therapy.

3.2 Improvements to integrating non-viral vectors

Non-viral vectors have found useful applications largely in the laboratory and pre-clinical settings but represent only 24% of all vectors used in clinical gene therapy trials. The fact that viruses have evolved over millennia to become effective infectious agents in humans understandably makes them superior in many aspects as gene transfer agents. The ultimate goal of designing synthetic non-viral vectors is to combine the positive traits of viruses without the negative traits of genotoxicity. Significant improvements have been made to methods of non-viral vector delivery (Conwell & Huang, 2005) with reported efficiencies that rival those achieved with viral transductions. Two classes of non-viral vectors may contribute to improved biosafety of gene therapy, namely episomally maintained vectors and integrating vectors with safer integration profiles. The ultimate goal of an ideal gene therapy vector in the context of treating many genetic diseases would be to ensure durable and regulated transgene expression either from an autonomously replicating artificial chromosome/stable plasmid or from a limited number of transgenes integrated into safe harbors in the genome. This section will review the progress in the developments of non-viral integrating vectors with safer integration profiles.

3.2.1 Transposase and recombinase

Transposases and recombinases are two classes of site-specific genome modifying agents. These enzymes recognise and bind to short stretches of DNA sequences within the vector and in the genome to mediate the integration of exogenous vector DNA into the genome. Analysis of the integration spectrum of transposases and recombinases identified some that mediate quasi-random and sequence specific integrations into the genome, a distinct advantage over randomly integrating viral vectors. Transposases and recombinases are also less immunogenic (Yant et al., 2000), have lower enhancer/promoter activity (Walisko et al., 2008) and have fewer epigenetic effects at genomic integration sites (Zhu et al., 2010), relative to viral vectors. Given their capacity to function in mammalian cells, these non-viral integrating systems evoke exciting possibilities for development into safer alternatives than randomly integrating vector systems. Several different classes and strains of transposases and recombinases have been discovered and studied as gene therapy agents. One major limitation is their relatively relaxed stringency of site-specific integrations which again raises the spectre of insertional mutagenesis. Therefore, a major effort has been directed at developing non-virally targeted gene integration systems with improved specificity. A note of caution is the low risk of unintended integration of the transposase or recombinase, which could have deleterious effects on the genome. Such risks may be minimised or abrogated by using mRNA rather than DNA to deliver the recombineering proteins. The next sections highlight advances and developments of the more commonly used transposases and recombinases.

3.2.1.1 Transposase – Sleeping Beauty, Piggy Bac, Tol2

Sleeping Beauty (SB) transposon, derived from *tc1/mariner* superfamily, is one of the most widely investigated transposase systems to date. SB transposase mediates genomic integration of vector sequences flanked by 2 inverted terminal repeats (ITR) at both transposon ends, preferentially into TA dinucleotides located within DNA segments with increased local bendability (Geurts et al., 2006), via a "cut-and-paste" mechanism. Integrations are quasi-random , without any preference for transcriptionally active regions (Huang et al., 2010). Optimised SB has a transposition efficiency ranging from 2.5 to 17% (Ortiz-Urda et al., 2003). Stable transgene integration using this system has enabled long term transgene expression in a variety of mammalian cells and animal models (Izsvák et al., 2009). Owing to the randomness of integrations, SB systems have been used also in the genetic screening and identification of potential oncogenes in *in vitro* and *in vivo* models. It is worth reiterating that these SB systems are different from those used in gene therapy applications. SB systems used in oncogene screening and discovery are deliberately modified *via* incorporation of strong transcriptional enhancers and splice acceptor sites to be potently mutagenic (Collier et al., 2005). Thus far, the use of SB as a gene therapy agent in animal models has not been associated with any tumorigenesis (Ohlfest et al., 2005). Inherent limitations of the SB system include limited cloning capacity, inhibition of transposition at high transposase concentrations and lack of targeting specificity of integrations.

Initial studies with naive SB system revealed their inherently low transposition efficiencies. Many modifications have since been introduced to create hyperactive versions of SB with increased transposition activity such as SB10 (Ivics et al., 1997), SB11 (Geurts et al., 2003) and SB100X (Mátés et al., 2009). The hyperactive SB100X, which was reported to have a 100-fold increased transposition activity, was discovered by high-throughput screening of mutants created by a PCR-based DNA shuffling strategy. Using these improved versions of SB, efficient transposition has been reported in a variety of human primary cells such as cord blood derived CD34+ hematopoietic progenitor cells (Xue et al., 2009) and primary T cells (Huang et al., 2010).

The issue of non-specific targeting by SB has been another prime focus of research aimed at inducing site-specific integration. An ideal modification would enable SB to direct transposition to a single pre-defined "safe harbor" in the genome. Skewing the random integration pattern of SB towards a more targeted profile would be hailed as an improvement. Several groups have attempted to do this by incorporating specific DNA-binding domains (DBD) either to the SB transposase (Yant et al., 2007), the transposon bearing the gene of interest (Ivics et al., 2007) or *via* a fused DBD-protein binding domain (PBD) that interacts with the transposase without modifying it (Ciuffi et al., 2006). The first strategy of fusing DBDs such as E2C (a synthetic zinc finger protein that recognizes an 18 bp target site in the 5′-untranslated region of the human *ERBB2* gene) and Gal-4 to the transposase has met with limited success. With the second strategy, Ivics and collaborators were able to demonstrate re-targeted integrations by incorporating a fusion of two DBDs to direct the transposon bearing the gene of interest to specific genomic sites where transposition could be mediated by the transposase (Ivics et al., 2007). The third strategy of utilizing a fusion of peptides to interact with the genomic locus of choice (*via* DBD) and the transposase (*via* PBD) without compromising transposase activity has also been reported by the same group (Ivics et al., 2007). However, it must be noted that none of these site targeting modifications has yet been successfully translated to human gene therapy applications, possibly due to the relatively poor efficiencies of re-targeting specificity.

The non-viral integrating SB system offers an alternative strategy for stably modifying cells for gene therapy applications. Their lack of propensity for integrating into active transcriptional units may make them safer than retroviral and lentiviral vectors. This has led to the idea of hybrid vectors that combine SB transposition with improved delivery by integrase defective lentiviruses (Vink et al., 2009). However, until effective solutions are developed to improve the specificity of integrations, the SB system may only have limited appeal for clinical gene therapy. The only human clinical trial (phase I/II, NIH-OBA no. 0804-922) utilizing the SB system is based on redirecting the specificity of T-cells by stable expression of CD19 specific-chimeric antigen receptors mediated by the SB11 transposase system (Hackett et al., 2010). However, caution should be exercised before more transposon-based systems are translated to clinical applications, especially in view of the unexpectedly high copy number of random integrations of transposase plasmid in human primary T cells (Huang et al., 2010).

Piggy Bac (PB) transposase, isolated from the cabbage looper moth (*Trichoplusia ni*) is another class of transposase which is active in human and murine cells (Ding et al., 2005). PB system has been effectively used to reprogramme induced pluripotent stem (iPS) cells (Woltjen et al., 2009) and to mutagenize mice for cancer gene discovery (Rad et al., 2010). PB demonstrated higher transposase activity than SB11 and could also be modified to incorporate DBD without loss of transposase activity (Wu et al., 2006). Several improved versions of PB have been reported. Liang et al. (Liang et al., 2009) demonstrated increased chromosomal transposition with a codon optimised PB and, more recently, reported the development of a hyperactive PB with a 7-fold increase in integration activity and showed its application for generating murine iPS cells (Yusa et al., 2011).

The Tol2 transposon of the hobo/Activator/Tam3 (hAT) family of elements derived from the medaka fish (*Orizyas latipes*) is active in human cells (Grabundzija et al., 2010). Like PB, Tol2 also tolerates overproduction inhibition and unlike the SB system has a large cloning capacity (up to 18 kb). However, both PB and Tol2 systems have significantly increased integrations into transcription start sites (TSS), CpG islands, DNaseI hypersensitivity and were able to alter transcriptional levels of neighboring genes close to integration sites in human T cells (Huang et al., 2010). This suggests a greater risk of insertional mutagenesis compared with the SB system. In this respect, the PB and Tol2 transposases may be better suited for applications where high frequencies of mutagenesis are desired, such as cancer gene discovery in mice (Rad et al., 2010).

3.2.1.2 PhiC31 phage integrase

The *Streptomyces lividans* bacteriophage derived phiC31 integrase, belonging to another class of site-specific recombinases (SSR) known as serine recombinases , works through a "cut-and paste" mechanism to mediate unidirectional integration of an attB (34 bp bacterial attachment site) bearing vector sequence to attP (39 bp phage attachment site) or pseudo attP sequences found in mammalian genomes. Unlike the reversible cyclization recombination (Cre) recombinase/flippase (flp) systems, phiC31 integrase-mediated genomic integration results in irreversible insertion of vector sequences flanked by attL and attR sequences which are refractory to further recombination by the integrase. The phiC31 integrase system has been effectively employed in recombinase mediated cassette exchange (RMCE) studies to insert transgenes into pre-integrated wild-type attP sites and also, more importantly, for stable gene transfer into endogenous pseudo attP sites in mammalian genomes. Its property of mediating irreversible unidirectional site-specific recombination into a limited number of chromosomal sites in human cells spurred intense interest as a relatively safer method for stable gene transfer for clinical applications. PhiC31 integrase has been successfully employed both *in vitro* and *in vivo* to induce stable expression of therapeutic transgenes. Ortiz-Urda et al. demonstrated functional correction of type VII collagen deficiency and laminin V deficiency in skin samples from patients with recessive dystrophic epidermolysis bullosa and junctional epidermolysis, respectively (Ortiz-Urda et al., 2002; Ortiz-Urda et al., 2003), Thyagarajan et al. generated ES lines with stable transgene expression (Thyagarajan et al., 2008) and Ishikawa et al. showed the possibility of correcting X-linked SCID deficiency by expressing IL2 receptor gamma chain in T cell-lines from SCID-X1 patients (Ishikawa et al., 2006). Successful correction of deficiencies of fumarylacetoacetate hydrolase (Held et al., 2005), alpha-1-antitrypsin, factor IX (Olivares et al., 2002) and dystrophin (Bertoni et al., 2006) have also been demonstrated in murine models. Experimental data and bioinformatic analyses point to 370 actual and potential genomic sites for phiC31 integrase-mediated integrations (Chalberg et al., 2006). The limited number of potential sequence-specific integrations coupled with the potential for long term gene expression suggests that phiC31 integrase could be a safer alternative to randomly integrating vectors. However, several studies have raised the possibility that phiC31 integrase could induce infrequent chromosomal translocations (Liu et al., 2006), possibly by promoting recombination between two endogenous pseudo attP sites in different chromosomes. Work done by our group (Sivalingam et al., 2010) suggests that the frequencies of chromosomal aberrations may differ in different cell types. Using spectral karyotyping, we observed translocations in only 4 of 300 metaphases of primary cells treated with phiC31 integrase, a frequency similar to the low background of chromosomal abnormalities reported in normal human somatic cells (Varella-Garcia et al., 2007). Moreover, chromosomal translocations have been observed *in vitro* in cells treated with vectors already approved for clinical trials such as the AAV vector (Miller et al., 2005), albeit without any pathological consequences *in vivo*. Concerns of potentially pathogenic chromosomal rearrangements have somewhat dampened interest in phiC31 integrase as an agent to be translated into clinical therapy. Although there is still a push to develop gene therapy vectors with impeccable safety profiles, our work suggests that phiC31 integrase has a relatively benign biosafety profile compared to randomly integrating retroviral and lentiviral vectors. Attempts to increase the site-specificity of phiC31 integrase include mutagenised versions of phiC31 integrase which display increased prevalence of integration at a pseudo attP site in chromosome 8p22 (Sclimenti et al., 2001) or other pseudo attP sites (Liesner et al., 2010), and versions with higher integration frequencies (Keravala et al., 2009). Thus, *ex vivo* gene therapy approaches utilising phiC31 integrase could be rendered even safer by using integrases with greater site-specificity and pre-screening gene modified cells, preferably with high-throughput methods, to exclude suspect cells and select cells with safe characteristics.

3.2.2 Targeted gene integration

Although transposases and SSRs integrate vectors non-randomly, some have questioned if these systems are truly sequence-specific or merely quasi-random as these systems are known to mediate integrations into degenerate sequences with very little homology to wild-type sequences. The terms site-directed or targeted gene integration could be used to describe modifications that are intended to direct integration to specific genomic regions recognised by the modifying agent which is usually a DNA-binding protein (DBP). Altering or skewing the integration preference of SSRs towards a particular locus is an apparent advantage as it reduces the risk of integrations into unfavourable and/or unsafe genomic regions. Gene targeting can be mediated by DNA-protein interactions or DNA-base pairing interactions. Naturally occurring DNA-binding proteins such as zinc finger proteins (ZFP) or viral peptides such as Rep have been deployed to favor DNA-protein interactions defined by their inherent specificities.

Several strategies have been proposed to achieve targeting specificity with DBPs. One approach is to tether a DBP to a recombinase by direct fusion or protein-protein interactions. This has the theoretical effect of enhancing local concentrations of the SSR at sites specified by the DBP and could more effectively restrict integration activity to a specific genomic region of choice. Care should be taken to ensure that the tethered SSR is not adversely compromised functionally. Another less frequently investigated approach relies on binding of the DBP to the vector sequence as a means of targeting vector sequences to the locus of interest (Izsvák et al., 2010). This section will review examples of targeted gene integration.

3.2.2.1 Targeting via DNA binding proteins

A classical example of targeted gene integration is observed with the AAV system which has been reported to mediate 70 to 85% of integrations into the AAVS1 site in human chromosome 19q13.3. Site-specific integration of AAV is attributed to viral Rep proteins (Rep68/Rep78) that recognize Rep binding elements in the inverted terminal repeats (ITRs) of AAV and in the AAVS1 site (Jang et al., 2005). This has led to the development of non-viral gene targeting using vector sequences flanked by AAV ITRs that can be recognised, nicked and integrated into AAVS1 sites by Rep proteins expressed in *trans* (Pieroni et al., 1998). Philpott and collaborators (Philpott et al., 2002) reported that a 138 bp P5 integration efficiency element within the ITR was sufficient for efficient Rep binding. More recently Feng et al. (Feng et al., 2006) demonstrated that efficient RBE binding and AAVS1 targeted integration could be achieved with vector sequences flanked by a 16 bp fragment within the ITR (RBEitr). Rep based non-viral systems mediate AAVS1-specific integrations in *in vitro* clonal cultures at frequencies ranging from 12 to 60% (Howden et al., 2008; Pieroni et al., 1998). On this basis, these systems have been tested and shown to operate *in vivo* (Liu, R. et al., 2010). In this sense, Rep protein may be regarded as a DBP that redirects vector sequences to a targeted genomic locus, notwithstanding the possibility for random integrations simultaneously. The persistent potential for random gene integrations coupled with the need for antibiotic selections to isolate cells with the desired targeted integrations and the relatively low targeting efficiencies are possible reasons why this strategy has not garnered much interest.

Several groups have explored the possibility of combining the integration mechanisms of transposons, HIV-1 integrase, phage integrase or SSRs with the desired DNA binding specificities of DBPs. Early gene targeting studies relied on the use of a handful of well studied naturally occurring DBPs such as yeast Gal4 (binds upstream activating sequences), *Escherichia coli* Lex A (binds to Lex A operator sequence) (Katz et al., 1996), phage λ repressor (binds phage λ operator sites) (Bushman, 1994) and murine transcription factors such as Zif268 (Bushman & Miller, 1997). Although Gal4, lex A and λ repressor proteins were instrumental in demonstrating the feasibility of targeted gene integrations *in vitro*, they were not adaptable to clinical applications as they lack physiological binding sites in the human genome. However, they have been used to bind vector sequences bearing their recognition elements and, fused with other endogenous DBPs, can be engineered to recognise elements in the human genome (Ivics et al., 2007). Other naturally occurring cellular DBPs such as scaffold attachment factor (SAF) (Ivics et al., 2007) and LEDGF (Ciuffi et al., 2006) also bind to several human genomic regions (without precise sequence recognition) and facilitate integration *in vitro*. Recent work by Gijsbers and collaborators showed the potential for redirecting lentiviral integrations into transcriptionally inactive regions by modifying the natural LEDGF/p75-viral integrase interactions (Gijsbers et al., 2010). Such retargeting strategies could potentially be adapted to engineer hybrid viral vectors with safer integration characteristics compared to current generations of viral vectors.

Amongst transcription factors, the zinc finger proteins (ZFP) are an especially favored class of DBPs, given that the human genome codes for an estimated 4500 ZFPs. An inherent limitation of naturally occurring ZFPs is their tendency to recognize short DNA sequences which may be present at many sites in the genome. This prompted engineering artificial ZFPs that could be tailored to bind to unique genomic sites. Advances in protein structure elucidation and high-throughput techniques for studying DNA-protein interactions have ushered in new possibilities of creating user-defined custom ZFPs to target specific loci in the human genome. Great expectations of the practical utility of customized ZFPs has spawned commercial investment in this technology which is the business platform of

Sangamo Biosciences which focuses on designing novel customized synthetic ZFPs for use as modulators of transcriptional control and as gene targeting agents in combination with nucleases (zinc finger nucleases). These artificial ZFPs could potentially retarget the integration spectrum of SSRs or viral integrases to enhance their biosafety.

Although tethering DBPs to recombinases and transposases has enriched targeted gene integrations, such chimeric systems continue to suffer from the disadvantage of non-directed integrations owing to residual activity of the recombinase/transposase and its inherent specificity. The holy grail of gene targeting is integration only at a single user defined safe harbour without incurring the disruptive consequences of insertional mutagenesis. This ideal may now be within reach with the advent of synthetic ZFPs. The combination of such synthetic ZFPs with existing recombinases and transposase has not yet been sufficiently evaluated. Recent years have also seen the development of other gene targeting systems based on homologous recombination which promise highly accurate gene integration but whose effectiveness has yet to be proven.

3.2.3 Site-specific homologous recombination

The transgene integration strategies discussed thus far rely on the activity of an enzyme or protein to direct and mediate the integration of vector DNA into the genome randomly or with limited specificities. Another highly site-specific strategy that has been utilized for many years to create transgenic cells and animals with targeted genome modifications exploits endogenous repair mechanisms of host cells to execute homologous recombination, thereby incorporating exogenous DNA into specific genomic sites. Effective homologous recombination requires transgenic DNA to be flanked by sequences homologous to the genomic sequences into which they are to be integrated. These exogenous DNA sequences are templates in the process of homologous recombination and are subsequently replicated along with the genomic locus during host cell divisions. The basal frequency of homologous recombination involving exogenous DNA is very low, occurring in 1 out of 10^5 - 10^7 treated cells. It was discovered that this frequency can be enhanced 1000-fold by creating site-specific nicks in the genome (Rouet et al., 1994), thereby stimulating DNA repair at these sites. DNA is repaired by one of two main mechanisms i.e. non-homologous end joining or homologous recombination, although variations of these mechanisms are also possible. Error prone non-homologous end joining results in genomic DNA repair without transgene integrations while homologous recombination may result in site-specific integration of the transgene into the desired locus. In the context of gene therapy, the prospect of exploiting homologous recombination is appealing as it holds the potential for targeted gene repair and precise transgene integration into safe genomic loci. A patient's cells could in theory be modified *ex vivo* to correct disease-causing mutations or to integrate a transgene for long term expression of a deficient or defective protein before being reimplanted into the same patients (autologous cell therapy). Recent advances exploring such strategies will be discussed in this section.

3.2.3.1 Meganucleases

A more efficient and reproducible strategy for gene editing or integration that has been the focus of recent research is the use of highly site-specific endonucleases to induce double stranded DNA breaks into specific genomic sites in order to stimulate deletions via non-homologous end joining or homologous recombination of exogenously delivered DNA into these sites. Three main classes of engineered endonucleases have emerged: zinc finger nucleases which are chimeras of ZFP and catalytic domain of *Fok* I restriction enzyme; chemical endonucleases which consist of chemical or peptidic cleavers fused with DNA recognising polymers; and meganucleases (homing endonucleases) which are capable of recognizing and cleaving target DNA sequences, usually 14 - 40 bp in length. HO endonuclease which mediates mating type switch in *Saccharomyces cerevisiae,* I-CreI and I-SceI meganucleases are examples of naturally occurring homing endonucleases. However, the applications of naturally occurring meganucleases have been limited either by the lack of recognition sites or by the presence of more than a single site in the human genome. The LAGLIDADG family of meganucleases includes I-SceI and I-CreI which are the largest and best characterised meganucleases, and are active as monomers or homodimers. Their catalytic cleavage centres are embedded within the DNA-binding domains and thus making non-specific cleavage very unlikely. Elucidation of the protein structures of endonucleases such as SceI and CreI have accelerated engineering of meganuclease variants with unique genomic recognition sites. Most effort have been directed to developing I-CreI and I-SceI variants with unique specificities and reduced off-target cleavage activity. Thus far two engineered meganucleases cleaving unique genomic loci in the human *XPC* (Arnould et al., 2007) and *Rag1* genes (Grizot et al., 2009) have been reported. Other improvements have been to engineer variant CreI (naturally homodimeric) meganuclease to function as obligate heterodimers (Fajardo-Sanchez et al., 2008) or as single-chain derivatives (Li et al., 2009). Computational approaches (Ashworth et al., 2006) have integrated structural and high throughput screening data to identify the cleavage properties of 18000 engineered meganucleases, based mostly on CreI meganuclease (Galetto et al., 2009).

Thus far, homologous recombination of transgenes with meganucleases has been demonstrated in only a few cell types and a comprehensive evaluation of their genotoxicity potentials has not been reported. The future development of engineered variants that collectively offer a wide spectrum of unique integration sites may be useful but will need careful evaluation. At present, there is a need to engineer endonucleases having user-defined specificities. This requirement may be more readily fulfilled with zinc finger nuclease technology given the potentially broader spectrum of genome-specific ZFPs that can be custom engineered.

3.2.3.2 Zinc finger nucleases

Zinc finger nucleases (ZFNs), first designed by Chandrasekaran and collaborators (Kim et al., 1996), are artificial chimeras composed of a tandem array of DNA-binding zinc finger proteins fused with the catalytic subunit of the non-specific *Fok*I restriction endonuclease *via* a short linker peptide. Naturally occurring zinc finger transcription factors, such as the murine Zif268 or human SP1, provide the framework in which each Cys2-His2 zinc finger that specifically recognises a 3-bp DNA sequence can be replaced to generate a novel ZFP capable in theory of binding to unique genomic sequences. Such polydactyl ZFPs have been assembled by modular assembly (Segal et al., 2003) by which individual zinc fingers are combined in a modular fashion to form a tandem array designed to recognize a selected DNA sequence. Another strategy is oligomerised pool engineering (OPEN) that takes into account the context dependence of sequence recognition and binding of each individual zinc finger as it may be influenced by its neighboring fingers (Maeder et al., 2008). Most recently, Sander and collaborators introduced yet another approach that takes into account context dependence of ZFPs. Termed the context dependent assembly (CoDA), this method involves first identifying two pairs of efficient ZFPs as identified by bacterial-2 hybrid assays. A 3-

finger ZFP array is next assembled using, as the central zinc finger, the finger that was common between the two pairs (Sander et al., 2011). ZFNs are designed as pairs to bind to adjacent nucleotide sequences on opposite strands. Their binding and localization at the intended locus induces dimerization and activation of *Fok*I endonuclease activity which induces double stranded DNA breaks at these specific sites. DNA breaks are repaired either by non-homologous end joining or by homology directed repair (presumably *via* synthesis dependent strand annealing). Initial concerns regarding the potential toxicity of off-target cleavage mediated by homodimers of *Fok*I catalytic monomers has been addressed by *Fok*I variants engineered to function as obligate heterodimers (Miller et al., 2007; Szczepek et al., 2007).

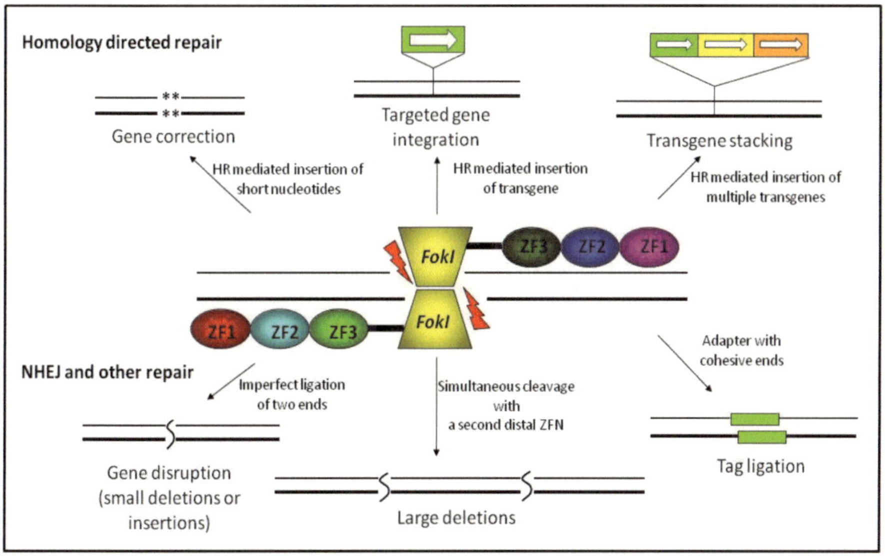

Fig. 6. Genome editing with ZFNs. Site-specific cleavage of genomic DNA by ZFNs can be repaired by homology-directed repair to correct or induce point mutations and to insert single or multiple transgenes (in the presence of donor molecule). Repair by NHEJ results in gene disruption *via* small insertions and/or deletions. Site-specific insertion of molecular tags and large genomic deletions may also be achieved with ZFN mediated cleavage of genomic DNA. (*Adapted from Urnov et al., 2010.*)

Two major applications of ZFNs to gene therapy are permanent gene disruption by insertions/deletions events during the error-prone non-homologous end joining repair or site-specific transgene insertion *via* repair by homologous recombination or homology-directed repair (figure 6). Since the turn of the millennium, ZFN technology has been harnessed to demonstrate feasibility of targeted gene corrections, transgene insertions and gene disruptions, in addition to pioneering a new approach for deriving transgenic plants and animals. ZFN technology has been used to derive transgenic crops with improved traits by mutagenesis of genes or targeted integration of herbicide resistance genes in species such as *Arabidopsis thaliana*, tobacco and *Zea mays* (Shukla et al., 2009; Townsend et al., 2009) and to derive specific gene knock-outs strains of mice and rats (Rémy et al., 2010). Given the ability to permanently disrupt specific genes, ZFNs have proved useful for elucidating gene functions during embryogenesis and development. Heritable targeted gene disruption has been demonstrated in human embryonic stem cells, *Danio rerio* and *Drosophilia* (Hockemeyer et al., 2009; McCammon & Amacher, 2010; Carroll et al., 2010). ZFN-mediated gene knock-out has been effectively employed to disrupt the *CCR5* locus in human hematopoietic stem cells as a possible therapeutic strategy to confer resistance to HIV-1 infection by adoptive cell therapy *in vivo* (Perez et al., 2008). This has led to the use of ZFN-modified T cells in three phase I human clinical trials - for glioblastoma (NCT01082926) and HIV-1 treatment (NCT00842634, NCT01044654) (Urnov et al., 2010). Targeted disruption of several other genes such as *Bax* and *Bak* has also been demonstrated in human cells (Cost et al., 2010). The ability to correct genetic mutations by base substitution and the theoretical potential for exquisitely precise site-specific gene insertions has opened a plethora of possibilities for gene therapy applications. Porteus and Baltimore first reported the possibilities of targeted ZFN mediated genome editing in human somatic cells with gene correction of a pre-integrated GFP reporter gene (Porteus & Baltimore, 2003). Work by Urnov et al. has also been influential in demonstrating efficient correction of a *IL2Rγ* gene mutation in human cells, pointing to the prospect of future therapy for SCID-X1 (Urnov et al., 2005). Others have shown the feasibility of integrating exogenous DNA up to 8 kb in size (Moehle et al., 2007), and into other human genomic sites such as *PIGA, PPP1R12C and POU5F1* in primary cells such as mesenchymal stromal cells (Benabdallah et al., 2010), cord blood derived CD34+ HSCs (Lombardo et al., 2007), embryonic stem cells and iPS cells (Hockemeyer et al., 2009).

A current limitation of ZFN technology for site-directed transgene insertion is concern about unintended genomic modifications and possible biological hazards therefrom. Although several groups have demonstrated that the likelihood of off-target genomic modifications is low, there has been no comprehensive genome-wide analysis to date to rigorously support these claims. Potential off-target interactions of ZFNs must be evaluated by genome-wide techniques such as CHIP-based methods combined with deep sequencing in order to detect rare integration events. Long term monitoring of ZFN-modified cells is essential, using small and large animal models to assess fully any potential genotoxicity. The current efficiency of targeted gene insertion using ZFNs is still relatively low and may not warrant its broad application in human gene therapy. This awaits more specific ZFNs with robust and efficient targeted genome modification activity. Several useful resources are currently available in the public domain to aid the design, construction and testing of specific ZFNs. Helpful information and software tools pertaining to ZFN design and construction as well as a collection of ZFN plasmids and reagents for constructing and testing ZFNs are readily available to the research community at The Zinc Finger Consortium (http://www.zincfingers.org). Information on individual C2H2 zinc fingers and engineered zinc finger arrays have been compiled into databases such as the Zinc Finger Database (ZiFDB; http://bindr.gdcb.iastate.edu/ZiFDB) (Fu et al., 2009). Web-based resources such as Zinc Finger Targeter (ZiFiT; http://bindr.gdcb.iastate.edu/ZiFiT/) (Sander et al., 2010) and more recently ZFNGenome (http://bindr.gdcb.iastate.edu/ZFNGenome) (Reyon et al., 2011) provide excellent tools to aid the identification of potential ZF binding sites in user supplied target regions. They include software that calculate strengths of predicted ZFNs to be engineered by modular assembly or the OPEN method and also give information regarding potential off-target binding sites. Furthermore, Sangamo Biosciences and several other groups have described assays to evaluate the functional specificities of user-designed ZFNs Recent improvements to ZFNs have also focused on deriving *Fok*I variants with increased cleavage activities, in an attempt to increase the rate of genome modifications

(Guo et al., 2010). Higher ZFN cleavage activity possibly due to increased protein stability was also achieved by conditioning cells to transient mild hypothermia (Doyon et al., 2010). We need better understanding of the factors that influence the efficiency of intracellular homologous recombination and how these can be exploited to obtain higher gene targeting efficiencies. More work is needed to identify and test safe harbors in the human genome and to design ZFNs targeting them. Lastly, improvements to vector designs such as CpG-free vectors, the use of suitable physiological promoters, codon-optimised transgenes and incorporation of relevant insulator and enhancer elements would be pertinent to achieve durable transgene expression and minimise risks of insertional gene mishaps.

An ideal gene-based treatment for some monogenic disorders would be to derive self-renewing cells expressing a corrected version of the defective gene *via* site-specific integration in a safe genomic locus. Such gene modified cells could be exhaustively evaluated for their genotoxic potential *ex vivo* before being administered into patients. Given the lexicon of site-specific ZFNs that is being developed, this could be a real possibility in the near future with ZFN-modified stem cells.

3.3 Episomal vectors

One of the most apparent advantages of extra-chromosomal vectors as gene transfer agents is the greatly decreased risk of insertional mutagenesis compared to integrating vectors. Episomal plasmids can be maintained at high copy number, have potentially higher transgene expression levels and are less likely to suffer transgene silencing or positional variegation effects associated with genomic integrations.

The essential characteristics of extra-chromosomal vectors are episomal maintenance, autonomous replication and segregation into daughter cells. Episomal vectors can be categorised as either viral based if they rely on viral origins of replication and other virally encoded proteins for replication and partitioning into daughter cells, or chromosome based, if they depend on elements derived from the human genome (figure 7). Examples of viral based episomal vectors include those based on plasmid replicons of viruses such as simian virus 40 (SV40), bovine papillomavirus (BPV) and Epstein Barr virus (EBV) or those based on plasmid replicons carrying limited viral components such as oriP/EBV nuclear antigen 1 (EBNA1). Chromosome based episomal vectors include the scaffold/matrix attachment region (S/MAR) based pEPI vectors and artificial chromosomes.

3.3.1 Viral based episomal vectors

Concerns relating to the oncogenic transforming properties of polyoma viruses such as SV40 and the restricted mode of replication afforded by BPV have deterred the use of such viral replicon based vectors. The EBNA/oriP episomal vector has been one of the more commonly used viral based episomal vector systems tested for gene therapy. It relies on the EBV origin of replication (oriP) and the trans-acting factor, EBNA-1, for episomal replication within eukaryotic cells. The origin of replication consists of the dyad symmetry (DS) element and the family of repeats (FR) elements which serve as binding sites for EBNA-1. Interaction of EBNA-1 with DS elements mediates episomal replication while interaction with FR elements ensures nuclear retention of oriP bearing plasmids. Long term transgene expression has been demonstrated with the use of EBNA/oriP plasmids both *in vitro* and *in vivo* (Saeki et al., 1998). A major drawback is the concern that EBNA-1 may have oncogenic effects (Schulz & Cordes, 2009) although this has been questioned by a single report that

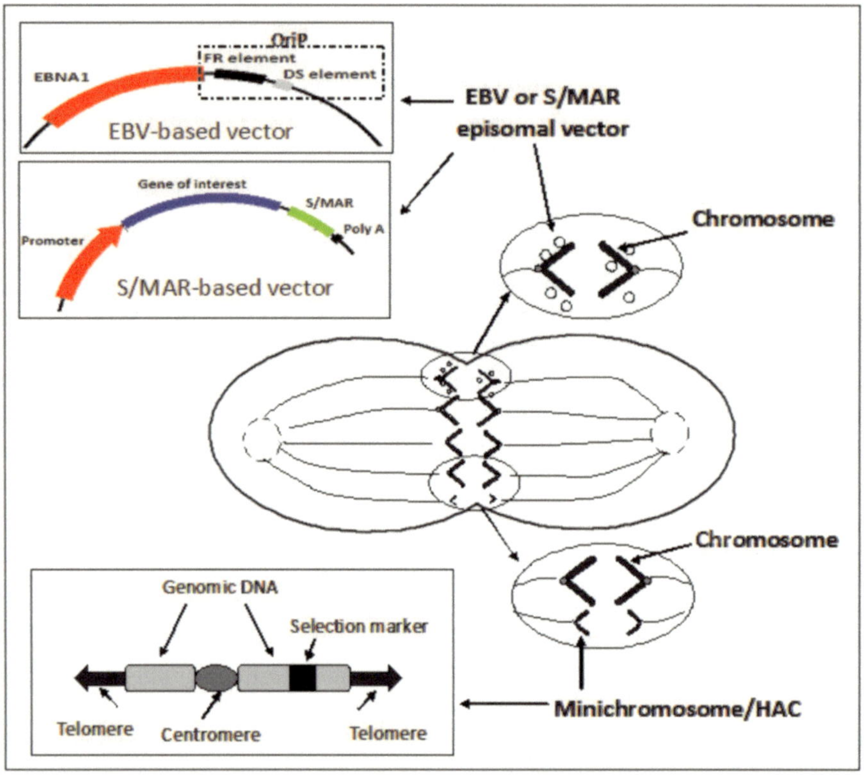

Fig. 7. Episomal vectors and artificial chromosomes. EBV-based episomal vectors require EBNA-1 and oriP elements for nuclear retention and episomal replication while S/MAR elements support the same functions in chromosome-based pEPI vectors. Nuclear retention for both types of vectors is mediated by tethering to subnuclear structures and transcriptionally active sites in the chromosomes. Mini-chromosomes or artificial chromosomes bearing selective genomic regions, centromeres, telomeres and selection marker can be assembled *de novo* and have been shown to segregate into daughter cells during mitosis. (*Redrawn from Lufino et al., 2008.*)

EBNA-1 does not activate cellular genes (Kang et al., 2001). Nevertheless, this prompted development of safer episomal vectors devoid of EBNA-1/oriP elements. Based on the known functions of DS/FR elements and EBNA-1, several groups investigated the functional features of episomal vectors substituted for these viral elements. Gerhardj et al. showed that episomal replication was possible even when the EBNA-1/oriP DS elements were replaced with small eukaryotic sequences (Gerhardt et al., 2006). Recently, Thomae and collaborators reported episomal replication and retention of an episomal plasmid (pCon) in which the DS elements were replaced with tet-operator sites and EBNA-1 replaced with a fusion protein comprised of the high mobility group protein, HGMA1a, which is known to interact with the cellular replication machinery (Thomae et al., 2008).These studies have shown the feasibility of developing episomal vectors devoid of EBNA-1/oriP elements but have yet to find favor as efficient and safer alternatives to existing EBNA-1/oriP episomal vectors. With their ultimate intended use in human clinical applications in view, the trend has now shifted to developing episomally replicating vectors exclusively composed of functional eukaryotic chromosomal elements devoid of foreign or viral elements.

3.3.2 Chromosome based episomal vectors

Three main approaches have been adopted in attempts to develop chromosome based episomal vectors: plasmid vectors with mammalian origins of replication, plasmid vectors with chromosomal S/MAR and mammalian artificial chromosomes.

Attempts to derive autonomously replicating plasmids by incorporating mammalian origins of replication had previously met with limited success, leading to speculation that epigenetic factors control the activation of mammalian origins of replication (Jackson et al., 2006).

The idea of deriving episomally maintained plasmids by incorporating S/MAR was based on the assumptions that mammalian replication origins are bound to the nuclear scaffold or matrix before the onset of DNA replication. S/MAR sequences function by tethering DNA to subnuclear structures and transcriptionally active sites in the chromosomes through the interaction with nuclear matrix protein scaffold attachment factor A (SAF-A) (Stehle et al., 2007) and are necessary for organization of chromatin loops that define the boundaries of chromatin domains (Jackson et al., 2006). The best characterised S/MAR based vectors are the pEPI vectors, which carry a 2kb- S/MAR element derived from human β-interferon gene cluster. These vectors are maintained at copy numbers of less than 10 per cell, replicate once per cell cycle and have been shown to be maintained episomally for several hundred generations in cell lines (Papapetrou et al., 2005), primary cells and animal models. Episomal replication is stringently dependent on transcription upstream from and into the 2kb-S/MAR element present within the plasmid during, but not after, episome establishment. Early generation S/MAR-based pEPI vectors have significant limitations associated with low rates of nuclear establishment, unintended genomic integrations, intrinsic vector instability, limited cloning capacity and loss of vector in dividing cells in the absence of initial selection pressure (Papapetrou et al., 2005).

Several improvements have since been made to pEPI vectors. Hasse and collaborators reported higher and persistent transgene expression *in vitro* and *in vivo* when they modified the pEPI vector to contain 60% reduced CpG DNA motifs and replaced the CMV promoter with EF1-alpha promoter (Haase et al., 2010). Another study looked into splitting pEPI vectors into a "mini-plasmid" containing prokaryotic vector sequences and a "mini-circle vector" comprised only of eukaryotic sequences including the transgene and a minimised S/MAR (Broll et al., 2010). The reduced size of S/MAR element allowed efficient and complete read-through of transcripts into the S/MAR regions and was associated with improved mRNA processing and higher expression levels. Furthermore, the use of plasmids devoid of prokaryotic sequences avoided the problems commonly associated with prokaryotic expression vectors such as heterochromatin formation, gene silencing and eventual loss from host cells (Haase et al., 2010).

Theoretically, artificial chromosomes would fit the role of ideal episomal vectors, given its very large cloning capacity, superior mitotic and meiotic stability and efficient segregation into daughter cells. Initial work on *Saccharomyces cervisiae* led to the discovery of yeast autonomously replicating sequences and subsequently, to yeast centromeres and telomeres which eventually enabled construction of yeast artificial chromosomes. This defined the path for constructing human artificial chromosomes (HACs) after human centromeres, telomeres and origins of replication had been identified and isolated as essential features for extra-chromosomal replication and retention. HACs can be constructed by a tedious process using a top-down or bottom-up approach. In the former, whole chromosomes in live cells are truncated by irradiation or telomere fragmentation into minichromosomes. The bottom-up approach assembles artificial chromosomes from isolated functional elements i.e. centromeres, telomeres and replication origins. Transgenes of interest are usually cloned into these artificial chromosomes by recombination using the Cre-recombinase/loxP or FLP/FRT systems (Kotzamanis et al., 2005). HAC and minichromosomes are delivered into cells by microcell mediated chromosome transfer (MMCT) or micro-injection. Several groups have demonstrated long-term transgene expression in several cell types modified with HACs and minichromosomes (Grimes et al., 2001). The major disadvantages of HAC are the difficulty of constructing and producing them and the low efficiency of intracellular delivery, given their very large size compared to other gene transfer vectors. Nevertheless, successful gene transfer of a 245 kb BAC vector has been demonstrated even with non-viral vectors based on a "LID vector" design comprised of lipofectin (L), integrin-targeting peptide (I) and DNA of interest (D), with efficiencies ranging from 10 -15% in 293 and MRC-5v2 cells. HACS are most efficiently delivered by MMCT. The efficiency of delivery and integrity of delivered chromosomes can be improved by the use of polycations such as poly-L-lysine and poly-ethylenimine. Viral delivery systems for extra-chromosomal vectors include vectors with EBV and CMV based amplicons, adenoviruses and HSV vectors.

Another class of gene transfer vectors capable of accommodating large genomic segments are the high-capacity extra-chromosomal vectors. These vectors drive the expression of genes of interest from a genomic DNA locus of extensive size that could be expected to be superior as well as to have greater fidelity of physiological control owing to the combined effects of regulatory elements, non-coding regions, chromatin opening elements and native promoters compared to cDNA expression from minimal promoters. Recent improvements in extra-chromosomal vectors include the development of large capacity F-factor based bacterial artificial chromosomes and P1-derived artificial chromosomes that incorporate EBV retentions systems (oriP and EBNA). Recent studies have also shown stable transgene expression from BAC vectors coupled with S/MAR elements (Lufino et al., 2008).

Episomal non-viral vectors represent a class of vectors that could function as efficient and safe gene therapy agents for persistent long term expression not only in *ex vivo* modified cells but also *in vivo*. The exciting possibility of utilizing them with adult and embryonic stem cells for *ex vivo* gene therapy warrants investigation. However, as with other gene transfer techniques, caution must be exercised to rigorously estimate the small but troubling risk of potentially random vector insertion (Wang et al., 2004).

3.4 Suicide genes as safety mechanisms for treatment modalities

The benefits of gene therapy for life threatening diseases for which there is currently no effective treatment justify their continued evaluation in clinical trials despite the known risks of iatrogenic complications. It is clear from the preceding sections that most research efforts have been directed at enhancing the biosafety of gene therapy vectors. An additional strategy to intervene and reverse adverse vector effects is to include secondary safety mechanisms capable of rapidly triggering the selective elimination of rogue transgenic cells. Suicide gene therapy or gene-directed enzyme prodrug therapy relies on the expression of transgene products from "suicide genes" that convert inactive prodrugs into cytotoxic drugs, thus selectively eliminating transgenic cells that express the suicide gene. Several suicide genes such as herpes simplex virus 1 thymidine kinase (HSV-TK), bacterial cytosine deaminase (CD), bacterial carboxypeptidase-G2 (CPDG2), purine nucleoside phosphorylase (PNP) and nitroreductase (NR) and their cognate prodrugs have been tested for their efficacy as agents of selective cell destruction (Denny, 2003). Problems such as suicide gene silencing, incomplete elimination of targeted cells, cytotoxicity to non-gene expressing cells and immune response to suicide genes have reduced the efficacy of such approaches. Continued improvements to existing suicide genes and prodrugs as well as development of novel genes capable of selective elimination of cells with reduced cytotoxicity to normal cells are necessary improvements to suicide gene therapy for clinical applications. Recent developments in suicide gene therapy strategies will be briefly discussed in this section.

3.4.1 HSV thymidine kinase

The HSV-TK suicide gene and its prodrug, gancyclovir (GCV) is one of the most extensively studied and the only clinically validated suicide gene/prodrug system. HSV-TK phosphorylates the non-toxic acyclic analogs of deoxyguanosine such as GCV and acyclovir (ACV) into a toxic form that becomes incorporated into DNA. This leads to eventual cell death by inhibiting DNA synthesis and disrupting DNA replication in sensitive cells. The use of HSV-TK has found broad applications *in vitro* as negative selection in homologous recombination studies and has been successfully used in phase I-II clinical trials for prevention of graft versus host disease following allogeneic stem cell transplantation (Lupo-Stanghellini et al., 2010). It has also been investigated extensively in cancer gene therapy to eliminate tumor cells. An on-going phase III clinical trial by Ark Therapeutics (www.arktherapeutics.com) is evaluating HSV-TK combined with surgery and chemotherapy in patients with high grade gliomas (cited by Preuß et al., 2010). However, there are certain disadvantages of the HSV-TK/GCV system. These include GCV toxicity at clinical doses, insensitivity of HSV-TK expressing cells to GCV due to inactive spliced HSV-TK variants (Garin et al., 2001), cellular toxicity of high levels of HSV-TK that phosphorylate endogenous thymidine (Balzarini et al., 2006) and the inherent immunogenicity of viral epitopes presented by HSV-TK protein (Berger et al., 2006). Several improvements have been made to improve the performance of HSV-TK such as reduced splice variants (Chalmers et al., 2001), improved GCV sensitivity (Black et al., 2001) and decreased affinity for endogenous thymidine (Balzarini et al., 2006). Notable HSV-TK variants with improved sensitivity to GCV include the SR39 (Black et al., 2001) and Q7530A (Mercer et al., 2002) mutants. Splice corrected versions of HSV-TK (scHSV-TK) have been derived by mutating internal splice sites within wild-type HSV-TK gene to prevent the emergence of GCV-resistant cells expressing inactive HSV-TK splice variants (Chalmers et al., 2001). Another recent development is the use of a codon-optimized HSV-TK A168H mutant, TK007 which causes faster and more robust GCV mediated killing of cells while having less non-specific cytotoxicity (Preuß et al., 2010) due to the reduced affinity for endogenous thymidine. These improved versions of HSV-TK could function effectively as benign suicide genes that would be activated to selectively eliminate implanted gene modified cells in the event of a serious adverse complication e.g. oncogenic transformation. However, outstanding issues such as immunogenicity of HSV-TK and the possibility of immune-mediated rejection of gene modified cells reiterate the need to investigate other novel human-based and possibly non-immunogenic suicide genes as better alternatives.

3.4.2 Suicide genes in development

The immunogenic nature of non-mammalian suicide genes such as HSV-TK and cytosine deaminase and the unintended immune mediated elimination of suicide gene expressing cells has prompted the search for novel human and/or non-immunogenic genes able to function as suicide genes. A human T-cell surface antigen, CD20, was one of the first human suicide genes to be investigated for its capacity to eliminate CD20 expressing T-cells using anti-CD20 antibodies. The CD20/anti CD20 mAb may be suitable for use in gene modified HSCs but requires high cellular expression of CD20 antigen and may also deplete cells normally expressing CD20 (Lupo-Stanghellini et al., 2010). Other systems that could be useful include the FK-506 binding protein (FKBP-FAS)/AP20187, AP1903 dimerization system that relies on the selective induction of apoptosis by expressing proapoptotic Fas-ligand molecules intracellularly, to be activated by non-toxic chemically induced dimerization of the FKBP-FAS molecules. Another notable non-immunogenic system (iCasp9) relies on activating apoptosis in selected cells by fusing the death domains of Caspase-9 with FKBP elements, which can be induced to dimerize and activate apoptosis (Tey et al., 2007). This system is currently being evaluated in an on-going clinical trial for graft versus host disease (cited by Lupo-Stanghellini et al., 2010).

In summary, the incorporation of safety switches in the form of suicide genes to eliminate gene modified cells would be essential and beneficial features in future clinical gene therapy. Ongoing efforts to develop suicide genes with increased prodrug sensitivity and reduced unintended toxicity, as well as exploring novel systems to selectively induce cell death ought to be helpful adjuncts to improve the biosafety of human gene therapy - currently mainly in clinical trials.

4. Challenges and future prospects

Although there have been major innovations and improvements to gene therapy in the past decade, the key challenges of sustained efficacy, biosafety and immunogenicity remain important challenges that need to be dealt with. Several early clinical trials have emphasized the primary need for increased transduction efficiencies and durable expression of delivered transgenes to achieve clinically meaningful treatment efficacy. Viral vectors now have significantly improved tissue specificity and transduction efficiencies. Delivery methods of non-viral vectors have also significantly advanced to attain near-comparable efficiencies. The use of *ex vivo* modified stem cells with self-renewing capacity *in vivo* may overcome the constraints of utilizing nondividing cells for *ex vivo* gene therapy for selected diseases. Continuous improvements are being integrated into vector designs to enable durable transgene expressions and minimise transgene silencing *in vivo*. Biosafety concerns of immunogenicity and insertional mutagenesis, although uncommon, are nonetheless barriers to clinical acceptance and there are ongoing concerted efforts to address these problems. It is important to ensure that improvised or novel vectors (viral or non-viral) are comprehensively tested and evaluated for their genotoxic potential. Absence of evidence is not evidence of absence of genotoxic risk. Genotoxicity risks should be evaluated using a range of tools to address interrogate cells at multiple levels i.e. transcriptome, genome, epigenome and chromosomes. High-throughput screening methods are highly desirable to increase the sensitivity and accuracy of characterization. Currently, integrating vectors are favoured choice given their ability to mediate high levels of and long-term transgene expression. The caveat is the random or quasi-random nature of gene integrations mediated by most currently used integrating vectors. The risks of insertional mutagenesis may be minimized by using episomally maintained vectors and by gene targeting strategies, ideally by targeted gene addition into a safe and unique genomic locus. At present such alternative strategies have not achieved sufficient efficacy to be translated into clinical applications. Continued efforts and greater resources therefore need to be channelled into developing episomal vectors and site-specific integrating vectors.

Whilst gene therapy aims primarily to correct inherent deficiencies in cells and organ systems, the emerging field of regenerative medicine offers the prospect of producing replacements for diseased or defective cells. Since Yamanaka and collaborators (Takahashi & Yamanaka, 2006) demonstrated the ability to convert somatic cells, such as fibroblasts, into induced pluripotent stem (iPS) cells by combined expression of *Oct4, Sox2, Klf4* and *c-Myc*, there has been a flurry of reports on the ability of other combinations of transcription factors and safer reprogramming methods to attain similar outcomes. In view of concerns of the need for genomic integration of the transcription factor genes for continued expression, others have adapted the use of episomal vectors, RNA and even peptide versions of the transcription factors to generate iPS cells. iPS cells have the potential to be differentiated into cells of the endoderm, ectoderm and mesoderm and could prove to be useful for treating diseases where replacement with fully functional surrogate cells or regenerating stem cells is a therapeutic option. Thus the field of regenerative medicine is an exciting field that could rival or complement present forms of gene and cell-based therapy in future.

5. Conclusion

Beginning in the 1960s, convergent advances in human genetics and recombinant DNA technology spawned the seductively compelling notion of gene therapy to cure, or at least, ameliorate diseases caused by defective genes. Almost half a century later, the initial enthusiasm and euphoria have been greatly tempered by the sober recognition that while gene therapy is simple in concept, it is highly complex and challenging in execution. The early promises of human gene therapy raised unrealistically high expectations that gene medicine was round the corner. Compounded by well publicised serious iatrogenic complications from a small number of clinical trials, a pall quickly descended on the field from the late 1990s that led many investigators to flee from a field of research that came to be perceived as both unfeasible and unfundable.

Gene therapy has now emerged from a much needed phase of reflection and correction. There is clear evidence that appropriately selected monogenic and acquired diseases can benefit from gene-based therapy. Notwithstanding that there remains a risk to certain viral vectors, the decision to reinitiate gene therapy trials for SCID-X1 (NCT01129544) is acknowledgement of what gene therapy may offer to diseases that are currently difficult to treat effectively or at reasonable cost. Failures of gene therapy should not discredit the field but ought to be opportunities to deepen scientific understanding of the complex processes demanded for therapeutic success. Safety is a key consideration, particularly with respect to genotoxicity. The confluence of autologous cell therapy with conventional gene therapy appears to be a promising approach. Cells that are first modified *ex vivo* lend themselves readily to comprehensive biosafety assessments that are not feasible with conventional *in vivo* gene therapy. The ability to thoroughly characterize cells for the desired phenotype, and for genotoxicity and other risks before *in vivo* implantation or administration should go some way to making such novel treatments safe.

(The authors were unable to cite all relevant publications owing to page limitations.)

6. References

Aiuti, A., Cattaneo, F., Galimberti, S., Benninghoff, U., Cassani, B., Callegaro, L., Scaramuzza, S., Andolfi, G., Mirolo, M. & Brigida, I. (2009). Gene therapy for immunodeficiency due to adenosine deaminase deficiency. *N Engl J Med*, Vol.360, No.5, pp. 447-458, ISSN 0028-4793

Apolonia, L., Waddington, S. N., Fernandes, C., Ward, N. J., Bouma, G., Blundell, M. P., Thrasher, A. J., Collins, M. K. & Philpott, N. J. (2007). Stable gene transfer to muscle using non-integrating lentiviral vectors. *Mol Ther*, Vol.15, No.11, pp. 1947-1954, ISSN 1525-0016

Appelt, J. U., Giordano, F. A., Ecker, M., Roeder, I., Grund, N., Hotz-Wagenblatt, A., Opelz, G., Zeller, W. J., Allgayer, H., Fruehauf, S. & Laufs, S. (2009). QuickMap: a public tool for large-scale gene therapy vector insertion site mapping and analysis. *Gene Ther*, Vol.16, No.7, pp. 885-893, ISSN 0969-7128

Arnould, S., Perez, C., Cabaniols, J. P., Smith, J., Gouble, A., Grizot, S., Epinat, J. C., Duclert, A., Duchateau, P. & Pâques, F. (2007). Engineered I-CreI derivatives cleaving sequences from the human XPC gene can induce highly efficient gene correction in mammalian cells. *J Mol Biol*, Vol.371, No.1, pp. 49-65, ISSN 0022-2836

Ashworth, J., Havranek, J. J., Duarte, C. M., Sussman, D., Monnat, R. J., Stoddard, B. L. & Baker, D. (2006). Computational redesign of endonuclease DNA binding and cleavage specificity. *Nature*, Vol.441, No.7093, pp. 656-659, ISSN 0028-0836

Avery, O. T., Macleod, C. M. & McCarty, M. (1944). Studies on the chemical nature of the substance inducing transformation of pneumococcal types: Induction of transformation by a desoxyribonucleic acid fraction isolated from pneumococcus type III. *J Exp Med*, Vol.79, No.2, pp. 137-158, ISSN 0022-1007

Balzarini, J., Liekens, S., Solaroli, N., El Omari, K., Stammers, D. K. & Karlsson, A. (2006). Engineering of a single conserved amino acid residue of herpes simplex virus type 1 thymidine kinase allows a predominant shift from pyrimidine to purine nucleoside phosphorylation. *J Biol Chem*, Vol.281, No.28, pp. 19273-19279, ISSN 0021-9258

Bauer, T. R., Allen, J. M., Hai, M., Tuschong, L. M., Khan, I. F., Olson, E. M., Adler, R. L., Burkholder, T. H., Gu, Y. C., Russell, D. W. & Hickstein, D. D. (2008). Successful treatment of canine leukocyte adhesion deficiency by foamy virus vectors. *Nat Med*, Vol.14, No.1, pp. 93-97, ISSN 1078-8956

Benabdallah, B. F., Allard, E., Yao, S., Friedman, G., Gregory, P. D., Eliopoulos, N., Fradette, J., Spees, J. L., Haddad, E., Holmes, M. C. & Beauséjour, C. M. (2010). Targeted gene addition to human mesenchymal stromal cells as a cell-based plasma-soluble protein delivery platform. *Cytotherapy*, Vol.12, No.3, pp. 394-399, ISSN 1465-3249

Berger, C., Flowers, M. E., Warren, E. H. & Riddell, S. R. (2006). Analysis of transgene-specific immune responses that limit the in vivo persistence of adoptively transferred HSV-TK-modified donor T cells after allogeneic hematopoietic cell transplantation. *Blood*, Vol.107, No.6, pp. 2294-2302, ISSN 0006-4971

Bertoni, C., Jarrahian, S., Wheeler, T. M., Li, Y., Olivares, E. C., Calos, M. P. & Rando, T. A. (2006). Enhancement of plasmid-mediated gene therapy for muscular dystrophy by directed plasmid integration. *Proc Natl Acad Sci U S A*, Vol.103, No.2, pp. 419-424, ISSN 0027-8424

Black, M. E., Kokoris, M. S. & Sabo, P. (2001). Herpes simplex virus-1 thymidine kinase mutants created by semi-random sequence mutagenesis improve prodrug-mediated tumor cell killing. *Cancer Res*, Vol.61, No.7, pp. 3022-3026, ISSN 0008-5472

Blaese, R. M., Culver, K. W., Miller, A. D., Carter, C. S., Fleisher, T., Clerici, M., Shearer, G., Chang, L., Chiang, Y., Tolstoshev, P., Greenblatt, J. J., Rosenberg, S. A., Klein, H., Berger, M., Mullen, C. A., Ramsey, W. J., Muul, L., Morgan, R. A. & Anderson, W. F. (1995). T lymphocyte-directed gene therapy for ADA- SCID: initial trial results after 4 years. *Science*, Vol.270, No.5235, pp. 475-480, ISSN 0036-8075

Bosticardo, M., Ghosh, A., Du, Y., Jenkins, N. A., Copeland, N. G. & Candotti, F. (2009). Self-inactivating retroviral vector-mediated gene transfer induces oncogene activation and immortalization of primary murine bone marrow cells. *Mol Ther*, Vol.17, No.11, pp. 1910-1918, ISSN 1525-0016

Boztug, K., Schmidt, M., Schwarzer, A., Banerjee, P. P., Díez, I. A., Dewey, R. A., Böhm, M., Nowrouzi, A., Ball, C. R., Glimm, H., Naundorf, S., Kühlcke, K., Blasczyk, R., Kondratenko, I., Maródi, L., Orange, J. S., von Kalle, C. & Klein, C. (2010). Stem-cell gene therapy for the Wiskott-Aldrich syndrome. *N Engl J Med*, Vol.363, No.20, pp. 1918-1927, ISSN 0028-4793

Broll, S., Oumard, A., Hahn, K., Schambach, A. & Bode, J. (2010). Minicircle performance depending on S/MAR-nuclear matrix interactions. *J Mol Biol*, Vol.395, No.5, pp. 950-965, ISSN 0022-2836

Bushman, F. D. (1994). Tethering human immunodeficiency virus 1 integrase to a DNA site directs integration to nearby sequences. *Proc Natl Acad Sci U S A*, Vol.91, No.20, pp. 9233-9237, ISSN 0027-8424

Bushman, F. D. & Miller, M. D. (1997). Tethering human immunodeficiency virus type 1 preintegration complexes to target DNA promotes integration at nearby sites. *J Virol*, Vol.71, No.1, pp. 458-464, ISSN 0022-538X

Carroll, D., Beumer, K. J. & Trautman, J. K. (2010). High-efficiency gene targeting in Drosophila with zinc finger nucleases. *Methods Mol Biol*, Vol.649, pp. 271-280, ISSN 1064-3745

Cartier, N., Hacein-Bey-Abina, S., Bartholomae, C. C., Veres, G., Schmidt, M., Kutschera, I., Vidaud, M., Abel, U., Dal-Cortivo, L., Caccavelli, L., Mahlaoui, N., Kiermer, V., Mittelstaedt, D., Bellesme, C., Lahlou, N., Lefrere, F.,

Blanche, S., Audit, M., Payen, E., Leboulch, P., l'Homme, B., Bougneres, P., Von Kalle, C., Fischer, A., Cavazzana-Calvo, M. & Aubourg, P. (2009). Hematopoietic stem cell gene therapy with a lentiviral vector in X-linked adrenoleukodystrophy. *Science*, Vol.326, No.5954, pp. 818-823, ISSN 0036-8075

Cavazzana-Calvo, M., Hacein-Bey, S., de Saint Basile, G., Gross, F., Yvon, E., Nusbaum, P., Selz, F., Hue, C., Certain, S., Casanova, J. L., Bousso, P., Deist, F. L. & Fischer, A. (2000). Gene therapy of human severe combined immunodeficiency (SCID)-X1 disease. *Science*, Vol.288, No.5466, pp. 669-672, ISSN 0036-8075

Chalberg, T. W., Portlock, J. L., Olivares, E. C., Thyagarajan, B., Kirby, P. J., Hillman, R. T., Hoelters, J. & Calos, M. P. (2006). Integration specificity of phage phiC31 integrase in the human genome. *J Mol Biol*, Vol.357, No.1, pp. 28-48, ISSN 0022-2836

Chalmers, D., Ferrand, C., Apperley, J. F., Melo, J. V., Ebeling, S., Newton, I., Duperrier, A., Hagenbeek, A., Garrett, E., Tiberghien, P. & Garin, M. (2001). Elimination of the truncated message from the herpes simplex virus thymidine kinase suicide gene. *Mol Ther*, Vol.4, No.2, pp. 146-148, ISSN 1525-0016

Chuah, M. K. L., Collen, D. & VandenDriessche, T. (2003). Biosafety of adenoviral vectors. Curr Gene Ther, Vol.3, No.6, pp. 527-543, ISSN 1566-5232

Ciuffi, A., Diamond, T. L., Hwang, Y., Marshall, H. M. & Bushman, F. D. (2006). Modulating target site selection during human immunodeficiency virus DNA integration in vitro with an engineered tethering factor. *Hum Gene Ther*, Vol.17, No.9, pp. 960-967, ISSN 1043-0342

Ciuffi, A., Ronen, K., Brady, T., Malani, N., Wang, G., Berry, C. C. & Bushman, F. D. (2009). Methods for integration site distribution analyses in animal cell genomes. Methods, Vol.47, No.4, pp. 261-268, ISSN 1046-2023

Collier, L. S., Carlson, C. M., Ravimohan, S., Dupuy, A. J. & Largaespada, D. A. (2005). Cancer gene discovery in solid tumours using transposon-based somatic mutagenesis in the mouse. *Nature*, Vol.436, No.7048, pp. 272-276, ISSN 0028-0836

Conwell, C. C. & Huang, L. (2005). Recent advances in non-viral gene delivery. *Adv Genet*, Vol.53, pp. 3-18, ISSN 0065-2660

Cornetta, K., Yao, J., Jasti, A., Koop, S., Douglas, M., Hsu, D., Couture, L. A., Hawkins, T. & Duffy, L. (2010). Replication-competent Lentivirus Analysis of Clinical Grade Vector Products. *Mol Ther*, ISSN 1525-0016

Cost, G. J., Freyvert, Y., Vafiadis, A., Santiago, Y., Miller, J. C., Rebar, E., Collingwood, T. N., Snowden, A. & Gregory, P. D. (2010). BAK and BAX deletion using zinc-finger nucleases yields apoptosis-resistant CHO cells. *Biotechnol Bioeng*, Vol.105, No.2, pp. 330-340, ISSN 0006-3592

De Oliveira, A. & Fraefel, C. (2010). Herpes simplex virus type 1/adeno-associated virus hybrid vectors. *The open virology journal*, Vol.4, pp. 109-122

Denny, W. A. (2003). Prodrugs for Gene-Directed Enzyme-Prodrug Therapy (Suicide Gene Therapy). *Journal of biomedicine & biotechnology*, Vol.2003, No.1, pp. 48-70, ISSN 1110-7243

Ding, S., Wu, X., Li, G., Han, M., Zhuang, Y. & Xu, T. (2005). Efficient transposition of the piggyBac (PB) transposon in mammalian cells and mice. *Cell*, Vol.122, No.3, pp. 473-483, ISSN 0092-8674

Doyon, Y., Choi, V. M., Xia, D. F., Vo, T. D., Gregory, P. D. & Holmes, M. C. (2010). Transient cold shock enhances zinc-finger nuclease-mediated gene disruption. *Nat Methods*, Vol.7, No.6, pp. 459-460, ISSN 1548-7091

Fajardo-Sanchez, E., Stricher, F., Pâques, F., Isalan, M. & Serrano, L. (2008). Computer design of obligate heterodimer meganucleases allows efficient cutting of custom DNA sequences. *Nucleic Acids Res*, Vol.36, No.7, pp. 2163-2173, ISSN 0305-1048

Farazi, T. A., Spitzer, J. I., Morozov, P. & Tuschl, T. (2011). miRNAs in human cancer. J Pathol, Vol.223, No.2, pp. 102-115, ISSN 0022-3417

Fazzari, M. J. & Greally, J. M. (2010). Introduction to epigenomics and epigenome-wide analysis. *Methods Mol Biol*, Vol.620, pp. 243-265, ISSN 1064-3745

Feng, D., Chen, J., Yue, Y., Zhu, H., Xue, J. & Jia, W. W. (2006). A 16bp Rep binding element is sufficient for mediating Rep-dependent integration into AAVS1. *J Mol Biol*, Vol.358, No.1, pp. 38-45, ISSN 0022-2836

Frank, K., Hogarth, D., Miller, J., Mandal, S., Mease, P., Samulski, R., Weisgerber, G. & Hart, J. (2009). Investigation of the cause of death in a gene-therapy trial. *N Engl J Med*, Vol.361, No.2, pp. 161-169, ISSN 0028-4793

Fu, F., Sander, J. D., Maeder, M., Thibodeau-Beganny, S., Joung, J. K., Dobbs, D., Miller, L. & Voytas, D. F. (2009). Zinc Finger Database (ZiFDB): a repository for information on

C2H2 zinc fingers and engineered zinc-finger arrays. *Nucleic Acids Res*, Vol.37, No.Database issue, pp. D279-D283, ISSN 0305-1048

Futreal, P. A., Coin, L., Marshall, M., Down, T., Hubbard, T., Wooster, R., Rahman, N. & Stratton, M. R. (2004). A census of human cancer genes. *Nat Rev Cancer*, Vol.4, No.3, pp. 177-183, ISSN 1474-175X

Gaspar, H., Parsley, K., Howe, S., King, D., Gilmour, K., Sinclair, J., Brouns, G., Schmidt, M., Vonkalle, C. & Barington, T. (2004). Gene therapy of X-linked severe combined immunodeficiency by use of a pseudotyped gammaretroviral vector. *The Lancet*, Vol.364, No.9452, pp. 2181-2187, ISSN 01406736

Garin, M. I., Garrett, E., Tiberghien, P., Apperley, J. F., Chalmers, D., Melo, J. V. & Ferrand, C. (2001). Molecular mechanism for ganciclovir resistance in human T lymphocytes transduced with retroviral vectors carrying the herpes simplex virus thymidine kinase gene. *Blood*, Vol.97, No.1, pp. 122-129, ISSN 0006-4971

Gerhardt, J., Jafar, S., Spindler, M. P., Ott, E. & Schepers, A. (2006). Identification of new human origins of DNA replication by an origin-trapping assay. *Mol Cell Biol*, Vol.26, No.20, pp. 7731-7746, ISSN 0270-7306

Gerrits, A., Dykstra, B., Kalmykowa, O. J., Klauke, K., Verovskaya, E., Broekhuis, M. J. C., de Haan, G. & Bystrykh, L. V. (2010). Cellular barcoding tool for clonal analysis in the hematopoietic system. *Blood*, Vol.115, No.13, pp. 2610-2618, ISSN 0006-4971

Geurts, A. M., Hackett, C. S., Bell, J. B., Bergemann, T. L., Collier, L. S., Carlson, C. M., Largaespada, D. A. & Hackett, P. B. (2006). Structure-based prediction of insertion-site preferences of transposons into chromosomes. *Nucleic Acids Res*, Vol.34, No.9, pp. 2803-2811, ISSN 0305-1048

Geurts, A. M., Yang, Y., Clark, K. J., Liu, G., Cui, Z., Dupuy, A. J., Bell, J. B., Largaespada, D. A. & Hackett, P. B. (2003). Gene transfer into genomes of human cells by the sleeping beauty transposon system. *Mol Ther*, Vol.8, No.1, pp. 108-117, ISSN 1525-0016

Gijsbers, R., Ronen, K., Vets, S., Malani, N., De Rijck, J., McNeely, M., Bushman, F. D. & Debyser, Z. (2010). LEDGF hybrids efficiently retarget lentiviral integration into heterochromatin. *Mol Ther*, Vol.18, No.3, pp. 552-560, ISSN 1525-0016

Giordano, F. A., Hotz-Wagenblatt, A., Lauterborn, D., Appelt, J. U., Fellenberg, K., Nagy, K. Z., Zeller, W. J., Suhai, S., Fruehauf, S. & Laufs, S. (2007). New bioinformatic strategies to rapidly characterize retroviral integration sites of gene therapy vectors. *Methods Inf Med*, Vol.46, No.5, pp. 542-547, ISSN 0026-1270

Grabundzija, I., Irgang, M., Mátés, L., Belay, E., Matrai, J., Gogol-Döring, A., Kawakami, K., Chen, W., Ruiz, P., Chuah, M. K. L., VandenDriessche, T., Izsvák, Z. & Ivics, Z. (2010). Comparative analysis of transposable element vector systems in human cells. *Mol Ther*, Vol.18, No.6, pp. 1200-1209, ISSN 1525-0016

Grimes, B. R., Schindelhauer, D., McGill, N. I., Ross, A., Ebersole, T. A. & Cooke, H. J. (2001). Stable gene expression from a mammalian artificial chromosome. *EMBO Rep*, Vol.2, No.10, pp. 910-914, ISSN 1469-221X

Grizot, S., Smith, J., Daboussi, F., Prieto, J., Redondo, P., Merino, N., Villate, M., Thomas, S., Lemaire, L., Montoya, G., Blanco, F. J., Pâques, F. & Duchateau, P. (2009). Efficient targeting of a SCID gene by an engineered single-chain homing endonuclease. *Nucleic Acids Res*, Vol.37, No.16, pp. 5405-5419, ISSN 0305-1048

Guo, J., Gaj, T. & Barbas, C. F. (2010). Directed evolution of an enhanced and highly efficient FokI cleavage domain for zinc finger nucleases. *J Mol Biol*, Vol.400, No.1, pp. 96-107, ISSN 0022-2836

Haase, R., Argyros, O., Wong, S. P., Harbottle, R. P., Lipps, H. J., Ogris, M., Magnusson, T., Vizoso Pinto, M. G., Haas, J. & Baiker, A. (2010). pEPito: a significantly improved non-viral episomal expression vector for mammalian cells. *BMC Biotechnol*, Vol.10, pp. 20

Hacein-Bey-Abina, S. (2003). LMO2-associated clonal T cell proliferation in two patients after gene therapy for SCID-X1. *Science*, Vol.302, No.5644, pp. 415-419, ISSN 0036-8075

Hacein-Bey-Abina, S., Garrigue, A., Wang, G. P., Soulier, J., Lim, A., Morillon, E., Clappier, E., Caccavelli, L., Delabesse, E., Beldjord, K., Asnafi, V., MacIntyre, E., Dal Cortivo, L., Radford, I., Brousse, N., Sigaux, F., Moshous, D., Hauer, J., Borkhardt, A., Belohradsky, B. H., Wintergerst, U., Velez, M. C., Leiva, L., Sorensen, R., Wulffraat, N., Blanche, S., Bushman, F. D., Fischer, A. & Cavazzana-Calvo, M. (2008). Insertional oncogenesis in 4 patients after retrovirus-mediated gene therapy of SCID-X1. *J Clin Invest*, Vol.118, No.9, pp. 3132-3142, ISSN 0021-9738

Hackett, P. B., Largaespada, D. A. & Cooper, L. J. (2010). A transposon and transposase system for human application. (1). *Mol Ther*, Vol.18, No.4, pp. 674-683, ISSN 1525-0016

Hanahan, D. & Weinberg, R. A. (2000). The hallmarks of cancer. *Cell*, Vol.100, No.1, pp. 57-70, ISSN 0092-8674

Held, P. K., Olivares, E. C., Aguilar, C. P., Finegold, M., Calos, M. P. & Grompe, M. (2005). In vivo correction of murine hereditary tyrosinemia type I by phiC31 integrase-mediated gene delivery. *Mol Ther*, Vol.11, No.3, pp. 399-408, ISSN 1525-0016

Hester, S. D., Reid, L., Nowak, N., Jones, W. D., Parker, J. S., Knudtson, K., Ward, W., Tiesman, J. & Denslow, N. D. (2009). Comparison of comparative genomic hybridization technologies across microarray platforms. *J Biomol Tech*, Vol.20, No.2, pp. 135-151, ISSN 1524-0215

Hockemeyer, D., Soldner, F., Beard, C., Gao, Q., Mitalipova, M., DeKelver, R. C., Katibah, G. E., Amora, R., Boydston, E. A., Zeitler, B., Meng, X., Miller, J. C., Zhang, L., Rebar, E. J., Gregory, P. D., Urnov, F. D. & Jaenisch, R. (2009). Efficient targeting of expressed and silent genes in human ESCs and iPSCs using zinc-finger nucleases. (1). *Nat Biotechnol*, Vol.27, No.9, pp. 851-857, ISSN 1087-0156

Howden, S. E., Voullaire, L. & Vadolas, J. (2008). The transient expression of mRNA coding for Rep protein from AAV facilitates targeted plasmid integration. *J Gene Med*, Vol.10, No.1, pp. 42-50, ISSN 1099-498X

Howe, S. J., Mansour, M. R., Schwarzwaelder, K., Bartholomae, C., Hubank, M., Kempski, H., Brugman, M. H., Pike-Overzet, K., Chatters, S. J., de Ridder, D., Gilmour, K. C., Adams, S., Thornhill, S. I., Parsley, K. L., Staal, F. J. T., Gale, R. E., Linch, D. C., Bayford, J., Brown, L., Quaye, M., Kinnon, C., Ancliff, P., Webb, D. K., Schmidt, M., von Kalle, C., Gaspar, H. B. & Thrasher, A. J. (2008). Insertional mutagenesis combined with acquired somatic mutations causes leukemogenesis following gene therapy of SCID-X1 patients. *J Clin Invest*, Vol.118, No.9, pp. 3143-3150, ISSN 0021-9738

Huang, X., Guo, H., Tammana, S., Jung, Y. C., Mellgren, E., Bassi, P., Cao, Q., Tu, Z. J., Kim, Y. C., Ekker, S. C., Wu, X., Wang, S. M. & Zhou, X. (2010). Gene transfer efficiency and genome-wide integration profiling of Sleeping Beauty, Tol2, and piggyBac transposons in human primary T cells. *Mol Ther*, Vol.18, No.10, pp. 1803-1813, ISSN 1525-0016

Huang, X., Haley, K., Wong, M., Guo, H., Lu, C., Wilber, A. & Zhou, X. (2010). Unexpectedly high copy number of random integration but low frequency of persistent expression of the Sleeping Beauty transposase after trans delivery in primary human T cells. *Hum Gene Ther*, Vol.21, No.11, pp. 1577-1590, ISSN 1043-0342

Ishikawa, Y., Tanaka, N., Murakami, K., Uchiyama, T., Kumaki, S., Tsuchiya, S., Kugoh, H., Oshimura, M., Calos, M. P. & Sugamura, K. (2006). Phage phiC31 integrase-mediated genomic integration of the common cytokine receptor gamma chain in human T-cell lines. *J Gene Med*, Vol.8, No.5, pp. 646-653, ISSN 1099-498X

Ivics, Z., Katzer, A., Stüwe, E. E., Fiedler, D., Knespel, S. & Izsvák, Z. (2007). Targeted Sleeping Beauty transposition in human cells. *Mol Ther*, Vol.15, No.6, pp. 1137-1144, ISSN 1525-0016

Ivics, Z., Hackett, P. B., Plasterk, R. H. & Izsvák, Z. (1997). Molecular reconstruction of Sleeping Beauty, a Tc1-like transposon from fish, and its transposition in human cells. *Cell*, Vol.91, No.4, pp. 501-510, ISSN 0092-8674

Izsvák, Z., Chuah, M. K. L., Vandendriessche, T. & Ivics, Z. (2009). Efficient stable gene transfer into human cells by the Sleeping Beauty transposon vectors. *Methods*, Vol.49, No.3, pp. 287-297, ISSN 1046-2023

Izsvák, Z., Hackett, P. B., Cooper, L. J. & Ivics, Z. (2010). Translating Sleeping Beauty transposition into cellular therapies: victories and challenges. *Bioessays*, Vol.32, No.9, pp. 756-767, ISSN 0265-9247

Jackson, D. A., Juranek, S. & Lipps, H. J. (2006). Designing nonviral vectors for efficient gene transfer and long-term gene expression. *Mol Ther*, Vol.14, No.5, pp. 613-626, ISSN 1525-0016

Jang, M. Y., Yarborough, O. H., Conyers, G. B., McPhie, P. & Owens, R. A. (2005). Stable secondary structure near the nicking site for adeno-associated virus type 2 Rep proteins on human chromosome 19. *J Virol*, Vol.79, No.6, pp. 3544-3556, ISSN 0022-538X

Kang, M. S., Hung, S. C. & Kieff, E. (2001). Epstein-Barr virus nuclear antigen 1 activates transcription from episomal but not integrated DNA and does not alter lymphocyte growth. *Proc Natl Acad Sci U S A*, Vol.98, No.26, pp. 15233-15238, ISSN 0027-8424

Katz, R. A., Merkel, G. & Skalka, A. M. (1996). Targeting of retroviral integrase by fusion to a heterologous DNA binding domain: in vitro activities and incorporation of a fusion protein into viral particles. *Virology*, Vol.217, No.1, pp. 178-190, ISSN 0042-6822

Keravala, A., Lee, S., Thyagarajan, B., Olivares, E. C., Gabrovsky, V. E., Woodard, L. E. & Calos, M. P. (2009). Mutational derivatives of PhiC31 integrase with increased efficiency and specificity. *Mol Ther*, Vol.17, No.1, pp. 112-120, ISSN 1525-0016

Kim, Y. G., Cha, J. & Chandrasegaran, S. (1996). Hybrid restriction enzymes: zinc finger fusions to Fok I cleavage domain. *Proc Natl Acad Sci U S A*, Vol.93, No.3, pp. 1156-1160, ISSN 0027-8424

Kim, Y. J., Kim, Y. S., Larochelle, A., Renaud, G., Wolfsberg, T. G., Adler, R., Donahue, R. E., Hematti, P., Hong, B. K., Roayaei, J., Akagi, K., Riberdy, J. M., Nienhuis, A. W., Dunbar, C. E. & Persons, D. A. (2009). Sustained high-level polyclonal hematopoietic marking and transgene expression 4 years after autologous transplantation of rhesus macaques with SIV lentiviral vector-transduced CD34+ cells. *Blood*, Vol.113, No.22, pp. 5434-5443, ISSN 0006-4971

Koboldt, D. C., Ding, L., Mardis, E. R. & Wilson, R. K. (2010). Challenges of sequencing human genomes. Brief Bioinform, Vol.11, No.5, pp. 484-498, ISSN 1467-5463

Kohn, D. B. & Candotti, F. (2009). Gene therapy fulfilling its promise. N Engl J Med, Vol.360, No.5, pp. 518-521, ISSN 0028-4793

Kotzamanis, G., Cheung, W., Abdulrazzak, H., Perez-Luz, S., Howe, S., Cooke, H. & Huxley, C. (2005). Construction of human artificial chromosome vectors by recombineering. *Gene*, Vol.351, pp. 29-38, ISSN 0378-1119

Laufs, S., Gentner, B., Nagy, K. Z., Jauch, A., Benner, A., Naundorf, S., Kuehlcke, K., Schiedlmeier, B., Ho, A. D., Zeller, W. J. & Fruehauf, S. (2003). Retroviral vector integration occurs in preferred genomic targets of human bone marrow-repopulating cells. *Blood*, Vol.101, No.6, pp. 2191-2198, ISSN 0006-4971

Li, Z., Dullmann, J., Schiedlmeier, B., Schmidt, M., von Kalle, C., Meyer, J., Forster, M., Stocking, C., Wahlers, A. & Frank, O. (2002). Murine leukemia induced by retroviral gene marking. *Science*, Vol.296, No.5567, pp. 497, ISSN 0036-8075

Li, H., Pellenz, S., Ulge, U., Stoddard, B. L. & Monnat, R. J. (2009). Generation of single-chain LAGLIDADG homing endonucleases from native homodimeric precursor proteins. *Nucleic Acids Res*, Vol.37, No.5, pp. 1650-1662, ISSN 0305-1048

Liang, Q., Kong, J., Stalker, J. & Bradley, A. (2009). Chromosomal mobilization and reintegration of Sleeping Beauty and PiggyBac transposons. *Genesis*, Vol.47, No.6, pp. 404-408, ISSN 1526-954X

Liesner, R., Zhang, W., Noske, N. & Ehrhardt, A. (2010). Critical amino acid residues within the φC31 integrase DNA-binding domain affect recombination activities in mammalian cells. *Hum Gene Ther*, Vol.21, No.9, pp. 1104-1118, ISSN 1043-0342

Liu, J., Jeppesen, I., Nielsen, K. & Jensen, T. G. (2006). Phi c31 integrase induces chromosomal aberrations in primary human fibroblasts. *Gene Ther*, Vol.13, No.15, pp. 1188-1190, ISSN 0969-7128

Liu, R., Li, Y., Hu, R., Jin, T., Deng, S., Liang, W., Zhang, N., Chen, J., Prud'homme, G. J., Jia, W. W., Ma, D. & Wang, Q. (2010). A site-specific genomic integration strategy for sustained expression of glucagon-like peptide-1 in mouse muscle for controlling energy homeostasis. *Biochem Biophys Res Commun*, Vol.403, No.2, pp. 172-177, ISSN 0006-291X

Lombardo, A., Genovese, P., Beausejour, C. M., Colleoni, S., Lee, Y. L., Kim, K. A., Ando, D., Urnov, F. D., Galli, C., Gregory, P. D., Holmes, M. C. & Naldini, L. (2007). Gene editing in human stem cells using zinc finger nucleases and integrase-defective lentiviral vector delivery. (1). *Nat Biotechnol*, Vol.25, No.11, pp. 1298-1306, ISSN 1087-0156

Lufino, M. M. P., Edser, P. A. H. & Wade-Martins, R. (2008). Advances in high-capacity extrachromosomal vector technology: episomal maintenance, vector delivery, and transgene expression. *Mol Ther*, Vol.16, No.9, pp. 1525-1538, ISSN 1525-0016

Lupo-Stanghellini, M., Provasi, E., Bondanza, A., Ciceri, F., Bordignon, C. & Bonini, C. (2010). Clinical impact of suicide gene therapy in allogeneic hematopoietic stem cell transplantation. *Hum Gene Ther*, Vol.21, No.3, pp. 241-250, ISSN 1043-0342

Maeder, M. L., Thibodeau-Beganny, S., Osiak, A., Wright, D. A., Anthony, R. M., Eichtinger, M., Jiang, T., Foley, J. E., Winfrey, R. J., Townsend, J. A., Unger-Wallace, E., Sander, J. D., Müller-Lerch, F., Fu, F., Pearlberg, J., Göbel, C., Dassie, J. P., Pruett-Miller, S. M., Porteus, M. H., Sgroi, D. C., Iafrate, A. J., Dobbs, D., McCray, P. B., Cathomen, T., Voytas, D. F. & Joung, J. K. (2008). Rapid "open-source" engineering of customized zinc-finger nucleases for highly efficient gene modification. *Mol Cell*, Vol.31, No.2, pp. 294-301, ISSN 1097-2765

Mátés, L., Chuah, M. K. L., Belay, E., Jerchow, B., Manoj, N., Acosta-Sanchez, A., Grzela, D. P., Schmitt, A., Becker, K., Matrai, J., Ma, L., Samara-Kuko, E., Gysemans, C., Pryputniewicz, D., Miskey, C., Fletcher, B., VandenDriessche, T., Ivics, Z. & Izsvák, Z. (2009). Molecular evolution of a novel hyperactive Sleeping Beauty transposase enables robust stable gene transfer in vertebrates. *Nat Genet*, Vol.41, No.6, pp. 753-761, ISSN 1061-4036

McCammon, J. M. & Amacher, S. L. (2010). Using zinc finger nucleases for efficient and heritable gene disruption in zebrafish. *Methods Mol Biol*, Vol.649, pp. 281-298, ISSN 1064-3745

Mercer, K. E., Ahn, C. E., Coke, A., Compadre, C. M. & Drake, R. R. (2002). Mutation of herpesvirus thymidine kinase to generate ganciclovir-specific kinases for use in cancer gene therapies. *Protein Eng*, Vol.15, No.11, pp. 903-911, ISSN 0269-2139

Miller, D. G., Rutledge, E. A. & Russell, D. W. (2002). Chromosomal effects of adeno-associated virus vector integration. *Nat Genet*, Vol.30, No.2, pp. 147-148, ISSN 1061-4036

Miller, D. G., Trobridge, G. D., Petek, L. M., Jacobs, M. A., Kaul, R. & Russell, D. W. (2005). Large-scale analysis of adeno-associated virus vector integration sites in normal human cells. *J Virol*, Vol.79, No.17, pp. 11434-11442, ISSN 0022-538X

Miller, J. C., Holmes, M. C., Wang, J., Guschin, D. Y., Lee, Y. L., Rupniewski, I., Beausejour, C. M., Waite, A. J., Wang, N. S., Kim, K. A., Gregory, P. D., Pabo, C. O. & Rebar, E. J. (2007). An improved zinc-finger nuclease architecture for highly specific genome editing. *Nat Biotechnol*, Vol.25, No.7, pp. 778-785, ISSN 1087-0156

Mitchell, R. S., Beitzel, B. F., Schroder, A. R. W., Shinn, P., Chen, H., Berry, C. C., Ecker, J. R. & Bushman, F. D. (2004). Retroviral DNA integration: ASLV, HIV, and MLV show distinct target site preferences. (1). *PLoS Biol*, Vol.2, No.8, pp. E234, ISSN 1544-9173

Modlich, U. (2005). Leukemias following retroviral transfer of multidrug resistance 1 (MDR1) are driven by combinatorial insertional mutagenesis. *Blood*, Vol.105, No.11, pp. 4235-4246, ISSN 0006-4971

Modlich, U., Bohne, J., Schmidt, M., von Kalle, C., Knöss, S., Schambach, A. & Baum, C. (2006). Cell-culture assays reveal the importance of retroviral vector design for insertional genotoxicity. *Blood*, Vol.108, No.8, pp. 2545-2553, ISSN 0006-4971

Modlich, U., Navarro, S., Zychlinski, D., Maetzig, T., Knoess, S., Brugman, M. H., Schambach, A., Charrier, S., Galy, A., Thrasher, A. J., Bueren, J. & Baum, C. (2009). Insertional transformation of hematopoietic cells by self-inactivating lentiviral and gammaretroviral vectors. (1). *Mol Ther*, Vol.17, No.11, pp. 1919-1928, ISSN 1525-0016

Moehle, E. A., Rock, J. M., Lee, Y. L., Jouvenot, Y., DeKelver, R. C., Gregory, P. D., Urnov, F. D. & Holmes, M. C. (2007). Targeted gene addition into a specified location in the human genome using designed zinc finger nucleases. *Proceedings of the National Academy of Sciences*, Vol.104, No.9, pp. 3055-3060, ISSN 0027-8424

Moldt, B., Staunstrup, N. H., Jakobsen, M., Yáñez-Muñoz, R. J. & Mikkelsen, J. G. (2008). Genomic insertion of lentiviral DNA circles directed by the yeast Flp recombinase. *BMC Biotechnol*, Vol.8, pp. 60

Montini, E., Cesana, D., Schmidt, M., Sanvito, F., Bartholomae, C., Ranzani, M., Benedicenti, F., Sergi, L., Ambrosi, A. & Ponzoni, M. (2009). The genotoxic potential of retroviral vectors is strongly modulated by vector design and integration site selection in a mouse model of HSC gene therapy. *J Clin Invest*, Vol.119, No.4, pp. 964-975, ISSN 0021-9738

Montini, E., Cesana, D., Schmidt, M., Sanvito, F., Ponzoni, M., Bartholomae, C., Sergi Sergi, L., Benedicenti, F., Ambrosi, A., Di Serio, C., Doglioni, C., von Kalle, C. & Naldini, L. (2006). Hematopoietic stem cell gene transfer in a tumor-prone mouse model uncovers low genotoxicity of lentiviral vector integration. *Nat Biotechnol*, Vol.24, No.6, pp. 687-696, ISSN 1087-0156

Nienhuis, A. W., Dunbar, C. E. & Sorrentino, B. P. (2006). Genotoxicity of retroviral integration in hematopoietic cells. *Mol Ther*, Vol.13, No.6, pp. 1031-1049, ISSN 1525-0016

Niidome, T. & Huang, L. (2002). Gene therapy progress and prospects: nonviral vectors. *Gene Ther*, Vol.9, No.24, pp. 1647-1652, ISSN 0969-7128

Ohlfest, J. R., Frandsen, J. L., Fritz, S., Lobitz, P. D., Perkinson, S. G., Clark, K. J., Nelsestuen, G., Key, N. S., McIvor, R. S., Hackett, P. B. & Largaespada, D. A. (2005). Phenotypic correction and long-term expression of factor VIII in hemophilic mice by immunotolerization and nonviral gene transfer using the Sleeping Beauty transposon system. *Blood*, Vol.105, No.7, pp. 2691-2698, ISSN 0006-4971

Olivares, E. C., Hollis, R. P., Chalberg, T. W., Meuse, L., Kay, M. A. & Calos, M. P. (2002). Site-specific genomic integration produces therapeutic Factor IX levels in mice. *Nat Biotechnol*, Vol.20, No.11, pp. 1124-1128, ISSN 1087-0156

Ortiz-Urda, S., Lin, Q., Yant, S., Keene, D., Kay, M. & Khavari, P. (2003). Sustainable correction of junctional epidermolysis bullosa via transposon-mediated nonviral gene transfer. (1). *Gene Ther*, Vol.10, No.13, pp. 1099-1104, ISSN 0969-7128

Ortiz-Urda, S., Thyagarajan, B., Keene, D. R., Lin, Q., Fang, M., Calos, M. P. & Khavari, P. A. (2002). Stable nonviral genetic correction of inherited human skin disease. *Nat Med*, Vol.8, No.10, pp. 1166-1170, ISSN 1078-8956

Ott, M. G., Schmidt, M., Schwarzwaelder, K., Stein, S., Siler, U., Koehl, U., Glimm, H., Kühlcke, K., Schilz, A., Kunkel, H., Naundorf, S., Brinkmann, A., Deichmann, A., Fischer, M., Ball, C., Pilz, I., Dunbar, C., Du, Y., Jenkins, N. A., Copeland, N. G., Lüthi, U., Hassan, M., Thrasher, A. J., Hoelzer, D., von Kalle, C., Seger, R. & Grez, M. (2006). Correction of X-linked chronic granulomatous disease by gene therapy, augmented by insertional activation of MDS1-EVI1, PRDM16 or SETBP1. *Nat Med*, Vol.12, No.4, pp. 401-409, ISSN 1078-8956

Papapetrou, E. P., Zoumbos, N. C. & Athanassiadou, A. (2005). Genetic modification of hematopoietic stem cells with nonviral systems: past progress and future prospects. *Gene Ther*, Vol.12 Suppl 1, pp. S118-S130, ISSN 0969-7128

Perez, E. E., Wang, J., Miller, J. C., Jouvenot, Y., Kim, K. A., Liu, O., Wang, N., Lee, G., Bartsevich, V. V., Lee, Y. L., Guschin, D. Y., Rupniewski, I., Waite, A. J., Carpenito, C., Carroll, R. G., S Orange, J., Urnov, F. D., Rebar, E. J., Ando, D., Gregory, P. D., Riley, J. L., Holmes, M. C. & June, C. H. (2008). Establishment of HIV-1 resistance in CD4+ T cells by genome editing using zinc-finger nucleases. *Nat Biotechnol*, Vol.26, No.7, pp. 808-816, ISSN 1087-0156

Peters, B., Dirscherl, S., Dantzer, J., Nowacki, J., Cross, S., Li, X., Cornetta, K., Dinauer, M. C. & Mooney, S. D. (2008). Automated analysis of viral integration sites in gene therapy research using the SeqMap web resource. *Gene Ther*, Vol.15, No.18, pp. 1294-1298, ISSN 0969-7128

Philpott, N. J., Gomos, J., Berns, K. I. & Falck-Pedersen, E. (2002). A p5 integration efficiency element mediates Rep-dependent integration into AAVS1 at chromosome 19. *Proc Natl Acad Sci U S A*, Vol.99, No.19, pp. 12381-12385, ISSN 0027-8424

Pieroni, L., Fipaldini, C., Monciotti, A., Cimini, D., Sgura, A., Fattori, E., Epifano, O., Cortese, R., Palombo, F. & La Monica, N. (1998). Targeted integration of adeno-associated virus-derived plasmids in transfected human cells. *Virology*, Vol.249, No.2, pp. 249-259, ISSN 0042-6822

Porteus, M. H. & Baltimore, D. (2003). Chimeric nucleases stimulate gene targeting in human cells. *Science*, Vol.300, No.5620, pp. 763, ISSN 0036-8075

Preuß, E., Treschow, A., Newrzela, S., Brücher, D., Weber, K., Felldin, U., Alici, E., Gahrton, G., von Laer, D., Dilber, M. S. & Fehse, B. (2010). TK.007: A novel, codon-optimized HSVtk(A168H) mutant for suicide gene therapy. *Hum Gene Ther*, Vol.21, No.8, pp. 929-941, ISSN 1043-0342

Rad, R., Rad, L., Wang, W., Cadinanos, J., Vassiliou, G., Rice, S., Campos, L. S., Yusa, K., Banerjee, R., Li, M. A., de la Rosa, J., Strong, A., Lu, D., Ellis, P., Conte, N., Yang, F. T., Liu, P. & Bradley, A. (2010). PiggyBac transposon mutagenesis: a tool for cancer gene discovery in mice. *Science*, Vol.330, No.6007, pp. 1104-1107, ISSN 0036-8075

Ramezani, A., Hawley, T. S. & Hawley, R. G. (2008). Combinatorial incorporation of enhancer-blocking components of the chicken beta-globin 5'HS4 and human T-cell receptor alpha/delta BEAD-1 insulators in self-inactivating retroviral vectors reduces their genotoxic potential. *Stem Cells*, Vol.26, No.12, pp. 3257-3266, ISSN 1066-5099

Raper, S. E., Chirmule, N., Lee, F. S., Wivel, N. A., Bagg, A., Gao, G. P., Wilson, J. M. & Batshaw, M. L. (2003). Fatal systemic inflammatory response syndrome in a ornithine transcarbamylase deficient patient following adenoviral gene transfer. *Mol Genet Metab*, Vol.80, No.1-2, pp. 148-158, ISSN 1096-7192

Reyon, D., Kirkpatrick, J. R., Sander, J. D., Zhang, F., Voytas, D. F., Joung, J. K., Dobbs, D. & Coffman, C. R. (2011). ZFNGenome: A comprehensive resource for locating zinc finger nuclease target sites in model organisms. *BMC Genomics*, Vol.12, No.1, pp. 83

Rouet, P., Smih, F. & Jasin, M. (1994). Expression of a site-specific endonuclease stimulates homologous recombination in mammalian cells. *Proc Natl Acad Sci U S A*, Vol.91, No.13, pp. 6064-6068, ISSN 0027-8424

Rémy, S., Tesson, L., Ménoret, S., Usal, C., Scharenberg, A. M. & Anegon, I. (2010). Zinc-finger nucleases: a powerful tool for genetic engineering of animals. *Transgenic Res*, Vol.19, No.3, pp. 363-371, ISSN 0962-8819

Saeki, Y., Wataya-Kaneda, M., Tanaka, K. & Kaneda, Y. (1998). Sustained transgene expression in vitro and in vivo using an Epstein-Barr virus replicon vector system combined with HVJ liposomes. *Gene Ther*, Vol.5, No.8, pp. 1031-1037, ISSN 0969-7128

Sander, J. D., Dahlborg, E. J., Goodwin, M. J., Cade, L., Zhang, F., Cifuentes, D., Curtin, S. J., Blackburn, J. S., Thibodeau-Beganny, S., Qi, Y., Pierick, C. J., Hoffman, E., Maeder, M. L., Khayter, C., Reyon, D., Dobbs, D., Langenau, D. M., Stupar, R. M., Giraldez, A. J., Voytas, D. F., Peterson, R. T., Yeh, J. R. J. & Joung, J. K. (2011). Selection-free zinc-finger-nuclease engineering by context-dependent assembly (CoDA). Nat Methods, Vol.8, No.1, pp. 67-69, ISSN 1548-7091

Sander, J. D., Maeder, M. L., Reyon, D., Voytas, D. F., Joung, J. K. & Dobbs, D. (2010). ZiFiT (Zinc Finger Targeter): an updated zinc finger engineering tool. *Nucleic Acids Res*, Vol.38, No.Web Server issue, pp. W462-W468, ISSN 0305-1048

Sarkis, C., Philippe, S., Mallet, J. & Serguera, C. (2008). Non-integrating lentiviral vectors. *Curr Gene Ther*, Vol.8, No.6, pp. 430-437, ISSN 1566-5232

Schambach, A., Galla, M., Maetzig, T., Loew, R. & Baum, C. (2007). Improving transcriptional termination of self-inactivating gamma-retroviral and lentiviral vectors. *Mol Ther*, Vol.15, No.6, pp. 1167-1173, ISSN 1525-0016

Schmidt, M., Schwarzwaelder, K., Bartholomae, C., Zaoui, K., Ball, C., Pilz, I., Braun, S., Glimm, H. & von Kalle, C. (2007). High-resolution insertion-site analysis by linear amplification-mediated PCR (LAM-PCR). *Nat Methods*, Vol.4, No.12, pp. 1051-1057, ISSN 1548-7091

Schulz, T. F. & Cordes, S. (2009). Is the Epstein-Barr virus EBNA-1 protein an oncogen? *Proc Natl Acad Sci U S A*, Vol.106, No.7, pp. 2091-2092, ISSN 0027-8424

Schäfer-Korting, M., Heilbronn, R. & Weger, S. (2010). Viral vectors for gene transfer: current status of gene therapeutics. *Handb Exp Pharmacol*, No.197, pp. 143-170, ISSN 0171-2004

Sclimenti, C. R., Thyagarajan, B. & Calos, M. P. (2001). Directed evolution of a recombinase for improved genomic integration at a native human sequence. *Nucleic Acids Res*, Vol.29, No.24, pp. 5044-5051, ISSN 0305-1048

Scollay, R. (2001). Gene therapy: a brief overview of the past, present, and future. *Ann N Y Acad Sci*, Vol.953, pp. 26-30, ISSN 0077-8923

Segal, D. J., Beerli, R. R., Blancafort, P., Dreier, B., Effertz, K., Huber, A., Koksch, B., Lund, C. V., Magnenat, L., Valente, D. & Barbas, C. F. (2003). Evaluation of a modular strategy for the construction of novel polydactyl zinc finger DNA-binding proteins. *Biochemistry*, Vol.42, No.7, pp. 2137-2148, ISSN 0006-2960

Shukla, V. K., Doyon, Y., Miller, J. C., DeKelver, R. C., Moehle, E. A., Worden, S. E., Mitchell, J. C., Arnold, N. L., Gopalan, S., Meng, X., Choi, V. M., Rock, J. M., Wu, Y. Y., Katibah, G. E., Zhifang, G., McCaskill, D., Simpson, M. A., Blakeslee, B., Greenwalt, S. A., Butler, H. J., Hinkley, S. J., Zhang, L., Rebar, E. J., Gregory, P. D. & Urnov, F. D. (2009). Precise genome modification in the crop species Zea mays using zinc-finger nucleases. *Nature*, Vol.459, No.7245, pp. 437-441, ISSN 0028-0836

Silver, J. & Keerikatte, V. (1989). Novel use of polymerase chain reaction to amplify cellular DNA adjacent to an integrated provirus. *J Virol*, Vol.63, No.5, pp. 1924-1928, ISSN 0022-538X

Sinn, P. L., Sauter, S. L. & McCray, P. B. (2005). Gene therapy progress and prospects: development of improved lentiviral and retroviral vectors--design, biosafety, and production. *Gene Ther*, Vol.12, No.14, pp. 1089-1098, ISSN 0969-7128

Sivalingam, J., Krishnan, S., Ng, W. H., Lee, S. S., Phan, T. T. & Kon, O. L. (2010). Biosafety assessment of site-directed transgene integration in human umbilical cord-lining cells. *Mol Ther*, Vol.18, No.7, pp. 1346-1356, ISSN 1525-0016

Smith, R. H. (2008). Adeno-associated virus integration: virus versus vector. *Gene Ther*, Vol.15, No.11, pp. 817-822, ISSN 0969-7128

Stehle, I. M., Postberg, J., Rupprecht, S., Cremer, T., Jackson, D. A. & Lipps, H. J. (2007). Establishment and mitotic stability of an extra-chromosomal mammalian replicon. *BMC Cell Biol*, Vol.8, pp. 33, ISSN 1471-2121

Stein, S., Ott, M. G., Schultze-Strasser, S., Jauch, A., Burwinkel, B., Kinner, A., Schmidt, M., Krämer, A., Schwäble, J., Glimm, H., Koehl, U., Preiss, C., Ball, C., Martin, H., Göhring, G., Schwarzwaelder, K., Hofmann, W. K.,Karakaya, K., Tchatchou, S., Yang, R., Reinecke, P., Kühlcke, K., Schlegelberger, B., Thrasher, A. J., Hoelzer, D., Seger, R., von Kalle, C. & Grez, M. (2010). Genomic instability and myelodysplasia with monosomy 7 consequent to EVI1 activation after gene therapy for chronic granulomatous disease. *Nat Med*, Vol.16, No.2, pp. 198-204, ISSN 1078-8956

Stephen, S. L., Sivanandam, V. G. & Kochanek, S. (2008). Homologous and heterologous recombination between adenovirus vector DNA and chromosomal DNA. *J Gene Med*, Vol.10, No.11, pp. 1176-1189, ISSN 1099-498X

Szczepek, M., Brondani, V., Büchel, J., Serrano, L., Segal, D. J. & Cathomen, T. (2007). Structure-based redesign of the dimerization interface reduces the toxicity of zinc-finger nucleases. *Nat Biotechnol,* Vol.25, No.7, pp. 786-793, ISSN 1087-0156

Takahashi, K. & Yamanaka, S. (2006). Induction of pluripotent stem cells from mouse embryonic and adult fibroblast cultures by defined factors. *Cell,* Vol.126, No.4, pp. 663-676, ISSN 0092-8674

Tatum, E. L. (1966). Molecular biology, nucleic acids, and the future of medicine. *Perspect Biol Med,* Vol.10, No.1, pp. 19-32, ISSN 0031-5982

Tenenbaum, L., Lehtonen, E. & Monahan, P. E. (2003). Evaluation of risks related to the use of adeno-associated virus-based vectors. Curr Gene Ther, Vol.3, No.6, pp. 545-565, ISSN 1566-5232

Tey, S. K., Dotti, G., Rooney, C. M., Heslop, H. E. & Brenner, M. K. (2007). Inducible caspase 9 suicide gene to improve the safety of allodepleted T cells after haploidentical stem cell transplantation. *Biol Blood Marrow Transplant,* Vol.13, No.8, pp. 913-924, ISSN 1083-8791

Thomae, A. W., Pich, D., Brocher, J., Spindler, M. P., Berens, C., Hock, R., Hammerschmidt, W. & Schepers, A. (2008). Interaction between HMGA1a and the origin recognition complex creates site-specific replication origins. *Proc Natl Acad Sci U S A,* Vol.105, No.5, pp. 1692-1697, ISSN 0027-8424

Thyagarajan, B., Liu, Y., Shin, S., Lakshmipathy, U., Scheyhing, K., Xue, H., Ellerström, C., Strehl, R., Hyllner, J., Rao, M. S. & Chesnut, J. D. (2008). Creation of engineered human embryonic stem cell lines using phiC31 integrase. *Stem Cells,* Vol.26, No.1, pp. 119-126, ISSN 1066-5099

Townsend, J. A., Wright, D. A., Winfrey, R. J., Fu, F., Maeder, M. L., Joung, J. K. & Voytas, D. F. (2009). High-frequency modification of plant genes using engineered zinc-finger nucleases. *Nature,* Vol.459, No.7245, pp. 442-445, ISSN 0028-0836

Urnov, F. D., Rebar, E. J., Holmes, M. C., Zhang, H. S. & Gregory, P. D. (2010). Genome editing with engineered zinc finger nucleases. *Nature Reviews Genetics,* Vol.11, No.9, pp. 636-646, ISSN 1471-0056

Urnov, F. D., Miller, J. C., Lee, Y. L., Beausejour, C. M., Rock, J. M., Augustus, S., Jamieson, A. C., Porteus, M. H., Gregory, P. D. & Holmes, M. C. (2005). Highly efficient endogenous human gene correction using designed zinc-finger nucleases. *Nature,* Vol.435, No.7042, pp. 646-651, ISSN 0028-0836

Varella-Garcia, M., Chen, L., Powell, R. L., Hirsch, F. R., Kennedy, T. C., Keith, R., Miller, Y. E., Mitchell, J. D. & Franklin, W. A. (2007). Spectral karyotyping detects chromosome damage in bronchial cells of smokers and patients with cancer. *Am J Respir Crit Care Med,* Vol.176, No.5, pp. 505-512, ISSN 1073-449X

Vasquez, K. M., Wang, G., Havre, P. A. & Glazer, P. M. (1999). Chromosomal mutations induced by triplex-forming oligonucleotides in mammalian cells. *Nucleic Acids Res,* Vol.27, No.4, pp. 1176-1181, ISSN 0305-1048

Vink, C. A., Gaspar, H. B., Gabriel, R., Schmidt, M., McIvor, R. S., Thrasher, A. J. & Qasim, W. (2009). Sleeping beauty transposition from nonintegrating lentivirus. *Mol Ther,* Vol.17, No.7, pp. 1197-1204, ISSN 1525-0016

Walisko, O., Schorn, A., Rolfs, F., Devaraj, A., Miskey, C., Izsvák, Z. & Ivics, Z. (2008). Transcriptional activities of the Sleeping Beauty transposon and shielding its genetic cargo with insulators. *Mol Ther,* Vol.16, No.2, pp. 359-369, ISSN 1525-0016

Walther, W. & Stein, U. (2000). Viral vectors for gene transfer: a review of their use in the treatment of human diseases. *Drugs,* Vol.60, No.2, pp. 249-271, ISSN 0012-6667

Wang, G. P., Berry, C. C., Malani, N., Leboulch, P., Fischer, A., Hacein-Bey-Abina, S., Cavazzana-Calvo, M. & Bushman, F. D. (2010). Dynamics of gene-modified progenitor cells analyzed by tracking retroviral integration sites in a human SCID-X1 gene therapy trial. *Blood*, Vol.115, No.22, pp. 4356-4366, ISSN 0006-4971

Wang, G. P., Garrigue, A., Ciuffi, A., Ronen, K., Leipzig, J., Berry, C., Lagresle-Peyrou, C., Benjelloun, F., Hacein-Bey-Abina, S., Fischer, A., Cavazzana-Calvo, M. & Bushman, F. D. (2008). DNA bar coding and pyrosequencing to analyze adverse events in therapeutic gene transfer. *Nucleic Acids Res*, Vol.36, No.9, pp. e49, ISSN 0305-1048

Wang, Z., Troilo, P. J., Wang, X., Griffiths, T. G., Pacchione, S. J., Barnum, A. B., Harper, L. B., Pauley, C. J., Niu, Z., Denisova, L., Follmer, T. T., Rizzuto, G., Ciliberto, G., Fattori, E., Monica, N. L., Manam, S. & Ledwith, B. J. (2004). Detection of integration of plasmid DNA into host genomic DNA following intramuscular injection and electroporation. *Gene Ther*, Vol.11, No.8, pp. 711-721, ISSN 0969-7128

Weber, E. L. & Cannon, P. M. (2007). Promoter choice for retroviral vectors: transcriptional strength versus trans-activation potential. *Hum Gene Ther*, Vol.18, No.9, pp. 849-860, ISSN 1043-0342

Wolff, J. & Lederberg, J. (1994). An early history of gene transfer and therapy. *Hum Gene Ther*, Vol.5, No.4, pp. 469-480, ISSN 1043-0342

Woltjen, K., Michael, I. P., Mohseni, P., Desai, R., Mileikovsky, M., Hämäläinen, R., Cowling, R., Wang, W., Liu, P., Gertsenstein, M., Kaji, K., Sung, H. K. & Nagy, A. (2009). piggyBac transposition reprograms fibroblasts to induced pluripotent stem cells. *Nature*, Vol.458, No.7239, pp. 766-770, ISSN 0028-0836

Wu, S. C. Y., Meir, Y. J. J., Coates, C. J., Handler, A. M., Pelczar, P., Moisyadi, S. & Kaminski, J. M. (2006). piggyBac is a flexible and highly active transposon as compared to sleeping beauty, Tol2, and Mos1 in mammalian cells. *Proc Natl Acad Sci U S A*, Vol.103, No.41, pp. 15008-15013, ISSN 0027-8424

Xue, X., Huang, X., Nodland, S. E., Mátés, L., Ma, L., Izsvák, Z., Ivics, Z., LeBien, T. W., McIvor, R. S., Wagner, J. E. & Zhou, X. (2009). Stable gene transfer and expression in cord blood-derived CD34+ hematopoietic stem and progenitor cells by a hyperactive Sleeping Beauty transposon system. *Blood*, Vol.114, No.7, pp. 1319-1330, ISSN 0006-4971

Yant, S. R., Meuse, L., Chiu, W., Ivics, Z., Izsvak, Z. & Kay, M. A. (2000). Somatic integration and long-term transgene expression in normal and haemophilic mice using a DNA transposon system. *Nat Genet*, Vol.25, No.1, pp. 35-41, ISSN 1061-4036

Yant, S. R., Huang, Y., Akache, B. & Kay, M. A. (2007). Site-directed transposon integration in human cells. *Nucleic Acids Res*, Vol.35, No.7, pp. e50, ISSN 0305-1048

Yusa, K., Zhou, L., Li, M. A., Bradley, A. & Craig, N. L. (2011). A hyperactive piggyBac transposase for mammalian applications. *Proc Natl Acad Sci U S A*, Vol.108, No.4, pp. 1531-1536, ISSN 0027-8424

Zhu, J., Park, C. W., Sjeklocha, L., Kren, B. T. & Steer, C. J. (2010). High-level genomic integration, epigenetic changes, and expression of sleeping beauty transgene. *Biochemistry*, Vol.49, No.7, pp. 1507-1521, ISSN 0006-2960

Zychlinski, D., Schambach, A., Modlich, U., Maetzig, T., Meyer, J., Grassman, E., Mishra, A. & Baum, C. (2008). Physiological promoters reduce the genotoxic risk of integrating gene vectors. *Mol Ther*, Vol.16, No.4, pp. 718-725, ISSN 1525-0016

8

Impacts of DNA Microarray Technology in Gene Therapy

Yadollah Omidi, Amir Ata Saei and Jaleh Barar
Research Center for Pharmaceutical Nanotechnology, Faculty of Pharmacy, Tabriz University of Medical Sciences, Tabriz, Iran

1. Introduction

Invention of microarray technology in the early 1990s revolutionized the genomic research, where it was exploited for global gene expression profiling through screening the expression of thousands of genes simultaneously (Watson et al., 1998). Northern blotting and reverse transcription polymerase chain reaction (RT-PCR) which were the traditional techniques for monitoring changes in mRNA levels were replaced with high density arrays, which proved to impart comprehensive data and to be better in the course of time.

Nowadays, microarrays are used for genotyping, large scale single nucleotide polymorphism analysis, comparative genomic hybridizations, identification of new genes, establishing genetic networks and as a more routine function, gene expression profiling (Bednar, 2000). Providing a unique tool for the determination of gene expression at transcriptomic level, it confers simultaneous measurement of large fractions of the genome which can facilitates the recognition of specific gene expression patterns associated with a certain disease or a specific pharmaceutical. Detection of the inimitable genomic signature of any active compound is deemed to be another important application of microarray technology, upon which "intrinsic genomic impacts" of any pharmacologically active agent can be clarified. And presumably, such toxicity predication may promise notable information about each individual resulting in unique patterns of gene expression that, in turn, exhibit individual specific responses to a particular toxic substance.

Basically, the discovery of diagnostic biomarkers has been the most promising feature of microarrays up to now and microarray technology has shown a great potential in predicting gene function and tracking the interactions among genetic networks too (Xiang & Chen, 2000). Microarray methodology has also been applied for analysis of proteins and metabolites, which are the principle controllers of gene expression, to verify the results at the molecular level. This in turn can extend our understanding of gene expression patterns and molecular pathways even though other techniques such as NMR, mass spectroscopy, gas and liquid chromatography can be employed for metabolite profiling. Having exploited such techniques, for example, the identity and quantity of different molecules can be determined in the CSF, urine or any other biological sample. Thus, by merging the classical techniques with new high-density microarray, the "omics" technology has been devised and implemented for investigation on genomics, proteomics, cytomics and metabolomics (Jares, 2006; Rosa et al., 2006). The microarray is by far one of the best tools for pursuing such impacts. For implementation of this technology, however, one needs to be familiar with the different methods used in microarray data analyses and the ways for more efficient applications of such methods to enhance the output of a microarray screening process. Fig.1 represents schematic steps of microarray (Saei & Omidi, 2011).

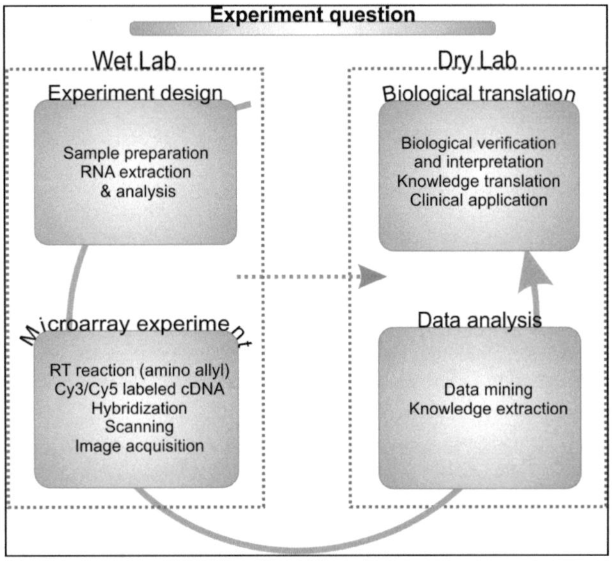

Fig. 1. Schematic steps of microarray, adapted with permission from (Saei & Omidi, 2011).

The main focus of this chapter is to provide the importance of DNA microarray technology in gene therapy, focusing on the application of DNA microarray technology (wet lab approach) and also giving simple descriptions on microarray data analysis as well as knowledge extraction (dry lab approach). In the next sections, we discuss some important information on the DNA microarray gene expression profiling.

2. DNA microarray technology

DNA microarrays consist of microscopic arrays of large sets of DNA sequences that are immobilized on solid substrates such as glass (slide array which are identical in dimensions to microscope slides) used as powerful tools for identification and/or quantification of many specific DNA sequences. Fig. 2 shows schematic illustration of spotted genes on a glass slide array.

For printing of arrays of the desired genes, glass slide arrays are commonly used. In practice, prior to spotting the genes, the surface of the microarray slides are uniformly coated with a chemical compound which is able to interact with and immobilize nucleic acids irreversibly and attach them onto the surface. Nucleic acids (e.g., clone library, cDNAs, PCR products, long oligonucleotides, microRNA) are then deposited on the coated surface using contact printing, after which the slides are further treated (using UV light or baking at 80°C) to crosslink the genes spots onto the slide surface. The printed slide arrays are normally stored (at room temperature and dark) until required for experimentation (Hobman et al., 2007).

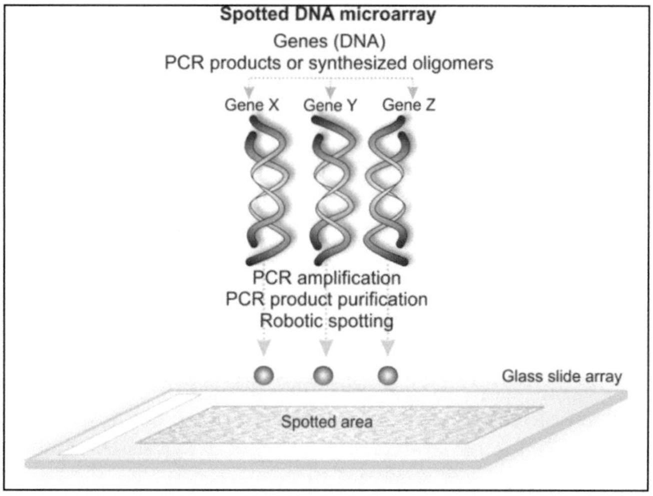

Fig. 2. Schematic illustration of spotted genes on a glass slide array. Glass slide arrays are produced by the robotic spotter that spots genes (e.g., PCR products, cDNAs, clone libraries or long oligonucleotides) onto coated glass slides. Each spot on the array represents a particular contiguous gene fragment, i.e. 40–70 nucleotides for oligonucleotide arrays, or several hundred nucleotides for PCR products, adapted with permission from (Saei & Omidi, 2011).

In DNA arrays, each spot on the array corresponds to a particular single gene. To spot greater numbers of genes on the slide arrays, the genes must be miniaturized and printed using tiny amount of biological material. The high throughput methods of sample preparation tend to be restricted in the amount of biological materials and concomitant with miniaturization of the array there has also been a trend towards decreasing the amount of biological material (e.g. RNA) used in the array experiments. Such approach can make the entire process much easier and more cost-effective. It should be also noticed that the fabrication of microarray screening systems are swiftly moving towards nanoarrays (Chen & Li, 2007), upon which some limitations of microarrays such as requirement for relatively large sample volumes and elongated incubation time can be resolved. We use the glass slide arrays commercially available by the Ocimum Bioslutions (www.ocimumbio.com/) mainly for gene expression profiling in cancer nanomedicine studies. The spotted glass slide arrays are now widely being used for research purposes as their fabrication is simple and cost-effective even though the spotting of genes tend not to be a simple approach by means of a printing machine (spotter). For printing the glass slide microarrays, the noncontact deposition and contact deposition methods have been widely used. The first uses ink-jet printing technology to deposit small droplets of liquid of pre-synthesized oligonucleotides or other biological materials onto a solid surface. The second uses physical deposition of small volumes of liquid from a metal pin onto the slide surface. Both of these technologies exploit microfluidics/nanofluidics approaches.

Basically, nucleic acid hybridization is the keystone of the DNA microarray technology. When denatured, single stranded nucleic acids are incubated together under certain conditions, hybridization can occur, upon which the formation of base paired duplex molecules can be prompted through G:C and/or A:T hydrogen bounds base paring. As a matter of fact the nucleic acids hybridization process may be influenced by the concentration and complexity of the sample, which also can be improved through manipulation of time, temperature and ionic strength of the hybridization buffer (Hobman et al., 2007). Maladjustment of these parameters may lead to some inadvertent mismatches in the nucleic acid duplex, resulting in undesired outcomes. Removal of mismatched hybrids is generally conducted under increasing stringency (i.e., by decreasing salt concentration and/or increasing temperature). Given that the removal of mismatched hybridization is difficult and may affect the end point results of the experiment, thus the more suitable experimental design with best variable adjustment should be considered (Hobman et al., 2007).

In general, some major applications and/or technologies of DNA microarrays are: 1) gene expression profiling, 2) pathogen detection and characterization, 3) comparative genome hybridization (CGH), 4) mutation and single nucleotide polymorphism (SNP) detection, 5) genotyping, 6) whole genome resequencing, 7) determining protein-DNA interactions using ChIP-chip (also known as ChIP-on-chip), 8) regulatory RNA studies, 9) alternative splicing detection (exon junction array), 10) RNA binding protein analysis, 11) microRNA studies, and 12) methylome analysis (DNA methylation profiling).

Recently, the US Food and Drug Administration (FDA) has conducted a project named "MicroArray Quality Control (MAQC)" upon which FDA aims to develop standards and quality control metrics which will eventually allow the use of microarray data in drug discovery, clinical practice and regulatory decision-making procedures. MAQC has gone to phase III now (i.e., MAQC-III, also called Sequencing Quality Control (SEQC)). The MAQC-III aims at: 1) assessing the technical performance of next-generation sequencing platforms, through generating benchmark datasets with reference samples, and 2) evaluating the advantages and limitations of various bioinformatics strategies in RNA and DNA analyses (Shi, 2008).

In practice, DNA microarray can be divided into two main dimensions, i.e., wet lab (Fig. 3A) and dry lab dimensions (Fig. 3B). The main steps of experimental approach for transcriptomics DNA microarray are shown in Fig. 3. Based on experiment question, the arrays are printed (Fig. 2) or the desired format of commercially available slide arrays are purchased. The wet lab experiments consists of: 1) sample preparation and total RNA extraction, 2) RT reaction and cDNA labeling (preparation for direct or indirect labeling, e.g., using aminoallyl tagged dUTP), 3) cyanine dyes (Cy3/Cy5) post labeling, 4) co hybridization of labeled cDNAs (Cy3-cDNA and Cy5-cDNA), 5) washing and scanning, 6) image acquisition, and 7) data analysis.

3. Wet lab experiments

3.1 Experimental design and sample preparation

A key to successful implementation of the DNA microarray technology is experimental design and quality of samples, i.e. the more accurate design, the more reliable microarray data. The user must make precise questions/hypotheses to be addressed through recruiting such technology, so are the statistical implications (e.g., replications, power analysis, clustering, principal component analysis (PCA), etc.). It has to be clarified that whether comparisons made on the microarray are to be direct or indirect (by making comparisons within or between slides, the so called type I/II experiments), and also whether experimental design needs to be single or multi-factorial (Shi, 2008).

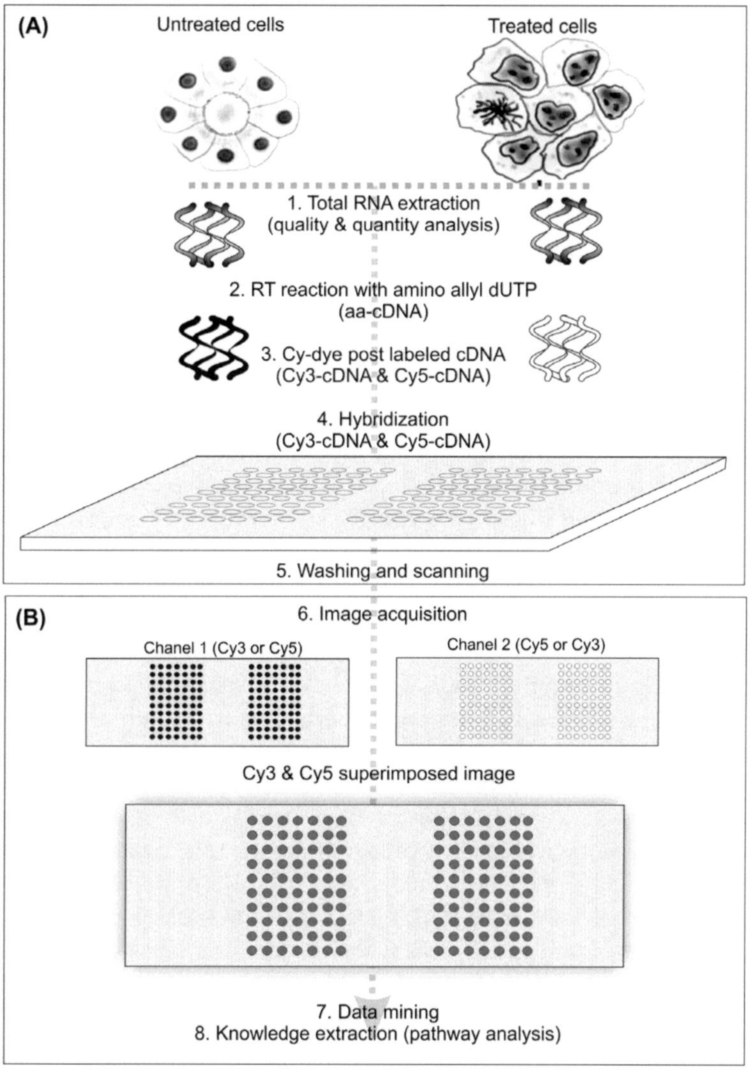

Fig. 3. Main steps of the experimental approach of transcriptomics DNA microarray for wet (A) and dry (B) lab experiments; adapted with permission from (Saei & Omidi, 2011).

In sample preparation, usually total RNA is isolated from the designated sample (e.g., animal/plant cells). Total RNA (10-20 µg), in the case of indirect labeling, is then converted to cDNA using tagged dNTPs (e.g., aminoallyl dUTP) and labeled with cyanine dyes (Cy3/Cy5) before hybridization to the array. Fundamentally, of critical importance to any successful transcriptomics experiment is believed to be the quality, quantity, and integrity of the isolated RNA (total RNA or mRNA) used in microarray experiments. Among various commercially available RNA isolation kits (e.g., from Sigma-Aldrich, Ambion, Qiagen, and Promega), we have successfully used TriReagent™ from Sigma-Aldrich Co. (Omidi et al., 2003). It should be evoked that most of these isolation kits are designed for quick, easy and reliable RNA extraction. Besides, in general, it is crucial to choose the best working protocol for RNA extraction considering vulnerability of RNA for degradation since the RNA even in the cell appears to show instability and short half-life to some extent. Successful use of commercially available kits such as RNAprotect™ (Ambion) and RNAlater™ (Qiagen) has been also reported. In the case of total RNA use, it should be noticed that only a small fraction of total RNA is mRNA, thus 10-20 µg of total RNA is commonly used to obtain sufficient mRNA for a transcriptomics microarray experiment. However, prior to conducting microarray experiment, the quality and quantity of the isolated total RNA has to be checked - the electrophoresed total RNA much be intact, showing 28s and 18s bands respectively at ~5 kbp and ~2 kbp using agarose gel electrophoresis, and the UV absorbance ratio (both for 260/280 and 260/230) must be about 1.8-2 using UV micro-spectrophotometers (e.g., Nanodrop™).

3.2 Labeling and hybridization

For labeling of samples, direct and indirect labeling of cDNA are widely used methods. In both approaches, the total RNA or mRNA is converted into cDNA by means of RT reaction (using either oligo dT priming to the 3' polyadenylation site, or random hexamer/nonamer). The main difference between these two approaches is direct or indirect incorporation of fluorescent dyes (e.g., cyanine dyes, CyDyes™ (Cy3 or Cy5), Alexa™ dyes) into the cDNA, i.e. direct incorporation of dye into the cDNA by RT reaction (direct labeling method), and indirect incorporation of dye through amino-allyl dUTP into the cDNA (indirect labeling method). Although the direct incorporation method is simple and rapid, it seems there is a bias of incorporation in this method so that the cDNA is labeled at higher efficiency by Cy3 than by Cy5. To resolve this issue, dye swap experiments in treated and untreated samples can be performed, in which in the replicate experiment the control sample is labeled with Cy3 instead of Cy5 and vice-versa for test sample; and comparing the results and analysis of combined outcome. The indirect labeling method display less biased dye incorporation, however its main disadvantage is that the protocols are more intricate and time consuming.
In our research center (http://nano.tbzmed.ac.ir/), we follow the protocol of the supplier "Ocimum Biosolutions". Briefly, after sticking the gas-tight sealing system (Gene Frame™), the hybridization buffer is preheated at 42°C for 10 min. The labeled cDNA is dissolved in an appropriate amount of hybridization buffer. The hybridization mixture is heated at 95°C for 3 min and subsequently cooled on ice for maximum 3 min. The appropriate volume of probe/hybridization solution is pipetted at one end of the frame and the polyester cover slip is carefully placed over the frame. The arrays are incubated at 42°C on a shaker in dark for 16-24 h. For washing, the following washing buffers (WB) are used: WB1 (2x saline-sodium citrate (SSC), 0.1 % sodium dodecyl sulfate (SDS)), WB2 (1 x SSC), WB3 (0.5x SSC). All washing steps are performed at room temperature for 3-5 min each step. All buffers should be filter sterilized. To dry the slide arrays, prior to scanning with a scanner, they are briefly gently centrifuged.

4. Data mining

A key point for translation of DNA microarray data into clinical application is data mining which is deemed to be the most confounding part. Data Mining is all about automating the process of searching for patterns in the data – it is an iterative process of discovery. As shown in Fig. 4, implementation of image processing and bioinformatics methodologies appears to be crucial for obtaining a sensible outcome from microarray data.

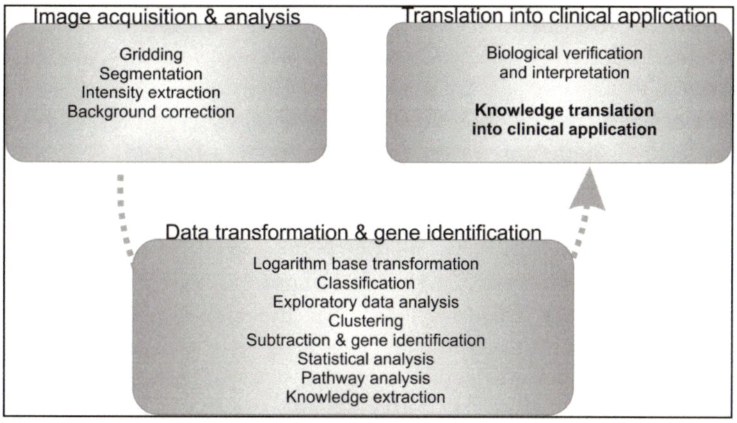

Fig. 4. Translation of DNA microarray data into clinical applications; adapted with permission from (Saei & Omidi, 2011).

Exploratory data analysis on microarray can help discover new patterns and networks in gene expression. The patterns that data mining discovers can have various forms including: trends in data over time, clusters of data defined by important combinations of variables, and finally evolution of these clusters over time. Patterns could be derived from analyzing the change in expression of the genes, and new insights could be gained into the underlying biology. Using the data retrieved from the microarray we can determine gene function in the cell, identify targets for new drug designation and reveal molecular networks and pathways

4.1 Image acquisition and primary analysis

Although the correct analysis and interpretation of microarray data is highly dependent upon image acquisition and data production, surprisingly less attention is usually given to such crucial steps which include: 1) scanning of the image, 2) spot recognition, 3) gridding 4) segmentation, and 5) intensity extraction.

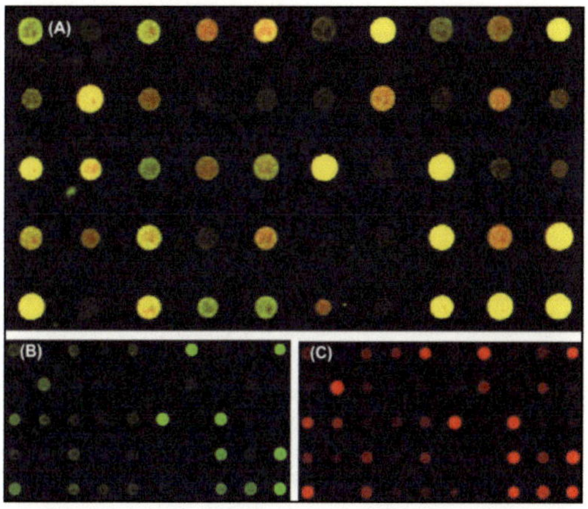

Fig. 5. Typical fluorescent images of hybridized cDNA microarray. A) Superimposed fluorescent image of Cy3-cDNA and Cy5-cDNA hybridization. B) Fluorescent images of Cy3 channel. C) Fluorescent images of Cy5 channel. Data are adapted with permission from (Barar et al., 2009).

Fig. 5 represents typical fluorescent images of hybridized cDNA microarray for superimposed image of Cy3- and Cy5-labeled cDNA as well as Cy3-labeled hybridized cDNA of untreated control cells and Cy5-labeled hybridized cDNA of treated cells.

For identification of each spot or gene on the slide, a grid has to be applied to the spots on the slide using appropriate softwares (e.g., we generally use TECAN scanner with ArrayPro™ software). However, a manual proofreading needs to be performed to ensure that all the spots on the array fall on the grid correctly (Lonardi & Luo, 2004). Once the gridding fulfilled, segmentation can be performed to separate the spots from the background and define the shape of each spot – there are always different shapes that do not have a constant diameter. Inside the circle is the signal we seek and outside is the background. Many methods are included in softwares for segmentation such as fixed circle segmentation (FCS), adaptive circle segmentation (ACS), adaptive shape segmentation (ASS) and histogram segmentation (HS). The selection of the best method largely depends on the quality of the produced images and personal interest and experience (Ahmed et al., 2004). As the name indicates, the FCS treats all spots equally. When almost all of the spots on the microarray are circular, the ACS has been proved to be the best approach, whereas ASS finds the shape which best fits the spot when the spots are not circular. The HS method considers pixel intensities in and around each spot to decide whether that specific pixel belongs to that spot (Ahmed et al., 2004; Bengtsson & Bengtsson, 2006; Lehmussola et al., 2006; Qin et al., 2005). After separation of the signal from the background, it comes to intensity extraction, after which the intensity ratios are calculated. To minimize the systematic errors, poor quality spots should be removed – that is any spot with intensity lower than the background plus two standard deviations should be excluded.

4.2 Normalization and transformation

Normalization and transformation of data is the first step after primary analysis and includes background subtraction, normalization, ratio calculation and log transformation (Geller et al., 2003; Quackenbush, 2002). Spotted arrays are routinely used for simultaneous analysis of gene expression in untreated control and treated cells. The mRNA extracted from untreated control is labeled with cy3, whereas mRNA obtained from treated cells is labeled with cy5. To minimize the impact of these two dyes and for verification of results, dye flipping appears to be a helpful strategy.

Cy3 and Cy5 data will be normalized individually and then the expression ratio (as logarithmic scale) will be calculated. The advantage of reporting $\log_2$ instead of the intact expression ratio is that in this way all the ratios fall between -1 and +1. Genes with a $\log_2$ of +1, have an upregulation factor of 2 and genes with a $\log_2$ of -1 have a downregulation factor of 2. Genes which possess constant expressions in the two samples will have a $\log_2$ of 0. Normalization is the most important process in transformation and compensates for the experimental variability of the data and assumes that all of the genes on an array or a subset of them have an average expression ratio of 1. In the scatter plot of cy5 versus cy3 intensities, most of the genes usually form a cluster along a straight line. Cy5 intensity is usually less than that of the Cy3. This is normally seen in the scatter plots with deviations from the one to one ratio.The slope of the line (Cy5 vs. Cy3) in the scatter plot should be one in the ideal case where there are no inconsistencies and/or all the variables are same for the two samples, but this is not usually the case. Normalization is, in fact, the calculation of the slope which best fits the line. This is usually performed using regression techniques which provide the slope value and helps removal of the unwanted effects, at the cost of losing some information such as the absolute expression values. The most often applied methods for the normalization of the dye bias include: 1) local mean, 2) global mean, 3) LOcally WEighed Scatter-plot Smoothing (LOWESS), and 4) bayesian analyses. We have effectively used the LOWESS normalization method. Fig. 6 represents a typical small array showing LOWESS based normalization of data as scatter plot.

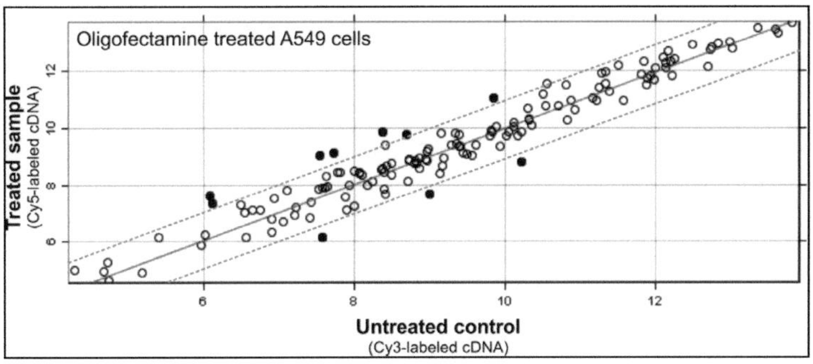

Fig. 6. A typical scatter plot for small array representing normalized data using LOWESS method. Data represent gene expression changes induced by Oligofectamine™ nanoliposome used for gene (antisense) delivery in A549 cells. White and Black circles respectively show unchanged and up-/down- regulated genes (with at least 2-fold changes). Data are adapted with permission from (Barar et al., 2009).

Now the question is how can we select a specific normalization method which best fits the structure of our data? In fact, the most simple normalization method is using housekeeping genes as reference points in the two chips and multiplying all the intensities by a constant until the expression of the controls get equal in the arrays under comparison (Quackenbush, 2001). The global normalization (total intensity normalization) assumes that the total amount of mRNA in a cell is fixed and the intensities of one chip are multiplied by a constant until the sum of the intensities of the genes in one chip equals the sum of the intensities in the other. This method is still a simple approach and does not remove the signal-dependent bias (Quackenbush, 2001). Regression techniques can be used instead of aforementioned methods for calculating the best-fit slope of the line (Kepler et al., 2002). If regression techniques for normalization are applied locally, it will be known as LOWESS which can be used to heal the nonlinearity in the data. LOWESS appears to be a powerful method in the normalization of the intensity-dependent dye bias and has shown to be good enough in many studies (Berger et al., 2004; Quackenbush, 2001). Once data were normalized, the expression ratio is calculated and then the $\log_2$ transformation is applied. To ensure about the quality of data produced, the expression of repeated genes on array as internal controls and the coefficient variation (CV) of normalized untreated controls of various experiments as external control can be checked.

4.3 Selection of differentially expressed genes and significance examination

The prime aim of a microarray analysis is to clarify the genes which have been differentially up or down regulated. The traditional method which was used for identifying the differentially expressed genes was setting a fixed cutoff threshold (usually in 2-fold) to infer significance. Genes with intensity ratio above or below the fixed ratio were said to be down or up regulated (Baggerly et al., 2001). This method is called fold change method (Draghici,

2002), but it is now believed to be inefficient due to the lack of a statistical basis. For example, if the condition under study changes the gene expression profile slightly, then this method will give no differentially regulated genes and as a result the sensitivity will be almost zero. In contrast to the former example, if the affecting parameter level is too high to produce the optimal detectable effect and the threshold is set at two, many genes will be selected as differentially regulated, the method will have low specificity and many genes will pass our filter as false positives (Cui & Churchill, 2003; Gusnanto et al., 2007). Another disadvantage is that, in microarray technology genes with little expression levels have a low signal to noise ratio, which can be demonstrated by the funnel shape at the bottom of the expression distribution in the scatter plot. It should be evoked that losing some data will be inevitable.

Another method for selecting differentially expressed genes is the unusual ratio which involves the selection of the genes for which the ratio of the experiment and control value is at certain distance that is usually taken ±2 standard deviation. In fact, the selected genes should have an "experiment: control" ratio of at least two standard deviations away from the related mean value. Basically, this procedure is accomplished by applying a z transformation to the log ratio values (Draghici, 2002).

4.4 Dimension reduction

A major problem in microarray analysis is the large number of dimensions. In gene expression experiments each gene and each experiment may represent one dimension. Visual analysis of the microarray data in the original format does not yield much because if a slide array (spotted with 1000 genes) is used to examine a particular disease in 10 patients, the resultant data will be of high dimensionality (which would be a matrix of 10 by 1000). To make the most of the data, feature reduction or dimension reduction is used which renders this possible by finding the minimum number of genes that can best describe data.

Dimensionality reduction algorithms can be classified into "feature selection" and "feature extraction". Feature selection is to select k dimensions, out of the original d dimensions, that can best represent the original data set. Feature extraction is to find a new set of k dimensions that are some combination of the original d dimensions. The most popular feature extraction algorithms may be the linear projection method such as PCA for unsupervised learning and linear discriminant analysis (LDA) for supervised learning. The number of dimensions after the methods are applied will be two as most analyses are performed in two dimensions x and y. There is a possibility of losing some weak but important data in this way as they cannot compete with the impact of more important features. The methods used in this section of analysis are PCA, correspondence analysis (CA), multi-dimensional scaling (MDS), and cluster analysis (Dugas et al., 2004; Nguyen, 2005; Shannon et al., 2003).

Of the dimension reduction methods, PCA is now mostly used method as a tool in exploratory data analysis and for making predictive models. PCA involves a mathematical procedure that transforms a number of possibly correlated variables into a smaller number of uncorrelated variables called principal components. The first principal component accounts for as much of the variability in the data as possible, and each succeeding component accounts for as much of the remaining variability as possible. PCA ignores the dimensions in which data do not vary much. PCA is closely related to factor analysis; indeed, some statistical packages deliberately conflate the two techniques.

4.5 Grouping methods

After performing multiple experiments under different conditions (e.g., number of patients or various time points), genes that reveal similar expression intensities can be grouped under a subset of conditions. Likewise based on the pattern of the distinguishing genes, boundaries between different subtypes (e.g., for cancer) can be set (Belacel et al., 2006). Grouping methods as "unsupervised method" or "supervised method" (the so called clustering and classification methods, respectively) can help identify co-expressed genes (Juan & Huang, 2007).

4.5.1 Unsupervised grouping: clustering

Unlike supervised methods, no data is provided in unsupervised methods that include hierarchical clustering, k means clustering and self-organizing maps (Au et al., 2004; Steinley, 2006). The efficiency of all these methods relies on whether high quality data has been produced.

Most clustering algorithms utilize a sort of distance metric (the distance between two expression vectors), based on which they group similar profiles together. This means that genes closer to each other in space are grouped together. They use either statistical correlation coefficient (from -1 to +1) or the Euclidean distance (the square root of the sum of the squared differences between corresponding feature values). The common measures of dissimilarity are "Euclidean distance" and "Manhattan distance" (Leung & Cavalieri, 2003; Quackenbush, 2001). Fig. 7 represents a schematic illustration for Euclidean distance clustering.

The Euclidean distance (*Ed*) and Manhattan distance (*Md*) are given by equations (1) and (2), respectively:

$$d_{Ed} = \sqrt{\sum_{i=1}^{n} (x_i - y_i)^2} \tag{1}$$

$$d_{Md} = \sum_{i=1}^{n} |x_i - y_i| \tag{2}$$

Where x_i and y_i are the measured expression values, respectively, for genes x and y in the experiment i, and n is the number of the experiments under the analysis.

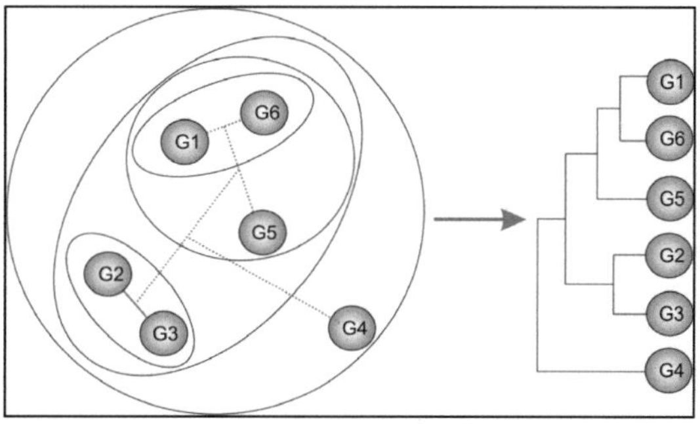

Fig. 7. Schematic illustration of Euclidean distance clustering of expressed genes (G); adapted from (Saei & Omidi, 2011).

The best way is to calculate the distance between a gene and the centroid of the cluster, however sometimes the distance between the gene and the nearest neighbor is calculated. Hierarchical clustering is a tree-like representation of data, which can be applied in two manners, "bottom-up" or "top-down" methods (Chipman & Tibshirani, 2006). The bottom-up method starts with each object representing one cluster of size 1 and at each following step, the two closest clusters are joined until all objects are in a single cluster of size *n*. The top-down method is the reverse phase of what was discussed and is usually of more interest when we aim to identify a few clusters (Chipman & Tibshirani, 2006). One major problem using the hierarchical clustering is that the number of the genes which undergo clustering should not exceed several thousands, because the process may fail or become time consuming since the algorithm calculates the distance between all genes. To resolve such problem, one of the solutions is to exclude the unchanged genes, or alternatively applying other methods such as K-means clustering which is faster than hierarchical clustering (Quackenbush, 2001). In fact, the K-means clustering uses the prior information about the expected number of the clusters (*k*) which can be obtained from principle component analysis. Each gene is randomly assigned to one of the clusters and then the distance between each gene with the centroid (average expression vector) of the clusters is calculated. If one gene is closer to the centroid of another cluster, it is moved to that cluster. The centroids are recalculated after the assignment of all the genes to their nearest centroids in an iterative process. This process continues until there is no change in the members of the clusters and the algorithm stops here (Steinley, 2006; Wilkin & Huang, 2008). Basically, the hierarchal clustering represents the relation of the genes to each other even though this is not the case with K-means clustering.

Self-organizing maps (SOMs) have been embedded with artificial neural networks (ANNs). And, based on the amount of the similarity of the expression vectors to reference, it is possible to clarify which gene belongs to which cluster. In contrast to other clustering algorithms, SOMs provide maps with the most similar clusters along each other's sides which make it a little bit different from K-means clustering (Covell et al., 2003).

One deficiency of the discussed algorithms is that a gene can only belong to just one cluster in the dataset, while a gene may be member of more than one cluster due to its different functions in the cell. An example to this can be those proteins that are the major players of complicated networks in the cell, e.g. second messengers of the cell transduction pathways or epidermal growth factor receptor (EGFR) which is known to play various roles in different cells. A fuzzy logic can be alternatively exploited to solve such problem, because it pursues clustering with overlapping. In fuzzy clustering, a gene may belong to different clusters with specific membership degrees between zero and one specified to each cluster. The sum of the membership degrees of each gene in fuzzy clustering is one (Dembele & Kastner, 2003).

As discussed above different clustering methods have different efficiencies and different algorithms and thus are likely to produce different results. Even two hierarchical clustering algorithms in two softwares are slightly different and do not completely match, thus the results vary from algorithm to algorithm and from software to software. This means one gene may be placed in different groups or clusters when applying different algorithms. Therefore, upon our experiences, it is recommended to apply various methods and different parameters to the data analysis and then, based on the result decide what to do. Function prediction is another technique which can be applied after cluster analysis (Joshi et al., 2004). Genes that behave similarly in response to different conditions are likely to have similar functions. Thus, the function of orphan genes (genes with unknown function) can be inferred from the known function of other genes placed in the same cluster.

4.5.2 Supervised grouping: classification, class prediction using the input data

In supervised methods the network is fed with some data for which the gene families are known. Thus based on the previous data provided for the network, it predicts that a new feature -that has not been used in the training step- belongs to a specific family (Peng, 2006; Wang et al., 2005). This is called "machine learning". The classifier is trained using the expression of all genes (which have passed the t-test or ANOVA for determination of the significance) as the input and then selects the features (genes) that contribute the most to your condition, and then classifier is validated on a set of sample that was not used in feature selection in the later step. For example, if you have two cancer subtypes you can easily classify the two subtypes and select the genes that are differentially expressed in one subtype and not in the other or using known genes you can classify the cancer subtypes. For comparison of more samples you need to find genes that are expressed differentially just in one subtype. To make a general model, one needs to apply cross-validation method (i.e., to split data into different training and prediction sets and to try the classifier) or leave-one-out method (i.e., crossing out one of the features and screening the effect of deletion on the dataset) to the data.

Supervised methods are almost good at pattern recognition and dividing the samples into groups, but so far have not shown to be effective enough in the new samples, i.e. when it comes to prediction they have lower efficiency. The supervised methods include neural networks, logistic regression and linear discriminant analysis (LDA) (Liao & Chin, 2007; Linder et al., 2007; Shen & Tan, 2005; Tai & Pan, 2007). Nearest neighbor classifier is one of the simplest classifiers (Shen & Hasegawa, 2008). If one has already performed a principal component analysis or clustering, then it will be possible to determine the most probable number of classes (as in K-means) in the data and the algorithm will work well.

For higher number of example it is better to use more advanced methods such as ANN which use the brain neurons' logic. In use of the classification methods, however, overfitting or overtraining of the classifier algorithm is a major problem, which means if the classifier is provided with too many parameters a false model may perfectly fit the data (Babyak, 2004; Hawkins, 2004). When the degrees of freedom in parameter selection are more than the information content, the ability of the model is diminished or destroyed. In machine learning, the algorithm is trained using some part of the data for which we know what the output will be. After training, the model should be able to predict the output for the other part of data for which the output is unknown. When overfitting happens, the performance of the model on training examples will increase, but the prediction power will be lower. Contrary to this, if the network is not complex enough it will fail to detect the signal. This is called underfitting. But a too complex network will fit even the noise, leading to overfitting which can produce excessive variance in the outputs and instead of capturing the desired pattern or trend in the data, it will memorize the training data (Babyak, 2004; Hawkins, 2004). The best way to chuck out overfitting is to use lots of training data. We should have at least 10 observations per variable. If one is looking at 30 variables, the model should be at least provided with 300 events. To avoid overfitting, it is also possible to use additional techniques such as cross-validation, weight decay, bayesian learning, early stopping and also model comparison (Babyak, 2004; Braga-Neto & Dougherty, 2004; Hawkins, 2004).

4.6 Pathway analysis

Pathway analysis should be towards functional enrichment to establish networks between genes and proteins. This may provide better understanding about the dynamics of gene expression that may grant a platform for reverse engineering of regulatory networks. Understanding the expression dynamics of gene networks helps us infer innate complexities and phenomenological networks among genes. Defining the true place of the genes in cell networks is indeed the foundation of our understanding of programming and functioning of living cells. Studying the regulation patterns of genes in groups, using clustering and classification methods helps us understand different pathways in the cell, their functions, regulations and the way one component in the system affects the other one. These networks can act as starting points for data mining and hypothesis generation, helping us reverse engineer (Guo et al., 2006; Li et al., 2007; Mircean et al., 2004; Park et al., 2007).

When the picture of gene interactions are established, the nodes with many connections in the network are thought to be of crucial role in the cell function and can be considered as probable specific targets for drug delivery or even design of new drugs (e.g., in the case with EGFR or other Tyrosine Kinase genes). These pathways can tell us where the drugs act and also where our carriers induce toxicity (Dewey, 2002). They also help us predict the function of unknown genes and investigate their true place in the pathways, where gene expression or metabolic changes have been produced due to mutations or changed environmental conditions. Using these techniques, the mechanisms underlying diseases can be discovered.

One of the methods used in pathway analysis is comparing the gene list to a pathway which gives a *p* value as a result. The scoring enrichment methods compare a list of the genes to that of a pathway and count the hits; the greater the number of the hits, the greater the score and the enrichment (Curtis et al., 2005). Other hit-counting methods used by MAPP Finder and Odds ratio are hit-counting methods which indicate the degree of enrichment (Doniger et al., 2003). GenMAPP, an open source package that allows users to visualize microarray and proteomics data in the context of biological pathways (freely available at http://www.genmapp.org/), represents biological pathways in a special file format called 'MAPPs' which are independent of the gene expression data. It is used to group genes by any organizing principle (e.g., apoptosis pathways). The gene set enrichment analysis (GSEA) is a novel method, which uses all the data on the microarray in the order of expression, determining whether an a priori defined set of genes shows statistically significant, concordant differences between two biological states (e.g. phenotypes) (Subramanian et al., 2005). This algorithm compares each gene, in turn, to the pathway or class, and enrichment score is specified (Subramanian et al., 2007). The GSEA and Z score analysis provide *p* values which are easy to interpret, but it is not clear whether these values are biologically relevant. As for other methods described above, using different criteria Z scores can yield different results, because they are sensitive to gene list and pathway length (Curtis et al., 2005).

In the gene ontology project (http://www.geneontology.org), the genes have been classified into a hierarchy, based on the similarities in functions. The Kyoto Encyclopedia of Genes and Genomes (KEGG) (http://www.genome.kp/kegg/) provides searchable pathways (Aoki & Kanehisa, 2005; Kanehisa, 2002). However, the major problem encountered is that there are many genes with unknown functions or pathways, thus attempt should be done in discovering more pathways and connecting them with existing ones. With the future data incorporated into the pathway analysis, there will sure be improvements in the information produced by the microarrays. One best approach for establishing relationships in the data is to focus mainly on the genes on which a large amount of data is available.

Reverse engineering of regulatory networks can be fulfilled using two methods, one of which is "time-series data" and second one is "steady-state data" of gene knockouts. In the first approach, the magnitude of expression of a certain gene at a certain time point is a function of expression amount of the other genes at all previous time points. In the second approach, the effects of deleting a certain gene on the expression of other genes are inspected and based on the regulation of the other genes the function of that certain gene is assessed. For example, if by deleting gene A, gene B is upregulated, then one can relatively think that gene A, either directly or indirectly, suppresses the expression of gene B. However, these methods and in particular reverse engineering still lack full applicability, because there is a need for more discovered sophisticated networks in the cells in order to identify the hidden role of different molecules in the circuitry of gene regulation (Curtis et al., 2005; Martin et al., 2007).

5. Microarray gene expression profiling blunders

Exploratory data analysis on microarray can help discover new patterns and networks in gene expression. Using the data retrieved from the microarray one can determine gene function in the cell, identify targets for new drug designation and reveal molecular networks and pathways (Lee et al., 2008).

In recent years, many methods have been devised which have now found critical applications in the analysis of the microarray data. The methods used to explore deep into the microarray data include the PCA, the singular value decomposition (SVD), the SOMs and the support vector machine (Nahar et al., 2007; Pandey et al., 2007; Wall et al., 2001; Xiao et al., 2003; Zhu et al., 2009). Some of these methods such as PCA and clustering methods are used for data reduction as the vast nature of the microarray data does not allow the analysis of the genes one by one and holism is also not possible (Leung & Cavalieri, 2003; Quackenbush, 2001). Most applicable methods are unsupervised, and do not require additional prior information to feed the algorithm. As our understanding and knowledge of the genes and their expression in different cells and tissues is increased, incorporation of the known data will empower the microarray data analysis which can help show some real potential of data. As the scientific demands grow, we will need more sophisticated bioinformatics and biostatistics tools to fulfill the different needs in the analysis of the microarray data. Distinguishing the truly differentially regulated genes from noises or other genes is a real challenge in the first steps, because the filtered data is going to be used as a basis for the next steps in data mining. Unfortunately there are more genes than conditions and this makes the analysis of the data difficult. To render the microarray data more reliable, one needs to use more stringent data cutoffs such as the Bonferonni correction (not the two-fold cutoff) as the selection measure of the differentially regulated genes and reducing the number of the false positives in the data set (Bland & Altman, 1995). It should be highlighted that obtaining microarray data appears to be easy, however the analysis of the data is usually tedious and time consuming (Loring, 2006), thus there should be special focus on the analysis of the microarray data. However, because of our poor understanding of cell pathways and molecular biology and also not incorporating the gene information when analyzing the data, we are not able to dig deep into the jam of data produced by microarrays. Another problem is that some sections of the analysis deal with genes one by one considering them as individuals, whereas others look at the data in a holistic way. After finding a responsible gene for a specific trait or function in the cell using microarray technology, other methods (e.g., RT-PCR, gene silencing, northern blotting) can be applied on the specific gene to assure that all the steps in the microarray analysis have been performed correctly. The reverse is also true; i.e. microarray can be used to verify the other techniques (Hembruff et al., 2005).

If microarray technology is to be employed in genomic impacts investigations of the gene delivery systems, then it should be noticed that microarrays are prone to many errors both in the experimental handling and data analysis steps. In fact, it should be perceived that all we have is the mere fluorescence intensity emitted from the two dyes and the ratio of the two intensities, steps which are vulnerable to many blunders. In different steps in a microarray analysis, multiple errors can be produced. These include the efficiency of RNA isolation, amount of mRNA used, cDNA generation, amplification, selective incorporation of cyanine dyes (i.e., Cy_3 or Cy_5), the quality of the array, hybridization and washing condition, spatial bias on the array during hybridization, scanning procedures, random errors and other variations in the conditions (Pounds, 2006). Because of these variations and errors, there exists a need for replicate experiments for normalizing the data, i.e., the more replicates in experiment, the less variance in the data. Taking the log of ratio of the intensities can eliminate the possible non-linearity in the data. Instead of using the 2-fold increase/decrease in the ratio intensities for identifying differentially regulated genes, some statistically based techniques (e.g., ANOVA and maximum likelihood analysis) can be applied (Bakewell & Wit, 2005; Churchill, 2004). It should be evoked that the result of a microarray experiment is largely dependent on statistical methods used and the results from two separate analyses do not usually concord because data analysis is a multiple step process, with each step being vulnerable to personal misunderstanding and bad interpretations and also because many combinations of the analytic methods are possible (Loring, 2006). One factor that contributes to the deterioration of the matter is that different laboratories often use different defined approaches to their analyses. Analyzing the data using different procedures makes the final results different. Each of these processes can be carried out using various methods, for example one can use hierarchical clustering, K-means clustering or self-organizing maps in the clustering step. As another example different linkage methods are available for hierarchical clustering that the analyst is free to choose from, each of them producing slightly different outcomes.

Recently some attempts have been performed to bring these divergent processes into one homogenous procedure. For overcoming the problem, the Microarray Gene Expression Data (MGED) society (http://www.mged.org) proposed standards termed as "Minimum Information About a Microarray Experiment (MIAME) standards" for homogenization of the microarray experiments and data handling (Whetzel et al., 2006). Many journals today require submissions to be in compliance with MIAME, upon which many experiments are now in concordance with MIAME in experimental design, implementation and data analysis. This may provide researchers a platform to share their data, to cooperate for better data analysis and comparison of experiments. The six most critical elements in MIAME are: 1) the raw data for each hybridization, 2) the final normalized data for the set of hybridizations, 3) the essential sample annotation including experimental factors and their values (e.g., compound and dose in a dose response experiment), 4) experimental design, 5) sufficient annotation of the array (e.g., gene identifiers, genomic coordinates, probe sequences or reference commercial array catalog number), and 6) the essential laboratory and data processing protocols; reader is directed to see (http://www.mged.org/ Workgroups/ MIAME/miame.html) for a review of these standards. Unfortunately, the variations in two separate experiments can also be due to the true variation in the samples. For optimal minimization of the errors and avoidance of irreproducible measurements in the microarray analyses, it is often recommended to conduct the experiment in three separate replicates. By further increasing the number of the repeats, the confidence level increases even though it is not usually practical due to economic issues. Basically, the order in which the data analysis methods are applied appears to be: 1) image analysis, 2) normalization, 3) clustering, 4) pathway analysis, 5) promoter analysis, 6) function prediction, and 7) classification (Allison et al., 2006; De, V et al., 2007; Olson, 2006).

6. Gene therapy trials and microarray technology

Gene therapy appears to be one of the most challenging fields even though gene therapy researches have been tarnished with the death of Jesse Gelsinger in 1999 (the first publicly identified person to die in a gene therapy trial). However, many positive phase II/III trials seem to accelerate these researches. Table 1 represents the latest state of the gene therapy clinical trials worldwide.

Phase	Number and percentage of clinical trials (1989-2010)
Phase I	995 (60.5%)
Phase I/II	308 (18.7%)
Phase II	267 (16.2%)
Phase II/III	13 (0.8%)
Phase III	57 (3.5%)
Phase IV	2 (0.1%)
Single subject	2 (0.1%)
Total	1644

Table 1. Gene therapy clinical trials worldwide, data are from (Edelstein, 2011).

For example, Contusugene ladenovec (Advexin™, INGN-201; Introgen Therapeutics Inc.) has been announced as a first-generation gene therapy for cancer, targeting the cancer suppressor gene p53. Based upon the phase III trial results showing fairly good responses of certain patients to Advexin™, it has been accepted to be reviewed by the European Medicines Agency. Having observed additive/synergistic effects in a variety of tumor types (non-small-cell lung carcinomas, squamous cell carcinoma of the head and neck, hepatocellular carcinoma, glioma, breast, prostate and colorectal cancers), researchers in the field of gene therapy hope that these advancements will eventually help restore gene-based treatment modalities alone and in combination with chemotherapy and radiation (Senzer & Nemunaitis, 2009). This is just a beginning of a "molecular big-bang", a domain of science which requires mechanistic investigations on early and late influences of gene-based modalities for their successful translation into clinical practice.

Of these gene therapy clinical trials, as shown in Table 1, about 4% have reached the final stage and it is expected to see several gene based medicines in clinic soon. About 64.5% and 8.7% of them respectively belong to cancer and cardiovascular gene therapies, which highlight importance of these diseases (Edelstein, 2011). Table 2 represents the latest state of the gene delivery vectors used for gene therapy clinical trials worldwide.

Gene delivery vector	Number and percentage of clinical trials (1989-2010)
Adenovirus	400 (23.8%)
Retrovirus	344 (20.5%)
Naked/Plasmid DNA	304 (17.7%)
Vaccinia virus	133 (7.9%)
Lipofection	109 (6.5%)
Poxvirus	93 (5.5%)
Adeno-associated virus	75 (4.5%)
Herpes simplex virus	56 (3.3%)
Lentivirus	29 (1.7%)
Other categories	82 (4.9%)
Unknown	55 (3.3%)

Table 2. Gene delivery vectors used for gene therapy clinical trials worldwide, data are from (Edelstein, 2011).

So far, DNA microarray technology has been employed for detection of unknown gene-based biomarkers in various diseases, and also for clinical diagnosis. For example, in 2010 Qin and Tian performed a microarray gene analysis of peripheral whole blood in normal adult male rats after long-term growth hormone (GH) gene therapy. They reported that 61 genes were found to be differentially ($p < 0.05$) expressed 24 weeks after receiving GH gene therapy. These genes were mainly associated with angiogenesis, oncogenesis, apoptosis, immune networks, signaling pathways, general metabolism, type I diabetes mellitus, carbon fixation, cell adhesion molecules, and cytokine-cytokine receptor interaction. The results imply that exogenous GH gene expression in normal subjects is likely to induce cellular changes in the metabolism, signal pathways and immunity. Based on such screening, these researchers claimed eight genes as candidate biomarkers (Qin & Tian, 2010).

Since genomedicines (e.g., antisense oligo deoxy nucleotides (As-ODN), RNA interference) can selectively block disease-causing genes, the responsible genes of diseases (e.g., cancer genes) have been chosen as potential targets even though undesired nonspecific side effects may tarnish the actual mechanism of gene therapy, blemishing clinical development of gene based therapeutics. Using DNA microarray technology, Cho et al. have conducted a systematic characterization of gene expression in cells exposed to antisense and showed that in a sequence-specific manner, antisense targeted to protein kinase A RIalpha alters expression of the clusters of coordinately expressed genes at a specific stage of cell growth, differentiation, and activation (Cho et al., 2001). These researchers showed that the genes defined the proliferation-transformation signature were down-regulated, however those genes defined the differentiation-reverse transformation signature were up-regulated in antisense-treated cancer cells and tumors. And based on such findings, they concluded that the defining As-ODNs on the basis of their effects on global gene expression may lead to identification of clinically relevant antisense therapeutics and can identify which molecular and cellular events might be important in complex biological processes.

A brief search of the relevant database of scientific literatures such as Medline, Toxnet and BIDS clearly reveals existence of a fairly large number of investigations upon gene delivery and/or targeting, while little works have been undertaken on cytogenomic impacts of such gene delivery vectors. It is still not totally clear what genomic impacts can be elicited by a particular genomedicine or even by its viral/non-viral carrier(s). Although, the gene/drug delivery systems are generally announced as inert materials, it seems that in many occasions they are not compatible in a genomic level. Thus, we may even face with new terminologies such as "functional excipients" which can inevitably impose non-specific intrinsic cytogenomic changes in target cells/tissues (Omidi et al., 2005a).

7. Genomic impacts of gene delivery systems

To date, the traditional chemotherapies have become an indispensable part of the cancer treatment procedures which almost always requires that the patient take high doses of multiple drugs. Thus, to avoid the inevitable occurrence of side effects, there is an emergent need for smart targeted delivery systems that provide lower toxicity and higher specificity - that will also be able to reduce the required dose of the drugs. Since gene therapy (using As-ODN, siRNA, aptamer, ribozyme, etc.) can target disease at genomic level, this approach has attained great attention. To deliver nucleic acids to target cells, gene carriers such as viral and nonviral vectors (Table 2) have been widely used to overcome systemic and subcellular barriers. In fact, such carriers like drug delivery systems can largely influence the pharmacokinetic properties (i.e., absorption, distribution, metabolism, and elimination) of drugs which are incorporated with designated carriers. Thus, there has been an increasing interest in design of delivery vehicles which are capable of delivering drugs (of any origin) inside cancer cells that is now an issue in design of molecular Trojan horses (Kim et al., 2008; Portney & Ozkan, 2006; Sawant et al., 2006).

It has been revealed that most gene delivery systems can nonspecifically induce alterations in the gene expression profile of the target cells (Omidi et al., 2005a); an impact which is either parallel with the therapeutic purpose or contrary to it or even null. From another viewpoint the individual effect of the carriers can be cut off into two categories (i.e., early and late impacts). For example, we have observed that most of the cationic gene delivery systems (e.g., linear and branched polyethylenimine (PEI), cationic lipids and dendrimers) are able to induce gene expression changes intrinsically (Hollins et al., 2007; Omidi et al., 2005b; Omidi, 2008). The determination of the early effects of a gene delivery system appears to be quite easy; however investigation on the late effects in a course of time is a cost demanding and time consuming trial. If a genomedicine is to enter clinic, there has to be some investigations to prove its safety. Time-series analysis can be a predictable section of these investigations. Up to now, many attempts have been made to design some gene delivery systems (viral and non-viral vectors). Some of these vectors include monoclonal antibodies, liposomes, metabolites, peptide hormones, cytokines, growth factors, viral and bacteriophage particles, nanoparticles and dendrimers. The choice of the carrier depends on the drug and also the cell to which the drug is going to be delivered. Almost all these carriers have suffered from either poor uptake and little transgene expression (non-viral vectors), or immunogenicity (viral vectors). With little efficacy of the carrier systems, some of them are still far from clinic and the gene therapy field needs a lot of time to reach the magic of genomedicines for treatment of diseases.

Viral vectors have a higher efficiency but their successful applications need more investigations. Expression of the recombinant viruses in the target cells is transient and can produce an inflammatory response in the patient. Another disadvantage of these vectors is that it is not known whether the re-administration is safe due to the immunological responses. Unfortunately the first volunteer, Jesse Gelsinger who was undergone a gene therapy with adenoviral vectors died due to the activated viruses in the phase I gene therapy trial in 1999 (Ferber, 2001). By far, as shown in Table 2, adenoviruses and retroviruses (viral vectors) and liposomes (nonviral vectors) have been the most frequently used viral vectors for gene therapy clinical trials. Molecular Trojans were introduced into the field of drug targeting, when the need for more specific drug targeting was felt. For brain drug delivery using molecular Trojan horses (Pardridge, 2008; Patel et al., 2009), different technologies are used including fusion protein technology, avidin biotin technology and Trojan horse liposome technology. Recently, tat protein transduction domain (PTD) as cell penetrating peptides have been used as molecular Trojans to cross biological barriers (Dietz & Bahr, 2004).

In non-viral vectors, DNA condensation and packaging (using cationic lipids or polymers) can protect gene based therapies against degradation by nucleases. These systems can also be equipped with specific ligands which help the carrier find its way in the hostile environment of the body through specific receptor-ligand interactions (Duzgunes et al., 2003; Nie et al., 2006; Putnam et al., 2001).

Ideally a targeted therapy should be specific, but assuming the vast variety of the proteins and receptors on the target cell surface, a substance may inadvertently bind to the cell surface receptors nonspecifically. Thus, we may witness many other interactions other than the desired one upon implementation of a drug or a target therapy system. A glucocorticoid, for example, can bind to myriad of cellular receptors and accordingly may have many nonspecific interactions. Hence it is not far from logic if we think that many of its interactions are still unknown. This may guide us towards a new field of science "nonspecific genomic/proteomic signature of chemicals" (the so called genomic impacts) (Hollins et al., 2007). Accordingly, screening the pseudo-targets of a substance or carrier can be of great help in choosing the best carrier for a molecule, as nonspecific signaling pathways can be induced by carriers alone. In this regard, implementation of microarray for development and approval of gene based medicines can assist us in establishing the genetic fingerprints of such modalities. In fact, now there is a growing hope that global gene expression profiling will replace histopathology and other traditional techniques used in toxicology and will become the primary tool for safety evaluation of drugs and their carriers. Comparison of the gene expression profiles between a healthy and mutant cell can be used to reveal the site of the interaction of a desired drug. Therefore, the detailed characterization of the genomic signature for each delivery system -both the complex and the vector- has to be performed in different cells, since different cells respond to stimuli in different ways (Omidi et al., 2005b). This clearly means that our future challenge will be finding and establishing the genomic signature for each carrier in specific cell lines -the way genes feel the toxicants and react against them and finally define the safety margins for them. This challenge requires implementation of high throughput microarray based screening methodology from bench works to data mining.

8. Final remarks

With many different attempts to translate gene therapy investigation into clinic, researchers in this field are still feeling the optimism that they felt years ago. In fact, although the initial burst of excitement over gene therapy hit inevitable hurdles, it appears that still we must work hard to learn more and more to provide improved treatments with minimal undesired side effects/impacts. For example, in cancer gene therapy, we have started learning which genes to choose (for suppression/stimulation), how to improve expression, and amplify their cancer-killing abilities by adding other approaches, such as cancer vaccines and chemotherapy. The entire music of life played by genes are yet to be fully understood, for which we need to get the practical and theoretical skills to comprehend the orchestral meaning of clusters of expressed genes in relation to a particular disease.

Now, we are just targeting a single or (at maximum) couple of biomarkers to fight a disease. This perception has to be improved through our understanding on entire picture of genomic expression of a biological function/disease in relation with so many others (genes/clusters of networked genes) that are directly/indirectly affecting the biological end point phenomena. Besides, a rapid, accurate, and reliable diagnostic method is necessary for identification of a disease for development of a suitable therapy, which consequently can reduce the mortality rate and also the cost of treatment. The recently developed molecular diagnostic assays (based on DNA-DNA or protein-DNA hybridization of clinical samples) appear to hopefully provide a robust platform, allowing effective diagnosis of different diseases with high speed, sensitivity, and specificity.

In the "functional genomics era", challenges on determination of proper analytical methods seem to be smoothly being shifted towards the post-analytical challenges, for which the microarray technology can provide a revolutionary analytical platform for concurrent analysis of thousands of genes in a single experiment. Such an approach confers enormous potential in the study of biological processes in health and disease. Based on recent FDA project on microarray (MAQC), this technology is going to become a potentially important tool in diagnostic applications and drug discovery too. In fact, the microarray based investigations have provided the vital impulse for biomedical experiments including: 1) identification of disease-causing genes in malignancies, 2) regulatory genes in the cell cycle mechanism, 3) investigation on genomic impacts of pharmacotherapies/gene therapies. The final point of these studies will guide us to translate our basic genomic knowledge into more sensible clinical practice, even for development of individual therapies, perhaps by identifying genes for new and unique potential drug targets and predicting drug responsiveness for individual patients. Given altogether, it seems we can use such technology for prevention strategies either to improve the health and life styles.

In the future, it is deemed that most of the investments on functional genomics will largely dependent upon research movement beyond the microarray based exploratory stages, so that new functional genomic pipeline demand sensible translation of a list of genes resulting from a microarray analysis. The real value and meaningful sense of gene expression changes need distinctive interpretation of a change by means of biological validation. Thus, the numerical verification of expression levels of thousands of genes need to be discovered, perhaps by finding biological relationships between the genes which require appropriate online systems to reveal new biological pathways in relation with clusters of the regulatory biomolecules. Unfortunately such an online tool has yet to be invented and till that comes into reality; the analysis of microarray data sets will be less rewarding. Other important issue seems to be the growing large size of microarray data and untapped information available in different data bases – the question is how we can extract the best results from existing data sets in relation with similar sets of data? Can we build an online network for such aim? It should be clarified that any set of microarray data has potential to be re-analyzed based upon many different integrative biological/clinical concepts.

9. References

Ahmed, A.A.; Vias, M.; Iyer, N.G.; Caldas, C. & Brenton, J.D. (2004). Microarray segmentation methods significantly influence data precision. *Nucleic Acids Res.*, Vol.32, No.5, (March 2004), pp. e50, ISSN 0305-1048

Allison, D.B.; Cui, X.; Page, G.P. & Sabripour, M. (2006). Microarray data analysis: from disarray to consolidation and consensus. *Nat.Rev.Genet.*, Vol.7, No.1, (January 2006), pp. 55-65, ISSN 1471-0056

Aoki, K.F. & Kanehisa, M. (2005). Using the KEGG database resource. *Curr.Protoc.Bioinformatics.*, Vol.Chapter 1 (October 2005), pp. Unit, ISSN 1934-3396

Au, N.H.; Cheang, M.; Huntsman, D.G.; Yorida, E.; Coldman, A.; Elliott, W.M.; Bebb, G.; Flint, J.; English, J.; Gilks, C.B. & Grimes, H.L. (2004). Evaluation of immunohistochemical markers in non-small cell lung cancer by unsupervised hierarchical clustering analysis: a tissue microarray study of 284 cases and 18 markers. *J.Pathol.*, Vol.204, No.1, (September 2004), pp. 101-109, ISSN 1096-9896

Babyak, M.A. (2004). What you see may not be what you get: a brief, nontechnical introduction to overfitting in regression-type models. *Psychosom.Med.*, Vol.66, No.3, (May 2004), pp. 411-421, ISSN 1534-7796

Baggerly, K.A.; Coombes, K.R.; Hess, K.R.; Stivers, D.N.; Abruzzo, L.V. & Zhang, W. (2001). Identifying differentially expressed genes in cDNA microarray experiments. *J.Comput.Biol.*, Vol.8, No.6, (2001), pp. 639-659, ISSN 1066-5277

Bakewell, D.J. & Wit, E. (2005). Weighted analysis of microarray gene expression using maximum likelihood. *Bioinformatics.*, Vol.21, No.6, (March 2005), pp. 723-729, ISSN 1367-4803

Barar, J.; Hamzeiy, H.; Mortazavi-Tabatabaei, S.A.; Hashemi-Aghdam, S.E. & Omidi, Y. (2009). Genomic signature and toxicogenomics comparison of polycationic gene delivery nanosystems in human alveolar epithelial A549 cells. *Daru*, Vol.17, No.3, (2009), pp. 139-147, ISSN 1560-8115

Bednar, M. (2000). DNA microarray technology and application. *Med.Sci.Monit.*, Vol.6, No.4, (July 2000), pp. 796-800, ISSN 1234-1010

Belacel, N.; Wang, Q. & Cuperlovic-Culf, M. (2006). Clustering methods for microarray gene expression data. *OMICS.*, Vol.10, No.4, (2006), pp. 507-531, ISSN 1536-2310

Bengtsson, A. & Bengtsson, H. (2006). Microarray image analysis: background estimation using quantile and morphological filters. *BMC.Bioinformatics.*, Vol.7 (2006), pp. 96, ISSN 1471-2105

Berger, J.A.; Hautaniemi, S.; Jarvinen, A.K.; Edgren, H.; Mitra, S.K. & Astola, J. (2004). Optimized LOWESS normalization parameter selection for DNA microarray data. *BMC.Bioinformatics.*, Vol.5, No.1, (December 2004), pp. 194, ISSN 1471-2105

Bland, J.M. & Altman, D.G. (1995). Multiple significance tests: the Bonferroni method. *BMJ*, Vol.310, No.6973, (January 1995), pp. 170, ISSN 0959-8138

Braga-Neto, U.M. & Dougherty, E.R. (2004). Is cross-validation valid for small-sample microarray classification? *Bioinformatics.*, Vol.20, No.3, (February 2004), pp. 374-380, ISSN 1367-4803

Cangelosi, R. & Goriely, A. (2007). Component retention in principal component analysis with application to cDNA microarray data. *Biol.Direct.*, Vol.2 (2007), pp. 2, ISSN 1745-6150

Chen, H. & Li, J. (2007). Nanotechnology: moving from microarrays toward nanoarrays. *Methods Mol.Biol.*, Vol.381 (2007), pp. 411-436,

Chipman, H. & Tibshirani, R. (2006). Hybrid hierarchical clustering with applications to microarray data. *Biostatistics.*, Vol.7, No.2, (April 2006), pp. 286-301, ISSN 1465 -4644

Cho, Y.S.; Kim, M.K.; Cheadle, C.; Neary, C.; Becker, K.G. & Cho-Chung, Y.S. (2001). Antisense DNAs as multisite genomic modulators identified by DNA microarray. *Proc.Natl.Acad.Sci.U.S.A*, Vol.98, No.17, (August 2001), pp. 9819-9823, ISSN 0027-8424

Churchill, G.A. (2004). Using ANOVA to analyze microarray data. *Biotechniques*, Vol.37, No.2, (August 2004), pp. 173-5, 177, ISSN 0736-6205

Covell, D.G.; Wallqvist, A.; Rabow, A.A. & Thanki, N. (2003). Molecular classification of cancer: unsupervised self-organizing map analysis of gene expression microarray data. *Mol.Cancer Ther.*, Vol.2, No.3, (March 2003), pp. 317-332, ISSN 1535-7163

Cui, X. & Churchill, G.A. (2003). Statistical tests for differential expression in cDNA microarray experiments. *Genome Biol.*, Vol.4, No.4, (2003), pp. 210, ISSN 1465-6914

Curtis, R.K.; Oresic, M. & Vidal-Puig, A. (2005). Pathways to the analysis of microarray data. *Trends Biotechnol.*, Vol.23, No.8, (August 2005), pp. 429-435, ISSN 0167-7799

De, B., V; Al-Mulla, F. & Pot, B. (2007). Methods for microarray data analysis. *Methods Mol.Biol.*, Vol.382 (2007), pp. 373-391, ISSN 1064-3745

Dembele, D. & Kastner, P. (2003). Fuzzy C-means method for clustering microarray data. *Bioinformatics.*, Vol.19, No.8, (May 2003), pp. 973-980, ISSN 1367-4803

Dewey, T.G. (2002). From microarrays to networks: mining expression time series. *Drug Discovery Today*, Vol.7, No.20, (October 2002), pp. s170-s175, ISSN 1359-6446

Dietz, G.P. & Bahr, M. (2004). Delivery of bioactive molecules into the cell: the Trojan horse approach. *Mol.Cell Neurosci.*, Vol.27, No.2, (October 2004), pp. 85-131, ISSN 1044-7431

Doniger, S.W.; Salomonis, N.; Dahlquist, K.D.; Vranizan, K.; Lawlor, S.C. & Conklin, B.R. (2003). MAPPFinder: using Gene Ontology and GenMAPP to create a global gene-expression profile from microarray data. *Genome Biol.*, Vol.4, No.1, (2003), pp. R7, ISSN 1465-6914

Draghici, S. (2002). Statistical intelligence: effective analysis of high-density microarray data. *Drug Discov.Today*, Vol.7, No.11 Suppl, (June 2002), pp. S55-S63, ISSN 1359-6446

Dugas, M.; Merk, S.; Breit, S. & Dirschedl, P. (2004). mdclust--exploratory microarray analysis by multidimensional clustering. *Bioinformatics.*, Vol.20, No.6, (April 2004), pp. 931-936, ISSN 1367-4803

Duzgunes, N.; De Ilarduya, C.T.; Simoes, S.; Zhdanov, R.I.; Konopka, K. & Pedroso de Lima, M.C. (2003). Cationic liposomes for gene delivery: novel cationic lipids and enhancement by proteins and peptides. *Curr Med Chem*, Vol.10, No.14, (2003), pp. 1213-20, ISSN 1568-0169

Edelstein, M. (2011). Gene therapy clinical trials worldwide In: *Wiley InterSciences*, (March 2011), Available from: http://www.wiley.com/legacy/wileychi/genmed/clinical/

Ferber, D. (2001). Gene therapy. Safer and virus-free? *Science*, Vol.294, No.5547, (2001), pp. 1638-42, ISSN 0036-8075

Geller, S.C.; Gregg, J.P.; Hagerman, P. & Rocke, D.M. (2003). Transformation and normalization of oligonucleotide microarray data. *Bioinformatics.*, Vol.19, No.14, (September 2003), pp. 1817-1823, ISSN 1367-4803

Guo, S.; Lu, J.; Subramanian, A. & Sonenshein, G.E. (2006). Microarray-assisted pathway analysis identifies mitogen-activated protein kinase signaling as a mediator of resistance to the green tea polyphenol epigallocatechin 3-gallate in her-2/neu-overexpressing breast cancer cells. *Cancer Res.*, Vol.66, No.10, (May 2006), pp. 5322-5329, ISSN 0008-5472

Gusnanto, A.; Calza, S. & Pawitan, Y. (2007). Identification of differentially expressed genes and false discovery rate in microarray studies. *Curr.Opin.Lipidol.*, Vol.18, No.2, (April 2007), pp. 187-193, ISSN 0957-9672

Hawkins, D.M. (2004). The problem of overfitting. *J.Chem.Inf.Comput.Sci.*, Vol.44, No.1, (January 2004), pp. 1-12, ISSN 0095-2338

Hembruff, S.L.; Villeneuve, D.J. & Parissenti, A.M. (2005). The optimization of quantitative reverse transcription PCR for verification of cDNA microarray data. *Anal.Biochem.*, Vol.345, No.2, (October 2005), pp. 237-249, ISSN 0003-2697

Hobman, J. L., Jones, A., and Constantinidou, C. (2007). Introduction to microarray technology, In: *Microarray technology through applications,* Falciani, F., pp. 1-52, Taylor & Francis Group, ISBN 9780415378536, New York

Hollins, A.J.; Omidi, Y.; Benter, I.F. & Akhtar, S. (2007). Toxicogenomics of drug delivery systems: Exploiting delivery system-induced changes in target gene expression to enhance siRNA activity. *J.Drug Target*, Vol.15, No.1, (January 2007), pp. 83-88, ISSN 1061-186X

Jares, P. (2006). DNA microarray applications in functional genomics. *Ultrastruct.Pathol.*, Vol.30, No.3, (May 2006), pp. 209-219, ISSN 0191-3123

Joshi, T.; Chen, Y.; Alexandrov, N. & Xu, D. (2004). Cellular function prediction and biological pathway discovery in Arabidopsis thaliana using microarray data. *Conf.Proc.IEEE Eng Med.Biol.Soc.*, Vol.4 (2004), pp. 2881-2884, ISSN 1557-170X

Juan, H.F. & Huang, H.C. (2007). Bioinformatics: microarray data clustering and functional classification. *Methods Mol.Biol.*, Vol.382 (2007), pp. 405-416, ISSN 1064-3745

Kanehisa, M. (2002). The KEGG database. *Novartis.Found.Symp.*, Vol.247 (2002), pp. 91-101, ISSN 1528-2511

Kepler, T.B.; Crosby, L. & Morgan, K.T. (2002). Normalization and analysis of DNA microarray data by self-consistency and local regression. *Genome Biol.*, Vol.3, No.7, (June 2002), pp. 1-12, ISSN 1465-6906

Kim, S.; Kim, J.H.; Jeon, O.; Kwon, I.C. & Park, K. (2008). Engineered polymers for advanced drug delivery. *Eur.J.Pharm.Biopharm.*, Vol.71, No.3, (October 2008), pp. 420-430, ISSN 0939-6411

Lee, J.K.; Williams, P.D. & Cheon, S. (2008). Data mining in genomics. *Clin.Lab Med.*, Vol.28, No.1, (March 2008), pp. 145-166, ISSN 0272-2712

Lehmussola, A.; Ruusuvuori, P. & Yli-Harja, O. (2006). Evaluating the performance of microarray segmentation algorithms. *Bioinformatics.*, Vol.22, No.23, (December 2006), pp. 2910-2917, ISSN 1367-4803

Leung, Y.F. & Cavalieri, D. (2003). Fundamentals of cDNA microarray data analysis. *Trends Genet.*, Vol.19, No.11, (November 2003), pp. 649-659, ISSN 0168-9525

Li, X.; Wang, H.; Touma, E.; Rousseau, E.; Quigg, R.J. & Ryaby, J.T. (2007). Genetic network and pathway analysis of differentially expressed proteins during critical cellular events in fracture repair. *J.Cell Biochem.*, Vol.100, No.2, (February 2007), pp. 527-543, ISSN 1097-4644

Liao, J.G. & Chin, K.V. (2007). Logistic regression for disease classification using microarray data: model selection in a large p and small n case. *Bioinformatics.*, Vol.23, No.15, (August 2007), pp. 1945-1951, ISSN 1367-4803

Linder, R.; Richards, T. & Wagner, M. (2007). Microarray data classified by artificial neural networks. *Methods Mol.Biol.*, Vol.382 (2007), pp. 345-372, ISSN 1064-3745

Lonardi, S. & Luo, Y. (2004). Gridding and compression of microarray images. *Proc.IEEE Comput.Syst.Bioinform.Conf.* (2004), pp. 122-130, ISSN 1471-2105

Loring, J.F. (2006). Evolution of microarray analysis. *Neurobiol.Aging*, Vol.27, No.8, (August 2006), pp. 1084-1086, ISSN 0197-4580

Martin, S.; Zhang, Z.; Martino, A. & Faulon, J.L. (2007). Boolean dynamics of genetic regulatory networks inferred from microarray time series data. *Bioinformatics.*, Vol.23, No.7, (April 2007), pp. 866-874, ISSN 1367-4803

Mircean, C.; Tabus, I.; Kobayashi, T.; Yamaguchi, M.; Shiku, H.; Shmulevich, I. & Zhang, W. (2004). Pathway analysis of informative genes from microarray data reveals that metabolism and signal transduction genes distinguish different subtypes of lymphomas. *Int.J.Oncol.*, Vol.24, No.3, (March 2004), pp. 497-504, ISSN 1019-6439

Nahar, J.; Ali, S. & Chen, Y.P. (2007). Microarray data classification using automatic SVM kernel selection. *DNA Cell Biol.*, Vol.26, No.10, (October 2007), pp. 707-712, ISSN 1044-5498

Nguyen, D.V. (2005). Partial least squares dimension reduction for microarray gene expression data with a censored response. *Math.Biosci.*, Vol.193, No.1, (January 2005), pp. 119-137, ISSN 0025-5564

Nie, Y.; Zhang, Z.R. & Duan, Y.R. (2006). Combined use of polycationic peptide and biodegradable macromolecular polymer as a novel gene delivery system: a preliminary study. *Drug Deliv.*, Vol.13, No.6, (November 2006), pp. 441-446, ISSN 1071-7544

Olson, N.E. (2006). The microarray data analysis process: from raw data to biological significance. *NeuroRx.*, Vol.3, No.3, (July 2006), pp. 373-383, ISSN 1545-5343

Omidi, Y. (2008). Microarray Analysis of the Toxicogenomics and the Genotoxic Potential of a Cationic Lipid-Based Gene Delivery Nanosystem in Human Alveolar Epithelial A549 Cells. *Toxicology Mechanisms and Methods*, Vol.18, No.4, (2008), pp. 369-378,

Omidi, Y.; Barar, J. & Akhtar, S. (2005a). Toxicogenomics of cationic lipid-based vectors for gene therapy: impact of microarray technology. *Curr.Drug Deliv.*, Vol.2, No.4, (October 2005), pp. 429-441, ISSN 1567-2018

Omidi, Y.; Hollins, A.J.; Benboubetra, M.; Drayton, R.; Benter, I.F. & Akhtar, S. (2003). Toxicogenomics of non-viral vectors for gene therapy: a microarray study of lipofectin- and oligofectamine-induced gene expression changes in human epithelial cells. *J.Drug Target*, Vol.11, No.6, (July 2003), pp. 311-323, ISSN 1567-2018

Omidi, Y.; Hollins, A.J.; Drayton, R.M. & Akhtar, S. (2005b). Polypropylenimine dendrimer-induced gene expression changes: the effect of complexation with DNA, dendrimer generation and cell type. *J.Drug Target*, Vol.13, No.7, (August 2005), pp. 431-443, ISSN 1061-186X

Pandey, G.; Yoshikawa, K.; Hirasawa, T.; Nagahisa, K.; Katakura, Y.; Furusawa, C.; Shimizu, H. & Shioya, S. (2007). Extracting the hidden features in saline osmotic tolerance in Saccharomyces cerevisiae from DNA microarray data using the self-organizing map: biosynthesis of amino acids. *Appl.Microbiol.Biotechnol.*, Vol.75, No.2, (May 2007), pp. 415-426, ISSN 0175-7598

Pardridge, W.M. (2008). Re-engineering biopharmaceuticals for delivery to brain with molecular Trojan horses. *Bioconjug.Chem.*, Vol.19, No.7, (July 2008), pp. 1327-1338, ISSN 1043-1802

Park, S.E.; Lee, M.J.; Yang, M.H.; Ahn, K.Y.; Jang, S.I.; Suh, Y.J.; Myung, H.; You, J.C. & Park, J.H. (2007). Expression profiles and pathway analysis in HEK 293 T cells overexpressing HIV-1 Tat and nucleocapsid using cDNA microarray. *J.Microbiol.Biotechnol.*, Vol.17, No.1, (January 2007), pp. 154-161, ISSN 1017-7825

Patel, M.M.; Goyal, B.R.; Bhadada, S.V.; Bhatt, J.S. & Amin, A.F. (2009). Getting into the brain : approaches to enhance brain drug delivery. *CNS.Drugs*, Vol.23, No.1, (2009), pp. 35-58, ISSN 1172-7047

Peng, Y. (June 2006). A novel ensemble machine learning for robust microarray data classification. *Comput.Biol.Med.*, Vol.36, No.6, (June 2006), pp. 553-573, ISSN 0010-4825

Portney, N.G. & Ozkan, M. (2006). Nano-oncology: drug delivery, imaging, and sensing. *Anal.Bioanal.Chem.*, Vol.384, No.3, (February 2006), pp. 620-630, ISSN 1618-2642

Pounds, S.B. (2006). Estimation and control of multiple testing error rates for microarray studies. *Brief.Bioinform.*, Vol.7, No.1, (March 2006), pp. 25-36, ISSN 1477-4054

Putnam, D.; Gentry, C.A.; Pack, D.W. & Langer, R. (2001). Polymer-based gene delivery with low cytotoxicity by a unique balance of side-chain termini. *Proc Natl Acad Sci U S A*, Vol.98, No.3, (2001), pp. 1200-5, ISSN 0027-8424

Qin, L.; Rueda, L.; Ali, A. & Ngom, A. (2005). Spot detection and image segmentation in DNA microarray data. *Appl.Bioinformatics.*, Vol.4, No.1, (2005), pp. 1-11, ISSN 1175-5636

Qin, Y. & Tian, Y.P. (2010). A microarray gene analysis of peripheral whole blood in normal adult male rats after long-term GH gene therapy. *Cell Mol.Biol.Lett.*, Vol.15, No.2, (June 2010), pp. 177-195, ISSN 1425-8153

Quackenbush, J. (2001). Computational analysis of microarray data. *Nat.Rev.Genet.*, Vol.2, No.6, (June 2001), pp. 418-427,

Quackenbush, J. (2002). Microarray data normalization and transformation. *Nat.Genet.*, Vol.32 Suppl (December 2002), pp. 496-501, ISSN 1061-4036

Rosa, G.J.; de, L.N. & Rosa, A.J. (2006). Review of microarray experimental design strategies for genetical genomics studies. *Physiol Genomics*, Vol.28, No.1, (December 2006), pp. 15-23, ISSN 1094-8341

Saei, A.A. & Omidi, Y. (2011). A glance at DNA microarray technology and applications. *BioImpacts*, Vol.1, No.2, (2011), pp. in press, ISSN 2228-5652

Sawant, R.M.; Hurley, J.P.; Salmaso, S.; Kale, A.; Tolcheva, E.; Levchenko, T.S. & Torchilin, V.P. (2006). "SMART" drug delivery systems: double-targeted pH-responsive pharmaceutical nanocarriers. *Bioconjug.Chem.*, Vol.17, No.4, (July 2006), pp. 943-949, ISSN 1043-1802

Senzer, N. & Nemunaitis, J. (2009). A review of contusugene ladenovec (Advexin) p53 therapy. *Curr.Opin.Mol.Ther.*, Vol.11, No.1, (February 2009), pp. 54-61, ISSN 1464-8431

Shannon, W.; Culverhouse, R. & Duncan, J. (2003). Analyzing microarray data using cluster analysis. *Pharmacogenomics.*, Vol.4, No.1, (January 2003), pp. 41-52, ISSN 1462-2416

Shen, F. & Hasegawa, O. (2008). A fast nearest neighbor classifier based on self-organizing incremental neural network. *Neural Netw.*, Vol.21, No.10, (December 2008), pp. 1537-1547, ISSN 0893-6080

Shen, L. & Tan, E.C. (2005). Dimension reduction-based penalized logistic regression for cancer classification using microarray data. *IEEE/ACM.Trans.Comput.Biol.Bioinform.*, Vol.2, No.2, (April 2005), pp. 166-175, ISSN 1545-5963

Shi, L. (2011). The MicroArray Quality Control (MAQC) Project: An FDA-Led Effort Toward Personalized Medicine In: *U.S.Food and Drug Administration,* (March 2011), Available from: http://www.fda.gov/downloads/ScienceResearch/BioinformaticsTools/MicroarrayQualityControlProject/ucm111050.pdf

Steinley, D. (2006). K-means clustering: a half-century synthesis. *Br.J.Math.Stat.Psychol.*, Vol.59, No.Pt 1, (May 2006), pp. 1-34, ISSN 0007-1102

Subramanian, A.; Kuehn, H.; Gould, J.; Tamayo, P. & Mesirov, J.P. (2007). GSEA-P: a desktop application for Gene Set Enrichment Analysis. *Bioinformatics.*, Vol.23, No.23, (December 2007), pp. 3251-3253, ISSN 1367-4803

Subramanian, A.; Tamayo, P.; Mootha, V.K.; Mukherjee, S.; Ebert, B.L.; Gillette, M.A.; Paulovich, A.; Pomeroy, S.L.; Golub, T.R.; Lander, E.S. & Mesirov, J.P. (2005). Gene set enrichment analysis: a knowledge-based approach for interpreting genome-wide expression profiles. *Proc.Natl.Acad.Sci.U.S.A*, Vol.102, No.43, (October 2005), pp. 15545-15550, ISSN 0027-8424

Tai, F. & Pan, W. (2007). Incorporating prior knowledge of gene functional groups into regularized discriminant analysis of microarray data. *Bioinformatics.*, Vol.23, No.23, (December 2007), pp. 3170-3177, ISSN 1367-4803

Wall, M.E.; Dyck, P.A. & Brettin, T.S. (2001). SVDMAN--singular value decomposition analysis of microarray data. *Bioinformatics.*, Vol.17, No.6, (June 2001), pp. 566-568, ISSN 1367-4803

Wang, A. & Gehan, E.A. (2005). Gene selection for microarray data analysis using principal component analysis. *Stat.Med.*, Vol.24, No.13, (July 2005), pp. 2069-2087, ISSN 0277-6715

Wang, Y.; Tetko, I.V.; Hall, M.A.; Frank, E.; Facius, A.; Mayer, K.F. & Mewes, H.W. (2005). Gene selection from microarray data for cancer classification--a machine learning approach. *Comput.Biol.Chem.*, Vol.29, No.1, (February 2005), pp. 37-46, ISSN 1476-9271

Watson, A.; Mazumder, A.; Stewart, M. & Balasubramanian, S. (1998). Technology for microarray analysis of gene expression. *Curr.Opin.Biotechnol.*, Vol.9, No.6, (December 1998), pp. 609-614, ISSN 0958-1669

Whetzel, P.L.; Parkinson, H.; Causton, H.C.; Fan, L.; Fostel, J.; Fragoso, G.; Game, L.; Heiskanen, M.; Morrison, N.; Rocca-Serra, P.; Sansone, S.A.; Taylor, C.; White, J. & Stoeckert, C.J., Jr. (2006). The MGED Ontology: a resource for semantics-based description of microarray experiments. *Bioinformatics.*, Vol.22, No.7, (April 2006), pp. 866-873, ISSN 1367-4803

Wilkin, G.A. & Huang, X. (2008). A practical comparison of two K-Means clustering algorithms. *BMC.Bioinformatics.*, Vol.9 Suppl 6 (2008), pp. S19, ISSN 1471-2105

Xiang, C.C. & Chen, Y. (2000). cDNA microarray technology and its applications. *Biotechnol.Adv.*, Vol.18, No.1, (March 2000), pp. 35-46, ISSN 0734-9750

Xiao, L.; Wang, K.; Teng, Y. & Zhang, J. (2003). Component plane presentation integrated self-organizing map for microarray data analysis. *FEBS Lett.*, Vol.538, No.1-3, (March 2003), pp. 117-124, ISSN 0014-5793

Zhu, Y.; Shen, X. & Pan, W. (2009). Network-based support vector machine for classification of microarray samples. *BMC.Bioinformatics.*, Vol.10 Suppl 1 (2009), pp. S21, ISSN 1471-2105

Hopes and Disillusions in Therapeutic Targeting of Intercellular Communication in Cancer

Kandouz, Mustapha
*Wayne State University School of Medicine, Department of Pathology
Detroit, MI,
USA*

1. Introduction

Although they tend to develop some independence upon malignant transformation, tumor cells and tumors remain"social" moieties. In many steps during tumor progression, tumor cells' interaction with each other and with their microenvironment is an essential element in their survival, growth and progression. This dependence on cell-cell interactions provides an opportunity for therapeutic interventions. In addition to long range interactions through growth factors, cytokines and other released molecules, the cells use various structures to interact directly, including gap junctions (GJ), tight junctions, adherens junctions and desmosomes.

Gap junction intercellular communication (GJIC), is a process involved in the transfer of second messengers such as cAMP, cGMP, glutamate, NAD+, IP_3, glutathione, and Ca^{++} ions, between cells, through channel structures called gap junctions (GJ). It is involved in various biological functions including regulation of cell growth, cell differentiation, and maintenance of tissue homeostasis (Wei et al. 2004). Structurally, gap junctions are formed by two head-to-head opposing hexameric transmembrane channels called connexons or hemichannels contributed by two interacting cells (Yeager and Harris 2007). The building units of connexons are the connexin proteins (Cxs), which are tetraspan integral membrane proteins (Nakagawa et al. 2010).

Expression and functional analysis of connexins and GJIC revealed that, in general, they are lost in cancer (Kandouz and Batist 2010) and their restoration has tumor inhibitory effects, which led to the concept that this type of intercellular communication plays a tumor suppressor role. Consequently, it early became clear that restoring GJIC and connexin expression, using different chemical treatments or by gene transfer, can be used to inhibit tumor cell growth (Fernstrom et al. 2002).

GJIC and Cxs have also been suggested to be involved during metastasis, although this role is still largely unclear. For example, on one hand connexin43 (Cx43) affects angiogenesis *in vitro* and *in vivo,* via an effect on proteins such as the Monocyte chemotactic protein-1 (MCP-1) and Interleukin-6 (McLachlan et al. 2006) , although this effect seems GJIC-independent (McLachlan et al. 2006) . On the other hand, Cx43-mediated GJIC facilitates metastatic homing to the lung via increased adhesion to endothelial cells (Elzarrad et al. 2008). GJIC as a result of overexpression of Cx43 in MDA-MET, an aggressive derivative of the metastatic breast cancer cell line MDA-MB-231, decreased cell invasion (Li et al. 2008a). Cx43 and Cx26 have been suggested to contribute to metastasis of breast cancer to the lymph nodes (Kanczuga-Koda et al. 2006).

However, although connexins and gap junctions are tightly associated, connexins are capable of functions of their own. The exact role of GJIC-dependent versus -independent functions of connexins is still ill-understood and sometimes even paradoxical (Mesnil et al. 2005) (Dbouk et al. 2009). For example, connexins seem to act as tumor suppressors as well as tumor facilitators in the breast (McLachlan et al. 2007). The above-mentioned role of Cx43 in angiogenesis seems GJIC-independent (McLachlan et al. 2006).

Visibly, more studies are needed to understand the complex role of GJIC and Cxs in cancer. This lack of information is a major obstacle to the full use of the therapeutic potential of Cxs and GJIC in cancer. Nevertheless, this obstacle didn't prevent from a attempting many creative and promising therapeutic strategies.

2. Connexins and GJIC in gene therapy: the bystander effect

A major limitation to cancer gene therapy is the often limited transfection efficiency of target cells. This is the specific aspect where the field of gap junctions has been particularly helpful, using a mechanism to amplify the cytotoxic signal originating from a limited population of target cells.

2.1 Bystander effect-mediated functions of connexins and GJIC

For the GJIC researchers, it quickly became clear that the ability of cells to transmit signaling moieties to their neighbors would offer an interesting opportunity. This strategy, based on a process called "bystander effect" (BE) (Figure 1), doesn't require the therapeutic agent to reach all tumor cells (van, I et al. 2002). Thanks to the BE, triggering the death process in a single cell could be amplified by transfer of the cytotoxic signaling molecules via the GJICs, resulting in similar changes and fate in interacting cells. A major mechanism of the BE involves direct gap junctional intercellular communication (GJIC) and changes in connexins' levels translate into changes in the BE potential (Asklund et al. 2003; Elshami et al. 1996; Yamasaki and Katoh 1988). Therefore, the BE is an important factor in the efficiency of cancer therapy (Mothersill and Seymour 2004), but its function requires direct intracellular contacts to undergo cytotoxicity. So far, a major application for the BE has been gene therapy. Many authors have shown a decade ago that the BE promotes the so-called "suicide gene therapy".

The first explorations of the BE therapeutic potential involved the use of enzyme/prodrug gene therapy approaches. In this therapy, target cells are made to express an enzyme that converts a prodrug inside the cell into the cytotoxic active drug that is transmitted to and kills the interacting cells. Two combinations of enzymes and prodrugs have been particularly tested: the bacterial cytosine deaminase (CD) with the antifungal drug 5-fluorocytosine (CD/5-FC) and, most widely, the herpes simplex virus thymidine kinase (HSVtk) with the antiherpetic ganciclovir (HSVtk/GCV) (Mesnil et al. 1996; Trinh et al. 1995). In the CD/5-FC system, CD converts 5-FC into the active cytotoxic form 5-fluorouracil (5-FU) (Mullen et al. 1992). While ganciclovir (GCV), a nucleoside analogue, is poorly metabolized by mammalian thymidine kinases, it is phosphorylated by the HSVtk and cellular kinases and thus converted into the nucleotide GCV triphosphate, a cytotoxic drug (Chen et al. 1994). The later works by incorporating into and blocking replication of DNA in dividing cells, resulting in induction of cell death (Thompson 1999). The phosphorylated form of GCV will be transmitted to neighboring cells via GJIC. For example, transfection of tumor cells expressing Cx43 with HSVtk will allow GCV to kill target as well as by-standing cells (Mesnil et al. 1996). GJIC and connexins have been shown to be involved during the BE-based HSV-tk/GCV therapy (Dilber et al. 1997; Vrionis et al. 1997; Elshami et al. 1996; Fick et al. 1995; Mesnil et al. 1996). BE using the UPRT/5-FU system (uracil phosphoribosyltransferase (UPRT) of E. coli origin and 5-fluorouracil (5-FU)) was found to be correlated to the level of Cx43 and GJIC (Kawamura et al. 2001). The extent of the role of GJIC and Cxs in BE-mediated cytotoxicity is most certainly underestimated. Many experimental therapeutic strategies make use of the BE but the role of GJICs or Cxs in their mechanism of action has not been investigated yet.

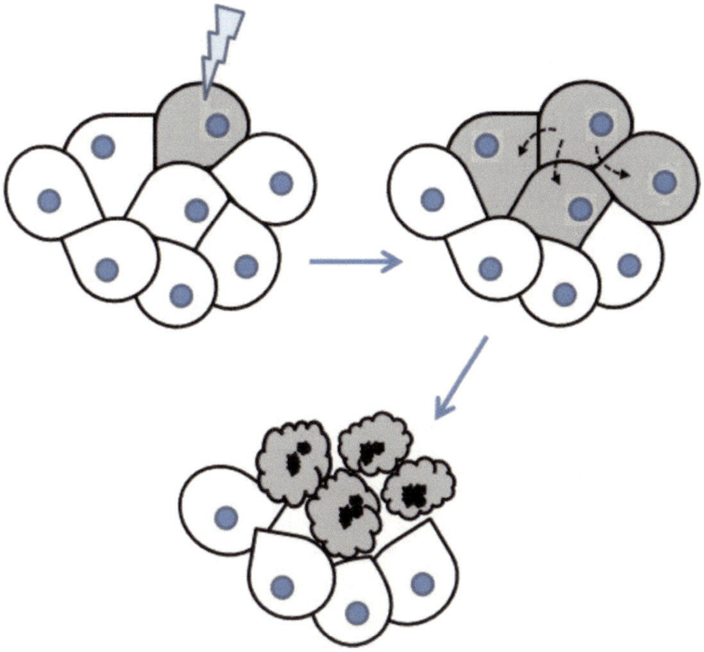

Fig. 1. Bystander Effect. A death signal, such as the one from the enzyme/prodrug system, triggered in a single cell is transmitted, through GJIC-dependent or -independent mechanisms, to neighboring cells. These bystanding cells are, in turn, destined to die without being directly targeted by the cytotoxic stimuli.

The efficacy of the enzyme/prodrug approach in vitro and in animal xenograft models has been demonstrated (Xu and McLeod 2001). However, there are many factors which immediately affect the efficacy of the approach. Although the % of cells expressing either HSVtk or CD has been shown to have some importance, the extent of contacts between cells was found to be the most crucial condition, as it requires contact between cells as well as their ability to transfer small cytotoxic molecules from one to another (Bi et al. 1993; Fick et al. 1995; Trinh et al. 1995). Using a murine breast cancer model transgenic for the activated rat neu oncogene under the control of the mouse mammary tumor virus long terminal repeat (MMTV-LTR), the efficacy of the HSVtk/GCV system has been shown in vivo.

However, this approach showed an incomplete antitumor potential, the limiting factors being low viral transduction efficiency and functionality of the BE and GJIC in mammary tumor cells (Sacco et al. 1996; Sacco et al. 1995).

As previously stressed, there is need for further deciphering of the respective roles played by GJIC, Cxs and the BE in these enzyme/prodrug systems in different cellular and cancer contexts. Characterizing the interdependence of the BE and GJIC in gene therapy systems could allow their more effective use. It has been reported that the BE resulting from the thymidine kinase/ganciclovir (tk/GCV) system requires functional GJIC while in the thymidine phosphorylase/5'-deoxy-5-fluorouridine (tp/DFUR) system, whereas thymidine phosphorylase (TP) converts 5'-deoxy-5-fluorouridine (5'-DFUR, doxifluridine) to 5-FU and its anabolite 5-fluoro-2'-deoxyuridine (5-FdUrd), the BE occurs via the cell culture medium and is independent of GJIC and apoptosis. Nevertheless, combining these two systems showed more BE than each system separately (Denning and Pitts 1997). It has also been reported that, in comparison to the HSVtk/GCV system, bystander killing resulting from the CD/5-FC system is GJIC-independent, and both communication-competent and -incompetent CD-transduced cells were killed dramatically more than bystander cells (Lawrence et al. 1998). Shared culture medium rather than direct cell-cell contacts were incriminated in the BE-mediated cell killing (Bai et al. 1999). Taken together, these findings particularly support the need for a better understanding of GJIC-independent BE to better rationalize the therapeutic use of this approach. This is particularly true when combining enzyme/prodrug targeting with connexin overexpression.

2.2 Role of apoptosis in the bystander effect cytotoxicity

The cytotoxic effects of these enzyme/prodrug systems via the BE are due to the induction of apoptosis (Hamel et al. 1996). GJIC can either mediate apoptotic cell death or potentiate the efficacy of pro-apoptotic agents. The BE allows these drugs or their signaling intermediates to reach by diffusion more cells than they would do alone (Peixoto et al. 2009) (Jensen and Glazer 2004; Udawatte and Ripps 2005). In fact, it has been shown that gap junctions remain open during the apoptotic process (Cusato et al. 2006). However, there are additional, less understood mechanisms for the role of gap junctions in BE cytotoxicity. In other respect, the BE can be instrumental in drug resistance. For instance, Src activation induces Cx43 tyrosine phosphorylation and GJIC decrease, resulting in resistance to Cisplatin (Peterson-Roth et al. 2009).

Therefore, one expected limitation to the enzyme/prodrug gene therapy approach would come from the fact that in cancer cells, many apoptosis-related signaling pathways are often aberrant. It has been shown for example that HSV-tk/GCV-induced BE is influenced by mutations in p53 (van, I et al. 2005), a tumor suppressor gene frequently mutated in cancer and which regulates apoptotic cell death. A study by Garcia-Rodríguez et al. showed a strong correlation of E-cadherin expression and the TK/GCV bystander effect and that increasing the expression of E-cadherin improved TK/GCV cytotoxicity and triggered a potent antitumoral effect in vivo, through reduction of the anti-apoptotic protein Bcl-2 (Garcia-Rodriguez et al. 2011a). Similarly, the efficacy of this gene therapy strategy could be undermined by certain treatment combinations. Treatment with dexamethasone significantly reduced their apoptotic response in glioma cells, as a result of diminished GJIC-dependent BE and efficacy of HSVtk gene therapy (Robe et al. 2005). This finding warns against future usage of dexamethasone as a symptomatic treatment if HSVtk gene therapy were to be attempted. Luckily, the outcome of this gene therapy strategy can also be improved by a multitude of other treatments (Robe et al. 2004) as will be discussed below.

3. Strategies to potentiate the bystander effect-based therapy

Attempts to use the BE in gene therapy studies are limited by the ability of target cells to communicate by gap junctions. Restoring GJIC to these cells in the enzyme/prodrug systems could not only bypass this limitation, it by itself has a gene therapy potential (Figure 2). Indeed, two different approaches have been used in the literature: 1) intratumoral delivery of Cx-encoding vectors that could either be used to enhance enzyme/prodrug gene therapy or potentiate the effect of pharmacological drugs, and 2) pharmacological induction of Cx expression and GJIC, which could be combined to enzyme/prodrug gene therapy.

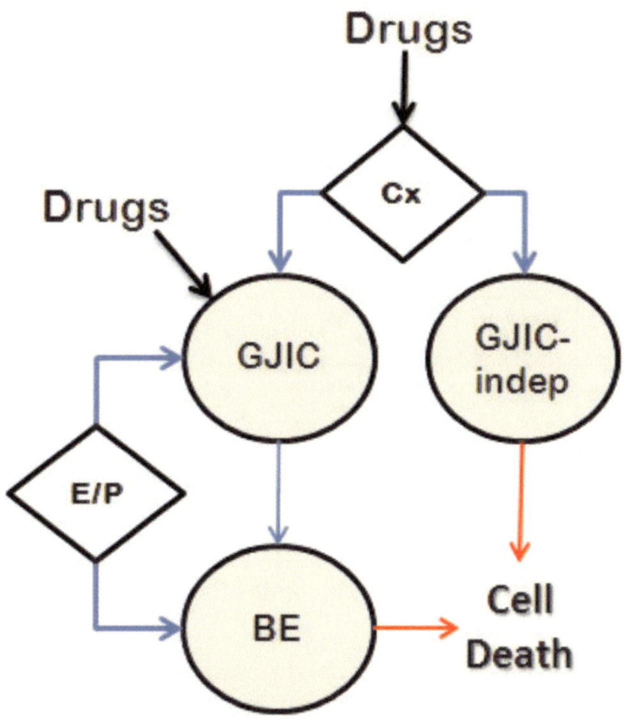

Fig. 2. Different GJIC, BE and/or Cx-based gene therapy approaches. Connexins (Cx) restoration could be performed either by direct gene delivery or by induction using pharmacological drugs. The Cx tumor suppressing effect is then either GJIC-dependent or independent (indep). Similarly, the BE-mediated cytotoxic effect of the enzyme/prodrug (E/P) approach could either be GJIC-dependent or independent. It could be improved by Cx restoration or by pharmacological intervention.

3.1 Combined enzyme/prodrug/connexin gene therapy

A major hurdle facing the enzyme/prodrug approach proved to be the loss of connexins and GJICs in the target cells, the malignant ones. Therefore, increasing the levels of Cxs and GJIC in cancer cells would result in a better response to BE-based gene therapy cytotoxicity. Transfecting cells with vectors encoding viral thymidine kinase and connexin genes has proven efficient in many studies (Cirenei et al. 1998; Ghoumari et al. 1998; Marconi et al. 2000; Tanaka et al. 2001a)(table 1).

Enzyme/Prodrug system	Connexin	Targeting Vector	Cell type	Reference
HSVtk/GCV	Cx43	Retroviral	Glioblastoma (U-87)	(Cirenei et al. 1998)
HSVtk/GCV	Cx43	Plasmid	Hepatocellular carcinoma cells (Hepa1-6)	(Ghoumari et al. 1998)
HSVtk/GCV	Cx43	A Herpes simplex viral vector (HSV)	Glioblastoma (U-87) and fibrosarcoma (L929)	(Marconi et al. 2000)
HSVtk/GCV	Cx26	Adenoviral multigenic	Bladder cancer (UM-UC-3 and UM-UC-14)	(Tanaka et al. 2001a)
HSVtk/GCV	Cx26	Retroviral	Pancreatic tumor cells (NP-9, NP-18, NP-31)	(Carrio et al. 2001)
HSVtk/GCV	Cx43	Plasmid	Cervical cancer (Hela)	(Tanaka et al. 2001c)
HSVtk/GCV	Cx43	Plasmid	Cervical cancer (Hela)	(Duflot-Dancer et al. 1998)
HSVtk/GCV	Cx43	Retroviral	Breast cancer (MDA-MB-435)	(Grignet-Debrus et al. 2000)

Table 1. Examples of gene therapy studies combining the enzyme/prodrug and Cx restoration approaches.

Nevertheless, enforced expression of Cxs might not always be sufficient to alleviate the inefficiency of the enzyme/prodrug system. For example, in a study of the efficacy of the HSVtk/GCV system combined with overexpression of Cx26 in a panel of pancreatic tumor cells, not all cell lines showed improved CJIC or bystander cytotoxicity (Carrio et al. 2001). Inability of Cx43 to properly localize at the cell surface prevented human colon tumor cells from being targeted by the BE and cytotoxicity of HSVtk (McMasters et al. 1998). The localization of Cx43 and the level of gap junctions functionality were also found to influence the BE in glioblastoma cells (Cottin et al. 2008). Therefore, a better understanding of the mechanisms involved in the stability and trafficking of connexins as well as the process of gap junction formation is needed. In particular, connexins' phosphorylation is an essential post-translational modification in their life cycle (Solan and Lampe 2009) and so are their stability and degradation by the lysosomal and proteasomal systems (Leithe and Rivedal 2007). For example, abnormal trafficking and lysosomal degradation can impede with the function of Cx43 (Qin et al. 2003a). Apigenin, a cancer chemopreventive flavonoid, was able to improve the effect of HSVtk only after concurrent transfection with the Cx43 gene, which suggests that, unlike other chemicals, it affects gap junction functionality rather than inducing connexin expression (Touraine et al. 1998). It has also been suggested that different connexins might have different abilities to modulate the BE. Cx32 and Cx26 were reported to be significantly more effective than Cx43 at mediating the BE in cocultures of connexin-expressing and HSVtk-expressing C6 glioma cells (Jimenez et al. 2006).

Another issue that is not completely elucidated is the importance of targeting tumor cells to express both the suicide gene and the connexin at the same time. It has been suggested that separate introduction of the HSVtk and connexin genes in tumor cells might have higher killing efficiency than simultaneous expression, as illustrated by transfection of HeLa cells with Cx43 and HSVtk genes (Tanaka et al. 2001c). Interestingly, the Cx-expressing cells induce the Cx-devoid cells to contribute to GJIC through an unknown mechanism (Tanaka et al. 2001b). This is an encouraging observation in view of the known heterogeneity of tumors or in situations where Cx-negative malignant cells are scattered within Cx-positive normal tissues (i.e. gliomas), which means that gene therapy targeting of these tumors with the enzyme/prodrug system might still be efficient even when only a small subpopulation of tumor cells expresses connexins.

3.2 Combined connexins delivery and pharmacological treatments.

Modulating GJIC and Connexins has been used to sensitize to chemotherapy using a variety of pharmacological drugs (Figure 2). For example, Cx32 expression enhanced the sensitivity of human renal cell carcinoma (RCC) cells to vinblastine (VBL) *in vitro* and *in vivo* (Sato et al. 2007c). Cx43 overexpression increased the sensitivity of the LNCaP prostate cancer cells to tumor necrosis factor alpha (TNFalpha), anti-Fas antibodies, and TRAIL (Wang et al. 2007). Overexpression of Cx26 improved the growth suppressive effect of doxorubicin in prostate cancer cells (Tanaka and Grossman 2004). Restoring Cx43 expression in human glioblastoma increased sensitivity to Etoposide, Paclitaxel (Taxol) and Doxorubicin, in a way that, paradoxically, seems GJIC-independent (Huang et al. 2001). Combining intratumoral injection of a Cx43-expressing vector and intravenous injection of Docetaxel (DTX) improved anti-tumor efficiency more than DTX alone (Fukushima et al. 2007). The overexpression of Cx26 resulted in increased GJIC and enhanced cytotoxic BE of gemcitabine, a nucleoside analogue drug whose phosphorylated form is transmitted through gap junctions, in pancreatic cancer cells both in vitro and in mice (Garcia-Rodriguez et al. 2011b). At low doses, PKI-166, a Her-2/Her-1 inhibitor and PP1, a Src family inhibitor, were shown to enhance the tumor-suppressive effect of Cx32 in human renal cell carcinoma Caki-2 cells, partly through GJIC (Fujimoto et al. 2005b; Fujimoto et al. 2005a). As a last example, Cx32 expression also significantly potentiated the cytotoxicity of vinorelbine (VBN), in lung adenocarcinoma A549 cells (Sato et al. 2007a).

3.3 Combined pharmacological restoration of connexins and gene therapy

In addition to exogenous delivery of connexins, their expression can be increased using pharmacological treatments that affect different levels of gene regulation. The strategy of restoring Cx expression to favor BE-mediated cytotoxicity is mainly confronted to a flagrant misunderstanding of the mechanisms of loss of Cx expression in cancer. Many transcriptional and post-transcriptional aberrations have been described so far but, as expected, none provide a ubiquitous explanation (Carystinos et al. 2003; Gao et al. 2007; Villares et al. 2009; Leithe and Rivedal 2007; Solan and Lampe 2009). Nevertheless, the available knowledge has significantly been used in a therapeutic perspective. Transcriptional silencing of Cx expression has been shown to involve epigenetic events such as promoter methylation and chromatin acetylation. Restoration of Cx32 in human RCC cells by 5-aza-2'-deoxycytidine (5-aza-CdR), a DNA demethylating agent, suppressed tumor growth in a xenograft model (Hagiwara et al. 2008). 4-phenylbutyrate (4-PB), a histone deacetylases inhibitor (HDACi), induced connexin expression and enhanced GJIC between pancreatic cancer cells in culture and potentiated HSVtk/GCV bystander killing effect in glioma cells (Ammerpohl et al. 2004; Ammerpohl et al. 2007). Other HDACi such as Trichostatin A (TSA) and sodium butyrate (NaBu), restored Cx43 expression and increased GJIC (Hernandez et al. 2006; Ammerpohl et al. 2007). It is not known if these HDACi would affect the outcome of the suicide gene therapy. Some of the compounds might also affect the BE independently of their gene expression-modulatory functions. N-butyrate, an inducer of histone hyperacetylation, was shown to enhance the GJIC and the BE in GJIC-deficient glioma cells independently from its HDACi function (Robe et al. 2004).

Post-transcriptional regulation of Cx expression via mRNA trafficking, stability, splicing and translation, are probably the least studied aspects of Cx life cycle and their impact in gene therapy improvement is still far-fetched. There is fortunately little more data on post-translational regulation, especially protein modification and degradation by proteasomal and lysosomal mechanisms (Kjenseth et al. 2010; Berthoud et al. 2004). Additional regulatory mechanisms include microRNA (Anderson et al. 2006) (Yang et al. 2007; Kedde et al. 2007). In addition, an active Cx43 pseudogene (PsiCx43) has been identified and found to be expressed in breast cancer cell lines but not in normal breast epithelial cells (Kandouz et al. 2004). Inhibition of this pseudogene using short interfering RNAs (siRNAs) can be used to restore Cx43 expression, thus improving chemosensitization of breast cancer cells (Bier et al. 2009). Although there are ways to specifically target these different pathways to restore Cx expression, it is not known whether this would succeed in enhancing the BE cytotoxicity.

In principle at least, connexins could also be targeted via various interaction partners that affect their localization, turnover and function such as the interaction of Cx30 with cytoskeletal (microtubules, actin filaments) and tight/adherens junction proteins (Carette et al. 2009; Qu et al. 2009) or the interaction of Cx43 with the Rab GAP-like protein CIP85 (Lan et al. 2005).

3.4 Combined pharmacological/gene therapy

Another strategy is the use of chemical inducers of Cx expression to improve the efficiency of the enzyme/prodrug gene therapy (Figure 2). The inhibition of ATP-sensitive potassium (KATP) channels with tolbutamide resulted in increased Cx43 and GJIC, enhancing the bystander effect in HSVtk/GCV therapy in U373 human glioma cells (Paino et al. 2010). All-trans retinoic acid was shown to induce Cx43 expression and to increase GJIC in tumor cell lines, resulting in an increased efficiency of the HSVtk/GCV-induced cytotoxicity in vitro and in vivo (Park et al. 1997). A similar result was observed after 8-bromo-cyclic-AMP treatment, (Carystinos et al. 1999; Kunishige et al. 1998). This approach has particularly been viewed as a chemopreventive one (King and Bertram 2005). The green tea flavonoid compound (-)Epicatechin, prevents tumor promoting chemicals such as the 12-O-tetradecanoylphorbol-13-acetate (TPA) from inhibiting GJIC (le-Agha et al. 2002). Resveratrol (3,5,4'-trihydroxy-stilbene), a natural polyphenol, provides a similar preventive effect against TPA and the insecticide DDT (Nielsen et al. 2000), and so do carotenoids (Zhang et al. 1991). It is yet to be examined whether these treatments could increase the cytotoxic potential of the HSVtk/GCV and other gene therapy systems, but we could already infer from the available data that pharmacologic upregulation of Cxs and gap junctions could be useful to combine with these gene therapy systems in clinical trials.

4. GJIC-independent and BE-independent connexin cytotoxic effects

Part of the reasons why the original strong faith in the strategy to target connexins in the treatment of human tumors has been shaken is due to the focus on the BE and GJIC only. However, it is now obvious that in many contexts, the tumor suppressor effect of Cxs' overexpression is GJIC-independent (Li et al. 2008b). Cx43 affect angiogenesis *in vitro* and *in vivo* (McLachlan et al. 2006) and improves the resistance to the chemotherapeutic agent cisplatin (CDDP) (Sato et al. 2009) in a GJIC-independent fashion. Cx26 regulates angiogenesis-related molecules by mechanisms that are both GJIC-dependent and -independent (Kalra et al. 2006; Qin et al. 2003b). GJIC-independent functions of Cx32 in blocking proliferation, invasion and metastasis in human renal cell carcinoma RCC cells, have also been reported (Sato et al. 2007b). Therefore, connexins could be used in gene therapy regardless of their ability to trigger BE or GJIC (Figure 2). The exact mechanisms and conditions where this strategy would be most effective are yet to be determined.

5. Targeting tumor cells through GJIC with their cellular environment

Another advantage of BE-based gene therapy strategies is that treatment could be aimed not only to the tumor cells but also to cellular partners within the microenvironment such as stromal and endothelial cells. For instance, when HSVtk-transduced endothelial cells and non-HSVtk-transduced tumor cells were co-cultured, treatment with GCV resulted in the BE-dependent death of both endothelial and tumor cells in vitro and in vivo (Trepel et al. 2009). Targeting human umbilical vein endothelial cells (HUVECs) with a Cx37-encoding adenovirus induced their death by apoptosis (Seul et al. 2004).

Although largely hypothetical at this point, we can envision a strategy where GJIC between tumor and stromal cells would be enforced to render tumor cells susceptible to cell killing. In other words, targeting tumor-associated endothelial cells for example, with delivery of connexins and an enzyme/prodrug system, could result in the demise of both the tumor and its irrigating blood vessels. Using a tridimensional model of cell culture, Benalalam et al. showed that GJIC between endothelial and tumor cells are required for antigenic peptide transfer to endothelial cells resulting in the latter's recognition and elimination by cytotoxic T cells (CTL) (Benlalam et al. 2009). Using the attraction of bone marrow-derived stem cells (BMSCs) for glioma cells, Huang et al. took advantage of GJIC between the two cell types to improve the efficiency of the HSVtk/GCV suicide gene therapy. Indeed, combining the expression of HSVtk by BMSCs and the expression of Cx43 by glioma cells enhanced the bystander effect and improved suicide gene therapy (Huang et al. 2009). Similarly, the formation of gap junctions between adipose-tissue derived human mesenchymal stem cells (AT-MSC) and human glioblastoma cells contributed to bystander cytotoxicity of HSVtk (Matuskova et al. 2009).

Paradoxically, GJIC-enabled bystander cells have been shown to confer protection against GCV to the very HSVtk-transduced cells that are the source of the cytotoxic signal. The impact of this observation on the therapeutic efficacy is not known. Indeed, as suggested by the authors of this study, it can either increase the efficacy of the treatment, by decreasing the demise of the HSVtk cells, thus prolonging their cytotoxic effect, or have an opposite effect by increasing their survival (Wygoda et al. 1997). Nevertheless, this observation shows that the so-called "bystander cells" and their ability to communicate by GJIC are an important element to take into consideration in the BE-based therapy. This applies to tumor cells as well as the stromal cells with which they communicate.

The therapeutic potential of the neural stem cells (NSCs) in the treatment of brain tumors have been demonstrated and, in many reports, have been shown to rely on bystander effect. NSCs are highly migrating cells able to cross the blood–brain barrier and which show tropism for tumor cells. Many studies showed that NSCs can be genetically modified to target tumor cells and the use of the cytosine deaminase (CD)/5-fluorocytosine (5-FC) system delivered particularly important results in medulloblastomas and gliomas (Aboody et al. 2000; Shimato et al. 2007; Kim et al. 2006) as well as breast or melanoma metastases to the brain (Joo et al. 2009; Aboody et al. 2006). Combined delivery of the CD/5-FC system with Interferon-β (IFN-β), known for its anti-tumor effects, showed a stronger bystander killing effect in glioma both in vitro and using an orthotopic xenograft in vivo model, where animals were intravenously infused with CD/IFN-β-expressing NSCs and administred with the prodrug 5-FC (Ito et al. 2010). Also, migratory HSVtk-transduced NSCs were able to kill untransduced glioma cells by a GJIC-mediated BE (Uhl et al. 2005).

An additional level of complexity is the formation of different types of GJICs between different cell types. Homotypic gap junction channels formed of identical connexons and heterotypic channels made of connexons containing different connexins (Vaney and Weiler 2000; Kapoor et al. 2004) can show different permeabilities (Weber et al. 2004; Bevans et al. 1998b). This implies that Cx-mediated gene therapy will necessitate an elaborate "customization" effort to target specific interactions and avoid non specific effects. For instance, transformed cells form GJICs between them that are independent of the GJICs formed within adjacent nontransformed cells, with apparently no heterologous communication (Yamasaki and Katoh 1988). Therefore, it is in principle possible to target cancer-specific GJIC compartments without affecting normal cells.

6. Clinical trials

Many clinical trials have been performed to validate the enzyme/prodrug gene therapy approach and test its effects. These include the trial of adenovirus mediated delivery of HSVtk combined with GCV treatment in operable primary or recurrent high-grade gliomas, which resulted in a clinically and statistically significant increase in mean patient survival (Immonen et al. 2004). A phase I dose escalation clinical trial was conducted in 11 men with localized recurrent and metastatic hormone-refractory prostate cancer. In this trial, an adenovirus vector carrying osteocalcin promoter-driven HSVtk was used to target both prostate cancer cells and their neighboring stromal cells and valacyclovir, another anti-herpetic prodrug converted to aciclovir, was given orally. The results showed a good tolerance with no serious adverse events but with local cell death in treated lesions in 63.6% of patients (Kubo et al. 2003). In another clinical phase I/II study, 36 prostate cancer patients with local recurrence after radiotherapy which received single or repeated cycles of adenoviral vector-mediated HSVtk/GCV intraprostatic gene therapy (Miles et al. 2001) showed no significant side effects and a significant increase in biological responses such as the mean serum PSA-doubling time (PSADT), prostate-specific antigen recurrence (PSAR), return to initial PSA (TR-PSA), and activated CD8(+) T cells present in the peripheral blood. In another phase I trial, nine courses of intraprostatic injections of adenoviral HSVtk followed by intravenous injection of GCV in 8 patients with local recurrence of prostate cancer after definitive hormonal therapy, showed no adverse events and a significant prolongation of the median serum PSADT. In five patients, decrease of PSA values was also observed (Nasu et al. 2007). Also, intraperitoneal administration of an HSVtk-encoding adenovirus and intravenous GCV showed significant efficacy in women with recurrent ovarian cancer (Alvarez et al. 2000). Finally, an adenoviral vector encoding the HSVtk gene was also used in a phase I trial where it has been introduced into the pleural cavity of patients with malignant mesothelioma in combination with systemic GCV treatments and showed good tolerance and detectable gene delivery (Sterman et al. 1998).

Most of these clinical trials focused on issues of tolerance of the therapy and efficacy of delivery. Although it is understood that these gene therapy attempts rely mainly on the BE, it is frustrating that no data is available that correlates these clinical results with the formation of gap junctions and Cx expression in the targeted tumors.

7. Conclusion

Bystander effect is a big step forward in attempts to use gene therapy in cancer treatment. The idea that one can kill more cells than initially targeted has been a revolutionary concept. However, the biggest challenge to the translation of this concept into an effective therapy has been the lack of information in many aspects surrounding the BE and the role of GJIC and connexins. As further basic science studies are performed, we will be able to comprehend the mechanisms of loss of Cx expression in cancer and how they could be alleviated. Whether and how these mechanisms could be used to improve gene therapy is, again, wide open to exploration. An immediate impact of these studies would be the analysis of tumors for GJIC or Cx expression to identify a subset of patients most likely to benefit from gene therapy using enzyme/prodrug systems such as HSVtk/GCV.

Other potential strategies could make use of the ability of gap junctions to transmit different types of cytotoxic signals. Radiotherapy for instance could benefit from this knowledge, based on the finding that death signals could be transmitted through BE from irradiated to nonirradiated cells (Azzam et al. 2001; Prise and O'Sullivan 2009). Radiation therapy could be combined with gene therapy interventions aimed at increasing GJIC which would amplify the cellular responsiveness to radiation therapy

The function of gap junction channels involves conductance and electrical and chemical gating that can be affected by many factors, including the nature and stoichiometry of the contributing connexins, ensuring selective permeability to various molecules (Saez et al. 2010; Nakagawa et al. 2010; Bevans et al. 1998a). In theory, BE-based gene therapy combined with Cx expression restoration would benefit from identifying Cxs with the best conductance in specific cancer settings. Furthermore, it would be possible to introduce specific mutations that would improve the conductance of BE cytotoxic molecules. Another possibility is to regulate opening and closure of gap junctional channels. The search for chemical inhibitors has delivered a series of drugs that result in either opening or closure of gap junctions (Salameh and Dhein 2005). Another approach involved the use of mimetic peptides that bind to connexin hemichannels, and modify their conductance (Evans and Leybaert 2007). Although it is yet to be assessed, targeting GJ opening and conductance properties could optimize the effect of the BE gene therapy. However, again, the relevance to cancer of channel gating functions of connexins versus GJIC-independent functions is a major unknown. Although this pharmacological approach is most likely to be successful in diseases such as arrhythmia or seizure, where hyperpolarization is a major issue, its possible impact in cancer therapy, especially in combination with gene therapy, should not be excluded.

Another issue of potential importance in improving the efficiency of the BE-based gene therapy is the nature of metabolites that could or could not be transmitted by BE as illustrated by the differential ability of pyrimidine nucleoside analogues such as GCV to pass the gap junctions and trigger cytotoxicity (Degreve et al. 1999). Enzyme/prodrug combinations involving pyrimidine analogues (BVDU, BVaraU) presented smaller bystander killing than the combination involving the purine analogue (GCV) (Grignet-Debrus et al. 2000).

In addition to connexins, another family of proteins called pannexins is increasingly being scrutinized for their ability to form gap junctions (D'hondt et al. 2009). Unless and until their role in cancer and GJIC has been clearly established, the only GJIC-based therapeutic strategies will likely keep focusing on connexins.

Finally, so far only clinical trials on localized malignancies have been conducted, such as direct intra-tumoral injection of the vector in glioma therapy. Future studies are necessary to develop intravenous delivery of viral vectors in the enzyme/prodrug gene therapy approach, to allow targeting of other cancers. In addition, these Phase I trials have mainly addressed safety, toxicity and gene delivery issues. Further assessment of the anti-tumor effects and the correlation with GJIC and connexin expression should absolutely be on the list of future clinical trials. Combinations of these gene therapy approaches with other cancer therapeutic modalities should also be considered.

In summary, the promises of the Bystander effect, GJIC and Connexin-based gene therapies are still alive. It is possible that the great enthusiasm for their potential was so high that it blinded us to the urgency of further examination of their mechanisms and regulations which, once performed, would much significantly improve the rationalization of the clinical application and outcome.

8. References

Aboody KS, Brown A, Rainov NG, Bower KA, Liu S, Yang W, Small JE, Herrlinger U, Ourednik V, Black PM, Breakefield XO and Snyder EY. (2000). *Proc Natl Acad Sci U S A,* 97, 12846-12851.

Aboody KS, Najbauer J, Schmidt NO, Yang W, Wu JK, Zhuge Y, Przylecki W, Carroll R, Black PM and Perides G. (2006). *Neuro Oncol,* 8, 119-126.

Alvarez RD, Gomez-Navarro J, Wang M, Barnes MN, Strong TV, Arani RB, Arafat W, Hughes JV, Siegal GP and Curiel DT. (2000). *Mol Ther,* 2, 524-530.

Ammerpohl O, Thormeyer D, Khan Z, Appelskog IB, Gojkovic Z, Almqvist PM and Ekstrom TJ. (2004). *Biochem Biophys Res Commun,* 324, 8-14.

Ammerpohl O, Trauzold A, Schniewind B, Griep U, Pilarsky C, Grutzmann R, Saeger HD, Janssen O, Sipos B, Kloppel G and Kalthoff H. (2007). *Br J Cancer,* 96, 73-81.

Anderson C, Catoe H and Werner R. (2006). *Nucleic Acids Res,* 34, 5863-5871.

Asklund T, Appelskog IB, Ammerpohl O, Langmoen IA, Dilber MS, Aints A, Ekstrom TJ and Almqvist PM. (2003). *Exp Cell Res,* 284, 185-195.

Azzam EI, de Toledo SM and Little JB. (2001). *Proc Natl Acad Sci U S A,* 98, 473-478.

Bai S, Du L, Liu W, Whittle IR and He L. (1999). *Biochem Biophys Res Commun,* 259, 455-459.

Benlalam H, Jalil A, Hasmim M, Pang B, Tamouza R, Mitterrand M, Godet Y, Lamerant N, Robert C, Avril MF, Neefjes J, Tursz T, Mami-Chouaib F, Kieda C and Chouaib S. (2009). *J Immunol,* 182, 2654-2664.

Berthoud VM, Minogue PJ, Laing JG and Beyer EC. (2004). *Cardiovasc Res,* 62, 256-267.

Bevans CG, Kordel M, Rhee SK and Harris AL. (1998a). *J Biol Chem,* 273, 2808-2816.

Bevans CG, Kordel M, Rhee SK and Harris AL. (1998b). *J Biol Chem,* 273, 2808-2816.

Bi WL, Parysek LM, Warnick R and Stambrook PJ. (1993). *Hum Gene Ther,* 4, 725-731.

Bier A, Oviedo-Landaverde I, Zhao J, Mamane Y, Kandouz M and Batist G. (2009). *Mol Cancer Ther,* 8, 786-793.

Carette D, Gilleron J, Decrouy X, Fiorini C, Diry M, Segretain D and Pointis G. (2009). *Traffic,* 10, 1272-1285.

Carrio M, Mazo A, Lopez-Iglesias C, Estivill X and Fillat C. (2001). *Int J Cancer,* 94, 81-88.

Carystinos GD, Kandouz M, Alaoui-Jamali MA and Batist G. (2003). *Mol Pharmacol,* 63, 821-831.

Carystinos GD, Katabi MM, Laird DW, Galipeau J, Chan H, Alaoui-Jamali MA and Batist G. (1999). *Clin Cancer Res,* 5, 61-68.

Chen SH, Shine HD, Goodman JC, Grossman RG and Woo SL. (1994). *Proc Natl Acad Sci U S A,* 91, 3054-3057.

Cirenei N, Colombo BM, Mesnil M, Benedetti S, Yamasaki H and Finocchiaro G. (1998). *Gene Ther,* 5, 1221-1226.

Cottin S, Ghani K and Caruso M. (2008). *Cancer Gene Ther,* 15, 823-831.

Cusato K, Ripps H, Zakevicius J and Spray DC. (2006). *Cell Death Differ,* 13, 1707-1714.

D'hondt C, Ponsaerts R, De SH, Bultynck G and Himpens B. (2009). *Bioessays,* 31, 953-974.

Dbouk HA, Mroue RM, El-Sabban ME and Talhouk RS. (2009). *Cell Commun Signal,* 7, 4.

Degreve B, De CE and Balzarini J. (1999). *Gene Ther,* 6, 162-170.

Denning C and Pitts JD. (1997). *Hum Gene Ther,* 8, 1825-1835.

Dilber MS, Abedi MR, Christensson B, Bjorkstrand B, Kidder GM, Naus CC, Gahrton G and Smith CI. (1997). *Cancer Res,* 57, 1523-1528.

Duflot-Dancer A, Piccoli C, Rolland A, Yamasaki H and Mesnil M. (1998). *Gene Ther,* 5, 1372-1378.

Elshami AA, Saavedra A, Zhang H, Kucharczuk JC, Spray DC, Fishman GI, Amin KM, Kaiser LR and Albelda SM. (1996). *Gene Ther,* 3, 85-92.

Elzarrad MK, Haroon A, Willecke K, Dobrowolski R, Gillespie MN and Al-Mehdi AB. (2008). *BMC Med,* 6, 20.

Evans WH and Leybaert L. (2007). *Cell Commun Adhes,* 14, 265-273.

Fernstrom MJ, Koffler LD, bou-Rjaily G, Boucher PD, Shewach DS and Ruch RJ. (2002). *Exp Mol Pathol,* 73, 54-60.

Fick J, Barker FG, Dazin P, Westphale EM, Beyer EC and Israel MA. (1995). *Proc Natl Acad Sci U S A,* 92, 11071-11075.

Fujimoto E, Sato H, Nagashima Y, Negishi E, Shirai S, Fukumoto K, Hagiwara H, Hagiwara K, Ueno K and Yano T. (2005a). *Life Sci,* 76, 2711-2720.

Fujimoto E, Yano T, Sato H, Hagiwara K, Yamasaki H, Shirai S, Fukumoto K, Hagiwara H, Negishi E and Ueno K. (2005b). *J Pharmacol Sci,* 97, 294-298.

Fukushima M, Hattori Y, Yoshizawa T and Maitani Y. (2007). *Int J Oncol,* 30, 225-231.

Gao FH, Wang Q, Wu YL, Li X, Zhao KW and Chen GQ. (2007). *Biochem Biophys Res Commun,* 356, 505-511.

Garcia-Rodriguez L, bate-Daga D, Rojas A, Gonzalez JR and Fillat C. (2011a). *Gene Ther,* 18, 73-81.

Garcia-Rodriguez L, Perez-Torras S, Carrio M, Cascante A, Garcia-Ribas I, Mazo A and Fillat C. (2011b). *Mol Cancer Ther,* 10, 505-517.

Ghoumari AM, Mouawad R, Zerrouqi A, Nizard C, Provost N, Khayat D, Naus CC and Soubrane C. (1998). *Gene Ther,* 5, 1114-1121.

Grignet-Debrus C, Cool V, Baudson N, Velu T and Calberg-Bacq CM. (2000). *Cancer Gene Ther,* 7, 1456-1468.

Hagiwara H, Sato H, Ohde Y, Takano Y, Seki T, Ariga T, Hokaiwado N, Asamoto M, Shirai T, Nagashima Y and Yano T. (2008). *Br J Pharmacol,* 153, 1373-1381.
Hamel W, Magnelli L, Chiarugi VP and Israel MA. (1996). *Cancer Res,* 56, 2697-2702.
Hernandez M, Shao Q, Yang XJ, Luh SP, Kandouz M, Batist G, Laird DW and aoui-Jamali MA. (2006). *Prostate,* 66, 1151-1161.
Huang Q, Liu XZ, Kang CS, Wang GX, Zhong Y and Pu PY. (2009). *Cancer Gene Ther.*
Huang RP, Hossain MZ, Huang R, Gano J, Fan Y and Boynton AL. (2001). *Int J Cancer,* 92, 130-138.
Immonen A, Vapalahti M, Tyynela K, Hurskainen H, Sandmair A, Vanninen R, Langford G, Murray N and Yla-Herttuala S. (2004). *Mol Ther,* 10, 967-972.
Ito S, Natsume A, Shimato S, Ohno M, Kato T, Chansakul P, Wakabayashi T and Kim SU. (2010). *Cancer Gene Ther,* 17, 299-306.
Jensen R and Glazer PM. (2004). *Proc Natl Acad Sci U S A,* 101, 6134-6139.
Jimenez T, Fox WP, Naus CC, Galipeau J and Belliveau DJ. (2006). *Cell Commun Adhes,* 13, 79-92.
Joo KM, Park IH, Shin JY, Jin J, Kang BG, Kim MH, Lee SJ, Jo MY, Kim SU and Nam DH. (2009). *Mol Ther,* 17, 570-575.
Kalra J, Shao Q, Qin H, Thomas T, aoui-Jamali MA and Laird DW. (2006). *Carcinogenesis,* 27, 2528-2537.
Kanczuga-Koda L, Sulkowski S, Lenczewski A, Koda M, Wincewicz A, Baltaziak M and Sulkowska M. (2006). *J Clin Pathol,* 59, 429-433.
Kandouz M and Batist G. (2010). *Expert Opin Ther Targets,* 14, 681-692.
Kandouz M, Bier A, Carystinos GD, Alaoui-Jamali MA and Batist G. (2004). *Oncogene,* 23, 4763-4770.
Kapoor P, Saunders MM, Li Z, Zhou Z, Sheaffer N, Kunze EL, Samant RS, Welch DR and Donahue HJ. (2004). *Int J Cancer,* 111, 693-697.
Kawamura K, Bahar R, Namba H, Seimiya M, Takenaga K, Hamada H, Sakiyama S and Tagawa M. (2001). *Int J Oncol,* 18, 117-120.
Kedde M, Strasser MJ, Boldajipour B, Oude Vrielink JA, Slanchev K, le SC, Nagel R, Voorhoeve PM, van DJ, Orom UA, Lund AH, Perrakis A, Raz E and Agami R. (2007). *Cell,* 131, 1273-1286.
Kim SK, Kim SU, Park IH, Bang JH, Aboody KS, Wang KC, Cho BK, Kim M, Menon LG, Black PM and Carroll RS. (2006). *Clin Cancer Res,* 12, 5550-5556.
King TJ and Bertram JS. (2005). *Biochim Biophys Acta,* 1719, 146-160.
Kjenseth A, Fykerud T, Rivedal E and Leithe E. (2010). *Cell Signal,* 22, 1267-1273.
Kubo H, Gardner TA, Wada Y, Koeneman KS, Gotoh A, Yang L, Kao C, Lim SD, Amin MB, Yang H, Black ME, Matsubara S, Nakagawa M, Gillenwater JY, Zhau HE and Chung LW. (2003). *Hum Gene Ther,* 14, 227-241.
Kunishige I, Samejima Y, Moriyama A, Saji F and Murata Y. (1998). *Anticancer Res,* 18, 3411-3419.
Lan Z, Kurata WE, Martyn KD, Jin C and Lau AF. (2005). *Biochemistry,* 44, 2385-2396.
Lawrence TS, Rehemtulla A, Ng EY, Wilson M, Trosko JE and Stetson PL. (1998). *Cancer Res,* 58, 2588-2593.
le-Agha N, Stahl W and Sies H. (2002). *Biochem Pharmacol,* 63, 2145-2149.
Leithe E and Rivedal E. (2007). *J Membr Biol,* 217, 43-51.
Li Z, Zhou Z and Donahue HJ. (2008a). *Clin Exp Metastasis,* 25, 265-272.
Li Z, Zhou Z, Welch DR and Donahue HJ. (2008b). *Clin Exp Metastasis,* 25, 893-901.

Marconi P, Tamura M, Moriuchi S, Krisky DM, Niranjan A, Goins WF, Cohen JB and Glorioso JC. (2000). *Mol Ther,* 1, 71-81.
Matuskova M, Hlubinova K, Pastorakova A, Hunakova L, Altanerova V, Altaner C and Kucerova L. (2009). *Cancer Lett.*
McLachlan E, Shao Q and Laird DW. (2007). *J Membr Biol,* 218, 107-121.
McLachlan E, Shao Q, Wang HL, Langlois S and Laird DW. (2006). *Cancer Res,* 66, 9886-9894.
McMasters RA, Saylors RL, Jones KE, Hendrix ME, Moyer MP and Drake RR. (1998). *Hum Gene Ther,* 9, 2253-2261.
Mesnil M, Crespin S, Avanzo JL and Zaidan-Dagli ML. (2005). *Biochim Biophys Acta,* 1719, 125-145.
Mesnil M, Piccoli C, Tiraby G, Willecke K and Yamasaki H. (1996). *Proc Natl Acad Sci U S A,* 93, 1831-1835.
Miles BJ, Shalev M, guilar-Cordova E, Timme TL, Lee HM, Yang G, Adler HL, Kernen K, Pramudji CK, Satoh T, Gdor Y, Ren C, Ayala G, Wheeler TM, Butler EB, Kadmon D and Thompson TC. (2001). *Hum Gene Ther,* 12, 1955-1967.
Mothersill C and Seymour CB. (2004). *Nat Rev Cancer,* 4, 158-164.
Mullen CA, Kilstrup M and Blaese RM. (1992). *Proc Natl Acad Sci U S A,* 89, 33-37.
Nakagawa S, Maeda S and Tsukihara T. (2010). *Curr Opin Struct Biol,* 20, 423-430.
Nasu Y, Saika T, Ebara S, Kusaka N, Kaku H, Abarzua F, Manabe D, Thompson TC and Kumon H. (2007). *Mol Ther,* 15, 834-840.
Nielsen M, Ruch RJ and Vang O. (2000). *Biochem Biophys Res Commun,* 275, 804-809.
Paino T, Gangoso E, Medina JM and Tabernero A. (2010). *Neuropharmacology,* 59, 480-491.
Park JY, Elshami AA, Amin K, Rizk N, Kaiser LR and Albelda SM. (1997). *Gene Ther,* 4, 909-917.
Peixoto PM, Ryu SY, Pruzansky DP, Kuriakose M, Gilmore A and Kinnally KW. (2009). *Biochem Biophys Res Commun,* 390, 38-43.
Peterson-Roth E, Brdlik CM and Glazer PM. (2009). *Cancer Res,* 69, 3619-3624.
Prise KM and O'Sullivan JM. (2009). *Nat Rev Cancer,* 9, 351-360.
Qin H, Shao Q, Igdoura SA, Alaoui-Jamali MA and Laird DW. (2003a). *J Biol Chem,* 278, 30005-30014.
Qin H, Shao Q, Thomas T, Kalra J, aoui-Jamali MA and Laird DW. (2003b). *Cell Commun Adhes,* 10, 387-393.
Qu C, Gardner P and Schrijver I. (2009). *Exp Cell Res,* 315, 1683-1692.
Robe PA, Jolois O, N'Guyen M, Princen F, Malgrange B, Merville MP and Bours V. (2004). *Int J Oncol,* 25, 187-192.
Robe PA, Nguyen-Khac M, Jolois O, Rogister B, Merville MP and Bours V. (2005). *BMC Cancer,* 5, 32.
Sacco MG, Benedetti S, Duflot-Dancer A, Mesnil M, Bagnasco L, Strina D, Fasolo V, Villa A, Macchi P, Faranda S, Vezzoni P and Finocchiaro G. (1996). *Gene Ther,* 3, 1151-1156.
Sacco MG, Mangiarini L, Villa A, Macchi P, Barbieri O, Sacchi MC, Monteggia E, Fasolo V, Vezzoni P and Clerici L. (1995). *Gene Ther,* 2, 493-497.
Saez JC, Schalper KA, Retamal MA, Orellana JA, Shoji KF and Bennett MV. (2010). *Exp Cell Res,* 316, 2377-2389.
Salameh A and Dhein S. (2005). *Biochim Biophys Acta,* 1719, 36-58.
Sato H, Fukumoto K, Hada S, Hagiwara H, Fujimoto E, Negishi E, Ueno K and Yano T. (2007a). *Cancer Chemother Pharmacol,* 60, 449-457.
Sato H, Hagiwara H, Ohde Y, Senba H, Virgona N and Yano T. (2007b). *J Membr Biol,* 216, 17-21.

Sato H, Iwata H, Takano Y, Yamada R, Okuzawa H, Nagashima Y, Yamaura K, Ueno K and Yano T. (2009). *J Pharmacol Sci,* 110, 466-475.
Sato H, Senba H, Virgona N, Fukumoto K, Ishida T, Hagiwara H, Negishi E, Ueno K, Yamasaki H and Yano T. (2007c). *Mol Carcinog,* 46, 215-224.
Seul KH, Kang KY, Lee KS, Kim SH and Beyer EC. (2004). *Biochem Biophys Res Commun,* 319, 1144-1151.
Shimato S, Natsume A, Takeuchi H, Wakabayashi T, Fujii M, Ito M, Ito S, Park IH, Bang JH, Kim SU and Yoshida J. (2007). *Gene Ther,* 14, 1132-1142.
Solan JL and Lampe PD. (2009). *Biochem J,* 419, 261-272.
Sterman DH, Treat J, Litzky LA, Amin KM, Coonrod L, Molnar-Kimber K, Recio A, Knox L, Wilson JM, Albelda SM and Kaiser LR. (1998). *Hum Gene Ther,* 9, 1083-1092.
Tanaka M, Fraizer GC, De La CJ, Cristiano RJ, Liebert M and Grossman HB. (2001a). *Gene Ther,* 8, 139-148.
Tanaka M and Grossman HB. (2004). *Oncol Rep,* 11, 537-541.
Tanaka T, Yamasaki H and Mesnil M. (2001b). *Mol Carcinog,* 30, 176-180.
Tanaka T, Yamasaki H and Mesnil M. (2001c). *Int J Cancer,* 91, 538-542.
Thompson TC. (1999). *Oncol Res,* 11, 1-8.
Touraine RL, Vahanian N, Ramsey WJ and Blaese RM. (1998). *Hum Gene Ther,* 9, 2385-2391.
Trepel M, Stoneham CA, Eleftherohorinou H, Mazarakis ND, Pasqualini R, Arap W and Hajitou A. (2009). *Mol Cancer Ther,* 8, 2383-2391.
Trinh QT, Austin EA, Murray DM, Knick VC and Huber BE. (1995). *Cancer Res,* 55, 4808-4812.
Udawatte C and Ripps H. (2005). *Apoptosis,* 10, 1019-1029.
Uhl M, Weiler M, Wick W, Jacobs AH, Weller M and Herrlinger U. (2005). *Biochem Biophys Res Commun,* 328, 125-129.
van D, I, Mulder NH, Sluiter WJ, Meijer C, de JS, Loncarek J, Mesnil M, de Vries EF, Vaalburg W and Hospers GA. (2005). *Oncol Res,* 15, 151-159.
van D, I, Mulder NH, Vaalburg W, de Vries EF and Hospers GA. (2002). *Curr Gene Ther,* 2, 307-322.
Vaney DI and Weiler R. (2000). *Brain Res Brain Res Rev,* 32, 115-120.
Villares GJ, Dobroff AS, Wang H, Zigler M, Melnikova VO, Huang L and Bar-Eli M. (2009). *Cancer Res,* 69, 6730-6737.
Vrionis FD, Wu JK, Qi P, Waltzman M, Cherington V and Spray DC. (1997). *Gene Ther,* 4, 577-585.
Wang M, Berthoud VM and Beyer EC. (2007). *J Cell Sci,* 120, 320-329.
Weber PA, Chang HC, Spaeth KE, Nitsche JM and Nicholson BJ. (2004). *Biophys J,* 87, 958-973.
Wei CJ, Xu X and Lo CW. (2004). *Annu Rev Cell Dev Biol,* 20, 811-838.
Wygoda MR, Wilson MR, Davis MA, Trosko JE, Rehemtulla A and Lawrence TS. (1997). *Cancer Res,* 57, 1699-1703.
Xu G and McLeod HL. (2001). *Clin Cancer Res,* 7, 3314-3324.
Yamasaki H and Katoh F. (1988). *Cancer Res,* 48, 3203-3207.
Yang B, Lin H, Xiao J, Lu Y, Luo X, Li B, Zhang Y, Xu C, Bai Y, Wang H, Chen G and Wang Z. (2007). *Nat Med,* 13, 486-491.
Yeager M and Harris AL. (2007). *Curr Opin Cell Biol,* 19, 521-528.
Zhang LX, Cooney RV and Bertram JS. (1991). *Carcinogenesis,* 12, 2109-2114.

10

Promising Role of Engineered Gene Circuits in Gene Therapy

Wei-dong Wang and Jinyi Lang
Department of Radiation Oncology, Sichuan Cancer Hospital
P.R. China

1. Introduction

Synthetic biology is concerned with applying the engineering paradigm of systems design to biological systems in order to produce predictable and robust systems with novel functionalities that do not exist in nature. The circuit-like connectivity of biological parts and their ability to collectively process logical operations was first appreciated nearly 50 years ago. This inspired attempts to describe biological regulation schemes with mathematical models and to apply circuit analogies from established frameworks in electrical engineering(McAdams & Arkin A,2000). Meanwhile, breakthroughs in genomic research and genetic engineering (e.g., recombinant DNA technology) were supplying the inventory and methods necessary to physically construct and assemble biomolecular parts. As a result, synthetic biology was born with the broad goal of engineering or "wiring" biological circuitry—be it genetic, protein, viral, pathway, or genomic—for manifesting logical forms of cellular control. Synthetic biology, equipped with the engineering-driven approaches of modularization, rationalization, and modeling, has progressed rapidly and generated an ever-increasing suite of genetic devices and biological modules.

synthetic biology is seeking to use and expand the mechanisms that control biological organisms using engineering approaches. These approaches will be applied on all scales of biological complexity: from the basic units to novel interactions between these units to novel multi-component modules that generate complex logical behaviour, and even to completely or partially engineered cells(McAdams & Shapiro,1995). Bringing the engineering paradigm to biology will allow us to apply existing biological knowledge to biotechnological problems in a much more rational and systematic way than has previously been possible, and at the same time to expand the scope of what can be achieved this way. The introduction of design principles such as modularity of parts, standardization of parts and devices according to internationally recognized criteria, and the adaptation of available abstract design procedures to biological systems, coupled to novel technological breakthroughs that allow the decoupling of design and fabrication, will fundamentally change our current concepts of how to manipulate biological systems. In this sense, synthetic biology is not primarily a "discovery science", but is ultimately about a new way of making things. By adapting natural biological mechanisms to the requirements of an engineering approach, the possibilities for re-assembling biological systems in a designed way will increase tremendously. While several of the fundamental scientific issues and current applied objectives of synthetic biology overlap with those in other, more mature fields, especially biotechnology and systems biology, synthetic biology should be properly seen as a completely new discipline, which brings a systematic, application-driven engineering perspective to biology. Just as in chemistry about a century ago, biology now seems poised to enter an era where significant advances in understanding will derive from a fruitful dialogue between theory and experiment, from analytical and synthetic efforts, and from interdisciplinary interaction with the chemical, physical, engineering and computational sciences. The potential for interaction with nanotechnology is especially apparent and appealing. It is often said that biology is the only existing nanotechnology that really works. But if we want to exploit this 'natural nanotechnology' for applied, engineering objectives, we will ultimately need to be able to intervene and to modify it at the level that synthetic biology is exploring. It can be anticipated that the major change that the field of synthetic biology will bring is the synergistic integration of existing disciplines: not just biology and engineering, but also computer modelling, information technology, control theory, chemistry and nanotechnology. Ulitmately, it is likely that the analytical and synthetic approaches to biology, as well as the in vitro and in vivo approaches, will fully complement each other.

Synthetic biology will revolutionize how we conceptualize and approach the engineering of biological systems. The vision and applications of this emerging field will influence many other scientific and engineering disciplines, as well as affect the next generation of cancer therapy. In this article, we discuss and analyze the recent advances in synthetic biology towards engineering complex living systems through novel assemblies of biological molecules. The discovery of mathematical logic in gene regulation in the 1960s (e.g. the lac operon; Monod and Jacob, 1961) and early achievements in genetic engineering that took place in the 1970s, such as recombinant DNA technology, paved the way for today's synthetic biology. Synthetic biology extends the spirit of genetic engineering to focus on whole systems of genes and gene products. The focus on systems as opposed to individual genes or pathways is shared by the contemporaneous discipline of systems biology, which analyzes biological organisms in their entirety. Synthetic biologists design and construct complex artificial biological systems using many insights discovered by systems biologists and share their holistic perspective. It is useful to apply many existing standards for engineering from well-established fields, including software and electrical engineering, mechanical engineering, and civil engineering, to synthetic biology. Methods and criteria such as standardization, abstraction, modularity, predictability, reliability, and uniformity greatly increase the speed and tractability of design. However, care must be taken in directly adopting accepted methods and criteria to the engineering of biology. We must keep in mind what makes synthetic biology different from all previous engineering disciplines. The insight gained from fully appreciating these differences is critical for developing appropriate standards and methods. Building biological systems entails a unique set of design problems and solutions. Biological devices and modules are not independent objects, and are not built in the absence of a biological milieu. Biological devices and modules typically function within a cellular environment. When synthetic biologists engineer devices or modules, they do so using the resources and machinery of host cells, but in the process also modify the cells themselves. A major concern in this process is our present inability to fully predict the functions of even simple devices in engineered cells and construct systems that perform complex tasks with precision and reliability. The lack of predictive power stems from several sources of uncertainty, some of which signify the incompleteness of available information about inherent cellular characteristics. The effects of gene expression noise, mutation, cell death, undefined and changing extracellular environments, and interactions with cellular context currently hinder us from engineering single cells with the confidence that we can engineer computers to do specific tasks. However, most applications or tasks we set to our synthetic biological systems are generally completed by a population of cells, not any single cell. In a synthetic system, predictability and reliability may be achieved in two ways: statistically by utilizing large numbers of independent cells or by synchronizing individual cells through intercellular communication to make each cell more predictable and reliable. More importantly, intercellular communication can coordinate tasks across heterogeneous cell populations to elicit highly sophisticated behavior(Khalil & Collins, 2010). Thus, it may be best to focus on multicellular systems to achieve overall reliability in performing complex tasks.

2. Recent advancements in synthetic biology

2.1 Engineering of artificial gene networks

Significant efforts were recently undertaken in the design of artificial genetic networks in prokaryotic and eukaryotic systems. Here, different genetic elements or 'parts' are (ultimately) rationally combined to 'devices' to realize specific cellular behaviors that have frequently analogies to elements from electric circuits such as switches and oscillators. We will outline recent efforts in the development of artificial gene networks.

2.1.1 Switches

A switch lets the cell adopt one of two possible states, depending either on the presence or absence of a chemical inducer or on two separate external stimuli (toggle switch) (Becskei et al.,2001). The latter behavior can be easily designed from any two repressors that reciprocally inhibit the transcription of their genes (Gardner et al.,2000). Switching between states can be achieved by intermittently inactivating the repressor that maintains the current state (such as adding a chemical inducer or increasing the temperature). Essentially, this property conveys a cell with a memory of its previous cultivation history and thus represents an epigenetic toggle switch. The former behavior requires positive feedback in the regulatory processes, such as (1) the positive autoregulation of a positive regulator's gene transcription or (2) the concomitant upregulation of an operon by external inducer and of the gene that encodes the transporter protein for entrance of the inducer. Besides the artificial design of such systems, this behavior is rather common in a number of well-characterized bacterial expression systems such as the bacterial lactose and arabinose systems (Atkinsonet al., 2003;Ozbudak et al.,2004;Vilar et al.,2003).

In addition, the switches can be engineered with a hysteretic character, so that the system switches into the 'ON' state at a higher concentration of external signal than is required to switch back to the 'OFF' state. This requires that the concentration of activator or active repressor can be made a function of the history of the cell, e.g. by adding another regulatory layer on top of the positive feedback element. This can be a concentration-dependent inactivation of a repressor that competes with an activator. Depending on the previous state of the cell, a given concentration of active repressor interacts with either high or low concentrations of activators, leading to a differentiation in response depending on the history (Kramer & Fussenegger, 2005).

2.1.2 Complex networks

An oscillator produces regular fluctuations in network elements such as reporter proteins. Oscillators have been realized in two ways: as ring oscillators ('repressilators') or as a combination of activation and repression elements. The ring oscillator consists of three repressor genes that are coupled to three corresponding promoters in such a way, that each repressor protein can turn off the synthesis of one other repressor protein. This design worked on single cell level, but not on culture-level, which probably has to do with the noise involved on gene expression level (Elowitz & Leibler,2000). However, by combining positive and negative regulation, it is possible to reduce the noise to such a degree that population-synchronized oscillation behavior over three periods can be observed in a turbidostat. Interestingly, such oscillating systems can be extended to include metabolite concentrations (Fung et al.,2005).

In order to execute ever more complex logical behavior, it will be important to be able to 'integrate' more and more signals into determining one or more cellular functions. This is facilitated by the high level of modularity in the regulatory elements of eukaryotic systems. This modularity makes them particularly amenable to design and can be used to implement a wide variety of logical behaviors for two and three signal inputs while exploiting only a limited number of genetic elements (Kramer et al.,2004).

2.1.3 Networks for intercellular communications

Creating macroscopically observable artificial functional behavior in a cell population requires some kind of synchronization. Such synchronization can be enforced by adding chemical inducers or by letting the cells themselves produce a signal in response to a change in a culture property. One example for such a property is cell density which can be communicated by quorum sensing, for example via the *luxR/luxI* system of *Vibrio fischeri* or via artificially engineered systems (Bulter et al., 2004).

The *luxR/luxI* system has been used to trigger a variety of population-density dependent responses, such as flipping of a toggle switch (Kobayashi et al., 2004) or programmed population control (You et al., 2004). The system has also been exploited to design spatial patterns of behavior that re-build aspects of multicellular systems: when producer cells send the autoinducer signal of the *lux* system via diffusion through a plate, cells at different distances from the senders experience differently steep gradients once the autoinducer reaches them. Alternatively, cells can be used to detect the differences in inducer concentration in resulting (quasi-)steady state. Networks can be designed which are able to detect these rather subtle differences in environmental conditions and which translate them into adequate cellular responses such as different pulses of reporter proteins or stable colorimetric patterns (Basu et al.,2004;Basu et al., 2005), introducing space as an additional design parameter into the synthetic biology realm.

2.1.4 Issues related to the design of genetic circuits

For the design of genetic networks, the availability of functional elements with specific properties (such as binding constants and degradation rates) that fit the design purpose is crucial. So far, we are only at the beginning of being able to easily measure, let alone program kinetic parameters, co-operativities or binding constants. Consequently, the design process remains–for the time being–an iterative process that still contains considerable elements of trial and error. Nevertheless, some work-around tools are available today in order to, at least crudely, shift certain characteristics from wild-type values to values that allow a desired behavior to be implemented. These include variations in gene dosage via changes in plasmid replicon, the increase of protein degradation rates by fusion to suitable protease sensitive tag-sequences, variations in the strength of RBSs (Yokobayashi et al.,2002) or drawing on the large number of mutants that are available for a number of model systems (such as phage λ, the *lac* system or the *tet* system). Alternatively, parameters can be adapted to the desired behavior by directed evolution, if a suitable assay is available. However, it is not really clear how such directed evolution assays can be easily tailored to screen for relatively subtle differences in properties important for optimized design. In summary, a primary task for the immediate future is to gain access to complete system parameter sets, which can then serve as the starting point to produce parts with parameter values that span suitable ranges.

2.2 Engineering of systems

Synthetic biology is a very young discipline that follows a powerful technological vision. However, there are no examples available where the whole approach has been implemented. Still, in some cases specific aspects of synthetic biology have been of critical importance. We will discuss the following examples: the design of an *E.coli* capable of image processing, refactoring of the phage T7, the design of novel polyketide antibiotics and the manufacturing of precursors for the anti-malaria drug artemisinin.

An original example for new applications that derives from the interface of engineering and life sciences, which came out of the iGEM student competition, is the image-processing *E.coli*. By designing proteins that couple light-detection to well-known *E.coli* regulatory circuits, first steps towards light-detecting pixel sizes of micrometer dimensions are possible (Levskaya et al., 2005).

A more fundamental aspect is covered by the work on the phage T7, which tries to help to answer the question whether it is indeed possible to refactor significant portions of small genomes. In other words, can we indeed modify those genomes according to the requirements of 'engineerability' such as monofunctionality of a part of the sequence and organization of the DNA into functional segments. Refactoring 10 kb of the T7 genome, representing about a quarter of the total genome, still produces functional phages, though their efficiency in propagation is reduced (Chan et al., 2005). This is an important validation of the synthetic biology approach, even though on a small scale. It remains to be seen whether the same concepts can be applied to more complex systems such as microbes.

Two examples for application of synthetic biology concepts come from the area of pharmaceutical production and involve primarily the opportunities offered by *de novo* DNA synthesis, such as the direct adaptation of codon usage, implementation of suitable regulatory circuitry and the possibility to modularize the DNA sequences by restriction sites to facilitate iterative optimizations. The first example involves the adaptation of polyketide synthesis to well studied *E.coli* production strains and the subsequent design of novel polyketides by semi-randomized recombination of polyketide synthase genes. These recombinations were easily enforced along the interfaces of the different functional modules that make up a synthase and resulted in a rather high success rate of detecting novel polyketides (Menzella et al., 2005).

Along similar lines, another project that very much catches the spirit of synthetic biology is the construction, from scratch, of a cheap terpenoid production pathway in *E.coli* leading to artemisinic acid, a precursor to the anti-malaria drug artemisinin. This goal essentially requires the design of an entirely new pathway in a suitable production organism. The corresponding pathway elements can be recruited from bacteria (*E.coli*), yeast (*Saccharomyces cerevisiae*) and plant (*Artemisa annua*), redesigned and functionally expressed in bacteria or yeast, effectively paving the road to a low-cost production route to effective malaria treatment (Martin et al.,2003;Ro et al.,2006).

Although the design of novel biological systems is only beginning, all ingredients of the engineering approach are visible: the role of *de novo* DNA synthesis, the design of well-behaved parts on the DNA and protein level, the organization of parts into the next functional level of devices and the corresponding abstractions and the attempt to introduce standardization, even though for the time being only on a parts level. With the design of ever more complex systems, the need to emphasize these elements will undoubtedly increase.

3. Design strategies of synthetic genetic circuits

Synthetic biology encompasses the building of novel biological entities for useful purposes and the corresponding endeavors can be subdivided into two distinct types of tasks: systems design and systems fabrication. Here, we will discuss the essential elements of these two tasks with a special focus on the computational and informatics requirements.

Fabrication deals with the transformation of design plans into actual physical instances. Today, this still involves a significant amount of cloning work, which should decrease in the future due to *de novo* DNA synthesis. The fabrication as such, is not expected to create a great demand for novel informatics tools.

In contrast, systems design consisting of forward-engineering of biological parts, devices or systems strongly relies on computing and informatics tools that assist the design process. Ultimately, it would be desirable to have computer aided design tools—CAD tools for biological engineering—in analogy to the respective software tools in the areas of mechanical or civil engineering. Using such software, the synthetic biology design engineer would try to improve the behavior of a biological system *in silico* by optimizing design parameters targeting a selected objective function. Design variants would be tested computationally by means of simulations.

Such design tools will be based on quantitative mechanistic models that reproduce biological behavior and–in order to be useful for forward-engineering design—would also have predictive power. In biology, we have not yet reached a level of understanding where such models can be developed on a large scale and consequently, true biological engineering is hardly possible until now (Endy & Brent, 2001). In fact, in most cases today, we are faced with highly uncertain or even unknown model topologies, mechanisms and parameters. The recent advances in the post-genomic research and especially in systems biology, however, provide hope that sooner or later we will be able to draw on a body of knowledge that allows for the envisioned directed engineering of biology (Endy & Brent, 2001). Ultimately, mathematical models developed for research purposes (e.g. in systems biology) will be employed as design models in synthetic biology. In contrast to the current lack of predictive models, tools for modeling and simulation exist in large numbers (Lemerle et al, 2005).

We envision that in the long run we will require models and design software for the following tasks: (1) sequence-based (*ab initio*) prediction of structure, function and interactions of macromolecules, in particular proteins and mRNA, (2) prediction of the dynamics of signaling and regulatory networks; and (3) prediction of the dynamics of metabolic networks. For each of these areas, we will shortly sketch the current status of development and also elaborate on future tasks.

3.1 Design of functions and interactions of macromolecules

We would like to predict—starting from a linear sequence of nucleotides or amino acids—2D (mRNA) and 3D structures of the respective macromolecules (RNA, proteins), as well as their function and their interaction parameters with other cellular components (DNA, metabolites, etc.). In other words, as outlined above we would like to have the possibility to modify sequences in a targeted manner to obtain, e.g. novel transcription factors (i.e. with altered binding constants or kinetics) or proteins with novel functions.

However today, as an example *de novo* protein structure prediction from a linear amino acids sequence can only be achieved for small protein domains at significant computational costs (Bradley et al.,2005; Misura et al.,2006). Nevertheless, starting from known structures of 'scaffold' proteins, design methods are available, which can be used to rationally modify the proteins' structure and function, i.e. to build completely new active sites into proteins or to redesign binding specificities of proteins. However, such design processes still go through several cycles of iterative improvement involving design, analysis, redesign, etc. where computational tools such as FoldX (Schymkowitz et al.,2005) are typically employed. In other words, the design of tailored catalytic activities on artificial proteins seems to be within reach, while quantitative prediction of enzymatic activity and selectivity from 3D protein structures in general is not yet feasible. For further information on the current status in modeling of protein structures and interactions, the reader is referred to a recent review (Schueler-Furman et al.,2005).

Based on structure models, molecular dynamics simulation have shown to be a versatile tool to investigate the dynamic behavior of complexes between DNA binding sites and respective DNA target sites (Marco et al., 2003;;Obika et al.,2003). These tools can also be employed to predict the effect of structural modulations on protein-ligand interactions in a way that would allow forward-engineering design of, e.g. DNA-binding specificity of transcription factors.

3.2 Design of signaling and regulatory networks

Artificial signaling and regulatory gene networks will need to be assembled for synthetic biology. Today, such circuits are still frequently assembled by intuition and optimized through several rounds of trial and error (Kærn et al.,2003) and the mathematical models are only developed once proper *in vivo* function has been demonstrated. Deterministic or stochastic models (or a combination of both) are then used to describe the observed dynamic behavior of the circuit.

Ideal, however, would be models that allow deriving *in silico* suggestions for optimal design strategies or debugging, prior to implementation of the circuit *in vivo* (Sprinzak & Elowitz, 2005). Such models should be able to capture the dynamic behavior of the gene networks. In cases where only small molecule numbers are involved (as in gene transcription or translation, where transcription factors and mRNA molecules only occur in low copy numbers), the models would also need to be able to reproduce the inherent stochasticity of such processes. This is imperative as it was shown that stochasticity in combination with certain system architectures can result in different system states (Pedraza & van

Oudenaarden,2005). A robust design of new devices and systems must exclude such eventualities.
In summary, to enable the envisioned forward-engineering (model-based) design of signaling and regulatory circuits, improvements are required in the following areas: It is necessary (1) to obtain an improved quantitative understanding of regulatory and signaling processes; (2) to develop effective rules (Wall et al.,2003) and standards for characterizing modules and (3) to improve multiscale simulation algorithms as the existing ones are limited in a way that the participating reactions have to occur on a comparative time scale and the participating reaction species have to fulfill certain population size requirements.

4. Genetic circuits and therapeutics

4.1 Drug target identification

Building up synthetic pathways and systems from individual parts is one way of identifying disease mechanisms and therapeutic targets. Another is to deploy synthetic biology devices to systematically probe the function of individual components of a natural pathway. To achieve post-transcriptional control over a target gene, the mRNA sequence of its 5′-UTR was designed to form a hairpin structure that sequesters the ribosomal binding site (RBS) and prevents ribosome access to it. Translational repression of this *cis*-repressed mRNA could then be alleviated by an independently regulated *trans*-activating RNA that targets the stem-loop for unfolding. Engineered riboregulators were used in a subsequent study to tightly regulate the expression of CcdB, a toxic bacterial protein that inhibits DNA gyrase, so as to gain a better understanding of the sequence of events leading to induced bacterial cell death(Dwyer,2007). These synthetic biology studies, in conjunction with systems biology studies of quinolones (antibiotics that inhibit gyrase), led to the discovery that all major classes of bactericidal antibiotics induce a common oxidative damage cellular death pathway(Kohanski,2008). This work provided new insights into how bacteria respond to lethal stimuli, and paved the way for the development of more effective antibacterial therapies.
Once a faulty pathway component or target is identified, whole-cell screening assays can be designed using synthetic biology strategies for drug discovery. As a demonstration of this approach, Fussenegger and colleagues(Weber,2008)developed a synthetic platform for screening small molecules that could potentiate a *Mycobacterium tuberculosis* antibiotic. Ethionamide, currently the last line of defense in the treatment of multidrug-resistant tuberculosis, depends on activation by the *M. tuberculosis* enzyme EthA for efficacy. Due to transcriptional repression of *ethA* by the protein EthR, however, ethionamide-based therapy is often rendered ineffective. To address this problem, the researchers designed a synthetic mammalian gene circuit, featuring an EthR-based transactivator of a reporter gene, and used it to screen for and identify EthR inhibitors that could abrogate resistance to ethionamide. Importantly, because the system is a cell-based assay, it intrinsically enriches for inhibitors that are nontoxic and membrane-permeable to mammalian cells, which are key drug criteria as *M. tuberculosis* is an intracellular pathogen. This framework, in which drug discovery is applied to whole cells that have been engineered with circuits that highlight a pathogenic mechanism, could be extended to other diseases and phenotypes.

4.2 Therapeutic treatment

Synthetic biology devices have additionally been developed to serve as therapies themselves. Entire engineered viruses and organisms can be programmed to target specific pathogenic agents and pathological mechanisms. In two separate studies(Lu,2009), for instance, engineered bacteriophages were deployed to combat antibiotic-resistant bacteria, by endowing them with genetic mechanisms that target and thwart bacteria's antibiotic evasion techniques. The first study was prompted by the observation that biofilms, in which bacteria are encapsulated in an extracellular matrix, have inherent resistance to antimicrobial therapies and are implicated sources of persistent infections. To more effectively penetrate this protective environment, T7 phage was engineered to express the biofilm matrix-degrading enzyme dispersin B (DspB) upon infection (Lu,2007). The two-pronged attack of phage-induced lysis fueling the creation and spread of matrix-degrading enzyme resulted in 99.997% removal of biofilm bacterial cells.

It was hypothesized that inhibition of certain bacterial genetic programs could help current antibiotic therapies achieve more effective activity. In this case, bacteriophages were deliberately designed to be non-lethal so as not to elicit resistance mechanisms; instead, non-lytic M13 phage was used to suppress the bacterial SOS DNA damage response by overexpression of its repressor, *lexA3*. The engineered bacteriophage significantly enhanced killing by three major classes of antibiotics in traditional cell culture and in *E. coli*-infected mice, potentiated killing of antibiotic-resistant bacteria, and importantly reduced the incidence of antibiotic-induced resistant cells.

Synthetically engineered viruses and organisms that are able to sense and link their therapeutic activity to pathological cues may be useful in the treatment of cancer, where current therapies often indiscriminately attack tumors and normal tissues. Adenoviruses, for instance, were programmed to couple their replication to the state of the p53 pathway in human cells(Ramachandra,2001). Normal p53 production would result in inhibition of a critical viral replication component, whereas a defunct p53 pathway, which is characteristic of tumor cells, would allow viral replication and cell killing. In another demonstration of translational synthetic biology applied to cancer therapy, Voigt and colleagues()developed cancer-targeting bacteria and linked their ability to invade the cancer cells to specific environmental signals. Constitutive expression of the heterologous *inv* gene (from *Yersinia pseudotuberculosis*) can induce *E. coli* cells to invade both normal and cancer human cell lines. So, to preferentially invade cancer cells, the researchers placed *inv* under the control of transcriptional operons that are activated by environmental signals specific to the tumor microenvironment. These engineered bacteria could be made to carry or synthesize cancer therapies for the treatment of tumors.

In addition to engineered therapeutic organisms, synthetic circuits and pathways can be used for the controlled delivery of drugs as well as for gene and metabolic therapy. In some cases, sophisticated, kinetic control over drug release in the body may yield therapeutic advantages and reduce undesired side effects. Most hormones in the body are released in time-dependent pulses. Glucocorticoid secretion, for instance, has a circadian and ultradian pattern of release, with important transcriptional consequences for glucocorticoid-responsive cells(Anderson,2006). Faithfully mimicking these patterns in the administration of synthetic hormones to patients with glucocorticoid-responsive diseases, such as rheumatoid arthritis, may decrease known side effects and improve therapeutic response. Periodic synthesis and release of biologic drugs can be autonomously achieved with synthetic oscillator circuits or programmed time-delay circuits(Weber,2007) In other cases, one may wish to place a limit on the amount of drug released by programming the synthetic system to self-destruct after a defined number of cell cycles or drug release pulses.

Gene therapy is beginning to make some promising advances in clinical areas where traditional drug therapy is ineffective, such as in the treatment of many hereditary and metabolic diseases. Synthetic circuits offer a more controlled approach to gene therapy, such as the ability to dynamically silence, activate, and tune the expression of desired genes. In one such example, a genetic switch was developed in mammalian cells that couples transcriptional repressor proteins and an RNA interference (RNAi) module for tight, tunable, and reversible control over the expression of desired genes. This system would be particularly useful in gene silencing applications, as it was shown to yield > 99% repression of a target gene. Additionally, the construction of non-native pathways offers a unique and versatile approach to gene therapy, such as for the treatment of metabolic disorders. Operating at the interface of synthetic biology and metabolic engineering, for instance, Liao and colleagues(Dean,2009) recently introduced the glyoxylate shunt pathway into mammalian liver cells and mice to explore its effects on fatty acid metabolism and, more broadly, whole-body metabolism. Remarkably, the researchers found that when transplanted into mammals the shunt actually increased fatty acid oxidation, evidently by creating an alternative cycle. Furthermore, mice expressing the shunt showed resistance to diet-induced obesity when placed on a high-fat diet, with corresponding decreases in total fat mass, plasma triglycerides, and cholesterol levels. This work offers a new synthetic biology model for studying metabolic networks and disorders, and for developing treatments for the increasing problem of obesity.

5. Challenges and future directions

Constructing a functional synthetic circuit requires assembling diverse genetic elements and getting them to work together. In general, combining disparate components requires the tuning of biochemical parameters such as affinities or rate constants, which is often difficult to implement in biological circuits. Characterization of a component may be valid in one context (locus, plasmid, strain, environment, and so on), but not in others. How can one design an operating circuit given these limitations? Several strategies have been applied. First, the use of tunable elements, such as transcription factors derived from tetR(Lutz,1997), allows external control over some parameters. Second, one can screen libraries of mutated components, or apply directed evolution in the laboratory, to optimize parameters. A third strategy is to use robust circuit designs that are inherently insensitive to unknown or variable parameters. Such designs are particularly interesting because they may have been selected by evolution for the very same property(Barkai,1997).

A related challenge is computational modelling of genetic circuits. Modelling is essential both for analysis of natural systems and also for design of synthetic ones. However, several problems complicate its application to cellular circuits. These include parameter sensitivity, the lack of effective rules to simplify complex circuits, and the difficulty of incorporating extrinsic noise. Because synthetic circuits are simpler and better characterized than their natural counterparts, they will probably offer ideal test systems to develop and refine models. The results should apply both to natural and synthetic circuits.

What are the goals of the synthetic circuit paradigm outlined here? One is to better understand natural circuits by building minimal replicas of those circuits, observing their dynamics in vivo, and comparing them to one another and to their natural counterparts.

The synthetic circuits presented above are highly simplified. However, as we gain confidence and expertise in our ability to build, model and analyse these circuits, we will be able to construct replicas of greater verisimilitude. Possible natural circuits that could be investigated this way include decision making in response to stress and DNA damage, as in the natural p53/mdm2 circuit(Vogelstein,2000), differentiation in response to extracellular signals, as in oocyte maturation(Xiong,2003), and regulated temporal oscillations, as in the cell cycle and circadian clock. Circuits that use the intrinsically noisy nature of the cell to create probabilistic behaviours are particularly compelling examples.

A second goal is to discover what other, non-natural, circuit designs are possible given realistic biological components, and which of those operate reliably in vivo. This will be achieved by building and characterizing a variety of alternative circuit designs in living cells. In this way, one may ask what advantages naturally evolved circuits have over synthetic ones. For example, the synthetic clock designs described earlier have not been discovered to occur in nature, suggesting that natural designs may confer better performance. At the same time, non-natural designs may prove useful for biotechnology applications.

Perhaps the most intriguing problem is how a circuit operates in the context of a complete organism. There are no dotted lines inside the cell isolating circuits from one another. The ultimate test for this synthetic approach is to delete natural circuits and replace them with synthetic counterparts within organisms. This will require synthetic circuits to interface with the rest of the cell. For example, by replacing the Drosophila circadian clock with synthetic versions we could learn more about the interaction of the circadian module with other functional subsystems in the organism. Even the most optimistic synthetic biologist would expect such circuits to be less functional than their natural counterparts. However, perhaps at this stage one can learn more by putting together a simple, if inaccurate, pendulum clock than one can by disassembling the finest Swiss timepiece.

6. Reference

Ahmad S. Khalil and James J. Collins. (2010).Synthetic Biology: Applications Come of Age. Nat Rev Genet. 11(5),pp.367-379.

Ander, M., et al. (2004).SmartCell, a framework to simulate cellular processes that combines stochastic approximation with diffusion and localisation: analysis of simple networks. *Syst. Biol*, 1, pp.129-138.

Anderson JC, Clarke EJ, Arkin AP, Voigt CA. (2006). Environmentally controlled invasion of cancer cells by engineered bacteria. *J Mol Biol.* 355,pp.619-27.

Arigoni, F., Talabot, F., Peitsch, M., Edgerton, M. D., Meldrum, E., (1998).A genome-based approach for the identification of essential bacterial genes. *Nat. Biotechnol. 16*, pp.851-856.

Atkinson, M.R., et al. (2003).Development of genetic circuitry exhibiting toggle switch or oscillatory behavior in *Escherichia coli*. *Cell*, 113, pp.597-607.

Barkai, N. & Leibler, S. (1997)Robustness in simple biochemical networks. Nature , 387, pp.913-917.

Basu, S., et al. (2005). A synthetic multicellular system for programmed pattern formation. *Nature*, 434, pp.1130-1134.

Basu, S., et al. (2004). Spatiotemporal control of gene expression with pulse-generating networks. *Proc. Natl Acad. Sci. USA*, 101, pp.6355-6360.

Becskei, A., et al. (2001). Positive feedback in eukaryotic gene networks: cell differentiation by graded to binary response conversion. *EMBO J*, 20, pp.2528-2535.

Blancafort, P., et al. (2004). Designing transcription factor architectures for drug discovery. *Mol. Pharmacol*, 66, pp.1361-1371.

Bradley, P., et al. (2005).Toward high-resolution *de novo* structure prediction for small proteins. *Science*, 309, pp.1868-1871.

Bulter, T., et al. (2004).Design of artificial cell-cell communication using gene and metabolic networks. *Proc. Natl Acad. Sci. USA*, 101, pp.2299-2304.

Cello, J., Paul, A. V., Wimmer, E., (2002). Chemical synthesis of poliovirus cDNA: generation of infectious virus in the absence of natural template. *Science, 297,* pp.1016–1018.

Chandonia, J.-M., Konerding, D. E., Allen, D.G., (2002). Computational structural genomics of a complete minimal organism. *Genome Informatics, 13,* pp.390–391.

Deamer, D., (2005). A giant step towards artificial life? *Trends Biotechnol. 23,* pp.336–338.

Dean JT, et al. (2009). Resistance to diet-induced obesity in mice with synthetic glyoxylate shunt. *Cell Metab.* 9,pp.525–36.

Dreier, B., et al. (2001).Development of zinc finger domains for recognition of the 5'-ANN-3' family of DNA sequences and their use in the construction of artificial transcription factors. *J. Biol. Chem,* 276, pp.29466–29478.

Dreier, B., et al. (2005).Development of zinc finger domains for recognition of the 5'-CNN-3' family DNA sequences and their use in the construction of artificial transcription factors. *J. Biol. Chem,* 280, pp.35588–35597.

Dueber, J. E., Yeh, B. J., Chak, K. & Lim, W. A. (2003).Reprogramming control of an allosteric signalling switch through modular recombination. Science, 301, pp.1904–1908.

Dueber, J.E., et al. (2003).Reprogramming control of an allosteric signaling switch through modular recombination. *Science,* 301, pp.1904–1908.

Dwyer DJ, Kohanski MA, Hayete B, Collins JJ. (2007).Gyrase inhibitors induce an oxidative damage cellular death pathway in Escherichia coli. *Mol Syst Biol.;*3:91.

Dwyer, M.A., et al. (2004).Computational design of a biologically active enzyme. *Science,* 304, pp.1967–1971.

Edwards, J.S., et al. (1999) Metabolic flux balance analysis. In Lee, S.Y. and Papoutsakis, E.T. (Eds.). *Metabolic Engineering,* , New York Marcel Dekker, pp. 13–57.

Elowitz, M.B. and Leibler, S. (2000).A synthetic oscillatory network of transcriptional regulators. *Nature,* 403, pp.335–338.

Endy, D. and Brent, R. (2001)Modelling cellular behaviour. *Nature,* 409, pp.391–395.

Fung, E., et al. (2005).A synthetic gene-metabolic oscillator. *Nature,* 435, pp.118–122.

Gossen, M. & Bujard, H. (1992).Tight control of gene expression in mammalian cells by tetracycline-responsive promoters. Proc. Natl Acad. Sci. USA, 89, pp.5547–5551.

Guet, C. C., Elowitz, M. B., Hsing, W. & Leibler, S. (2002).Combinatorial synthesis of genetic networks. Science, 296, pp.1466–1470.

Howard, P.L., et al. (2003).Redirecting tyrosine kinase signaling to an apoptotic caspase pathway through chimeric adaptor proteins. *Proc. Natl Acad. Sci. USA,*100, 11267–11272.

Hutchison, C. A., III, Peterson, S. N., Gill, S. R., Cline, R. T., (1999).Global transposon mutagenesis and a minimal *mycoplasma* genome. *Science, 286,* pp.2165–2169.

Ji, Y., Zhang, B., von Horn, S.F., Warren, P. *et al.,* (2001).Identification of critical staphylococcal genes using conditional phenotypes generated by antisense RNA. *Science, 293,* pp.2266–2269.

Kobayashi, K., Ehrlich, S. D., Albertini, A., Amati, G. *et al.,* (2003).Essential *Bacillus subtilis* genes. *Proc. Natl. Acad. Sci. USA, 100,* pp.4678–4683.

Kohanski MA, Dwyer DJ, Wierzbowski J, Cottarel G, Collins JJ. (2008).Mistranslation of membrane proteins and two-component system activation trigger antibiotic-mediated cell death. *Cell.;*135. pp.679–90.

Koonin, E. V., (2000).How many genes can make a cell: the minimal-geneset concept. *Annu. Rev. Genomics Hum. Genet., 1,* pp.99–116.

Kramer, B.P. and Fussenegger, M. (2005).Hysteresis in a synthetic mammalian gene network. *Proc. Natl Acad. Sci. USA,* 102, pp.9517–9522.

Kramer, B.P., et al. (2004).BioLogic gates enable logical transcription control in mammalian cells. *Biotechnol. Bioeng,*87, pp.478–484.

Lee, D.Y., et al. (2006).WebCell: a web-based environment for kinetic modeling and dynamic simulation of cellular networks. *Bioinformatics*, 22, pp.1150-1151.

Lemerle, C., et al. (2005).Space as the final frontier in stochastic simulations of biological systems. *FEBS Lett*,579, pp.1789-1794.

Liu, H., Schmidt, J. J., Bachand, G. G., Rizk, S.S. *et al.*, (2003).Control of a biomolecular motor-powered nanodevice with an engineered chemical switch. *Nat. Mater., 1*, pp.173-177.

Looger, L.L., et al. (2003).Computational design of receptor and sensor proteins with novel functions. *Nature*, 423, pp.185-190.

Lu TK, Collins JJ. (2007). Dispersing biofilms with engineered enzymatic bacteriophage. *Proc Natl Acad Sci U S A.*;104. pp.11197-202.

Lu TK, Collins JJ. (2009).Engineered bacteriophage targeting gene networks as adjuvants for antibiotic therapy. *Proc Natl Acad Sci U S A.* 106.pp.4629-34.

Luisi, P. L., Oberholzer, T., Lazcano, A., (2002). The notion of a DNA minimal cell: a general discourse and some guidelines for an experimental approach. *Helvet. Chim. Acta, 85*, pp.1759-1777.

Lutz, R. & Bujard, H. (1997).Independent and tight regulation of transcriptional units in Escherichia coli via the LacR/O, the TetR/O and AraC/I1-I2 regulatory elements. *Nucleic Acids Res.* 25, pp.1203-1210.

Marco, E., et al. (2003).Assessment by molecular dynamics simulations of the structural determinants of DNA-binding specificity for transcription factor Sp1. *J. Mol. Biol*, 328, pp.9-32.

Martin, V.J.J., et al. (2003).Engineering a mevalonate pathway in *Escherichia coli* for production of terpenoids. *Nat. Biotechnol*,21, pp.796-802.

McAdams HH, Shapiro L. (1995). Circuit simulation of genetic networks. *Science.* 269. pp.650-6.

Menzella, H.G., et al. (2005).Combinatorial polyketide biosynthesis by *de novo* design and rearrangement of modular polyketide synthase genes. *Nat. Biotechnol*,23, pp.1171-1176.

Misura, K.M.S., et al. (2006).Physically realistic homology models built with ROSETTA can be more accurate than their templates. *Proc. Natl Acad. Sci. USA*, 103, pp.5361-5366.

Obika, S., et al. (2003).Sequence specific DNA binding of Ets-1 transcription factor: molecular dynamics study on the Ets domain-DNA complexes. *J. Mol. Biol* 331, pp.345-359.

Ozbudak, E.M., et al. (2004).Multistability in the lactose utilization network of *Escherichia coli. Nature*, 427, 737-740.

Park, S. H., Zarrinpar, A. & Lim, W. A. (2003).Rewiring MAP kinase pathways using alternative scaffold assembly mechanisms. Science, 299, pp.1061-1064.

Patil, K., et al. (2005).Evolutionary programming as a platform for in silico metabolic engineering. *BMC Bioinformatics*, 6, pp.308.

Paulsson, J. (2004).Summing up the noise in gene networks. Nature, 427, pp.415-418.

Pedraza, J.M. and van Oudenaarden, (2005).A. Noise propagation in gene networks. *Science*, 307, pp.1965-1969.

Perkel, J. M., (2004).Investigating molecular motors step by step: recent discoveries begin to answer how dyneins, kinesins, and myosins actually work. *Scientist, 18*, pp.19-31.

Pharkya, P., et al. (2004).OptStrain: a computational framework for redesign of microbial production systems. *Genome Res*,14, pp.2367-2376.

Ramachandra M, et al. (2001).Re-engineering adenovirus regulatory pathways to enhance oncolytic specificity and efficacy. *Nat Biotechnol.*;19.pp.1035-41.

Rasmussen, S., Chen, L., Deamer, D., Krakauer, D.C. *et al.*, (2004).Transitions from nonliving to living matter. *Science, 303*, pp.963-965.

Ro, D.K., et al. (2006).Production of the antimalarial drug precursor artemisinic acid in engineered yeast. *Nature*, 440, pp.940–943.

Rosenfeld, N., Elowitz, M. B. & Alon, U. (2002).Negative autoregulation speeds the response times of transcription networks. J. Mol. Biol., 323, pp.785–793.

Schilling, C.H., et al. (2000).Theory for the systemic definition of metabolic pathways and their use in interpreting metabolic function from a pathway-oriented perspective. *J. Theor. Biol*,203, pp.229–248.

Schueler-Furman, O., et al. (2005).Progress in modeling of protein structures and interactions. *Science*, 310, pp.638–642.

Schuster, S., et al. (1999).Detection of elementary flux modes in biochemical networks: a promising tool for pathway analysis and metabolic engineering. *Trends Biotechnol*,17, pp.53–60.

Schymkowitz, J., et al. (2005).The FoldX web server: an online force field. *Nucleic Acids Res*, 33, pp.W382–W388.

Segal, D.J., et al. (1999).Toward controlling gene expression at will: selection and design of zinc finger domains recognizing each of the 5'-GNN-3' DNA target sequences. *Proc. Natl Acad. Sci. USA*, 96, pp.2758–2763.

Sera, T. and Uranga, C. (2002).Rational design of artificial zinc-finger proteins using a nondegenerate recognition code table. *Biochemistry*, 41, pp.7074–7081.

Smith, H. O., Hutchison, C. A. III, Pfannkoch, C., Venter, J.C., (2003).Generating a synthetic genome by whole genome assembly: FX174 bacteriophage from synthetic oligonucleotides. *Proc. Natl. Acad. Sci. USA*, *100*, pp.15440–15445.

Sprinzak, D. and Elowitz, M.B. (2005). Reconstruction of genetic circuits. *Nature*, 438, pp.443–448.

Stavreva DA, et al. (2009). Ultradian hormone stimulation induces glucocorticoid receptor-mediated pulses of gene transcription. *Nat Cell Biol.* 11. pp.1093–102.

Varma, A. and Palsson, B.O. (1994). Stoichiometric flux balance models quantitatively predict growth and metabolic by-product secretion in wild-type *Escherichia coli* W3110. *Appl. Environ. Microbiol*,60, pp.3724–3731.

Vilar, J.M.G., et al. (2003).Modeling network dynamics: the lac operon, a case study. *J. Cell. Biol*, 161, pp.471–476.

Vogelstein, B., Lane, D. & Levine, A. J. (2000). Surfing the p53 network. Nature, 408, pp.307–310.

Wall, M.E., et al. (2003). Design principles for regulator gene expression in a repressible gene circuit. *J. Mol. Biol*,332, pp.861–876.

Weber W, et al. (2008).A synthetic mammalian gene circuit reveals antituberculosis compounds. *Proc Natl Acad Sci U S A.* 105. pp.9994–8.

Weber W, et al. (2007). A synthetic time-delay circuit in mammalian cells and mice. *Proc Natl Acad Sci U S A.* 104. pp.2643–8.

Xiong, W. & Ferrell, J. E. Jr (2003). A positive-feedback-based bistable 'memory module' that governs a cell fate decision. Nature, 426, pp.460–465.

Yasuda, R., Noji, H., Kinosita, K., Yoshida, M., (1998).F1-ATPase is a highly efficient molecular motor that rotates with discrete 120° steps. *Cell*, *93*, pp.1117–1124.

Yokobayashi, Y., et al. (2002).Directed evolution of a genetic circuit. *Proc. Natl Acad. Sci. USA*, 99, pp.16587–16591.

You, L., et al. (2004). Programmed population control by cell–cell communication and regulated killing. *Nature*, 428, pp.868–871.

Zhang, R., Ou, H.-Y., Zhang, C.T., (2004).DEG: a database of essential genes. *Nucleic Acids Res. 32*, pp.D271–272.

11

Comparison of DNA Delivery and Expression Using Frequently Used Delivery Methods

Sara A. Collins[1,2], David Morrissey[1], Simon Rajendran[1], Garrett Casey[1], Martina F. Scallan[2], Patrick T. Harrison[3], Gerald C. O'Sullivan[1] and Mark Tangney[1]

[1]*Cork Cancer Research Centre, Mercy University Hospital and Leslie C. Quick Jnr. Laboratory, University College Cork, Cork,*
[2]*Department of Microbiology, University College Cork, Cork,*
[3]*Department of Physiology and Biosciences Institute, University College Cork, Cork, Ireland*

1. Introduction

Ensuring an appropriate level and duration of expression is essential in achieving an efficient and safe gene therapy. The delivery of the therapeutic gene to target cells has to be sufficiently high to elicit a response, and minimum therapeutic thresholds may vary dramatically between therapeutic strategies. Delivery modalities can be broadly grouped into biological, chemical or physical methods. Biological modalities used in our laboratory include the viral vectors Adeno-Associated Virus and replication incompetent Adenovirus; physical modalities currently being studied include electroporation and sonoporation, while commercially available lipofection reagents are also widely used. Non-viral methods delivering plasmid DNA are argued to present a relatively safe alternative to viral vectors. They are less immunogenic, toxicity is generally very low, plasmid DNA has greater potential for delivery of larger genetic units and large-scale production is relatively easy. Physical methods such as electroporation have been utilised effectively for *in vivo* plasmid delivery to accessible tissues (Collins, C. G. et al. 2006; Mir 2008). Like electroporation, low intensity ultrasound, or sonoporation, can induce transient permeabilisation of the cell membrane and facilitates intracellular delivery of plasmid DNA (Larkin et al. 2008; Rome et al. 2008).

However, all the described methods have associated problems; the transfer of naked DNA is typically an inefficient process, with cell & tissue damage caused by administration of physical and chemical modalities, while adenoviral-mediated gene transfer is complicated by a host immune response to both the vector and transduced target cells (Jooss et al. 1998; Heller et al. 2008). In addition, only transient transgene expression is typically achieved by these approaches. Proposed causes of transient expression include loss of DNA due to cell turnover, immune responses against transfected cells and/or expressed proteins, and inhibition of transcription through host cell methylation of microbial DNA sequences (Prosch et al. 1996; Scheule 2000). AAV vectors have been shown not to elicit strong immune responses in general (Jooss, Ertl et al. 1998) (although immune responses against AAV have been reported following liver administration (Manno et al. 2006)) and the levels of transgene expression following AAV mediated delivery have been shown to increase post delivery in heart, brain and muscle tissues *in vivo* (Lo et al. 1999; Vassalli et al. 2003; Collins, S. A. et al. 2008; Collins, S. A. et al. 2010). However, transduction is receptor dependant and rAAV has a size limit for DNA carrying capacity. Also, for therapeutic purposes, immediate gene expression is generally desirable. The optimal length of time for gene expression varies between therapeutic strategy and disease. For cancer gene therapy for example, short-lived transgene expression for cytokine production may be sufficient for immune sensitisation and containment of tumours (Collins, C. G., Tangney et al. 2006), while sustained secretion of therapeutic molecules is preferable with anti-angiogenic therapies (Malecki et al. 2005; Buhles et al. 2009).

The optimal gene delivery method for a given therapy will be dependant on tissue location, and type, as well as therapeutic strategy. While certain studies have been reported comparing the efficiencies from different vectors (Wang, A. Y. et al. 2004; Kealy et al. 2009), given the paucity of information regards direct comparisons between various delivery techniques, especially in the cancer setting, this study assesses the level and duration of reporter gene expression within target murine tissues when delivered by a range of commonly used gene delivery techniques; electroporation, sonoporation, lipofection, Adenovirus and Adeno-Associated Virus.

2 Materials and methods

2.1 DNA constructs

pCMV-luc plasmid, which expresses firefly luciferase under the transcriptional control of the cytomegalovirus (CMV) promoter, was purchased from Promega (Wisconsin, USA). pCMV-LacZ plasmid, which expresses β-Galactosidase under the transcriptional control of the CMV promoter, was purchased from Plasmid Factory (Bielefeld, Germany). Plasmid concentration was determined using the Nanodrop spectrophotometer (ND-1000 Spectrophotometer, Labtech Int, East Sussex, UK). Replication incompetent recombinant Adenovirus 5 particles encoding the luciferase gene under the transcriptional control of the CMV promoter were a kind gift from Prof. Andrew Baker, University of Glasgow, they were generated and titrated as described previously (Waddington et al. 2008). Replication incompetent Adenovirus 5 particles encoding the β-galactosidase gene under the transcriptional control of the CMV promoter were a kind gift from the Regenerative Medicine Institute, NUI Galway, they were generated and titrated as described previously (Sharif et al. 2006). An AAV plasmid expressing firefly luciferase under the transcriptional control of the cytomegalovirus (CMV) promoter was constructed by first excising the firefly *luciferase* gene from pGL3 (Promega Medical Supply Company, Dublin, Ireland) using Nco1 and Xba1, and cloning the Klenow enzyme treated fragment into the EcoRI and Xba1 sites of pAAV-MCS plasmid (Stratagene, Agilent, Dublin) downstream of the CMV promoter. Inserts were confirmed by sequencing (MWG Biotech) and restriction enzyme analysis. This plasmid and the commercially available pAAVLacZ (Stratagene) were used to generate rAAV using the AAV Helper-Free System (Stratagene, Agilent, Dublin). The rAAV were purified using the Virakit AAV Purification Kit (Virapur, San Diego, USA) per manufacturer's instructions. Purified recombinant AAV-2 preparations were titrated using real time PCR. The samples were first pre-treated with DNase. For DNase digestion, 1 μl of the viral sample was incubated with 350 Unit of DNase in a final volume of 10 μl at 37 °C for 30 min followed by inactivation at 65 °C for 10 min. 1 μl of Proteinase K (10mg/ml) was added to each sample and it was incubated at 50 °C for 60 min followed by inactivation at 95 °C for 20 min. PCR was performed using the Lightcycler FastStart DNA Master Sybr Green system (Roche Molecular Biochemicals, Mannheim, Germany). PCR was carried out in a final volume of 20 µl using 0.5 µl of each primer (0.25 µM), 3 mM MgCl2 and 2 µl of the template. The PCR was performed in a lightcycler (Roche) with a 10 min pre-incubation at 95 °C followed by 40 cycles of 15 s at 95 °C, 4 s at 56 °C, 4 s at 72 °C. PCR products were subjected to melting curve analysis using the light cycler system to exclude the amplification of unspecific products. The PCR products were analysed by conventional agarose gel electrophoresis. Primers were synthesized by MWG Biotech, Germany. The following primers were used to detect the CMV promoter sequence, forward: 5′ aaatgggcggtaggcgtgta 3′, reverse: 5′ gatcggtcccggtgtcttct 3′. A fragment of length 124 bp is expected using the primers.

2.2 Cell lines and tissue culture

Murine JBS fibrosarcoma tumour cells (Collins, C. G., Tangney et al. 2006) and murine CT26 colonic adenocarcinoma cells (obtained from ATCC) were maintained in culture at 37 °C in a humidified atmosphere of 5 % CO2, in Dulbecco's Modified Essential Medium (GIBCO, Invitrogen Corp., Paisley, Scotland) supplemented with 10 % iron-supplemented donor calf serum (Sigma Aldrich Ireland, Ireland), 300 µg/ml L-glutamine, and 10 mM HEPES (1-Piperazineethane sulfonic acid, 4-(2-hydroxyethyl) monosodium salt), (Sigma Aldrich Ireland, Ireland) pH 7.4. The murine MGC8 gastric carcinoma cell line was kindly provided by Dr. Robert Kammerer, Ludwig-Maximilians-University, Germany (Nockel et al. 2006), and was maintained in RPMI (Roswell Park Memorial Institute- Gibco) medium supplemented with 10 % iron-supplemented donor calf serum (Sigma Aldrich Ireland, Ireland) and 1mM sodium pyruvate (Sigma Aldrich Ireland, Ireland). Cell densities were determined by visual count using a haemocytometer. Cells were at 80 % confluency on the day of transduction *in vitro*. Cell viability was confirmed by Trypan Blue Dye Exclusion (Sigma Aldrich Ireland, Ireland) to be > 95 % for tumour inoculation.

2.3 *In vitro* gene delivery

The efficacies of the different delivery methods *in vitro* were determined using the JBS, CT26 and MGC8 cell lines. Transductions were carried out accordingly to manufacturers' protocols or under optimal conditions where appropriate. Electroporation: 10 µg pCMV-Luc or pCMV-LacZ DNA was added to 1 X 10^6 cells in 100 µl ZAP buffer (250 mM sucrose, 10 mM K_2HPO_4 1 mM $MgCl_2$ ph 7.4). Electroporations were carried out in a 1.0 mm cuvette and the conditions used were 8 X 0.1 ms pulses of 140 V with a 0.1 sec pulse interval. Cells were incubated at room temperature for 15 min. Following the addition of growth medium the treated cells were seeded into a tissue culture dish and incubated for 24 h at 37 °C, 5 % CO_2. Ultrasound: 1 X 10^6 cells were seeded in a 6-well tissue culture dish 3 h prior to treatment. Prior to US application, the medium was replaced with serum free medium and 10 µg of the pCMV-Luc or pCMV-LacZ plasmid was added. The US conditions used were 1.0 W/cm^2, 20 % duty cycle, 2 min. Cells were incubated for 15 min before replacing serum free medium with supplemented medium and cells incubated for 24 h at 37 °C 5 % CO_2. Lipofectamine2000: Cells were seeded in a 12-well plate in complete medium 24 h before transfection. On the day of transfection cells were 80 % confluent. Prior to transfection, the cells were rinsed and incubated in serum free medium. 1.6 µg pCMV-Luc or pCMV-LacZ DNA was complexed to Lipofectamine2000 (Invitrogen, Biosciences Ltd, Dublin, Ireland), according to manufacturer's instructions and incubated with cells for 4 h. Serum free medium was then replaced with complete medium and cells incubated for 24 h 37 °C, 5% CO_2. AAV: Growth medium was removed and replaced with 0.5 ml AAV permissive growth medium (DMEM, 0.5 mM Tyrphostin (Calbiochem, Merck, UK; (Mah et al. 1998)) per well. The plates were incubated for 2 h at 37 °C, 5 % CO_2. Permissive medium was subsequently removed and cells washed twice with 0.5 ml/well DMEM. 5 X 10^8 genome copies (GC) of AAVCMVLuc or 3.5 X 10^{10} GC of AAVCMVLacZ in a 0.5 ml volume of transduction medium (DMEM, 2 % FBS) was added to individual wells containing the permissive cells. The plates were incubated for 2 h at 37 °C, 5 % CO_2 with gentle rocking at 30 min intervals during the incubation. 0.5 ml post infection medium (DMEM, 18 % FBS) was added to each well and incubated at 37 °C, 5 % CO_2 for a further 24 h. Ad: 1.5 X 10^9 viral particles (VP) of AdCMVLuc or 4.5 X 10^8 VP of AdCMVLacZ in 0.5 ml transduction medium (DMEM, 2 % FBS) was added to individual wells of 6-well plates containing the cells. Plates were incubated for 2 h at 37 °C, 5 % CO_2 with gentle rocking at 30 min. 0.5 ml post infection medium (DMEM, 18 % FBS) was added to each well and incubated at 37 °C, 5 % CO_2 for a further 24 h.

2.4 *In vitro* luciferase assay

Treated cells were analysed for luciferase activity using the Luciferase Assay System (Promega MSC, Dublin) 24 hr post transfection. Treated cells were counted and resuspended to 10^4 cells in 50 µl DMEM medium. 50 µl 1X lysis buffer was added to each of the samples and incubated for 5 min at room temperature. 100 µl Luciferase assay reagent was then added to each sample and the luminescence was measured with a Junior LB 9509 luminometer (Berthold Technology, Promega MSC, Dublin).

2.5 *In vitro* β-galactosidase assay

Treated cells were analysed for β-Galactosidase activity using the Roche β-Gal Staining set (Roche Diagnostics GmbH, Penzberg, Germany) as per the manufacturer's protocol. Briefly, cells were washed with PBS, and incubated in fixative (2% formaldehyde, 0.2 % gluteraldehyde in PBS) for 15 min. Cells were incubated in staining solution o/n at 37 °C. Cells were analysed in PBS under a light microscope and transfection efficiency (% stained cells) was calculated from 10 random viewing fields per well.

2.6 DNA/RNA extraction

Transfections were carried out as previously outlined with the CMVLacZ constructs. At 24 hr post transfection, cells were harvested for simultaneous DNA/RNA extraction using the Qiagen Allprep DNA/RNA Kit (Qiagen Crawley, West Sussex). Briefly, treated cells were counted and resuspended in 350 µl of Buffer RLT containing β-mercaptoethanol and vortexed. The DNA and RNA extraction was carried out as per the manufacturer's protocol. 5 µg RNA was treated with DNase 1 (DNAfree, Ambion) to remove contaminating genomic DNA. cDNA synthesis was carried out using 500 ng of the DNase treated RNA with the Qiagen Omniscript RT kit, per manufacturer's instructions. The resulting cDNA was brought to a 50 µl volume using nuclease free water.

2.7 Quantitative real-time PCR

PCR was performed using the Lightcycler FastStart DNA Master Sybr Green system (Roche). PCR was carried out in a final volume of 20 µl using 0.5 µl of each primer (0.25 µM),

3 mM $MgCl_2$. PCR was performed in a lightcycler (Roche) with a 15 min pre-incubation at 95 °C followed by 40 cycles of 15 s at 95 °C, 5 s at 60 °C, 5 s at 72 °C. PCR products were subjected to melting curve analysis using the light cycler system to exclude the amplification of unspecific products. PCR products were analysed by conventional agarose gel electrophoresis. Primers were synthesized by MWG Biotech. The following primers were used to detect the *LacZ* sequence, forward: 5' GCGTGGATGAAGACCAGC 3' and reverse: 5' CGAAGCCGCCCTGTAAAC 3'. A standard curve was generated using the pCMV-LacZ plasmid DNA, ranging from 5 X 10^3 to 5 X 10^7 plasmid copies. 50 ng of DNA or 5 µl of cDNA reaction from each delivery method was used for the real time PCR detection of LacZ.

2.8 Animals and tumour induction

All murine experimentation was approved by the University College Cork Animal Ethics Committee. Mice were obtained from Harlan Laboratories (Oxfordshire, England). They were kept at a constant room temperature (22 °C) with a natural day/night light cycle in a conventional animal colony. Standard laboratory food and water were provided *ad libitum*. Before experiments, the mice were afforded an adaptation period of at least 14 days. Female Balb/C mice in good condition, without fungal or other infections, weighing 16–22 g and of 6–8 weeks of age, were included in experiments. For routine tumour induction, 2 × 10^6 JBS cells suspended in 200 µl of serum free DMEM were injected subcutaneously into the flank.

2.9 *In vivo* gene delivery

Mice were randomly divided into experimental groups and subjected to specific experimental protocols. For tumour experiments, mice were treated at a tumour volume of approximately 100 mm^3 in volume (5-7 mm major diameter). For liver transfection, a 1 cm subcostal incision was made over the liver and the peritoneum opened. The proximal portion of the liver was exposed and DNA administered as described below. The wound was closed in two layers, peritoneal and skin, using 4/0 prolene sutures (Promed, Killorglin, Ireland). For muscle experiments, a single intramuscular injection was carried out into the right or left quadriceps muscle of the animal. Mice were anaesthetized during all treatments by intraperitoneal (IP) administration of 200 µg xylazine and 2 mg ketamine.

For plasmid delivery by electroporation, a custom-designed applicator with 2 needles 4 mm apart was used, with both needles placed central to the tissue. Tissue was injected between electrode needles with plasmid DNA in sterile injectable saline in an injection volume of 50 µl. Concentration of plasmid was adjusted to administer 4 x 10^{12} gene copy numbers. After 80 seconds, square-wave pulses (1200 V/cm 100 µsec x 1 and 120 V/cm 20 msec, 8 pulses) were administered in sequence using a custom designed pulse generator (Cliniporator (IGEA, Carpi, Italy).

For plasmid delivery by ultrasound, tissue was injected with plasmid DNA as above. The ultrasound probe was then applied to the tissue and ultrasonic waves delivered at 1.0 W/cm^2, 20 % duty cycle for 5 min (Sonoporator, Sonidel, Dublin, Ireland).

For plasmid delivery using Lipofection, tissue was injected with plasmid DNA/Lipofectamine 2000 complex in an injection volume of 100 µl. Concentration of plasmid was adjusted to administer 4 x 10^{12} gene copies.

Viral vector particles were administered by direct intratumoural, intramuscular or intra-hepatic injection in a volume of 50 µl. 2 X 10^8 - 2 X 10^9 GC of replication incompetent recombinant AAV2 particles, or 1 x 10^9 VP of replication incompetent recombinant Adenovirus 5 particles were used per administration.

2.10 Whole body luciferase imaging

In vivo luciferase activity from tissues was analysed at set time points post-transfection as follows: 80 µl of 30 mg/ml firefly luciferin (Biosynth, Basil, Switzerland) was injected IP (for muscle and liver experiments) and/or intratumourally. Mice were anaesthetised as before. Ten minutes post-luciferin injection, live anaesthetised mice were imaged for 3 min at high sensitivity using an intensified CCD camera (IVIS Imaging System, Xenogen, UK). The exposure conditions were maintained at identical levels so that all measurements would be comparable. Data analysis was carried out on the Living Image 2.5 software package (Xenogen, UK). Luminescence levels were calculated using standardised regions of interest (ROIs) for all three anatomical areas. Actual levels were obtained by subtracting the corresponding ROI of an untransfected mouse to account for background luminescence. For comparison between vectors, luminescence was represented as p/sec/cm^2/sr/gene copy.

2.11 Statistical analysis

The primary outcome variable of the statistical analyses was luminescence per cell per gene copy administered in each cell line or luminescence per gene copy administered in each organ measured at each time point. The principal explanatory variables were the delivery modalites used. *In vivo* luminescence was analysed as continuous. At specified time points, a two-sampled t-test was used to compare mean luminescence per gene copy administered for each delivery modality. Microsoft Excel 11.0 (Microsoft) and GraphPad Prism Version 4.0 (GraphPad Prism Software Inc, San Diego, CA, USA) were used to manage and analyze data. Statistical significance was defined at the standard 5 % level.

3. Results

3.1 Comparison of transgene expression levels *in vitro*

Reporter gene expression was analysed following *in vitro* delivery of CMV firefly luciferase gene cassette by the various delivery systems to JBS fibrosarcoma cells. The optimal protocol for each delivery method was utilised in all *in vitro* experiments. Data were standardised by reporting results for each system as expression/cell at time of administration/gene copy administered. The results displayed in Figure 1a correspond to expression from viable cells at time of assay (24 h post-delivery) and cell cytotoxicity relating to transfection is not taken into account. Cell death resulted in 99.8 % and 89 % cells exposed to US and EP respectively, while no significant cell death was observed in the course of Ad, AAV or Lipofectamine transfections (data not shown). Reproducible levels of luciferase expression per cell per gene copy resulted from the various methods with expression from AAV achieving the highest levels (AAV > Ad > Lipo > EP > US).

In order to assess consistency across cell lines, delivery to a range of tumour cell models was examined. Efficiencies arising from Lipofectamine, Ad and AAV delivery to JBS was compared with those from CT26 and MGC8 (Nockel, van den Engel et al. 2006). Cancer cell type-specificity was clearly observed for each vector (Figure 1b). AAV also achieved the highest levels of expression in CT26 cells as with JBS cells. However, AAV failed to transduce MGC8 cells. There were also considerable relative differences observed in Lipofectamine transfected cells ($p < 0.05$), while Ad delivery resulted in expression in all cell lines, albeit with statistically significant variation between each ($p < 0.05$).

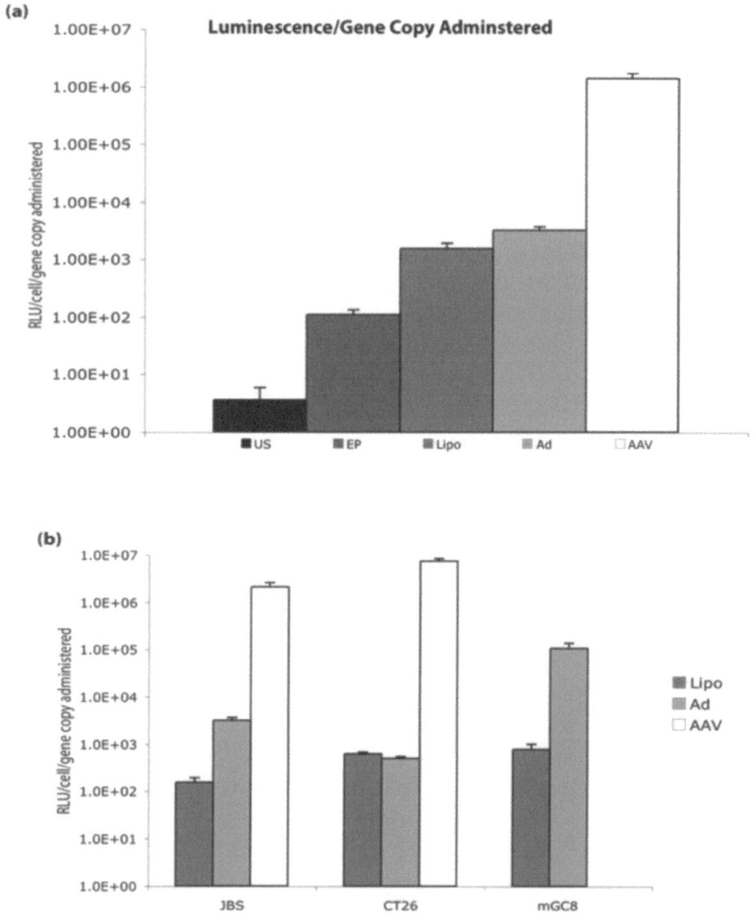

Fig. 1. *In vitro* transfection/transduction (a) Comparison of transgene expression in JBS cells *in vitro* pCMV-Luc was delivered to JBS cells *in vitro* using US, EP or Lipofection, while the corresponding CMVLuc cassette was delivered via Ad (AdCMVLuc) or AAV2 particles (AAVCMVLuc). Luciferase expression was assayed 24 h post-delivery and expressed as relative light units (RLU) per cell per gene copy. Data represent the mean ± S.E. of triplicate values. Intra-modality differences were statistically different in all cases ($p \leq 0.02$). (b) Cell line specificity in transfection/transduction Average luminescence arising from Lipo, Ad and AAV delivery to JBS, CT26 and mGC8 are shown. There was significant variation between cell line efficiencies for each vector (Ad $p< 0.05$; Lipo $p< 0.05$; AAV $p < 0.0001$). AAV failed to transduce MGC8 cells. Data represent the mean ± S.E. of triplicate values.

3.2 Analysis of DNA delivery and transcription efficiencies *in vitro*

The CMV-*LacZ* gene cassette was delivered to JBS cells *in vitro* using each of the delivery methods. To determine percentages of cells transfected/transduced by each method, treated cells were fixed 24 h post delivery and stained for β-Galactosidase activity. The number of positive cells was expressed as a percentage of the total number of cells (Figure 2a). Viral and chemical methods of delivery resulted in significantly higher proportions of reporter gene expressing cells in comparison with the physical methods (ultrasound and electroporation) ($p < 0.02$), possibly reflecting the high cell death rates associated with these systems. Again, AAV resulted in the highest number of transduced cells in comparison with other methods.

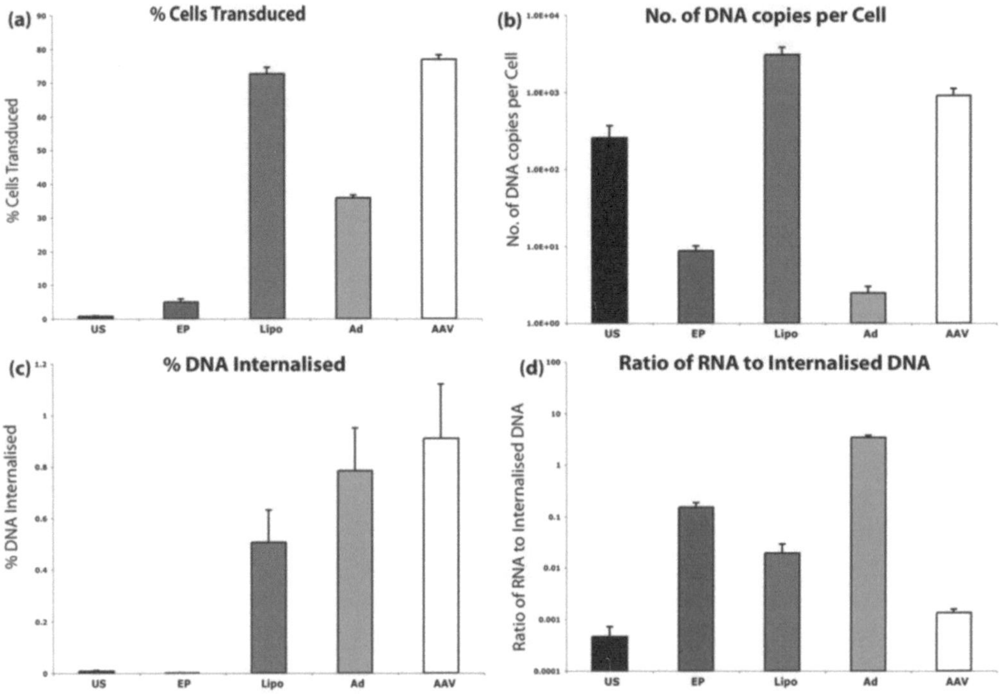

Fig. 2. *In vitro* DNA delivery and transcription efficiencies (a) Percentage of transgene-expressing cells pCMV-LacZ was delivered to JBS cells *in vitro* using US, EP or Lipo, while the corresponding CMVLacZ cassette was delivered via Ad (AdCMVLacZ) or AAV2 particles (AAVCMVLacZ). β-Galactosidase expression was assayed 24 h post-delivery and expressed as % cells transfected/transduced. (b) Number of transgene copies per cell The number of transgene copies in total DNA from a known number of cells was quantified using real time PCR 24 h post-delivery and expressed as the number of transgene copies per cell. (c) Efficiency of DNA delivery to cells The number of transgene copies in total DNA was quantified using real time PCR and was expressed as a percentage of the total number of copies administered for each delivery method. (d) Transcription Efficiency Quantitative real time PCR was used to determine the number of copies of transgene mRNA 24 h post-delivery. This was expressed as a percentage of the number of internalised DNA copies. For (a-d) data represent the mean ± S.E. of triplicate values.

In order to assess and compare DNA entry efficiency and subsequent transcription efficiencies for each delivery method, LacZ reporter gene DNA and mRNA was quantified by PCR. Prior to DNA/RNA extraction at 24 h post delivery, the number of cells was determined using trypan blue exclusion. The total number of LacZ DNA copies was expressed per cell at 24 h (Figure 2b). The highest number of DNA copies per cell was observed with Lipo, followed by AAV, which were both significantly higher than US, EP and Ad methods ($p<0.02$). Lipofection delivery does not involve physical generation of pores required by the other plasmid methods for delivery, nor is it dependent on the presence of cell surface receptors (e.g. CAR), which may be poorly expressed in certain cancers, which may in turn explain the poor Ad uptake by JBS cells observed here. The efficiency of DNA entry to cells was also calculated by comparing the number of transgene copies in extracted DNA and expressing it as a percentage of the number of transgene copies initially administered (Figure 2c). Results correlated with the above % cell transfection data, with viral and chemical methods displaying the highest efficiencies of gene delivery to cells in comparison with the physical modalities ($p<0.02$). There was no significant difference between AAV, Ad and Lipo methods ($p>0.05$).

Transcription efficiency was determined using qPCR analyses on LacZ DNA and mRNA (Figure 2d). The number of copies of transgene mRNA 24 h post-delivery was expressed as a percentage of the number of internalised DNA copies. Ad resulted in significantly higher ratio of mRNA:DNA compared with all other delivery methods ($p<0.01$). There was no significant difference in transcription efficiencies between the remaining delivery methods. With US and Lipo, while these methods may efficiently mediate delivery of plasmid DNA to the cytoplasm, subsequent trafficking to the nucleus and transgene transcription is not ensured. For AAV, the low level observed can be attributed to the rate limiting step associated with AAV mediated expression, involving synthesis of double stranded DNA from the single stranded genome prior to transcription (Ferrari et al. 1996). EP transcription efficiency was also significantly higher than US, AAV and Lipo ($p<0.02$). The combination of high and low voltage pulses used for electroporation here is believed to create transient pores in both the cell and nuclear membranes enhancing DNA entry and subsequent nuclear localisation (Gothelf & Gehl ; Chang 1992).

3.3 Duration of transgene expression in tumour, liver and skeletal muscle *in vivo*

In vivo luciferase expression was examined from murine liver, quadriceps muscles and subcutaneous JBS tumour (following consistent results with the JBS cell line *in vitro*) using IVIS whole body imaging at various time-points up to 250 days post delivery with Ad, AAV or plasmid. Vector related luminescence expressed as a percentage of maximum expression observed for that vector is graphed in Figure 3. Background thresholds for each vector varied as a result of expressing per gene copy or as a percentage of maximum, and while imaging continued for the full duration of experiments, values below background are not shown. All plasmid methods (Lipo, US and EP) displayed similar time-points of maximal luminescence within the first month (data not shown), and only EP is shown as representative for plasmid.

Luminescence from plasmid and Ad reduced dramatically within 48 h post delivery to tumour and liver (Figure 3), and both plasmid and Ad reduced to background levels from day 7 in tumour, and day 14 (EP) or day 21 (Ad) in liver. Day 5 was the earliest practical time point for imaging of AAV for reasons including safety guidelines for animal experimentation with this vector. AAV-related expression also decreased in tumour, to background levels by day 16-post administration. However, a different pattern of transgene expression was observed for AAV in liver and quadriceps muscle, with an overall increase in luminescence over time. When muscle related expression was examined with plasmid, prolonged sustained luminescence was observed, with equivalent expression seen at day 370 and day 18 post electroporation (data not shown). However, unlike plasmid, complete loss of Ad mediated luciferase activity was observed when muscle was examined, with Ad expression increasing up to day 7, before reducing to background levels by day 21.

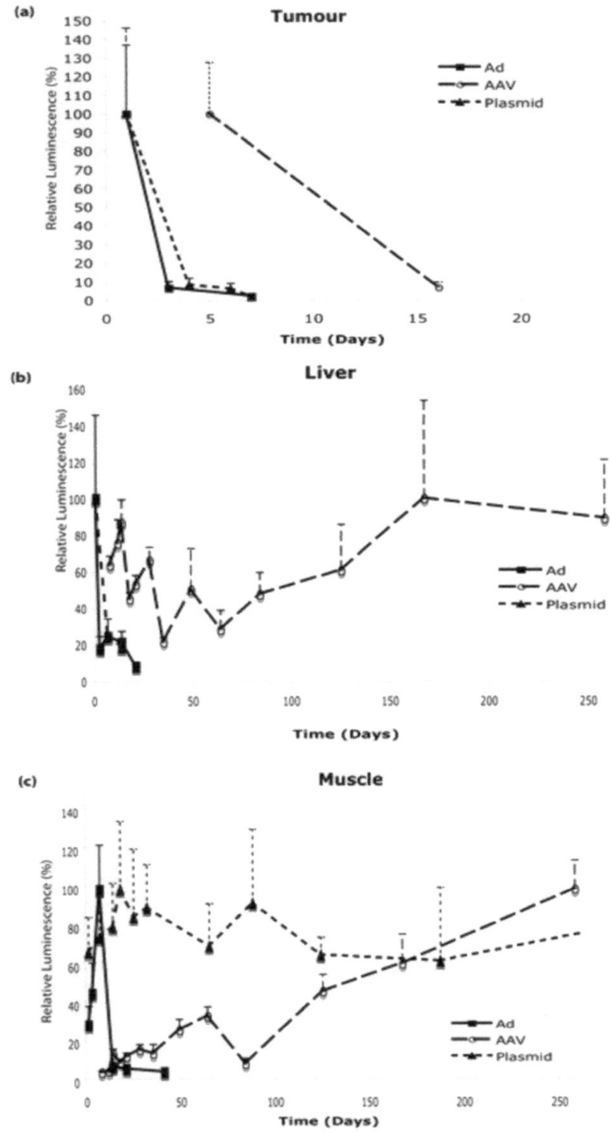

Fig. 3. Vector specific kinetics of transgene expression in tumour, liver and muscle *In vivo* luciferase expression from (a) tumour, (b) liver and (c) muscle was assessed using live whole body imaging (IVIS) at various time-points up to 250 days post delivery (n ≥ 3). Relative average luminescence as a percentage of maximum expression for each vector is shown. Values below appropriate background for each vector are not shown. Data represent the mean ± S.E.

3.4 Comparisons between transgene expression levels in tumour, liver and skeletal muscle *in vivo*

To directly compare *in vivo* expression levels between vectors, the time-point of maximum luminescence in a given tissue within one month post gene delivery was used. Luminescence/gene copy in JBS tumour, liver and quadriceps muscles from each vector at the appropriate time-point is displayed in Figure 4.

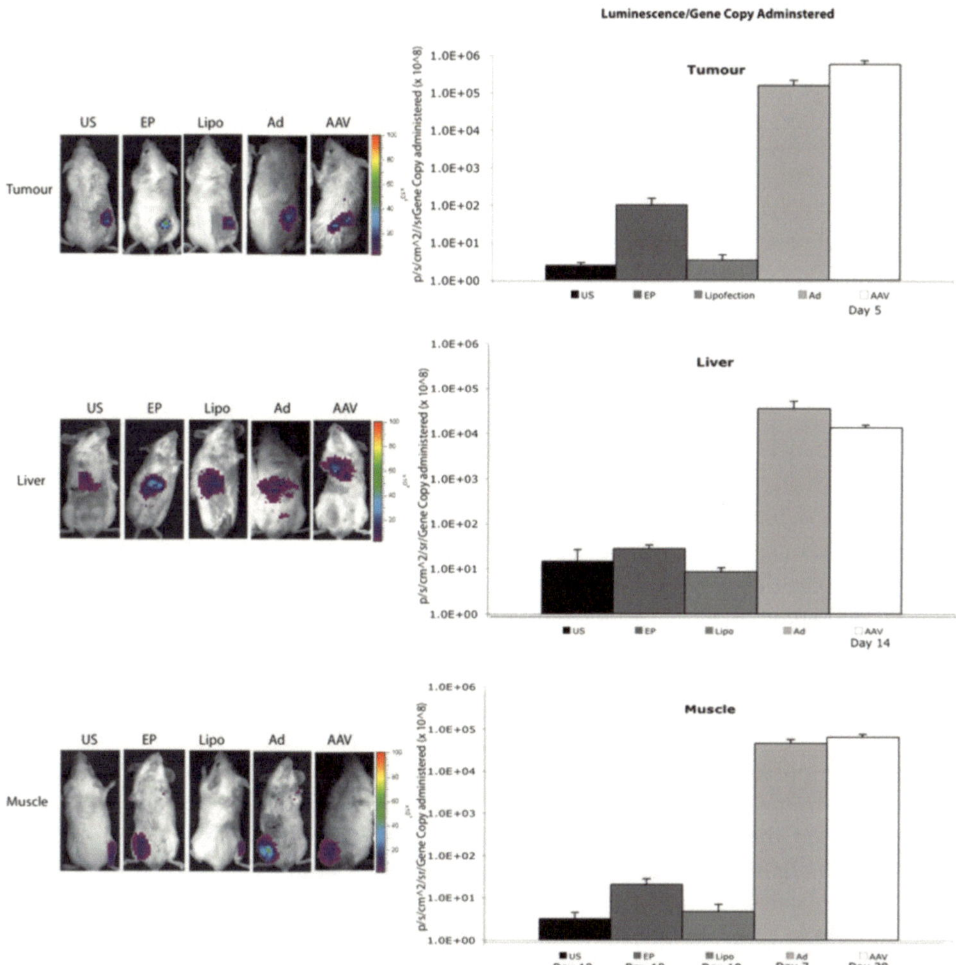

Fig. 4. *In vivo* transfection efficiency Vector constructs were examined *in vivo* in murine subcutaneous JBS tumour, liver and quadriceps muscle (n ≥ 3). Luciferase expression *in vivo* was assessed using IVIS whole body imaging, and maximum gene expression level achieved within 1 month post administration is reported in all cases, corresponding to 24 h unless otherwise stated. Resulting average luminescence per gene copy is shown. Data represent the mean ± S.E.

It can be seen that the intra-modality pattern of expression differed from that observed *in vitro*, with AAV and Ad resulting in the highest expression in all tissues *in vivo*, while EP provided the highest non-viral mediated expression. Significant intra-tissue variation in luciferase activity was observed for all vectors (Figure 5). Tumour produced the highest luminescence for EP and both viral vectors, while liver produced highest expression from US and Lipo. The least consistent results (largest standard error of the mean) were observed with the mechanical methods US and EP. It should be noted that firefly luciferase associated luminescence is dependent on the availability of luciferin substrate and oxygen to cells, which may vary between tissues. However, excess substrate was administered in all experiments in an attempt to achieve saturation levels, and the finding that each vector displayed unique intra-tissue patterns of expression supports the validity of the findings.

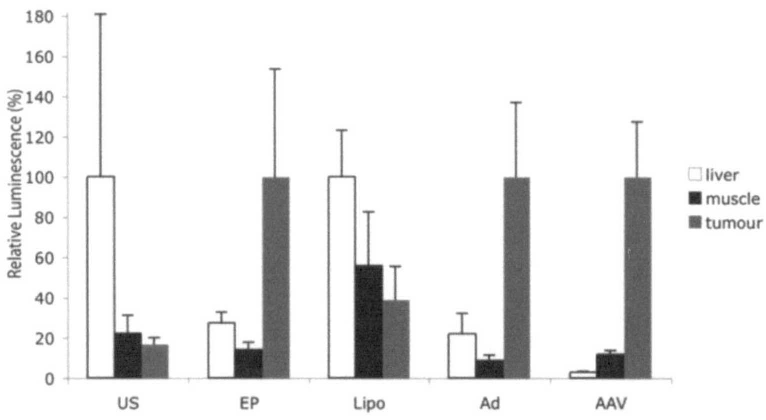

Fig. 5. Intra-tissue variations in reporter gene expression *In vivo* luminescence from liver, muscle or JBS tumour is represented according to the method of gene delivery. Relative average luminescence as a percentage of maximum expression (time-points as per figure 3) for each vector is shown. Data represent the mean ± S.E (n ≥ 3).

4. Discussion

The method employed to deliver genes of interest is the primary parameter related to expression in a target tissue, and consequently has important therapeutic implications. Our findings delineate the relative efficiencies of five well-described delivery modalities, and highlight target organ/tissue specific variations in transfection capability. Furthermore the kinetics of gene expression arising from each modality were compared.

In order for data to be generated *in vitro*, it was necessary to employ different parameters for various delivery methods. Different quantities of DNA and cell numbers were used, and tyrphostin was added to medium to aid in *in vitro* AAV transduction. Attempts to standardise these experimental parameters produced no reportable data, as a result of total cell killing and/or lack of transfection. Numerical results were instead standardised post experimentation, and all *in vitro* results were reported as expression/administered cell/gene copy administered. We standardized the quantity of vector employed in each case by utilising total vector copy numbers for all vectors, as per Materials and Methods. As such, both viable and non-viable gene constructs are factored in results, and take into account non-infectious viral particles and naked plasmid DNA, which does not successfully enter cells (e.g. due to degradation by extracellular nucleases). Determination and use of productive viral vector particle numbers increases resulting efficiency rates of DNA cell entry (data not shown).

Given the mechanism of AAV single-stranded DNA virus transduction of cells, it is likely that at the time of measurement of AAV-transduced cells *in vitro* (24 h), second strand synthesis was not completed and protein production had yet to reach maximum levels. The majority of cells were killed by the physical methods *in vitro*, most likely due to heat and physical stresses. Given the distance from clinical reality of the *in vivo* tissue situation, and the known cytotoxic effects of the non-viral modalities examined here, *in vitro* experiments do not accurately represent the more cell protective environment of tissue, since three-dimensional structural architecture, blood flow etc. are not represented. Furthermore, *in vivo* targets are not homogenous populations, particularly in the case of tumours, and gene expression observed from tumours most likely does not represent expression solely from tumour cells, as various stromal and phagocytic cells may also take up DNA.

Uniform conditions were used for all tissues in this study. In the absence of titrations to determine the precise optimal parameters for each method for each target cell or tissue, we cannot rule out that the relative differences reported between vectors *in vitro* may change following targeted optimisation for each vector.

Considerable variation in transgene expression was observed between modalities and cell types. Lipofectamine consistently transfected all cell types examined *in vitro*. It does not have the same cell killing effects associated with EP and US nor is it dependent on cell surface receptors for internalisation like the viral methods. Ad transduced all cell types examined with varying degrees of efficiency, correlating with the ubiquitous expression of the CAR receptor at different levels in cells (Lyons et al. 2006). The finding that AAV2 was unable to transduce all cancer cell types examined, is consistent with a lack of expression of its primary receptor, heparin sulfate proteoglycans (HSPG), which may be absent or deleted on certain tumour types (Summerford & Samulski 1998), and/or CD9, which can mediate AAV-2 infection in certain cancer cells in the absence of HSPG (Kurzeder et al., 2007). The HSPG and CD9 status of the tumour cell lines used in this study is unknown. Several serotypes of AAV exist and corresponding tissue tropism varies considerably (Wu et al. 2006). The AAV2 serotype examined here is known to transduce a wide range of tissue types, including liver and muscle, albeit at a lower efficiency than other serotypes more specific for individual cell types. Therefore, use of an AAV serotype with a high tropism for the target tissue would be expected to produce efficiencies higher than reported here for AAV, in addition to providing a level of selectivity in terms of vector safety. "Cross-packaging" strategies to generate pseudotyped AAV vectors, where AAV2 vector genome is packaged together with capsid proteins of a different serotype, have been shown to improve target specificity and efficiency (Harding et al. 2006; Nathwani et al. 2008).

In vitro analyses at 24 h	**% Cell Transfection**	**DNA Delivery**	**Copy Number**	**Transcription Efficiency**	**Net Expression**
AAV	High	High	High	Low *	High
US	Low	Low	Medium	Low	Low
EP	Low	Low	Low	Medium	Medium
Lipo	High	Medium	High	Low/Medium	Medium
Ad	Medium	High	Low	High	Medium/High

* As measured at 24 h

Table 1. Relative efficiencies of DNA delivery and subsequent expression *in vitro*.

Efficient reporter gene expression requires cell and nuclear DNA molecule entry, followed by transcription, translation and enzymatic activity on substrate. We analysed various steps for each delivery modality *in vitro*. Table 1 highlights the combined findings from *in vitro* analyses of DNA delivery, transcription and expression efficiencies. It is evident from these studies that while cell entry is an obvious prerequisite, the efficiency of nuclear localisation and transcription may be the major rate limiting step for all methods, as exemplified by the high expression observed with viruses examined here, both capable of mediating their entry to the nucleus. With plasmids, poor nuclear uptake through the restrictive nuclear membrane pore limits expression even when high copy numbers are delivered to the cytosol (e.g. lipofection). The inclusion of nuclear localisation sequences to plasmid DNA has been shown to improve plasmid transgene expression (Manam et al. 2000). Regional variation in cell mitotic rates may also affect plasmid nuclear uptake and subsequent gene expression *in vivo*, particularly in tumours. Reporter gene associated luminescence was utilised *in vivo* as a measure of transfection efficiency of these vectors. Since multiple factors influence transgene expression *in vivo*, differences in luminescence observed between tissues may reflect variations in cell turnover, CMV promoter activity or local immune activity, in addition to the above described *in vitro* factors.

There were significant inter-vector and inter-tissue variations in the times at which highest luminescence values were observed *in vivo*. Since maximum luciferase expression levels afforded by AAV were not observed for many months post transduction of muscle and liver, reporter gene expression levels observed for each modality at times of maximal expression within the first month post administration were used to provide indicative expression levels for comparison purposes here. Firefly luciferase protein has previously been shown to have a short half-life *in vivo*, in the region of 1 - 4 hours, and any luminescence detected in our experiments was due to recently transcribed gene (Baggett et al. 2004). Both Ad and plasmid-based gene delivery systems have previously been shown to provide short-term gene expression in several tissues (Jooss, Ertl et al. 1998; Wang, L. et al. 2005). Increasing expression profiles for AAV2 have previously been reported (Lo, Qu et al. 1999; Vassalli, Bueler et al. 2003), and sustained AAV expression is proposed to be mediated by episomal persistence of the vector (Flotte et al. 1994). Since all the vector systems examined in this study are non-integrating, loss of transgene with cell division may be the major reason for reductions in expression loss in transfected/transduced cells, especially in rapidly growing tumours. Inhibition of transcription through host cell methylation of viral promoter DNA sequences can also lead to transient expression (Di Ianni et al. 1999; Al-Dosari et al. 2006). Given that luciferase transcription from all constructs examined in this study relied upon the CMV promoter, such activity is likely to have been involved with all vectors examined in tumour and liver. While Ad delivered transgene expression levels in skeletal muscle have been demonstrated to reduce as a result of immune clearance of transfected cells (Jooss, Ertl et al. 1998), muscle related expression has been shown to increase over time with both AAV and plasmid vectors, albeit in a gene product dependent manner, with certain proteins eliciting silencing immune responses (Mir et al. 1999; Yuasa et al. 2002). Luciferase protein has low immunogenicity, and immune responses are believed not to occur in mice (Davis et al. 1997).

While the patterns of luciferase expression from Ad and plasmid were similar in tumour and liver, this was not the case for muscle. It has previously been demonstrated with Ad gene delivery to muscle, that associated Ad transduction of Dendritic Cells resulted in presentation of transgene as antigen and subsequent T cell elimination of transgene expressing muscle cells (Jooss, Ertl et al. 1998). When we examined Ad mediated expression in quadriceps of athymic mice, no reduction was evident for up to 2 months, unlike in immunocompetent Balb/C mice where luminescence was absent from day 21-post muscle transduction (figure 3d). This suggests the involvement of T-cell inactivation of adenoviral-transduced cells in immunocompetent mice. Plasmid electroporation, on the other hand, has been shown not to elicit such transgene silencing immune responses (Vicat et al. 2000), and presents an attractive option in achieving long-term gene expression, especially in light of recent improvements in plasmid vectors (Gill et al. 2009).

Although Ad provided the highest immediate gene expression in all tissues, the potential for high level expression from AAV is highlighted in this study, with AAV2 providing expression in the same order of magnitude as Ad within the first month post administration, increasing to higher levels over time. Sustained transgene expression is desirable for many therapies and there is also potential to overcome transient expression from plasmids by inclusion of integrating transposon or S/MAR elements (Gill, Pringle et al. 2009). EP yielded the highest transfection among the non-viral techniques, in all tissues, unlike *in vitro* where lipofection displayed optimum efficiency of plasmid delivery, validating the common use of lipofection for *in vitro* laboratory transfections. Identical EP conditions were used for all experiments in this study. However, EP parameters can be optimised for specific tissue/cell types, and higher efficiencies than reported here might be achieved by use of cell-specific parameters (Mir 2008). This may also be true for sonoporation. Sonoporation is the least characterised of these plasmid delivery systems, and the finding that gene expression resulted in all situations examined, albeit it lower than the other non-viral methods, indicates potential for this strategy, especially given the attractive possibility of focusing ultrasound beams externally on internal organs. However, the lack of consistent levels of transfection observed (figure 4) highlight the need for technological improvement. Use of US in combination with 'micro-bubble' technology may increase the efficacy of transfection and enable localisation of systemically administered DNA complex through focussed US mediated sonoporation (Shimamura et al. 2004).

Overall, the data generated here clearly define the relative efficiencies of the various delivery systems in a wide range of tissues *in vivo*, and a range of tumour cell lines *in vitro*, providing the researcher with valuable information to aid in design of experimentation and clinically applicable strategies for gene therapies. Vectors achieve gene delivery with different efficiencies depending on the target cells. As such, the optimal conditions for delivery to one target may differ completely to another target. This study aims at comparing the maximum protein produced by the vectors, but this does not mean that with further optimization, it is not possible to achieve a higher level of expression.

5. Conclusion

The results clearly define the relative efficiencies of these delivery systems in a range of situations, providing researchers with valuable information to support vector choice in therapeutic strategy design.

6. Acknowledgment

We thank Prof. Andrew Baker of the University of Glasgow and Martina Harte of the Regenerative Medicine Institute Galway for providing rAd particles. This work was supported in part by grants from Cancer Research Ireland (CRI07TAN) and Science Foundation Ireland (06/RF/BIC055 and 07/RF/BIMF542).

7. References

Al-Dosari, M., Zhang, G., Knapp, J. E. & Liu, D. (2006). "Evaluation of viral and mammalian promoters for driving transgene expression in mouse liver." *Biochem Biophys Res Commun* 339(2): 673-8

Baggett, B., Roy, R., Momen, S., Morgan, S., Tisi, L., Morse, D. & Gillies, R. J. (2004). "Thermostability of firefly luciferases affects efficiency of detection by in vivo bioluminescence." *Mol Imaging* 3(4): 324-32

Buhles, A., Collins, S. A., van Pijkeren, J. P., Rajendran, S., Miles, M. C., O'Sullivan, G. C., O'Hanlon, D. M. & Tangney, M. (2009). "Anti-metastatic effects of viral and non-viral mediated Nk4 delivery to tumours." *Genet Vaccines Ther* 7(1): 5

Chang, D. C. (1992). *Structure and Dynamics of electric field-induced membrane pores as revealed by raid-freezing electron microscopy*. San Diego, Academic Press, Inc.

Collins, C. G., Tangney, M., Larkin, J. O., Casey, G., Whelan, M. C., Cashman, J., Murphy, J., Soden, D., Vejda, S., McKenna, S., Kiely, B., Collins, J. K., Barrett, J., Aarons, S. & O'Sullivan, G. C. (2006). "Local gene therapy of solid tumors with GM-CSF and B7-1 eradicates both treated and distal tumors." *Cancer Gene Ther* 13(12): 1061-7

Collins, S. A., Buhles, A., Scallan, M. F., Harrison, P. T., O'Hanlon, D. M., O'Sullivan, G. C. & Tangney, M. (2010). "AAV2-mediated in vivo immune gene therapy of solid tumours." *Genet Vaccines Ther* 8: 8

Collins, S. A., Guinn, B. A., Harrison, P. T., Scallan, M. F., O'Sullivan, G. C. & Tangney, M. (2008). "Viral vectors in cancer immunotherapy: which vector for which strategy?" *Curr Gene Ther* 8(2): 66-78

Davis, H. L., Millan, C. L. & Watkins, S. C. (1997). "Immune-mediated destruction of transfected muscle fibers after direct gene transfer with antigen-expressing plasmid DNA." *Gene Ther* 4(3): 181-8

Di Ianni, M., Terenzi, A., Perruccio, K., Ciurnelli, R., Lucheroni, F., Benedetti, R., Martelli, M. F. & Tabilio, A. (1999). "5-Azacytidine prevents transgene methylation in vivo." *Gene Ther* 6(4): 703-7

Ferrari, F. K., Samulski, T., Shenk, T. & Samulski, R. J. (1996). "Second-strand synthesis is a rate-limiting step for efficient transduction by recombinant adeno-associated virus vectors." *J Virol* 70(5): 3227-34

Flotte, T. R., Afione, S. A. & Zeitlin, P. L. (1994). "Adeno-associated virus vector gene expression occurs in nondividing cells in the absence of vector DNA integration." *Am J Respir Cell Mol Biol* 11(5): 517-21

Gill, D. R., Pringle, I. A. & Hyde, S. C. (2009). "Progress and prospects: the design and production of plasmid vectors." *Gene Ther* 16(2): 165-71

Gothelf, A. & Gehl, J. (2010) "Gene Electrotransfer to Skin; Review of Existing Literature and Clinical Perspectives." *Curr Gene Ther* 10(4): 287-99

Harding, T. C., Dickinson, P. J., Roberts, B. N., Yendluri, S., Gonzalez-Edick, M., Lecouteur, R. A. & Jooss, K. U. (2006). "Enhanced gene transfer efficiency in the murine striatum and an orthotopic glioblastoma tumor model, using AAV-7- and AAV-8-pseudotyped vectors." *Hum Gene Ther* 17(8): 807-20

Heller, L. C., Jaroszeski, M. J., Coppola, D. & Heller, R. (2008). "Comparison of electrically mediated and liposome-complexed plasmid DNA delivery to the skin." *Genet Vaccines Ther* 6(1): 16

Jooss, K., Ertl, H. C. & Wilson, J. M. (1998). "Cytotoxic T-lymphocyte target proteins and their major histocompatibility complex class I restriction in response to adenovirus vectors delivered to mouse liver." *J Virol* 72(4): 2945-54

Kealy, B., Liew, A., McMahon, J. M., Ritter, T., O'Doherty, A., Hoare, M., Greiser, U., Vaughan, E. E., Maenz, M., O'Shea, C., Barry, F. & O'Brien, T. (2009). "Comparison of viral and nonviral vectors for gene transfer to human endothelial progenitor cells." *Tissue Eng Part C Methods* 15(2): 223-31

Kurzeder C, Koppold B, Sauer G, Pabst S, Kreienberg R, Deissler H. (2007). "CD9 promotes adeno-associated virus type 2 infection of mammary carcinoma cells with low cell surface expression of heparan sulphate proteoglycans." *Int J Mol Med* 19(2):325-33.

Larkin, J. O., Casey, G. D., Tangney, M., Cashman, J., Collins, C. G., Soden, D. M. & O'Sullivan, G. C. (2008). "Effective tumor treatment using optimized ultrasound-mediated delivery of bleomycin." *Ultrasound Med Biol* 34(3): 406-13

Lo, W. D., Qu, G., Sferra, T. J., Clark, R., Chen, R. & Johnson, P. R. (1999). "Adeno-associated virus-mediated gene transfer to the brain: duration and modulation of expression." *Hum Gene Ther* 10(2): 201-13

Lyons, M., Onion, D., Green, N. K., Aslan, K., Rajaratnam, R., Bazan-Peregrino, M., Phipps, S., Hale, S., Mautner, V., Seymour, L. W. & Fisher, K. D. (2006). "Adenovirus type 5 interactions with human blood cells may compromise systemic delivery." *Mol Ther* 14(1): 118-28

Mah, C., Qing, K., Khuntirat, B., Ponnazhagan, S., Wang, X. S., Kube, D. M., Yoder, M. C. & Srivastava, A. (1998). "Adeno-associated virus type 2-mediated gene transfer: role of epidermal growth factor receptor protein tyrosine kinase in transgene expression." *J Virol* 72(12): 9835-43

Malecki, M., Kolsut, P. & Proczka, R. (2005). "Angiogenic and antiangiogenic gene therapy." *Gene Ther* 12 Suppl 1: S159-69

Manam, S., Ledwith, B. J., Barnum, A. B., Troilo, P. J., Pauley, C. J., Harper, L. B., Griffiths, T. G., 2nd, Niu, Z., Denisova, L., Follmer, T. T., Pacchione, S. J., Wang, Z., Beare, C. M., Bagdon, W. J. & Nichols, W. W. (2000). "Plasmid DNA vaccines: tissue distribution and effects of DNA sequence, adjuvants and delivery method on integration into host DNA." *Intervirology* 43(4-6): 273-81

Manno, C. S., Pierce, G. F., Arruda, V. R., Glader, B., Ragni, M., Rasko, J. J., Ozelo, M. C., Hoots, K., Blatt, P., Konkle, B., Dake, M., Kaye, R., Razavi, M., Zajko, A., Zehnder, J., Rustagi, P. K., Nakai, H., Chew, A., Leonard, D., Wright, J. F., Lessard, R. R., Sommer, J. M., Tigges, M., Sabatino, D., Luk, A., Jiang, H., Mingozzi, F., Couto, L., Ertl, H. C., High, K. A. & Kay, M. A. (2006). "Successful transduction of liver in hemophilia by AAV-Factor IX and limitations imposed by the host immune response." *Nat Med* 12(3): 342-7

Mir, L. M. (2008). "Application of electroporation gene therapy: past, current, and future." *Methods Mol Biol* 423: 3-17

Mir, L. M., Bureau, M. F., Gehl, J., Rangara, R., Rouy, D., Caillaud, J. M., Delaere, P., Branellec, D., Schwartz, B. & Scherman, D. (1999). "High-efficiency gene transfer into skeletal muscle mediated by electric pulses." *Proc Natl Acad Sci U S A* 96(8): 4262-7

Nathwani, A. C., Cochrane, M., McIntosh, J., Ng, C. Y., Zhou, J., Gray, J. T. & Davidoff, A. M. (2009). "Enhancing transduction of the liver by adeno-associated viral vectors." *Gene Ther 16: 60-69*

Nockel, J., van den Engel, N. K., Winter, H., Hatz, R. A., Zimmermann, W. & Kammerer, R. (2006). "Characterization of gastric adenocarcinoma cell lines established from CEA424/SV40 T antigen-transgenic mice with or without a human CEA transgene." *BMC Cancer* 6: 57

Prosch, S., Stein, J., Staak, K., Liebenthal, C., Volk, H. D. & Kruger, D. H. (1996). "Inactivation of the very strong HCMV immediate early promoter by DNA CpG methylation in vitro." *Biol Chem Hoppe Seyler* 377(3): 195-201

Rome, C., Deckers, R. & Moonen, C. T. (2008). "The use of ultrasound in transfection and transgene expression." *Handb Exp Pharmacol*(185 Pt 2): 225-43

Scheule, R. K. (2000). "The role of CpG motifs in immunostimulation and gene therapy." *Adv Drug Deliv Rev* 44(2-3): 119-34

Sharif, F., Hynes, S. O., McMahon, J., Cooney, R., Conroy, S., Dockery, P., Duffy, G., Daly, K., Crowley, J., Bartlett, J. S. & O'Brien, T. (2006). "Gene-eluting stents: comparison of adenoviral and adeno- associated viral gene delivery to the blood vessel wall in vivo." *Hum Gene Ther* 17(7): 741-5

Shimamura, M., Sato, N., Taniyama, Y., Yamamoto, S., Endoh, M., Kurinami, H., Aoki, M., Ogihara, T., Kaneda, Y. & Morishita, R. (2004). "Development of efficient plasmid DNA transfer into adult rat central nervous system using microbubble-enhanced ultrasound." *Gene Ther* 11(20): 1532-9

Summerford, C. & Samulski, R. J. (1998). "Membrane-associated heparan sulfate proteoglycan is a receptor for adeno-associated virus type 2 virions." *J Virol* 72(2): 1438-45

Vassalli, G., Bueler, H., Dudler, J., von Segesser, L. K. & Kappenberger, L. (2003). "Adeno-associated virus (AAV) vectors achieve prolonged transgene expression in mouse myocardium and arteries in vivo: a comparative study with adenovirus vectors." *Int J Cardiol* 90(2-3): 229-38

Vicat, J. M., Boisseau, S., Jourdes, P., Laine, M., Wion, D., Bouali-Benazzouz, R., Benabid, A. L. & Berger, F. (2000). "Muscle transfection by electroporation with high-voltage and short-pulse currents provides high-level and long-lasting gene expression." *Hum Gene Ther* 11(6): 909-16

Waddington, S. N., McVey, J. H., Bhella, D., Parker, A. L., Barker, K., Atoda, H., Pink, R., Buckley, S. M., Greig, J. A., Denby, L., Custers, J., Morita, T., Francischetti, I. M., Monteiro, R. Q., Barouch, D. H., van Rooijen, N., Napoli, C., Havenga, M. J., Nicklin, S. A. & Baker, A. H. (2008). "Adenovirus serotype 5 hexon mediates liver gene transfer." *Cell* 132(3): 397-409

Wang, A. Y., Peng, P. D., Ehrhardt, A., Storm, T. A. & Kay, M. A. (2004). "Comparison of adenoviral and adeno-associated viral vectors for pancreatic gene delivery in vivo." *Hum Gene Ther* 15(4): 405-131043-0342 (Print)

Wang, L., Dobrzynski, E., Schlachterman, A., Cao, O. & Herzog, R. W. (2005). "Systemic protein delivery by muscle-gene transfer is limited by a local immune response." *Blood* 105(11): 4226-34

Wu, Z., Asokan, A. & Samulski, R. J. (2006). "Adeno-associated virus serotypes: vector toolkit for human gene therapy." *Mol Ther* 14(3): 316-27

Yuasa, K., Sakamoto, M., Miyagoe-Suzuki, Y., Tanouchi, A., Yamamoto, H., Li, J., Chamberlain, J. S., Xiao, X. & Takeda, S. (2002). "Adeno-associated virus vector-mediated gene transfer into dystrophin-deficient skeletal muscles evokes enhanced immune response against the transgene product." *Gene Ther* 9(23): 1576-88

Part 3

Potential Applications of Gene Therapy in Future

12

Preclinical and Clinical Aspects of Gene Therapy in Myocardial Infarction

Saurabh Bharti, Ashok Kumar Sharma,
Bhaskar Krishnamurthy and Dharamvir Singh Arya
Department of Pharmacology,
All India Institute of Medical Sciences,
New Delhi,
India

1. Introduction

Clinical occurrence of acute myocardial infarction (AMI) has substantially increased over the last decade. More than 50% of the cases of coronary heart disease alone are covered under AMI. Thus, the prevalence of AMI poses a serious health care burden, demanding for more strategic approaches. Exploration in molecular mechanisms underlying myocardial infarction (MI) has radically improved over the last half century. Novel pathways have not only provided in-depth knowledge of mechanistic approach to understand the pathophysiology of MI but also offer new strategies for its treatment. Currently, polypharmacy comprising β-blockers, angiotensin converting enzyme (ACE) inhibitors, angiotensin receptor blockers (ARB) and aspirin are generally adopted for treating patients of MI. Surgical interventions include stenting procedures and percutaneous coronary interventions. Despite availability of these pharmacological and surgical therapies, they are associated with limitations encompassing side effects, recurrence, non-compliance and interactions with other drugs. The early mortality rate from AMI is about 30%, with more than half of these deaths occurring before the stricken individual reaches the hospital (AHA report, 2003). Therefore looking towards the 21st century, now the question arises, can we bring an ideal therapy for treatment of human MI where all the side effects, interaction and compliance issues can be eliminated? The answer might lie in an emerging area known as gene therapy. Cardiovascular gene therapy is one of those areas where administration of a particular gene would result in long term gene expression and preclude the heart from various insults. In general an ideal gene therapy should have multifaceted approach such as 1) It should be specific for the myocardial tissue 2) it should not cause potential adverse effects 3) it should not disrupt the vital genes 4) it should not increase the risk of other diseases such as predisposition to cancer and finally 5) it should be long enough to sustain and to prevent any recurrence of the disease. Most recent exciting development in gene therapy includes formation of new blood vessels and improved blood flow to ischemic tissues induced by growth factors such as VEGF, HGF, FGF and PDGF. Furthermore, improved calcium handing through SERCA2a, phospholamban, parvalbumin and S100A1 proteins offers a viable and attractive approach in the treatment of heart failure. In addition, modulation of β-adrenergic receptor signaling through β2 adrenergic receptor overexpression, GRK2/βARKct and Adenlyl cyclase 6 has yielded encouraging results in experimental models of MI. Thereafter, various cardiovascular diseases where gene therapy has made its mark in pre-clinical studies are angiogenesis for myocardial ischemia, re-stenosis and bypass graft failure. Gene therapy with its specificity on myogenesis, cell cycle activation anti-oxidant and anti-apoptotic pathways upregulates the cellular defense system and provides augmented cardioprotective response to injury and cardiac remodeling. Success in animal models and in early phases of clinical trials of gene therapy in myocardial ischemic reperfusion setting further validates imminent use of gene therapy. Mechanistically, gene therapy for MI must be aimed at activating key molecular pathways in myocardium that significantly alleviate the cardiac injury by inducing neo-angiogenesis, strengthening anti-oxidant status of the myocardium, inhibiting necrosis/apoptotic pathways, inhibiting mitochondrial permeability transition pore and most importantly preserving the integrity of myocardium (remodeling).

This chapter will basically focus on the significant results of gene therapy obtained in myocardial ischemia reperfusion injury in pre-clinical studies, phase I/II clinical trials and their future implications to make gene therapy a completely bench to bed-side approach.

2. Preclinical aspect

2.1 Role of angiogenesis in gene therapy

Perhaps, the most highly investigated and promising application of gene therapy which has shown indispensable results in animal models of myocardial infarction is angiogenesis. Angiogenesis occurs as a result of multiple growth factors participating in the formation of new blood vessels. Growth factors including vascular endothelial growth factor (VEGF), hepatocyte growth factor (HGF), fibroblast growth factor (FGF) and platelet derived growth factor (PDGF), either alone or in combination, result in induction of angiogenesis. Therefore gene therapy can act in very specific and targeted manner, i.e. either to activate the pathways which up-regulate endogenous growth factors like hypoxia inducible factor-1 alpha (HIF-1α), to inhibit endogenous anti-angiogenic processes or to induce growth factors exogenously. The various angiogenic growth factors which have shown significant results in animal models of myocardial infarction are as follows:

2.1.1 VEGF

Family comprises of five isoforms viz. VEGF-A, VEGF-B, VEGF-C, VEGF-D and placental growth factor. The major function of VEGF is to regulate coronary vasculature development, blood vessel physiology, vasodilation, proliferation and migration of endothelial and smooth muscle cells.

2.1.2 HGF

HGF shows its diversified action through coupling with c-Met receptor following tyrosine kinase activation. HGF is a pleiotropic factor which promotes neo-vascularization, migration and proliferation of endothelial cells and inhibits apoptosis. In addition; morphogenesis, mitogenesis, motogenesis and neurite extension are the other effects shown by HGF.

2.1.3 FGF

Family comprises of 22 distinct polypeptide growth factors and seven single-chain tyrosine receptor kinases. FGF is also known as heparin binding growth factor because of its higher affinity towards heparin and heparan sulfate. FGF displays its activities through auto-phosphorylation via dimerization of its receptor. FGF actively participates in both the phases of angiogenesis/arteriogenesis i.e. early invasive phase and late maturative phase. Functionally, it is involved in migration and proliferation of endothelial and smooth muscle cells, production of proteases and vessel maturation.

2.1.4 PDGF

Family comprises of five isoforms viz. PDGF-A, PDGF-B, PDGF-C, PDGF-D and PDGF-AB heterodimer; and acts through two distinct receptors namely α and β. Its function is to regulate cell growth and division. PDGF is a potent mitogen for smooth muscle cells of mesenchymal origin.

Growth Factors	Species	Outcome	References
VEGF-165	Rats, rabbits	Increased neovascularization and improved fractional shortening after MI	Bull et al., 2003; Hao et al., 2007; Ruixing et al., 2006.
VEGF-165	Porcine	Increased myocardial blood flow, increased vasodilation with adenosine, improved wall thickening and strain, improved wall motion, increased ejection fraction and increased myocardial viability	Choi et al., 2006; Ferrarini et al., 2006; Jacquier et al., 2007; Tio et al., 1999; Zhang et al., 2002.
VEGF-121	Rats, porcine	Increased collateral circulation following MI	Lee et al., 2000; Mack et al., 1998.
VEGF-B186	Pigs, rabbits	improved myocardial perfusion and ejection fraction	Lahteenvuo et al., 2009
VEGF-C	Piglets	augmented collateral formation and decreased wall thickening after MI	Patila et al., 2006
VEGF-D	Porcine	improved perfusion when administered through a catheter mediated intra myocardial gene transfer method	Rutanen et al., 2004
VEGF gene constructs	Rat, mouse	Reduced infarct size and induction of angiogenesis	Lee et al., 2003; Su et al., 2002; Yockman et al., 2009
HGF	Rats, dogs	Induction of angiogenesis	Aoki et al., 2000; Funatsu et al., 2002; Wang et al., 2006a
HGF	Mice, Swine, canine, porcine	Improved remodeling, decreased apoptosis, improved mobilization of stem cells for cardiac repair, decreased fibrotic scar formation and improved contractility of the heart	Ahmet et al., 2002; Ahmet et al., 2003; Cho et al., 2008; Jayasankar et al., 2003; Jin et al., 2004; Li et al., 2003; Taniyama et al., 2002; Yang et al., 2007; Yang et al., 2010

Growth Factors	Species	Outcome	References
HGF + ultrasound mediated micro bubble destruction	Rat	Increased angiogenesis, limitation of infarct size, and prevention of LV remodeling	Kondo et al., 2004
FGF	Pig	Improved blood flow and MI by enhancing collateral formation	Post et al., 2006
FGF-2	Pigs	Improved LV functions and increased arteriogenesis	Horvath et al., 2002
FGF-4	Pigs	increased perfusion and decreased LV dysfunction	Gao et al., 2004
FGF-5	Pigs	Improved blood flow, Reduced pacing-induced regional myocardial dysfunction	Giordano et al., 1996; Suzuki et al., 2005
PDGF-AB	Rat	Promoted angiogenesis and minimized the extent of myocardial infarction	Edelberg et al., 2002
PDGF + basic FGF	Rat	Promoted angiogenesis with more stable capillaries	Hao et al., 2004a
PDGF-BB + VEGF-A165	Rat	Stimulated angiogenesis both at the capillary and arteriolar levels and transiently counteracted cardiac remodelling after MI	Hao et al., 2004b
PDGF	Rat	Improved cardiac function	Zheng et al., 2004
PDGF	Rats	Improved post-infarction ventricular function without pulmonary toxicity	Hsieh et al., 2006
PDGF-BB + FGF-2	Pigs	Enhanced myocardial collateral growth and significantly restored myocardial perfusion and function	Lu et al., 2007
PDGF-BB	Rats	Significantly decreased MI	Krausgrill et al., 2009

Table 1. The examples of various growth factors in myocardial infarction.

2.2 Role of oxidative stress in gene therapy

The human cells are replete with a number of molecules that function as antioxidants, i.e. which protect the cells from a group of molecules known as pro-oxidants. Anti-oxidants are molecules that are capable of inhibiting the oxidation of other molecules. In this process, they themselves get oxidized. On the other hand, pro-oxidants either generate free radicals or inhibit the anti-oxidant systems, thus predisposing the cell to oxidative damage. Oxidative stress represents a condition characterized by an imbalance between the pro-oxidant and anti-oxidant systems within the cell, leading to oxidative damage to the cell; ultimately leading to lipid peroxidation, protein degradation and DNA damage and has been implicated in a vast variety of disorders; atherosclerosis, diabetes, myocardial infarction, myocardial ischemia-reperfusion injury, hypertension, heart failure, cardiomyopathy and rheumatoid arthritis being just a few of them. Examples of ROS include radicals like superoxide, hydroxyl, alkoxyl and peroxyl; and non-radicals like hydrogen peroxide, hypochlorous acid and organic hydroperoxides.

The observation that the level of antioxidants is increased during periods of oxidative stress has led to the finding that the synthesis of antioxidants is increased at the times of oxidative stress. This has led to the concept that administration of genes for antioxidants can combat the role of oxidative stress and thus protect cells and tissues from damage. Various studies and clinical trials have been carried out in this regard and the role of gene therapy for antioxidants in myocardial ischemia prevention has been established in animal models. The intramyocardial delivery of heme oxygenase-1(HO-1) into the left ventricle of rats using AAVs (Adeno-Associated Virus) several weeks before myocardial infarction resulted in approximately 80% decrease in infarct size in association with decreases in oxidative stress, inflammation, and interstitial fibrosis and was accompanied by postinfarction recovery and normalization of ventricular dimensions (Melo et al., 2002). Similar results were obtained after transfer of gene for extracellular superoxide dismutase (EC-SOD); wherein recombinant adeno virus transfer into the myocardium of conscious rabbits of the gene encoding EC-SOD, three days before the induction of myocardial ischaemia by a 30-minute coronary artery occlusion using a balloon occluder, afforded cardioprotection with a decrease in the region at risk and infarct size as compared to controls (Li et al., 2001). Its intracellular counterparts (Mn-SOD and Cu/Zn-SOD) have also been shown to decrease infarct size following ischaemia-reperfusion injury, as well as decrease apoptosis and delay induction of NF-κB (Michiels et al., 1994; Chen et al., 1998). Thioredoxins are potent antioxidants that decrease p38MAPK signaling and superoxide anion generation and hence, combat oxidative stress. Trx-1 gene therapy administered post-MI has been shown to promote angiogenesis, decrease apoptosis, reduce ventricular remodeling, and improve ejection fraction in diabetic rats (Samuel et al., 2010). Below are mentioned some important anti-oxidants which have shown remarkable results in experimental models of myocardial infarction.

2.2.1 HEME oxygenase-1 (HO-1)

Heme oxygenase cleaves the heme ring at the alpha-methene bridge to form biliverdin, iron and carbon monoxide. Its activity is highest in the spleen, where old RBCs are sequestered and destroyed, leading to liberation of hemoglobin and its subsequent separation into heme and globin. It has three isoforms: HO-1 (which is also referred to as heat-shock protein 32K or HSP-32K) is inducible in response to oxidative stress, hypoxia, heavy metals, cytokines and a variety of other compounds. HO-1 has also been suggested to induce VEGF formation. HO-2 is constitutive and is expressed under normal or homeostatic conditions. HO-3, unlike the other two isoforms, is not catalytically active, but has been postulated to work in oxygen sensing. AAV delivery of HO-1 performed in MI-rat models demonstrated an increase in cardiac remodeling and an improvement in cardiac function (Melo et al., 2002). Studies performed in animals with human heme oxygenase-1 (hHO-1) administered 6 - 8 weeks prior to induction of ischaemia resulted in decreased mortality at 1 year, along with a decrease in infarct size, reduction in ventricular thinning, decreased inflammation stress and interstitial fibrosis, decreased lipid peroxidation, and was accompanied by post-infarction recovery and normalization of ventricular functions (Melo et al., 2002).

2.2.2 Superoxide dismutase (SOD)

The enzyme superoxide dismutase (EC: 1.15.1.1) was first discovered by Fridowich and McCord (McCord & Fridovich, 1988). It scavenges the superoxide ($O^{-2.}$) radical and causes its dismutation into water and hydrogen peroxide by the following reaction –

$$2O^{-2.} + 2H \rightarrow H_2O_2 + O_2$$

The enzyme has three isoforms – 1. Cytosolic (Cu/Zn-SOD) or SOD-1, dependent on copper and zinc (Cao, et al., 2008). 2. Mitochondrial (Mn-SOD) or SOD-2, dependent on manganese (Borgstahl, et al., 1996) and 3. Extracellular (EC-SOD) or SOD-3. The genes for these are located on chromosomes 21q22.1, 6q25.3 and 4p15.3 respectively. Cu/Zn-SOD is dimeric and the other two are tetrameric in structure. All of them have improved left ventricular function and increased survival in rat ischaemia-reperfusion models (Michiels et al., 1994, Chen et al., 1998; Li, et al., 2001). Studies on EC-SOD in rat ischaemia-reperfusion models have demonstrated decreased myocardial stunning and infarct size (Li et al., 2001). Mn-SOD and eNOS administered together have also led to decreased infarct size in animal ischaemia-reperfusion models (Abunasra et al., 2001).

2.2.3 Thioredoxins

Thioredoxins are another group of antioxidant proteins that are ubiquitously found in many organisms and are encoded by the TNX gene in humans (Wollman et al., 1988). They have a 12 kDa tertiary structure, that contains a dithiol-disulfide active site and facilitate the reduction of other proteins by a cysteine thiol-disulfide exchange. The amino acid sequence of thioredoxins is characterized by two vicinal cysteines in a CXXC motif which provide the enzyme the ability to reduce various substrates, such as ribonucleases, chorionic gonadotrophins, coagulation factors, glucocorticoid receptors and insulin. The thioredoxins also act as electron donors to peroxidases and ribonucleotide reductase (Arner & Holmgren, 2000).

The summary of the researches carried out on antioxidant gene therapy in MI is summarized in the table 2.

Gene	Model	Outcome	References
HO-1	Rat I/R	Decrease in infarct size. Decrease in oxidative stress, inflammation and interstitial fibrosis. Post-infarction recovery with normalization of ventricular dimensions	Melo et al., 2002
SOD	Rat I/R	Decreased stunning. Decreased infarct size following I/R injury. Improved left ventricular function. Increased survival	Michiels et al., 1994 & Chen et al., 1998, Li et al., 2001
TRX-1	Post-MI diabetic rats	Angiogenesis. Decreased apoptosis. Decreased ventricular remodeling. Improved ejection fraction.	Samuel et al., 2010
SPHK1	Rats	Improved systolic and diastolic functions of the heart and improved peak contraction velocity	Jin et al., 2007

Table 2. Examples of various anti-oxidants studied for gene therapy.

Gene	Species	Outcome	Reference
Bcl-2	Rabbits	Reduced apoptosis, reduced ventricular dilatation and decreased wall thinning	Chatterjee et al., 2002
Apoptosis repressor gene	Rabbits	Inhibition of apoptosis, decreased LV dilatation with preserved ejection fraction	Chatterjee et al., 2003
Cardio-trophin-1 (CT-1)	Mouse	Decreased apoptosis, decreased infarct size, decreased caspase-3 activation and improved ventricular pressure indices	Ruixing et al., 2007
Akt	Rats	Limitation of infarct size, improved myocardial contractility and reduced infarct size	Cittadini et al., 2006; Miao et al., 2000
sTNFR1 (TNF-α antagonist)	Mice	Reduced infract size and improved cardiac function	Sugano et al., 2004
HSP 20	Rats	Improved LV end systolic and end diastolic pressures, reduced apoptosis and decreased infarct size	Zhu et al., 2005
HSP 70	Rabbits	Decreased infarct size	Okubo et al., 2001
HSP 72	Rats	Decreased apoptosis and prevented MI	Suzuki et al., 2002
Kallikrein gene	Rats	Decreased apoptosis, endothelial dysfunction and preservation of cardiac output	Agata et al., 2002
Sonic hedgehog homolog (Shh)	Mice, Rats	Preserved ventricular function by enhancing neovascularization, reduced apoptosis and fibrosis	Kusano et al., 2005
Troponin I type 3 interacting kinase	Mice	Decreased MI and inhibition of remodeling	Lai et al., 2008
Leukemia inhibitory factor (LIF)	Rats	Preservation of rat myocardium post-MI	Berry et al., 2004
Cluster of Differentiation 151 (CD151)	Pigs and rats	Promoted neovascularization and improved cardiac function	Wang et al., 2006b, Zuo et al., 2009
p38 kinase + active MAP kinase kinase 3b	Rats	Reduced infarct size, decreased apoptosis, increased capillary density, decreased fibrosis and improved ejection fraction	Tenhunen et al., 2006

Table 3. The examples of various proteins involved in apoptosis studied for gene therapy.

2.3 Role of apoptosis in gene therapy

Apoptosis means programmed cell death. It is a physiological phenomenon that normally occurs during the embryonic development in humans and also serves as a protective response in case of irreparable DNA damage to avoid the multiplication of defective cells. Two various pathways are involved in induction of apoptosis. The extracellular pathway involves stimulation of death receptors that transduce signals to the nucleus to activate caspases. The intracellular pathway involves increase in the permeability of the inner mitochondrial membrane that causes leakage of pro-apoptotic molecules like cytochrome c into the cytoplasm that directly activate the caspases. The end-result is the activation of caspases that digest the protein cytoskeleton of the cell. The distinct family of Bcl proteins is involved in apoptosis, with Bcl-2 and Bcl-x acting as anti-apoptotic factors; while Bax and Bak act as pro-apoptotic factors.

The pathways of apoptosis provide an excellent target for gene therapy as inhibition of apoptosis allows the cells to survive. Gene therapies with pro-apoptotic molecules and genes that transcribe proteins that suppress the anti-apoptotic proteins have been tried in animal models with sufficiently encouraging results, which are yet to be supplemented by results from clinical trials (Table 3).

2.4 Role of calcium signaling in gene therapy

The handling of Ca^{2+} during excitation–contraction (EC) coupling is an important feature of the cardiomyocyte contraction. In cardiomyocytes, EC coupling begins with the initiation of action potential, whereby, Ca^{2+} enters the cell through voltage-gated L-type Ca^{2+}channels and triggers the ryanodine receptor (RyR) to extrude Ca^{2+} from the sarcoplasmic reticulum (SR) into the cytosol. This Ca^{2+}induced Ca^{2+} release trigger is a crucial step in cardiomyocyte contraction through Ca^{2+} binding to troponin C within the myofilaments of the sarcomere. Furthermore, it is again imperative to remove the Ca^{2+} from the cytosol to initiate the relaxation of sarcomere which is mainly dependent on sarco/endoplasmic reticulum Ca^{2+}-ATPase 2a (SERCA2a) and sarcolemmal Na^{+}–Ca^{2+}exchanger (NCX). Moreover, distortion of Ca^{2+} handling in cardiomyocytes occurs due to decreased SR Ca^{2+} store and a prolonged Ca^{2+} transient, which is generally a consequence of increased NCX, reduction in SERCA2a, decreased phospholamban (PLN)/SERCA2a ratio and increased open probability of the RyR. In addition, these abnormalities in Ca^{2+} handling cause dysfunctional contractile performance and may increase the risk of cardiac arrhythmias and cardiac remodeling. Because myocardial contractility is dependent on ventricular Ca^{2+} handling, therefore, genetic modification of molecules involved in dysfunctional cardiomyocyte Ca^{2+} handling could be a viable and attractive target in the treatment of heart failure. The major proteins which participate in handling of calcium during cardiomyocyte contraction are discussed briefly:

2.4.1 Sarco/endoplasmic reticulum Ca2+-ATPase (SR Ca^{2+}-ATPase, SERCA)

SERCA, a calcium ATPase (type P-ATPase) exists in the SR within muscle cells and transfers Ca^{2+} from the cytosol of the cell to the SR at the cost of ATP hydrolysis during muscle relaxation. There are three isoforms of SERCA viz. SERCA1-3, which have been shown to play distinct roles in various cells. Of the three isoforms available SERCA2 plays a significant role in calcium handling during myocyte contraction. Of note, SERCA2a activity is reduced in heart failure, resulting in decreased calcium uptake and impaired relaxation. Furthermore, SERCA2a activity in myocytes is controlled by phospholamban (PLN), a small inhibitory peptide that inhibits SERCA2a in its dephosphorylated form; whereas phosphorylated PLN reduces this inhibition. Therefore, SERCA2a gene therapy would aim to increase SERCA2a activity, which in turn would increase calcium uptake and thus improve diastolic relaxation. In addition it would also increase contractile reserve because of higher SR calcium concentration.

2.4.2 Phospholamban (PLN)

PLN is a protein which is encoded by the PLN gene in humans. The important function of PLN is to regulate Ca^{2+} pump in skeletal and cardiac muscle cells. It has been observed that dephosphorylated phospholamban (PLB) inhibits SERCA2a activity, while proteins such as calcium-calmodulin-dependent protein kinase (CAMkinase) and protein kinase A (PKA) cause phosphorylation of PLB to relieve this inhibition. This cross-talk between PLB and SERCA2a controls the calcium content of the SR and normal myocardial contractility. The role of PLB in cardiac Ca^{2+} handling has been elucidated through PLB-knockout mice; that displayed enhanced Ca^{2+} kinetics and showed significantly increased cardiac contractility. Paradoxically, PLB overexpressing mice showed impaired Ca^{2+} cycling associated with depressed contractile parameters. Thus, PLB plays a nodal role in the regulation of SR Ca^{2+} homeostasis through its potent action on SERCA2a activity which in turn leads to slower cytosolic Ca^{2+} decay and prolonged diastolic relaxation.

2.4.3 Parvalbumin

Parvalbumin is a calcium-binding albumin protein that resides in fast-contracting muscles (highest levels), in the brain and some endocrine tissues. Gene therapy with parvalbumin, a Ca^{2+} sequestering protein, potentially provides an energy-independent removal of cystosolic calcium and thus improves the functioning of the heart. Adenovirus (AdV) parvalbumin delivery in hypothyroid rat hearts led to an increased rate of calcium removal and an improved rate of diastolic relaxation. Thus, parvalbumin may constitute a potentially attractive mode of correcting the prolonged diastolic Ca^{2+} decay generally seen in heart failure without further energy deprivation. Likewise, AdV-parvalbumin delivery to isolated cardiomyocytes from dog hearts after thoracic aortic coarctation resulted in improved relaxation kinetics but depressed sarcomere shortening at higher parvalbumin concentrations. This was probably due to inadvertant calcium removal during systole. Although potentially promising target for gene therapy in heart failure, further studies addressing the impact of long-term parvalbumin expression in relevant models of HF is warranted to clarify its role.

2.4.4 S100A1

S100A1 belongs to the S100 protein family (the largest Ca^{2+} binding protein subfamily) and appears to play multiple and inimitable roles in cardiomyocyte Ca^{2+} handling. It is highly expressed in the heart and localized to SR, sarcomere and the mitochondria. It is demonstrated by some researchers that myocardial levels of S100A1 are decreased in heart failure. So, S100A1 gene delivery to cardiomyocytes may result in an increased isometric contraction followed by an increase in the amount of Ca^{2+} pumped into the SR. Adrenergic receptor stimulation in the presence of S100A1 overexpression enhanced maximal contractile performance. Furthermore, S100A1 decreases the Ca^{2+} concentration during diastole and augments Ca^{2+} release during systole by regulating both RyR and SERCA2a. In addition, S100A1 also augments SERCA2a activity during the relaxation phase and improves diastolic relaxation.

Target Gene	Species	Outcome	References
SR CA^{2+} ATPASE	Isolated cardio myocytes	In vitro restored the contractile function of cardiomyocytes isolated from failing human hearts.	del Monte et al., 1999
	Rats	Improved systolic and diastolic function along with improved survival (63% versus 9%).	del Monte et al., 2001a
		Improved left ventricular systolic pressure, enhanced ventricular pressure rise decline (dp/dt), normalized rate of isovolumic relaxation.	del Monte et al., 2001b
	SERCA2a	Adenoviral gene transfer of SERCA2a in a rat model of heart failure (aortic banding) improved left ventricular function.	Miyamoto et al., 2000
PHOSPHO LAMBAN	Mice	Impaired Ca^{2+} cycling associated with depressed contractile parameters .	Kadambi et al., 1996
	Human myocardial cells	Improvement in contraction and relaxation velocities.	del Monte et al., 2002
	Silencing of PLB sheep	Improved SERCA activity, improved systolic and diastolic LV function.	Kaye et al., 2007
	Mice	Enhanced Ca^{2+} kinetics.	Kiriazis et al., 2000
PARV ALBUMIN	Dog cardio myocytes	Improved relaxation kinetics but depressed sarcomere shortening at higher parvalbumin concentrations.	Hirsch et al., 2004
S100A1	Cardiomyocytes	Increase of isometric contraction followed by an increase in the amount of Ca^{2+} pumped into the SR.	Remppis et al., 1996
	Mice	Substantially worsened LV function, transaortic constriction and MI with significantly lower survival.	Most et al., 2006
	Intracoronary delivery of AAV6-S100A1Post-MI rat heart	LV dysfunction and HF was evident initially and 2 months after gene delivery, S100A1-treated HF rats presented with significantly enhanced cardiac function and a reversal of LV remodeling compared to control HF rats.	Pleger et al., 2007
	AdV-mediated S100A1 gene transfer to failing rat cardiomyocytes	Restoration of disturbed Ca^{2+} handling by increasing reuptake of SR Ca^{2+} during the relaxation phase and a lowering of the RyR-mediated Ca^{2+} leak.	Most et al., 2004

Table 4. The examples of various proteins involved in calcium signaling studied for gene therapy.

2.5 Role of cell cycle activation in gene therapy

The normal cell passes through the stages of G1-S-G2-M in that orderly sequence as a part of the cell cycle; with a quiescent G0 phase before entering the S phase from G1. This cell cycle is highly subject to strict regulation by a number of molecules that either enhance or retard the progression of the cycle. The two important check-points G1-S and G2-M demand the requirement of a group of proteins called cyclins to overcome them; that do so by combining with a group of cyclin-dependent kinases (CDKs). The expression of cyclins is enhanced by dephosphorylation of Rb protein; mutations in which are found to be responsible for the ocular tumour retinoblastoma. Similarly, the CDKs are inhibited by the proteins of the Cip/Kip family as well as those of the p16/INK4a locus. A major role is also played by p53 protein, that halts the cell cycle, allowing time for the DNA damage to be rectified; if successful, terminates its own action by inducing autocatalysis through induction of MdM2 and if the DNA damage cannot be repaired, initiates apoptosis. Cell cycle activation is another promising application of gene therapy which results in the induction of endogenous myocardial regeneration. In various pre-clinical set ups it has resulted in activation of the cardiomyocyte cell cycle, thereby limiting the infarct size and improving LV dysfunction. The cyclins and the CDKs are the various candidate genes, the induction of which permits the cell to overcome the endogenous checkpoints and continue with the replication, thus allowing the cardiomyocyte growth. Studies in animals have yielded encouraging results, as listed in the following table; while clinical trials in humans are still awaited (Table 5).

Target Gene	Species	Outcome	Reference
Cyclin -A2	Rats	Increased border-zone myofilament density and improved myocardial function	Woo et al., 2006
CDK4	Rats	Improved left ventricular function	Tamamori-Adachi et al., 2008

Table 5. The examples of proteins involved in cell cycle studied for gene therapy.

2.6 Role of β-adrenergic system in gene therapy

β-adrenergic receptor blockers have been shown to exert favorable effects in heart-failure patients. Numerous clinical and experimental studies have shown that molecular targeting of various proteins within the cardiac beta-adrenergic receptor (β-ARs) pathway may be beneficial in heart failure. Chronic heart failure due to MI is associated with increased sympathetic discharge. However, this increased sympathetic activity is compensated mechanistically, but is more injurious in the long term. The β-adrenergic system is affected by multiple modifications including β-AR down-regulation, up-regulation of β-AR kinases and increased Gi function leading to β-AR desensitization and decreased β-AR signaling activity in heart failure. Several gene-based experiments tested and established that cardiac functions are improved or enhanced by genetic manipulation of the myocardial β-AR system.

2.6.1 β2-adrenergic receptor overexpression

Although β2-AR overexpression in mouse hearts results in improved systolic and diastolic function; but at significantly high levels, mice developed fibrotic cardiomyopathy and heart failure. Moreover, β2 signaling stimulates cell-survival and protects myocyte damage from apoptosis. This fact led to the use of β2-AR gene delivery in various experimental models of heart failure (Table 6).

2.6.2 Inhibition of G protein-coupled receptor kinases (GRKs)

Homologous desensitization (agonist dependent) is mediated by G protein–coupled receptor kinases (GRKs). GRK-2 upregulation is responsible for β-AR desensitization in heart failure and these kinases dampen the interaction between β-receptors and their G proteins. In addition, β-ARKct is a peptide within the carboxy terminus of GRK2 that inhibits GRK-2 mediated β-AR desensitization. βARKct gene transfer to isolated failing human cardiomyocytes improved their contractile function.

2.6.3 Adenylatecyclase type 6

β-AR stimulation activates adenylate cyclase (AC) through G-protein activation and AC then activates protein kinases to exert its downstream effects. AC6 is the predominant cardiac isoform and its overexpression in cardiac tissue leads to increased left ventricle contractility and function.

Target Gene	Species	Outcome	References
β-ARs	AdVβ-AR intracoronary delivery mice	Enhanced cardiac function.	Shah et al., 2000
Inhibition of GRK-2by βARKct gene transfer	Isolated failing human cardiomyocytes	Improved their contractile function.	Jameel & Zhang, 2009
	Intracoronary delivery of AdV-βARKct in mice	Improved cardiac function post-MI.	Iaccarino et al., 1998
Adenylate cyclase type 6	AdV-AC6 gene delivery in pigs	Improved LV contractility and function.	Lai et al., 2004

Table 6. Proteins involved in β-adrenergic system studied for gene therapy.

3. Clinical aspects

The human quest and efforts to expand the boundaries of his knowledge into the arena of gene therapy is endless. Genes responsible for cardiovascular events or diseases, myocardial

Clinical Trial	Sample size = n	Outcome	References
Intramyocardial injection of adenovirus (Ad.VEGF-121) by thoracotomy & CABG / by minimally invasive thoracotomy	21	Both groups showed reduction in angina but no improvement in exercise duration. Proper conclusions could not be drawn due to absence of control group.	Rosengart et al., 1999
Injection of ph.VEGF-165 into LV myocardium by minimally invasive thoracotomy	5 20	Reduction in angina and nitroglycerine use in 60 days in all 5 patients. Results limited because of a small sample size and absence of controls. Reduction in angina and nitroglycerine use in 90 days in 16 out of 20 patients. Results limited due to absence of controls.	Losordo et al., 1998
Administration of VEGF-165	20	Significant symptomatic improvement in patients with inoperable CAD	Symes et al., 1999
Catheter-mediated VEGF plasmid/liposome (P/L) gene transfer	15	Catheter-mediated intracoronary gene transfer performed after angioplasty significantly prevents restenosis and myocardial ischemia.	Laitinen et al., 2000
Percutaneous catheter-based gene transfer of naked plasmid DNA for VEGF-2 to LV myocardium	19	Decrease in angina & improvement in symptoms. Drawback: sample size is low.	Losordo et al., 2002

Table 7. Clinical trials for gene therapy in myocardial infarction. Ad.VEGF-121: Adenovirus encoding Vascular Endothelial Growth Factor-121; ph.VEGF-165: Plasmid vector encoding Vascular Endothelial Growth Factor-165; Ad.FGF-4: Adenovirus encoding Fibroblast Growth Factor-4; LV: Left ventricle; LacZ: Z gene of lac operon; HIF-α: Hypoxia-Inducible Factor-α.

infarction in particular, have been identified and targeted as a means of curative approach. An example can be illustrated of the study conducted by Doney and his colleagues (Doney et al., 2009) who identified an allele of rs9939609 gene, also referred to as FTO (Fat mass and obesity associated) gene. This gene increased the risk of Type II diabetes mellitus, an atherogenic lipid profile (including decreased high density lipoprotein and increased triglycerides) and myocardial infarction. This allele presents a target which if suitably replaced by the wild type can decrease the risks for all the above conditions.

One of the main drawbacks for designing gene therapy for myocardial infarction is the ethical concerns pertaining to the selection of participants. The participants are among those who have suffered an attack of myocardial infarction and conducting studies on such a cohort of patients with a risk of failure of therapy raises a substantial debate. Apart from this, the set-up for these studies also demands technical and financial support on a tremendously large scale. It is for these very precise reasons that a large number of these studies have not yet been conducted so far and hence the relative paucity of these studies in literature as compared to other studies. However the recent advances in the study of human genome and identification of genes associated with the risk factors, pathogenesis as well as outcome of myocardial infarction, has given a great impetus for designing clinical trials for gene therapy. As a result, a good number of trials are currently underway, for instance, the endocardial gene therapy with VEGF-D for severe coronary heart disease.

Apart from the ethical and financial constraints, there are practical difficulties as well, for instance, the delivery of viral particles in to the human body may stimulate the immune system that stimulates the T lymphocytes and cytokines to clear the virus. The naked DNA administered may be lysed by DNAses present in the serum. The permeability of the naked DNA across cell membranes is also restricted, necessitating the requirement for intracellular transfer. On the other hand, an intravenous injection may result in transfection of other tissues apart from the heart and lodgement of the vectors in other organs such as the lung or kidney. To circumvent these possibilities, the technology required for gene transfer needs to be highly advanced and sophisticated to ensure that the vector containing the therapeutic gene transfects only the desired myocardial cells. An example of such technology is the UTMD (ultrasound targeted microbubble destruction), in which ultrasound contrast agents used as gas microbubbles, are packed with the therapeutic gene containing DNA and are destroyed within the myocardium by subjecting them to high ultrasound frequency. A very high number of clinical trials have not been conducted for gene therapy in MI. Some of the clinical trials that have been undertaken in this regard are enlisted in table 7.

4. Limitations of gene therapy

As with most experimental therapies, safety of gene therapy for ischemic heart disease is of paramount importance. Though clinical trials have shown short-term safety, long-term surveillance over a period of decades is lacking. The question still remains as to which therapy benefits what sub-population of patients. Inclusion of a wide selection of patients in studies over time may lead to improvement in subgroups of patients if not the entire population. Confounding factors such as use of concurrent medications and concurrent medical conditions lead to difficulty in standardizing groups of patients. Objective end points of assessment need to be used uniformly as exercise testing may be subjective and is victim to high variability in the same patient on different days. Frequency of testing for objective improvements may need to be ramped up as the effects of therapeutic genes may have abated at the time of a single test. Another surprising factor that confounded results of clinical trials was a strong placebo effect. This might be minimized when objective and not subjective end points are used when assessing outcomes. Drug related issues such as the dose, gene transfection efficiency, pharmacokinetics and pharmacodynamics of individual therapies are valid as these may differ in different populations of patients. Also cost-effectiveness analysis has to be considered, as production of gene therapy vectors itself is cumbersome, requires specialized equipment and personnel and the administration of gene therapy is invasive in nature. Besides, specific gene therapy may not compare favourably to available pharmacological agents in use to treat ischemic heart disease in terms of cost-benefit ratio.

5. Conclusions and future directions

As of now, the applications of gene therapy for treatment of human diseases, including cardiovascular conditions, though appears to be extremely promising and fascinating, is, in the true sense of the term, still in its infancy. A vast magnitude of studies, not only on humans, but further studies on animal models, are still necessary to validate the practical efficacy of this widely-sought-after approach. Overcoming the practical difficulties discussed above is not an easy task and a tremendous amount of finance and infrastructure is an inevitable requirement to achieve this goal. In spite of that, there still remains a possibility that the gene therapeutically administered may not be expressed in the target individual, subject to an inability of the vectors to reach the target tissue, metabolism of the vectors by the immune system or the presence of other intracellular substances that may exert a negative regulation on the gene expression.

It is possible that extensive use of small animals for pre-clinical research may have led to excessive enthusiasm too early. Gene therapy testing on larger animals may provide a better insight into the true efficacy of specific therapies.

However, these shortcomings should not prove to be a permanent obstacle as the prospects offered by the advent of gene therapy have been extremely fascinating. The elucidation of the human genome has exposed a vast array of genes that are responsible for umpteen number of diseases; such as cystic fibrosis, familial hypercholesterolemia, Lesch-Nyhan syndrome, Alzheimer's disease, Parkinson's disease, Duchenne muscular dystrophy, multiple sclerosis and others. These genes offer potential candidates for regulation that can alter the course of the disease as against the current medications available that mainly provide symptomatic relief. Thus, the future for gene therapy appears to be very bright. A good political establishment to provide the necessary infrastructure and monetary support might go a long way to circumvent the existing shortcomings and empower gene therapy to grow as the most preferred and successful therapeutic approach to most of the diseases that were considered incurable till the past few decades.

6. References

Abunasra, H.J.; Smolenski, R.T.; Morrison, K. et al. (2001). Efficacy of adenoviral gene transfer with manganese superoxide dismutase and endothelial nitric oxide synthase in reducing ischaemia and reperfusion injury. *European Journal of Cardio-Thoracic Surgery* 20, 153–158.

Agata, J.; Chao, L. & Chao, J. (2002). Kallikrein gene delivery improves cardiac reserve and attenuates remodeling after myocardial infarction. *Hypertension* 40, 653–659.

Ahmet, I.; Sawa, Y.; Iwata, K. et al. (2002). Gene transfection of hepatocyte growth factor attenuates cardiac remodeling in the canine heart: a novel gene therapy for cardiomyopathy. *The Journal of Thoracic and Cardiovascular Surgery* 124, 957–963.

Ahmet, I.; Sawa, Y.; Yamaguchi, T. et al. (2003). Gene transfer of hepatocyte growth factor improves angiogenesis and function of chronic ischemic myocardium in canine heart. *The Annals of Thoracic Surgery* 75, 1283–1287.

American Heart Association, 2003, Heart and Stroke facts 2002: Statistical supplement. Dallas, USA

Aoki, M.; Morishita, R.; Taniyama, Y. et al. (2000) Angiogenesis induced by hepatocyte growth factor in non-infarcted myocardium and infarcted myocardium: upregulation of essential transcription factor for angiogenesis, ets. *Gene Therapy* 7, 417–27.

Arner, E. & Holmgren, A. (2000). Physiological functions of thioredoxin and thioredoxin reductase. *European Journal of Biochemistry* 267, 6102 – 6109.

Berry, M.F.; Pirolli, T.J.; Jayasankar, V. et al. (2004). Targeted overexpression of leukemia inhibitory factor to preserve myocardium in a rat model of postinfarction heart failure. *The Journal of Thoracic and Cardiovascular Surgery* 128, 866–875.

Borgstahl, G.E.; Parge, H.E.; Hickey, M.J. et al. (1996). Human mitochondrial manganese superoxide dismutase polymorphic variant Ile58Thr reduces activity by destabilizing the tetrameric interface. *Biochemistry* 35, 4287 - 4297.

Bull, D.A.; Bailey, S.H.; Rentz, J.J. et al. (2003) Effect of Terplex/ VEGF-165 gene therapy on left ventricular function and structure following myocardial infarction. VEGF gene therapy for myocardial infarction. *Journal of Controlled Release* 93, 175–181.

Cao, X.; Antonyuk, S.V.; Seetharaman, S.V. et al. (2008). Structures of the G85R variant of SOD1in familial amyotrophic lateral sclerosis. *Journal of Biological Chemistry* 283, 16169 - 16177.

Kumar, V.; Abbas, A.K.; Fausto, N. & Aster, J.C. (2010). Cellular Responses to Stress and Toxic Insults: Adaptation, Injury and Death. *Robbins and Cotran's Pathologic Basis of Disease*, Ed. 8, pp22-24, ISBN 978-81-312-2491-5; Pennsylvania, USA.

Chatterjee, S.; Stewart, A.S.; Bish, L.T. et al. (2002). Viral gene transfer of the antiapoptotic factor Bcl-2 protects against chronic postischemic heart failure. *Circulation* 106 (12 Suppl 1), I212–I217.

Chatterjee, S.; Bish, L.T.; Jayasankar, V. et al. (2003). Blocking the development of postischemic cardiomyopathy with viral gene transfer of the apoptosis repressor with caspase recruitment domain. *The Journal of Thoracic and Cardiovascular Surgery* 125, 1461–1469.

Chen, Z.; Siu, B.; Ho, Y. et al. (1998). Overexpression of MnSOD protects against Myocardial Ischemia/Reperfusion Injury in Transgenic Mice. *Journal of Molecular and Cellular Cardiology* 30, 2281 – 2289.

Cho, K.R.; Choi, J.S.; Hahn, W. et al. (2008). Therapeutic angiogenesis using naked DNA expressing two isoforms of the hepatocyte growth factor in a porcine acute myocardial infarction model. *European Journal of Cardio-thoracic Surgery* 34, 857–863.

Choi, J.S.; Kim, K.B.; Han, W. et al. (2006). Efficacy of therapeutic angiogenesis by intramyocardial injection of pCK-VEGF165 in pigs. *The Annals of Thoracic Surgery* 82, 679–686.

Cittadini, A.; Monti, M.G.; Iaccarino, G. et al. (2006). Adenoviral gene transfer of Akt enhances myocardial contractility and intracellular calcium handling. *Gene Therapy* 13, 8–19.

del Monte F, Harding SE, Schmidt U. et al. (1999). Restoration of contractile function in isolated cardiomyocytes from failing human hearts by gene transfer of SERCA2a. *Circulation* 100, 2308–2311.

del Monte, F.; Williams, E.; Lebeche, D. et al. (2001a). Improvement in survival and cardiac metabolism after gene transfer of sarcoplasmic reticulum Ca(2+)-ATPase in a rat model of heart failure. *Circulation* 104, 1424–1429.

del Monte, F.; Hajjar, R.J. & Harding, S.E. (2001b). Overwhelming evidence of the beneficial effects of SERCA gene transfer in heart failure. *Circulation Research* 88, E66–E67.

del Monte, F.; Harding, S.E.; Dec, G.W. et al. (2002). Targeting phospholamban by gene transfer in human heart failure. *Circulation* 105, 904-907.

Doney, A.S.; Dannfald, J.; Kimber, C.H. et al. (2009). The FTO gene is associated with an Atherogenic Lipid Profile and Myocardial Infarction in patients with type 2 diabetes mellitus. *Circulation: Cardiovascular Genetics* 2, 255 - 259.

Edelberg, J.M.; Lee, S.H.; Kaur, M. et al. (2002). Platelet-derived growth factor-AB limits the extent of myocardial infarction in a rat model: feasibility of restoring impaired angiogenic capacity in the aging heart. *Circulation* 105, 608-613.

Ferrarini, M.; Arsic, N.; Recchia, F.A. et al. (2006). Adeno-associated virus-mediated transduction of VEGF165 improves cardiac tissue viability and functional recovery after permanent coronary occlusion in conscious dogs. *Circulation Research* 98, 954–961.

Funatsu, T.; Sawa, Y.; Ohtake, S. et al. (2002). Therapeutic angiogenesis in the ischemic canine heart induced by myocardial injection of naked complementary DNA plasmid encoding hepatocyte growth factor. *The Journal of Thoracic and Cardiovascular Surgery* 124, 1099–1105.

Gao, M.H.; Lai, N.C.; McKirnan, M.D. et al. (2004). Increased regional function and perfusion after intracoronary delivery of adenovirus encoding fibroblast growth factor 4: report of preclinical data. *Human Gene Therapy* 15, 574–587.

Giordano, F.J.; Ping, P.; McKirnan, M.D. et al. (1996). Intracoronary gene transfer of fibroblast growth factor-5 increases blood flow and contractile function in an ischemic region of the heart. *Nature Medicine* 2, 534–539.

Hao, X.; Månsson-Broberg, A.; Gustafsson, T. et al. (2004a). Angiogenic effects of dual gene transfer of bFGF and PDGF-BB after myocardial infarction. *Biochemical and Biophysical Research Communications* 315, 1058-1063.

Hao, X.; Månsson-Broberg, A.; Blomberg, P. et al. (2004b). Angiogenic and cardiac functional effects of dual gene transfer of VEGF-A165 and PDGF-BB after myocardial infarction. *Biochemical and Biophysical Research Communications* 322, 292-296.

Hao, X.; Mansson-Broberg, A.; Grinnemo, K.H. et al. (2007). Myocardial angiogenesis after plasmid or adenoviral VEGF-A (165) gene transfer in rat myocardial infarction model. *Cardiovascular Research* 73, 481–487.

Hirsch, J.C.; Borton, A.R.; Albayya, F.P. et al. (2004). Comparative analysis of parvalbumin and SERCA2a cardiac myocytegene transfer in a large animal model of diastolic dysfunction. *American Journal of Physiology. Heart and Circulatory Physiology* 286, H2314-2321.

Horvath, K.A.; Doukas, J.; Lu, C.Y. et al. (2002). Myocardial functional recovery after fibroblast growth factor 2 gene therapy as assessed by echocardiography and magnetic resonance imaging. *The Annals of Thoracic Surgery* 74, 481–486.

Hsieh, P.C.; MacGillivray, C.; Gannon, J. et al. (2006). Local controlled intra myocardial delivery of platelet-derived growth factor improves post infarction ventricular function without pulmonary toxicity. *Circulation* 114, 637-644.

Iaccarino, G.; Tomhave, E.D.; Lefkowitz, R.J. et al. (1998). Reciprocal in vivo regulation of myocardial G protein-coupled receptor kinase expression by β-adrenergic receptor stimulation and blockade. *Circulation* 98, 1783–1789.

Jacquier, A.; Higgins, C.B.; Martin, A.J. et al. (2007). Injection of adeno associated viral vector encoding vascular endothelial growth factor gene in infarcted swine myocardium: MR measurements of left ventricular function and strain. *Radiology* 245, 196–205.

Jameel, M.N. & Zhang, J. (2009). Heart failure management: the present and the future. *Antioxidants and Redox Signaling* 11, 1989-2010.

Jayasankar, V.; Woo, Y.J.; Bish, L.T. et al. (2003). Gene transfer of hepatocyte growth factor attenuates postinfarction heart failure. *Circulation* 108 (Suppl 1), II230–II236.

Jin, H.; Wyss, J.M.; Yang, R. et al. (2004). The therapeutic potential of hepatocyte growth factor for myocardial infarction and heart failure. *Current Pharmaceutical Design* 10, 2525–2533.

Jin, Z.Q.; Zhang, J.; Huang, Y. et al. (2007). A sphingosine kinase 1 mutation sensitizes the myocardium to ischemia/reperfusion injury. *Cardiovascular Research* 76, 41-50.

Kadambi, V.J.; Ponniah, S.; Harrer, J.M. et al. (1996). Cardiac-specific overexpression of phospholamban alters calcium kinetics and resultant cardiomyocyte mechanics in transgenic mice. *Journal of Clinical Investigation* 97, 533-539.

Kaye, D.M.; Preovolos, A.; Marshall, T. et al. (2007). Percutaneous cardiac recirculation-mediated gene transfer of an inhibitory phospholambanpeptide reverses advanced heart failure in large animals. *Journal of the American College of Cardiology* 50, 253-260.

Kiriazis, H. & Kranias, E.G. (2000). Genetically engineered models with alterations in cardiac membrane calcium-handling proteins. *Annual Review of Physiology* 62, 321-351.

Kondo, I.; Ohmori, K.; Oshita, A. et al. (2004). Treatment of acute myocardial infarction by hepatocyte growth factor gene transfer: the first demonstration of myocardial transfer of a "functional" gene using ultrasonic microbubble destruction. *Journal of the American College of Cardiology* 44, 644–653.

Krausgrill, B.; Vantler, M.; Burst, V. et al. (2009). Influence of cell treatment with PDGF-BB and reperfusion on cardiac persistence of mononuclear and mesenchymal bone marrow cells after transplantation into acute myocardial infarction in rats. *Cell Transplantation* 18, 847-853.

Kusano, K.F.; Pola, R.; Murayama, T. et al. (2005). Sonic hedgehog myocardial gene therapy: tissue repair through transient reconstitution of embryonic signaling. *Nature Medicine* 11, 1197–204.

Lahteenvuo, J.E.; Lahteenvuo, M.T.; Kivela, A. et al. (2009). Vascular endothelial growth factor-B induces myocardium-specific angiogenesis and arteriogenesis via vascular endothelial growth factor receptor-1- and neuropilin receptor-1-dependent mechanisms. *Circulation* 119, 845–856.

Lai, N.C.; Roth, D.M. & Gao, M.H. (2004). Intracoronaryadenovirus encoding adenylyl cyclase VI increases leftventricular function in heart failure. *Circulation* 110, 330–336.

Lai, Z.F.; Chen, Y.Z.; Feng, L.P. et al. (2008). Overexpression of TNNI3K, a cardiac-specific MAP kinase, promotes P19CL6-derived cardiac myogenesis and prevents myocardial infarction-induced injury. *American Journal of Physiology. Heart and Circulatory Physiology* 295, H708–716.

Laitinen, M.; Hartikainen, J. & Eranen, J. (2000). Catheter-mediated VEGF-gene transfer to human coronary artery after angioplasty. *Human Gene Therapy* 110, 263 – 270.

Lee, L.Y.; Patel, S.R.; Hackett, N.R. et al. (2000). Focal angiogen therapy using intramyocardial delivery of an adenovirus vector coding for vascular endothelial growth factor 121. *The Annals of Thoracic Surgery* 69, 14–23

Lee, M.; Rentz, J.; Bikram, M. et al. (2003). Hypoxia-inducible VEGF gene delivery to ischemic myocardium using water-soluble lipopolymer. *Gene Ther*apy 10, 1535–1542.

Li, Q.; Bolli, R.; Qiu, Y. et al. (2001). Gene Therapy with Extracellular Superoxide Dismutase protects conscious rabbits against Myocardial Infarction. *Circulation* 103, 1893 - 1898.

Li, Y.; Takemura, G.; Kosai, K. et al. (2003). Postinfarction treatment with an adenoviral vector expressing hepatocyte growth factor relieves chronic left ventricular remodeling and dysfunction in mice. *Circulation* 107, 2499–506.

Losordo, D.W.; Vale, P.R.; Hendel, R.C. et al. (2002). Phase 1/2 placebo-controlled, double-blinded, dose-escalating trial of myocardial VEGF-2 Gene Transfer by Catheter Delivery in patients with chronic Myocardial Infarction. *Circulation* 105, 2012-2018.

Losordo, D.W.; Vale, P.R.; Symes, J.F. et al. (1998). Gene therapy for myocardial angiogenesis: initial clinical results with direct injection of ph.VEGF-165 as a sole therapy for myocardial ischemia. *Circulation* 98, 2800 - 2804.

Lu, H.; Xu, X.; Zhang, M. et al. (2007). Combinatorial protein therapy of angiogenic and arteriogenic factors remarkably improves collaterogenesis and cardiac function in pigs. *Proceedings of the National Academy of the Sciences of the USA*. 104, 12140-12145.

Mack, C.A.; Patel, S.R.; Schwarz, E.A. et al. (1998). Biologic bypass with the use of adenovirus-mediated gene transfer of the complementary deoxyribonucleic acid for vascular endothelial growth factor 121 improves myocardial perfusion and function in the ischemic porcine heart. *The Journal of Thoracic and Cardiovascular Surgery* 115, 168–176.

Maines, M.D. (1988). Heme oxygenase: Function, multiplicity, regulatory mechanisms, and clinical application. *FASEB J* 2, 557 - 2568.

McCord, J.M. & Fridovich, I. (1988). Superoxide dismutase, the first twenty years (1968 - 1988). *Free Radical Biology and Medicine* 5, 363 - 369.

Melo, L.G.; Agarwal, R.; Zhang, L. et al. (2002). Gene Therapy Strategy for Long-Term Myocardial Protection using Adeno-Associated Virus- Mediated Delivery of Heme Oxygenase gene. *Circulation* 105, 602 - 607.

Miao, W.; Luo, Z.; Kitsis, R.N. et al. (2000). Intracoronary, adenovirus-mediated Akt gene transfer in heart limits infarct size following ischemia–reperfusion injury in vivo. *Journal of Molecular and Cellular Cardiology* 32, 2397–402.

Michiels, C.; Raes, M.; Toussaint, O. et al. (1994). Importance of SE-glutathione peroxidase, catalase and Cu/Zn-SOD for cell survival against oxidative stress. *Free Radical Biology and Medicine* 17, 235 - 248.

Miyamoto, M.I.; del Monte, F.; Schmidt, U. et al. (1996). Altered expression of the Ca(2+)-binding protein S100A1 in human cardiomyopathy. *Biochimica et Biophysica Acta* 1313, 253–257.

Miyamoto, M.I.; del Monte, F.; Schmidt, U. et al. (2000). Adenoviral gene transfer of SERCA2a improves left-ventricular function in aortic-banded rats in transition to heart failure. *Proceedings of the National Academy of the Sciences of the USA* 97, 793-798.

Most, P.; Pleger, S.T.; Volkers, M. et al. (2004). Cardiac adenoviral S100A1 gene deliveryrescues failing myocardium. *Journal of Clinical Investigation* 114, 1550 -1563.

Most, P.; Seifert, H.; Gao, E. et al. (2006). Cardiac S100A1 protein levels determine contractile performance and propensity toward heart failure after myocardial infarction. *Circulation* 114, 1258 -1268.

Nabel, E.G.; Plautz, G.; Boyce, F.M. et al. (1989). Recombinant gene expression in vivo within endothelial cells of the arterial wall. *Science* 244, 1342-1344.

Okubo, S.; Wildner, O.; Shah, M.R. et al. (2001). Gene transfer of heat-shock protein 70 reduces infarct size in vivo after ischemia/reperfusion in the rabbit heart. *Circulation* 103, 877–881.

Patila, T.; Ikonen, T.; Rutanen, J. et al. (2006). Vascular endothelial growth factor C-induced collateral formation in a model of myocardial ischemia. *The Journal of Heart and Lung Transplantation* 25, 206–213.

Pleger, S.T.; Most, P.; Boucher, M. et al. (2007). Stable myocardial-specific AAV6-S100A1 gene therapy results in chronic functional heart failure rescue. *Circulation* 115, 2506–2515.

Post, M.J.; Sato, K.; Murakami, M. et al. (2006). Adenoviral PR39 improves blood flow and myocardial function in a pig model of chronic myocardial ischemia by enhancing collateral formation. *American Journal of Physiology. Regulatory, Integrative and Comparative Physiology* 290, R494–500.

Remppis, A.; Greten, T.; Schafer, B.W. et al. (1996). Altered expression of the Ca(2+)-binding protein S100A1 in human cardiomyopathy. *Biochimica et Biophysica Acta* 1313, 253–257.

Rosengart, T.K.; Lee, L.Y.; Patel, S.R. et. al. (1999). Angiogenesis gene therapy: Phase I assessment of direct intramyocardial administration of an adenovirus vector expressing VEGF-121 cDNA to individuals with clinically significant coronary artery disease. *Circulation* 100, 468–474.

Ruixing, Y.; Jiaquan, L.; Jie, C. & Dezhai, Y. (2006). Intravenous administration of vascular endothelial growth factor improves cardiac performance and inhibits cardiomyocyte apoptosis. *Growth Factors* 24, 209–217.

Ruixing, Y.; Jinzhen, W.; Dezhai, Y. et al. (2007). Cardioprotective role of cardiotrophin- 1 gene transfer in a murine model of myocardial infarction. *Growth Factors* 25, 286–294.

Rutanen, J.; Rissanen, T.T.; Markkanen, J.E. et al. (2004). Adenoviral catheter-mediated intramyocardial gene transfer using the mature form of vascular endothelial growth factor-D induces transmural angiogenesis in porcine heart. *Circulation* 109, 1029–1035.

Samuel, S.M.; Thirunavukkarasu, M.; Penumathsa, S.V. et al. (2010) Thioredoxin-1 gene therapy enhances angiogenic signaling and reduces ventricular remodeling in infarcted myocardium of diabetic rats. *Circulation* 121, 1244-55.

Shah, A.S.; Lilly, R.E.; Kypson, A.P. et al. (2000). Intracoronary adenovirus-mediated delivery and overexpression of the beta (2)-adrenergic receptor in the heart prospects for molecular ventricular assistance. *Circulation* 101, 408–14.

Su, H.; Arakawa-Hoyt, J. & Kan, Y.W. (2002). Adeno-associated viral vector-mediated hypoxia response element-regulated gene expression in mouse ischemic heart model. *Proceedings of the National Academy of the Sciences of the USA* 99, 9480–9485.

Sugano, M.; Tsuchida, K.; Hata, T. et al. (2004). In vivo transfer of soluble TNF-alpha receptor 1 gene improves cardiac function and reduces infarct size after myocardial infarction in rats. *FASEB J* 18, 911–913.

Suzuki, G.; Lee, T.C.; Fallavollita, J.A. et al. (2005). Adenoviral gene transfer of FGF-5 to hibernating myocardium improves function and stimulates myocytes to hypertrophy and reenter the cell cycle. *Circulation Research* 96, 767–775.

Suzuki, K.; Murtuza, B.; Sammut, I.A. et al. (2002). Heat shock protein 72 enhances manganese superoxide dismutase activity during myocardial ischemia-reperfusion injury, associated with mitochondrial protection and apoptosis reduction. *Circulation* 106 (12 Suppl 1), 1270–1276.

Symes, J.F.; Losordo, D.W.; Vale, P.R. et. al. (1999). Gene therapy with vascular endothelial growth factor for inoperable coronary artery disease. *The Annals of Thoracic Surgery* 68, 830 - 837.

Tamamori-Adachi, M.; Takagi, H.; Hashimoto, K. et al. (2008). Cardiomyocyte proliferation and protection against post-myocardial infarction heart failure by cyclin D1 and Skp2 ubiquitin ligase. *Cardiovascular Research* 80, 181-90.

Taniyama, Y.; Morishita, R.; Aoki, M. et al. (2002). Angiogenesis and antifibrotic action by hepatocyte growth factor in cardiomyopathy. *Hypertension* 40, 47–53.

Tenhunen, O.; Soini, Y.; Ilves, M. et al. (2006). p38 Kinase rescues failing myocardium after myocardial infarction: evidence for angiogenic and anti-apoptotic mechanisms. *FASEB J* 20, 1907–1909.

Tio, R.A.; Tkebuchava, T.; Scheuermann, T.H. et al. (1999). Intramyocardial gene therapy with naked DNA encoding vascular endothelial growth factor improves collateral flow to ischemic myocardium. *Human Gene Therapy* 10, 2953–2960.

Wang, W.; Yang, Z.J.; Ma, D.C. et al. (2006a). Induction of collateral artery growth and improvement of post-infarct heart function by hepatocyte growth factor gene transfer. *Acta Pharmacologica Sinica* 27, 555–560.

Wang, L.; Yang, J.; Liu, Z.X. et al. (2006b). Gene transfer of CD151 enhanced myocardial angiogenesis and improved cardiac function in rats with experimental myocardial infarction. *Zhonghua Xin Xue Guan Bing Za Zhi* 34, 159–163.

Wollmann, E.E.; d'Auriol, L.; Rimsky, L. et al. (1988). Cloning and expression of a cDNA of human thioredoxin. *Journal of Biological Chemistry* 263, 15506 - 15512.

Woo, Y.J.; Panlilio, C.M.; Cheng, R.K. et al. (2006). Therapeutic delivery of cyclin A2 induces myocardial regeneration and enhances cardiac function in ischemic heart failure. *Circulation* 114, I206–I213.

Yang, Z.; Wang, W.; Ma, D.; et al. (2007). Recruitment of stem cells by hepatocyte growth factor via intracoronary gene transfection in the postinfarction heart failure. *Science China Life Sciences* 50, 748–752.

Yang, Z.J.; Chen, B.; Sheng, Z. et al. (2010). Improvement of heart function in postinfarct heart failure swine models after hepatocyte growth factor gene transfer: comparison of low-, medium- and high-dose groups. *Molecular Biology Reports* 37, 2075–2081.

Yla-Hertella, S. & Martin, J.F. (2000). Cardiovascular gene therapy. *Lancet* 355, 213–222.

Yockman, J.W.; Choi, D.; Whitten, M.G. et al. (2009). Polymeric gene delivery of ischemia-inducible VEGF significantly attenuates infarct size and apoptosis following myocardial infarct. *Gene Therapy* 16, 127–135.

Zhang, D.; Gai, L.; Fan, R. et al. (2002). Efficacy and safety of therapeutic angiogenesis from direct myocardial administration of an adenoviral vector expressing vascular endothelial growth factor 165. *Chinese Medical Journal* 115, 643–648.

Zheng, J.; Shin, J.H.; Xaymardan, M. et al. (2004). Platelet-derived growth factor improves cardiac function in a rodent myocardial infarction model. *Coronary Artery Disease* 15, 59-64.

Zhu, Y.H.; Ma, T.M. & Wang, X. (2005). Gene transfer of heat-shock protein 20 protects against ischemia/reperfusion injury in rat hearts. *Acta Pharmacologica Sinica* 26, 1193–2000.

Zuo, H.; Liu, Z.; Liu, X. et al. (2009). CD151 gene delivery after myocardial infarction promotes functional neovascularization and activates FA signaling. *Molecular Medicine* 15, 307–315.

13

Gene Therapy for Therapeutic Angiogenesis

Rudolf Kirchmair
Dept. of Internal Medicine, Angiology
Medical University Innsbruck
Austria

1. Introduction

Cardiovascular diseases still represent the leading cause of death in the western world. Coronary artery disease (CAD) affects over 5% of the US population and is responsible for nearly 7 millions of in-patient procedures every year (1). Peripheral arterial disease (PAD), with a prevalence of 3-30%, also is a very common disease (2). PAD can be classified according to the severity of clinical symptoms into Fontaine-stages I-IV. In Fontaine-stage I patients are clinically asymptomatic and this stage is the most common form of PAD (70-80%). Patients with Fontaine II (10-20%) suffer from intermittent claudication that might be life-style limiting and require therapy like percutaneous transluminal angioplasty (PTA). A smaller portion (3-5%) of PAD patients have critical limb ischemia (CLI) characterized by rest pain (Fontaine III) or ulcer (Fontaine IV). The incidence of CLI is estimated to be 500-1000 per 1 Million but prognosis is very bad. One year after diagnosis only 45 % of patients are alive without major amputation and effective revascularization with relieve of symptoms can only be achieved in 25% of patients. Therefore, new therapeutic strategies are urgently needed for these patients.

2. Preclinical data

Generation of new blood vessels can be achieved by sprouting of new vessels out of the pre-existing capillary plexus (angiogenesis), by generation of new arteries (arteriogenesis) or by circulating endothelial progenitor cells (vasculogenesis) (3). Several factors have been characterized which induce growth of new blood vessels, the most prominent being vascular endothelial growth factor (VEGF) and members of the fibroblast growth factor (FGF) family. In animal models of hindlimb and myocardial ischemia beneficial effects on blood perfusion and blood vessel density of these (and other) factors as well as of progenitor cells could be demonstrated (4) (5). This therapeutic concept was named "therapeutic angiogenesis" and application of angiogenic factors via gene therapy vectors like plasmids or adenoviruses was superior to protein application probably due to longer lasting expression of respective cytokines.

3. Therapeutic angiogenesis: gene therapy trials in PAD patients

Due to promising data in preclinical studies the concept of therapeutic angiogenesis was tested in clinical trials in PAD and CAD patients. While first phase-1 studies in PAD patients were promising phase-II studies in patients with intermittent claudication were negative (see summary for clinical trials in PAD patients in table 1). Obviously especially patients with CLI respond to therapy with angiogenic factors and gene therapy seems to have a benefit over therapy with respective proteins.

Trial	Factor	Patients	Effects	Reference
Phase-1	VEGF-165 plasmid i.m.	n=6; CLI (Buerger's)	Increase ABI, collaterals; improvement ulcer, pain	Isner et al 1998 (6)
Phase-1	VEGF-165 plasmid i.m.	n=9; CLI	Increase ABI, collaterals; improvement ulcer, pain, walking time	Baumgartner et al 1998 (7)
PREVENT I Phase-1	E2F decoy, bypass graft ex-vivo	n=41; bypass OP	Reduction bypass-stenosis, - occlusion and - revision	Mann et al 1999 (8)
Phase-1	FGF-2 protein i.a.	n=13; claudication	Increase calf blood flow	Lazarous et al 2000 (9)
Phase-1	FGF-2 protein i.v.	n=24; claudication	No improvement of walking time, proteinuria	Cooper et al 2001(10)
Phase-1	FGF-1 Plasmid i.m.	n=66; CLI	Improvement TcPO2, ABI, pain, ulcer	Comerota et al 2002 (11)
TRAFFIC Phase-2	FGF-2 protein i.a.	n=195; claudication	Improvement walking time, ABI day 90, not 180	Lederman et al 2002 (12)
RAVE Phase-2	VEGF-121 adenovirus i.m.	n=105; claudication	No improvement of walking time	Rajagopalan et al 2003 (13)
Phase-1	VEGF-165 plasmid i.m.	n=21; CLI	Improvement ABI, collaterals, ulcer, pain	Shyu et al 2003 (14)
Phase-1/2	FGF-4 adenovirus i.m.	n=13, CLI	Improvement pain	Matyas et al 2005(15)
PREVENT III Phase-3	E2F decoy, bypass graft ex-vivo	n=1138 bypass operation	Secondary bypass patency improved; primary endpoint (time to bypass occlusion) negative	Conte et al 2006(16)

Trial	Factor	Patients	Effects	Reference
Phase-1/2	HGF plasmid i.m.	n=6; CLI	Improvement pain, ABI, TcPO2, ulcer	Morishita et al 2006(17)
Phase-1/2	FGF-2 gelatine-hydrogel	n=7; CLI	Improvement walking time, TcPO2, ABI, pain	Marui et al 2007(18)
DELTA-1 Phase-2	Del-1 plasmid i.m.	n=105; claudication	No improvement walking time, ABI	Grossman et al 2007(19)
Phase-1	HIF-1α/VP16 adenovirus i.m.	n=41; CLI	Improvement pain, ulcer	Rajagopalan et al 2007(20)
WALK Phase-2	HIF-1α/VP16 adenovirus i.m.	n=289 claudication	No difference in walking time	ACC 2009

Abbreviations: CLI, critical limb ischemia; ABI, ankle/brachial index; E2F, transcription factor E2F; HGF, hepatocyte growth factor; Del-1, developmentally regulated endothelial locus 1; HIF-1 α, hypoxia inducible factor-1 α ; Buerger's, thrombangitis obliterans Winiwater-Buerger; i.m., intra-muscular; i.v., intra-venous; i.a., intra-arterial; TcPO2, transcutaneous oxygen tension

Table 1. Therapeutic angiogenesesis in PAD.

Trial	Factor	Patients	Outcome
VEGF PVD Mäkinen et al (22)	VEGF-165 adenovirus or plasmid/liposome i.a. after PTA	n=54; claudication, CLI	Increase of vascular density
Groningen Kusumanto et al (23)	VEGF-165 plasmid i.m.	n=54; CLI	Improvement ABI, ulcers
TALISMAN Nikol et al (24)	FGF-1 plasmid i.m.	n=112; CLI	Reduction of amputations; primary endpoint (healing of ulcers) not reached
HGF-STAT Powell et al (25)	HGF plasmid i.m.	n=106; CLI	Improvement TcPO2
TAMARIS, Phase 3 AHA 2010	FGF-1 plasmid i.m.	n=525; CLI	Primary endpoint (major amputation or death) not reached

Abbreviations: ABI, ankle/brachial index; i.m., intra-muscular; i.v., intra-venous; i.a., intra-arterial; TcPO2, transcutaneous oxygen tension

Table 2. Therapeutic Angiogenesis in PAD:-larger placebo-controlled, double-blinded trials.

The last years several placebo-controlled double-blinded trials have been published which showed beneficial effects in CLI patients after i.m.plasmid gene therapy with VEGF, FGF1 or hepatocyte growth factor (HGF) (Tab. 2). Especially the TALISMAN study could demonstrate a reduction in amputation rate. Regarding potential adverse effects these studies did not show evidence of increase of cancer rates or proliferative retinopathy. (21)

The positive results of the TALISMAN study on reduction of amputation rate and mortality in CLI patients by FGF1 gene therapy was the basis for a large phase 3 study. Over 500 CLI patients were treated with FGF1 gene therapy versus placebo. The primary outcome after 12 months was a combined endpoint of major amputation above the ankle or death. The results of this trial, called TAMARIS, were presented at the AHA meeting, November 2010, in Chicago, USA. There was no difference in mortality and major amputation between FGF1 gene therapy and placebo. Also secondary endpoints were not different and there was no increase in occurrence of malignant diseases or proliferative retinopathy. The difference between the positive results in phase 2 (TALISMAN) and negative results in phase 3 (TAMARIS) were explained by a type-1 error (finding by chance) in the phase-2 study. It will be interesting to see the publication of the TAMARIS trial to further discuss the reasons for this negative trial and the different results of this trial and phase 2 TALISMAN.

4. Therapeutic angiogenesis: gene therapy trials in CAD patients

Several angiogenic cytokines (especially VEGF-A and FGF4) were tested in patients with severe chronic CAD in whom revascularization by angioplasty or bypass surgery was no further option and who suffered from severe angina and limited exercise tolerance (for recent excellent reviews please also see (26, 27). As observed in PAD-patients phase-1 and phase-2 studies showed feasibility of these therapies and signs of bioactivity. Specifically, gene therapy (adenovirus, administered intra-coronary) with FGF4 showed a trend toward increase in exercise time in the AGENT (Angiogenic Gene Therapy) trial and the subsequent phase-2 AGENT 2 trial showed reduction in reversible perfusion defect size (however not statistically significant due to one outlier in the placebo group). The phase-3 AGENT 3 and AGENT 4 trials were stopped early when an interim analysis of the AGENT 3 cohort indicated that the primary endpoint (change in exercise treadmill test after 12 weeks) was unlikely to differ between FGF4 and placebo. A pooled analysis of AGENT 3 and 4 however revealed that women and patients >65 years with severe angina had statistically significant improvement in angina class and exercise test. A subsequent gene therapy trial in women with CAD was stopped, apparently due to slow enrollment.

Also VEGF gene therapy was tested in CAD patients in randomized studies. In the Kuopio Angiogenesis Trial (KAT) no difference in restenosis rate (primary endpoint) was observed after intra-coronary VEGF gene therapy (plasmid liposome or adenovirus), however after 6 months increased myocardial perfusion was found after adenoviral VEGF application. In the Euroinject One study VEGF plasmid was injected intra- myocardial into regions with perfusion defects. The primary endpoint, improvement of myocardial perfusion was not reached, however, VEGF improved regional wall motion score.

For summary of controlled trials on therapeutic angiogenesis in CAD patients see table 3.

5. Future perspectives

The negative results of phase-3 trials AGENT and TAMARIS raise important question about therapeutic angiogenesis and gene therapy. What is the reason that therapeutic angiogenesis with factors like VEGF or FGF did improve outcomes in a variety of animal models but failed to improve human disease? One explanation is that often young animals were used

Trial	**Factor**	**Patients**	**Effects**	**Reference**
Phase-1/2	VEGF-2 plasmid i.myoc.	n=19; CCS3-4, RA, NR	Improvement angina class	Losordo et al 2002(28)
AGENT Phase-1/2	Adenovirus-FGF4; i.coro.	n=79; CCS2-3	Trend toward increase in exercise time	Grines et al 2002 (29)
AGENT 2 Phase-2	Adenovirus-FGF4; i.coro.	n=52; CCS2-4, RA, NR	Improvement of perfusion defects by SPECT (not sign.)	Grines et al 2003 (30)
VIVA Phase-2	VEGF protein i.coro., i.v.	n=178; RA, NR	Improvement angina class, no effect on exercise time	Henry et al 2003(31)
KAT Phase-2	VEGF-165 adenovirus or plasmid/liposome i.coro.	n=103; stable angina	Improvement in myocardial perfusion, no effect on restenosis	Hedman et al 2003(32)
EUROINJECT-ONE Phase-2	VEGF-165 Plasmid i.myoc.	n=80; CCS3-4, RA, NR	Improvement wall motion, no effect on myocardial perfusion	Kastrup et al 2005(33)
REVASC Open label	Adenovirus VEGF-121 i.myoc. (thoracotomy)	n=65; CCS2-4, RA, NR	Improvement in exercise time at 26 weeks, not at 12 weeks	Stewart et al 2006(34)
AGENT3/4 Phase-3	Adenovirus-FGF4; i.coro.	n=532; CCS2-4, RA, (AGENT4: NR)	Enrollment stopped after interim analysis, primary endpoint negative. Improvement angina and exercise time in women, older patients with severe symptoms	Henry et al 2007(35)

Abbreviations: CCS, Canadian cardiovascular society; i.coro., intra-coronary; i.myoc., intra-myocardial; i.v., intra-venous; NR, nonrevascularizable; RA, refractory stable angina;

Table 3. Controlled trials on therapeutic angiogenesis in CAD patients.

whereas in humans usually patients of older age and a variety of co-morbidities are affected. Additionally, transfection efficacy of gene therapy vectors, even of adenoviruses, is lower in humans than in animals and precise dosing of vectors is not possible due to the fact that transgene expression cannot be precisely quantified. Another open question is the selection of gene therapy vectors-adenoviruses usually have adverse effects, especially immunogenicity, whereas plasmid vectors are safe but have low transfection efficacy. Dose and duration of therapy is another question. One dose of a vector that expresses the transgene for days to weeks might not be sufficient to treat a disease that evolved over the time-course of many years. Also patient selection might have been a problem: usually "no-option" patients were included in these studies, e.g. patients with large ischemic ulcers in the case of CLI (Rutherford class 6). Maybe patients with less severe disease, like patients with Rutherford class 5 or patients who would be treated additionally with revascularization procedures would benefit more from therapeutic angiogenesis. Endpoint selection is another critical point as some functional outcome measurements like severity of angina are subjective and might be affected by the placebo effect. Cell-based therapies have shown positive effects in CAD and PAD (36, 37)-maybe a combined therapeutic strategy consisting of cell application and gene therapy with angiogenic factors would result in better outcome.

6. References

[1] Nikol, S. 2008. Gene therapy of cardiovascular disease. *Curr Opin Mol Ther* 10:479-492.

[2] Norgren, L., Hiatt, W.R., Dormandy, J.A., Nehler, M.R., Harris, K.A., Fowkes, F.G., Bell, K., Caporusso, J., Durand-Zaleski, I., Komori, K., et al. 2007. Inter-Society Consensus for the Management of Peripheral Arterial Disease (TASC II). *Eur J Vasc Endovasc Surg* 33 Suppl 1:S1-75.

[3] Carmeliet, P. 2000. Mechanisms of angiogenesis and arteriogenesis. *Nat Med* 6:389-395.

[4] Losordo, D.W., and Dimmeler, S. 2004. Therapeutic angiogenesis and vasculogenesis for ischemic disease: part I: angiogenic cytokines. *Circulation* 109:2487-2491.

[5] Losordo, D.W., and Dimmeler, S. 2004. Therapeutic angiogenesis and vasculogenesis for ischemic disease: part II: cell-based therapies. *Circulation* 109:2692-2697.

[6] Isner, J.M., Baumgartner, I., Rauh, G., Schainfeld, R., Blair, R., Manor, O., Razvi, S., and Symes, J.F. 1998. Treatment of thromboangiitis obliterans (Buerger's disease) by intramuscular gene transfer of vascular endothelial growth factor: preliminary clinical results. *J Vasc Surg* 28:964-973; discussion 973-965.

[7] Baumgartner, I., Pieczek, A., Manor, O., Blair, R., Kearney, M., Walsh, K., and Isner, J.M. 1998. Constitutive expression of phVEGF165 after intramuscular gene transfer promotes collateral vessel development in patients with critical limb ischemia. *Circulation* 97:1114-1123.

[8] Mann, M.J., Whittemore, A.D., Donaldson, M.C., Belkin, M., Conte, M.S., Polak, J.F., Orav, E.J., Ehsan, A., Dell'Acqua, G., and Dzau, V.J. 1999. Ex-vivo gene therapy of human vascular bypass grafts with E2F decoy: the PREVENT single-centre, randomised, controlled trial. *Lancet* 354:1493-1498.

[9] Lazarous, D.F., Unger, E.F., Epstein, S.E., Stine, A., Arevalo, J.L., Chew, E.Y., and Quyyumi, A.A. 2000. Basic fibroblast growth factor in patients with intermittent claudication: results of a phase I trial. *Journal of the American College of Cardiology* 36:1339-1344.

[10] Cooper, L.T., Jr., Hiatt, W.R., Creager, M.A., Regensteiner, J.G., Casscells, W., Isner, J.M., Cooke, J.P., and Hirsch, A.T. 2001. Proteinuria in a placebo-controlled study of basic fibroblast growth factor for intermittent claudication. *Vasc Med* 6:235-239.

[11] Comerota, A.J., Throm, R.C., Miller, K.A., Henry, T., Chronos, N., Laird, J., Sequeira, R., Kent, C.K., Bacchetta, M., Goldman, C., et al. 2002. Naked plasmid DNA encoding fibroblast growth factor type 1 for the treatment of end-stage unreconstructible lower extremity ischemia: preliminary results of a phase I trial. *J Vasc Surg* 35:930-936.

[12] Lederman, R.J., Mendelsohn, F.O., Anderson, R.D., Saucedo, J.F., Tenaglia, A.N., Hermiller, J.B., Hillegass, W.B., Rocha-Singh, K., Moon, T.E., Whitehouse, M.J., et al. 2002. Therapeutic angiogenesis with recombinant fibroblast growth factor-2 for intermittent claudication (the TRAFFIC study): a randomised trial. *Lancet* 359:2053-2058.

[13] Rajagopalan, S., Mohler, E.R., 3rd, Lederman, R.J., Mendelsohn, F.O., Saucedo, J.F., Goldman, C.K., Blebea, J., Macko, J., Kessler, P.D., Rasmussen, H.S., et al. 2003. Regional angiogenesis with vascular endothelial growth factor in peripheral arterial disease: a phase II randomized, double-blind, controlled study of adenoviral delivery of vascular endothelial growth factor 121 in patients with disabling intermittent claudication. *Circulation* 108:1933-1938.

[14] Shyu, K.G., Chang, H., Wang, B.W., and Kuan, P. 2003. Intramuscular vascular endothelial growth factor gene therapy in patients with chronic critical leg ischemia. *Am J Med* 114:85-92.

[15] Matyas, L., Schulte, K.L., Dormandy, J.A., Norgren, L., Sowade, O., Grotzbach, G., Palmer-Kazen, U., Rubanyi, G.M., and Wahlberg, E. 2005. Arteriogenic gene therapy in patients with unreconstructable critical limb ischemia: a randomized, placebo-controlled clinical trial of adenovirus 5-delivered fibroblast growth factor-4. *Hum Gene Ther* 16:1202-1211.

[16] Conte, M.S., Bandyk, D.F., Clowes, A.W., Moneta, G.L., Seely, L., Lorenz, T.J., Namini, H., Hamdan, A.D., Roddy, S.P., Belkin, M., et al. 2006. Results of PREVENT III: a multicenter, randomized trial of edifoligide for the prevention of vein graft failure in lower extremity bypass surgery. *J Vasc Surg* 43:742-751; discussion 751.

[17] Morishita, R., Aoki, M., Hashiya, N., Makino, H., Yamasaki, K., Azuma, J., Sawa, Y., Matsuda, H., Kaneda, Y., and Ogihara, T. 2004. Safety evaluation of clinical gene

therapy using hepatocyte growth factor to treat peripheral arterial disease. *Hypertension* 44:203-209.

[18] Marui, A., Tabata, Y., Kojima, S., Yamamoto, M., Tambara, K., Nishina, T., Saji, Y., Inui, K., Hashida, T., Yokoyama, S., et al. 2007. A novel approach to therapeutic angiogenesis for patients with critical limb ischemia by sustained release of basic fibroblast growth factor using biodegradable gelatin hydrogel: an initial report of the phase I-IIa study. *Circ J* 71:1181-1186.

[19] Grossman, P.M., Mendelsohn, F., Henry, T.D., Hermiller, J.B., Litt, M., Saucedo, J.F., Weiss, R.J., Kandzari, D.E., Kleiman, N., Anderson, R.D., et al. 2007. Results from a phase II multicenter, double-blind placebo-controlled study of Del-1 (VLTS-589) for intermittent claudication in subjects with peripheral arterial disease. *Am Heart J* 153:874-880.

[20] Rajagopalan, S., Olin, J., Deitcher, S., Pieczek, A., Laird, J., Grossman, P.M., Goldman, C.K., McEllin, K., Kelly, R., and Chronos, N. 2007. Use of a constitutively active hypoxia-inducible factor-1alpha transgene as a therapeutic strategy in no-option critical limb ischemia patients: phase I dose-escalation experience. *Circulation* 115:1234-1243.

[21] Tongers, J., Roncalli, J.G., and Losordo, D.W. 2008. Therapeutic angiogenesis for critical limb ischemia: microvascular therapies coming of age. *Circulation* 118:9-16.

[22] Makinen, K., Manninen, H., Hedman, M., Matsi, P., Mussalo, H., Alhava, E., and Yla-Herttuala, S. 2002. Increased vascularity detected by digital subtraction angiography after VEGF gene transfer to human lower limb artery: a randomized, placebo-controlled, double-blinded phase II study. *Mol Ther* 6:127-133.

[23] Kusumanto, Y.H., van Weel, V., Mulder, N.H., Smit, A.J., van den Dungen, J.J., Hooymans, J.M., Sluiter, W.J., Tio, R.A., Quax, P.H., Gans, R.O., et al. 2006. Treatment with intramuscular vascular endothelial growth factor gene compared with placebo for patients with diabetes mellitus and critical limb ischemia: a double-blind randomized trial. *Hum Gene Ther* 17:683-691.

[24] Nikol, S., Baumgartner, I., Van Belle, E., Diehm, C., Visona, A., Capogrossi, M.C., Ferreira-Maldent, N., Gallino, A., Wyatt, M.G., Wijesinghe, L.D., et al. 2008. Therapeutic angiogenesis with intramuscular NV1FGF improves amputation-free survival in patients with critical limb ischemia. *Mol Ther* 16:972-978.

[25] Powell, R.J., Simons, M., Mendelsohn, F.O., Daniel, G., Henry, T.D., Koga, M., Morishita, R., and Annex, B.H. 2008. Results of a double-blind, placebo-controlled study to assess the safety of intramuscular injection of hepatocyte growth factor plasmid to improve limb perfusion in patients with critical limb ischemia. *Circulation* 118:58-65.

[26] Gupta, R., Tongers, J., and Losordo, D.W. 2009. Human studies of angiogenic gene therapy. *Circ Res* 105:724-736.

[27] Beohar, N., Rapp, J., Pandya, S., and Losordo, D.W. 2010. Rebuilding the damaged heart: the potential of cytokines and growth factors in the treatment of ischemic heart disease. *J Am Coll Cardiol* 56:1287-1297.

[28] Losordo, D.W., Vale, P.R., Hendel, R.C., Milliken, C.E., Fortuin, F.D., Cummings, N., Schatz, R.A., Asahara, T., Isner, J.M., and Kuntz, R.E. 2002. Phase 1/2 placebo-controlled, double-blind, dose-escalating trial of myocardial vascular endothelial growth factor 2 gene transfer by catheter delivery in patients with chronic myocardial ischemia. *Circulation* 105:2012-2018.

[29] Grines, C.L., Watkins, M.W., Helmer, G., Penny, W., Brinker, J., Marmur, J.D., West, A., Rade, J.J., Marrott, P., Hammond, H.K., et al. 2002. Angiogenic Gene Therapy (AGENT) trial in patients with stable angina pectoris. *Circulation* 105:1291-1297.

[30] Grines, C.L., Watkins, M.W., Mahmarian, J.J., Iskandrian, A.E., Rade, J.J., Marrott, P., Pratt, C., and Kleiman, N. 2003. A randomized, double-blind, placebo-controlled trial of Ad5FGF-4 gene therapy and its effect on myocardial perfusion in patients with stable angina. *J Am Coll Cardiol* 42:1339-1347.

[31] Henry, T.D., Annex, B.H., McKendall, G.R., Azrin, M.A., Lopez, J.J., Giordano, F.J., Shah, P.K., Willerson, J.T., Benza, R.L., Berman, D.S., et al. 2003. The VIVA trial: Vascular endothelial growth factor in Ischemia for Vascular Angiogenesis. *Circulation* 107:1359-1365.

[32] Hedman, M., Hartikainen, J., Syvanne, M., Stjernvall, J., Hedman, A., Kivela, A., Vanninen, E., Mussalo, H., Kauppila, E., Simula, S., et al. 2003. Safety and feasibility of catheter-based local intracoronary vascular endothelial growth factor gene transfer in the prevention of postangioplasty and in-stent restenosis and in the treatment of chronic myocardial ischemia: phase II results of the Kuopio Angiogenesis Trial (KAT). *Circulation* 107:2677-2683.

[33] Kastrup, J., Jorgensen, E., Ruck, A., Tagil, K., Glogar, D., Ruzyllo, W., Botker, H.E., Dudek, D., Drvota, V., Hesse, B., et al. 2005. Direct intramyocardial plasmid vascular endothelial growth factor-A165 gene therapy in patients with stable severe angina pectoris A randomized double-blind placebo-controlled study: the Euroinject One trial. *J Am Coll Cardiol* 45:982-988.

[34] Stewart, D.J., Hilton, J.D., Arnold, J.M., Gregoire, J., Rivard, A., Archer, S.L., Charbonneau, F., Cohen, E., Curtis, M., Buller, C.E., et al. 2006. Angiogenic gene therapy in patients with nonrevascularizable ischemic heart disease: a phase 2 randomized, controlled trial of AdVEGF(121) (AdVEGF121) versus maximum medical treatment. *Gene Ther* 13:1503-1511.

[35] Henry, T.D., Grines, C.L., Watkins, M.W., Dib, N., Barbeau, G., Moreadith, R., Andrasfay, T., and Engler, R.L. 2007. Effects of Ad5FGF-4 in patients with angina: an analysis of pooled data from the AGENT-3 and AGENT-4 trials. *J Am Coll Cardiol* 50:1038-1046.

[36] Schachinger, V., Erbs, S., Elsasser, A., Haberbosch, W., Hambrecht, R., Holschermann, H., Yu, J., Corti, R., Mathey, D.G., Hamm, C.W., et al. 2006. Intracoronary bone marrow-derived progenitor cells in acute myocardial infarction. *N Engl J Med* 355:1210-1221.

[37] Walter, D.H., Krankenberg, H., Balzer, J.O., Kalka, C., Baumgartner, I., Schluter, M., Tonn, T., Seeger, F., Dimmeler, S., Lindhoff-Last, E., et al. 2011. Intraarterial Administration of Bone Marrow Mononuclear Cells in Patients With Critical Limb Ischemia: A Randomized-Start, Placebo-Controlled Pilot Trial (PROVASA). *Circ Cardiovasc Interv* 4:26-37.

14

Cancer Gene Therapy - Developments and Future Perspectives

David A Good[1,2], Wei Duan[3], Jozef Anné[4] and Ming Q Wei[1]
[1]*Division of Molecular Medicine and Gene Therapy, Griffith Health Institute, Schoolof Medical Science, Gold Coast campus, Griffith University, Qld,*
[2]*School of Physiotherapy, Australian Catholic University, McAuley Campus, Banyo, Qld,*
[3]*School of Medicine, Deakin University, Waurn Ponds, VIC.,*
[4]*Rega Institute for Medical Research, Minderbroedersstraat 10, Leuven,*
[1,2,3]*Australia*
[4]*Belgium*

1. Introduction

Cancer is the second leading cause of death in the Western world. Whilst there are many therapies which can significantly improve patient outcomes, there is still no definitive "cure" for cancer. Over the last decade we have witnessed gene therapy developing at a very fast pace representing a potential new and more effective modality for the treatment of cancer. By the end of 2010, over 1060 gene therapy protocols have been proposed or trialled in the clinical setting for various cancers; this figure represents over 64% of all gene therapy trials in humans in the United States. From many of these trials modest therapeutic responses have been reported, however, unequivocal proof of clinical efficacy is still to be seen. In 2003, the first commercially produced gene based product was manufactured by Shenzhen SiBiono GeneTech. Gendicine™, a replication-incompetent recombinant human Ad5-p53, was approved by the Chinese State Food and Drug Administration to treat head and neck squamous cell carcinoma. Again in 2006, Shanghai Sunway Biotech, commercially released a conditionally replicative adenovirus therapy, Oncorine™[8]. However, it is fair to say that cancer gene therapy has yet to realise its full potential.

2. The gene therapy vector systems

An important feature for any successful gene therapy protocol is the vector system. To date, a number of vectors have been developed, including both viral and non-viral based therapy systems (Table 1). Each of these vectors possesses a number of unique features and each has its own advantages and disadvantages. The most promising existing vectors are the replication-competent oncolytic viral vector based gene therapy systems, particularly the adenoviruses[9, 10].

Vector	Advantages	Disadvantages
Adenovirus	Easy to produce, Can achieve high titre, High efficiency of gene transfer	Large DNA virus, many viral genes, often Immunogenic
Adeno-associated virus	Relatively easy to produce, Has ability for gene integration	Wide type Adenovirus contamination
Retrovirus	Can be made through packaging cells, Has ability for gene integration	Low efficiency of gene transfer, dividing cells only
Herpesvirus	Has Neurotropic affinity, Can be applied to Neurons or Glioma	Large DNA virus, many viral genes, Immunogenic
Viral replicons: Semliki Forest virus	Easy production, less immunogenic	Difficult to purify
Non-viral vectors	Simple, easy to make and easy to use	Low efficiency

Table 1. List of commonly used vectors for cancer gene therapy as well as their advantages and disadvantages

3. Viral vector systems

3.1 Adenoviral vectors

Adenovirus vector (AV) is the most commonly studied and most widely used system in cancer gene therapy. It is of particular use for cancer gene therapy applications, where temporary gene expression is acceptable or even beneficial. There are several serotypes, but the currently employed AVs in clinical trials are mostly based on serotype 5. These vectors can replicate highly and have demonstrated efficient gene transfer into various types of cancer cells[11]. Two AVs related gene therapy products have been approved for clinical use in patients suffering from head and neck cancers in China, replication-incompetent recombinant human Ad5-p53[12], and the other is a conditionally replicative adenovirus therapy.

Several other adenoviruses, based on canine, porcine, bovine, ovine and avian adenoviruses have been developed. The ovine AV is based on serotype 7 and was developed in Australia. Preclinical testing of ovine AV on prostate cancer in animal models has shown therapeutic efficacy[13].

Unfortunately, AVs contain many viral genes which encode for major proteins that elicit a strong host immune response. Of particular concern is the release of cytotoxic T lymphocytes that lyse cells expressing the recombinant genes. Newer generations of AV vector have been designed to overcome some of these problems and initial results are encouraging. New techniques involved in removing the recombinant viral genes and transfecting the non-recombinant plasmid with a helper virus and then separating the helper virus with sedimentation techniques have been developed. Improvements in helper virus have also been trialled that reduces "floxed" helper virus production 1000-fold, but this method still has a 1% wide type (WT) contamination thus still allowing the possibility of *in vivo* recombination. With regard to AV-mediated cancer treatment, high-level tumour transduction remains a key developmental hurdle. To this end, AV vectors possessing infectivity enhancement and targeting capabilities should be evaluated in the most stringent model systems possible. Advanced AV-based vectors with imaging, targeting and therapeutic capabilities have yet to be fully realized; however, the feasibilities leading to this accomplishment are within close reach[14].

3.2 Adeno-associated virus (AAV)-based vectors

AAV-based vectors have been shown to be non-toxic and undergo widespread cellular uptake in preclinical evaluation[15]. A recent study has compared five different AAV strains and amongst them, serotype 2 was proven to be the most efficient killers of tumour cells. In another study, serotype 8 AAV vector encoding a soluble vascular endothelial growth factor (VEGF) receptor was able to halt tumour growth in several rodent glioma models. However, difficulties in the development of packaging cell lines for AAV, as well as bulk production and vector purification have been reported as problematic[16]. A new system was developed recently to scale up and bulk production of AAV from insect cells which may solve some of these existing problems[16].

3.3 Retroviral vectors

The earliest system that was developed for gene therapy was the murine Moloney leukaemia virus (MoMLV)-based retroviral vector. More than 23% of all gene therapy trials in patients for various diseases have used a replication-defective or competent MoMLV vector system. This vector's unique ability to transduce dividing cells[17] makes it an ideal choice of vector for continuously dividing and fast growing tumours, such as gliomas. However, poor vector penetration and lack of vector migration away from the injection site is usually seen[18]. To overcome this effect, replication competent MoMLV was developed. A 2005 publication showed complete transduction of human U87 glioma xenografts in nude mice after a single intracranial (*i.c.*) injection of replication-competent MoMLV[19]. In this study, viral envelope was stained positively in glioma cells away from the injection sites. Most importantly, no virus was detected in any non-tumour tissue which is good indication of strict tumour specificity.

Potential limitations of retroviral vector systems are related to their ability to activate cellular oncogenes and inactivate tumour suppressor genes by insertional mutagenesis. One study used MoMLV to transduce bone marrow stem cells for the therapy of severe combined immune deficiency syndrome (SCID), following treatment 4 out of 11 children subsequently developed leukaemia[20]. In addition to improving safety, there are also studies that have shown that dissemination of the vectors in solid tumours still needed to be improved in order to reach clinical efficacy.

Lentiviral vectors are a more recently developed and complicated retroviral vector, based on the Human or Bovine Immunodeficiency Virus. They have all the unique features of MoMLV and have been shown to transduce post mitotic cells *in vitro* and *in vivo*[21]. Studies with the Human Immunodeficiency Virus (HIV)-based vectors have shown efficient gene transfer in tumour models. An understandable reluctance in the use of potentially pathogenic HIV vectors in humans has been seen, although a clinical trial assessing use of lentiviral vector for the therapy of AIDS is underway[22]. To reduce the risk of seroconversion in human patients several bovine based vector systems have been developed, which have the advantage of less or no pathogenicity in humans. We have also developed a bovine lentiviral vector system based on the Jembrana Disease virus (JDV)[23, 24]. JDV only causes disease in a specific species of cattle in the Jembrana district in Bali,

Indonesia, but does not affect humans. Pathological changes in cattle include intense non-follicular lympho-proliferation by reticulum and lymphoblastoid cells in lymphoid organs. Protein and genome sequence studies have confirmed that JDV has a genome of 7732 nucleotides and structure and organisation similar to other members of the lentivirus family. More importantly, JDV possesses several features in common with HIV that are very attractive as a vector, including a high replication rate and the ability to efficiently integrate into chromosomes of non-dividing and terminally differentiated cells.

3.4 Herpesvirus-based vectors

Vectors based on herpesviruses are well-developed and have progressed to clinical trials. As with other viral vectors, replication-defective vectors have not shown much potential. The first replication competent vector was based on a mutant strain, where the vectors are deleted from the main neurovirulence gene r34.5, thus restricting its ability to replicate in adult central nervous system and to form latency. However, later study showed that the mutant strain which had the deletion of the r34.5 gene also had reduced capacity for replication inside tumour cells[25]. New vectors were developed with a deletion of the ICP47 gene which does not appear to impact on efficient replication.

Pre-existing immunity may pose a problem that limits the clinical efficacy of herpesvirus-based vectors. This immunity prevents the transduction of peripheral organs and also can cause liver toxicity. However, a recent mutant strain-secreting cytokine granule macrophage colony stimulatory factor (GM-CSF) or IL-12 was shown to be effective in liver cancer therapy in a murine model which likely involves both direct viral oncolysis and actions of specific immune effector cells[26].

3.5 Viral replicons and transposons

Semliki Forest virus (SFV) subgenomic replicons (i.e. non toxic replication) have been developed that allow stable expression of a required gene e.g. beta-galactosidase (beta-Gal) in mammalian cell lines. Studies showed that expression remained high (approximately 150 pg per cell) throughout cell passages[27].

Since construction of the Sleeping Beauty transposon from defective copies of a Tc1/*mariner* fish element[28], new vertebrate genetic manipulation tools (i.e. transposase enzymes) have become available for gene therapy. This particular transposase in the system binds to the inverted repeats of salmonid transposons that surround the insertion gene and mediate precise 'cut and paste' into fish, mouse and human chromosomes. Potential problems with the use of transposons for gene therapy may arise from having no 'off' switch for the transposase and the relatively low quantities of integrated product, either of which would make retroviral intergrase a more suitable or alternative enzyme for chromosomal integration.

3.6 Targeted viral vectors

While efforts have been focused on the continuing refinement of various vector systems, several obstacles remain, primarily the low efficiency of gene delivery into target tumour cells. The vascular endothelial wall is a significant physical barrier prohibiting access of systemically administered vectors to the tumour cell. To overcome this obstacle, strategies are currently being developed to take advantage of transcytosis pathways through the endothelium. An AV vector targeted to the transcytosing transferrin receptor pathway, using the bifunctional adapter molecule has been constructed[29]. The transcytosed AV virions retain the ability to infect cells, establishing the feasibility of this approach. However, efficiency of AV trafficking via this pathway is poor. Other efforts are directed towards exploring other transcytosing pathways such as the melanotransferrin pathway, the poly-IgA receptor pathway, or caveolae-mediated transcytosis pathways. There are hopes to develop mosaic AV vectors incorporating both targeting ligands directed to such transcytosis pathways as well as ligands mediating subsequent targeting and infection of tumour cells present beyond the vascular wall[30].

3.7 Viral vector-associated multifunctional particles (MFPs)

Nanotechnology has recently been incorporated into viral vector systems in the form of multifunctional particles (MFPs). Nanotechnology is defined as the development of devices of 100 nm or smaller, having unique properties due to their scale. The devices that are being developed generally incorporate inorganic or biological material. In this regard, the coupling of inorganic nano-scale materials to targeted AV vectors has much potential for tumour targeting, imaging and amplified tumour killing capacities. For example, magnetic nano-particles have recently received much attention due to their potential application in clinical cancer treatment; targeted drug delivery and magnetic resonance imaging (MRI) contrast agents[31]. However, despite the useful functionalities that might derive from metal nanoparticle systems, the lack of targeting strategies has limited their application to locoregional disease. Thus, tumour-selective delivery is the key to improve therapeutic applications of this technology.

AAV has been developed with MFP, by virtue of genetic capsid modifications, to incorporate additional functionalities, such as modified fibres, combined with imaging motifs on the pIX protein, to simultaneously target tumour cells while monitoring viral replication and spread. Herpes simplex virus thymidine kinase (HSV TK) has been incorporated at pIX site of the AAV capsid. This enzyme is compatible with available PET imaging ligands such as ^{18}F-penciclovir, providing an imaging system for viral replication that can directly be translated for clinical applications. Interestingly, HSV TK is an enzyme that has utility in so-called suicide gene therapy, in which the expressed enzyme converts a substrate such as ganciclovir to its phosphorylated metabolite, which can then be further phosphorylated by cellular kinases to a toxic metabolite, causing cell death[32]. Also, tumour cells expressing this gene product induce the death of adjacent cells via the so-called 'bystander effect', thus representing an 'amplifying strategy' as mentioned above.

3.8 Oncolytic virus

An oncolytic virus is a virus that has the ability to infect cancer cells and cause oncolysis. It is with obvious reasons that these types of viruses have received much attention in the field of cancer therapy as they can result in direct destruction of the tumour cells. Initial research into the anticancer potential of oncolytic viruses examined naturally occurring oncolytic viruses including adenovirus, poliovirus and Coxsackie virus[33-36]. However, these studies highlighted a number of limitations with naturally occurring oncolytic viruses including uncontrolled infection, incomplete oncolysis and the development of an immune response[33, 35]. The stimulation of the immune system prevented the virus from destroying the cancer and therefore reduced the efficacy of the treatment. Due to these limitations many researchers discontinued their research into naturally occurring oncolytic viruses.

Recent advances in genetic modification techniques of oncolytic viruses have again awoken researchers' interest into these agents for cancer therapy. There are now many different oncolytic viruses currently being trailed as potential therapeutic agents (Table 2)(reviewed in [37]). The first to be produced for the clinic was ONYX-015 which has been shown to be a safe anticancer agent[38, 39].

Name	Oncolytic virus strain	Type of tumour
ONYX-015	Adenovirus	Head & neck Ovarian Primary & secondary liver tumours Pancreatic
CV706	Adenovirus	Prostate
CV787	Adenovirus	Prostate
G207	HSV	Glioma
NV1020	HSV	Colorectal Liver metastases
Vaccinia-GM-CSF	Vaccinia	Melanoma
PV701	NDV	Advanced solid tumour
1716	HSV	Glioma Melanoma

Table 2. List of oncolytic viruses used in clinical trials (*adapted from* [37]).

4. Limitation of viral vectors

Although both viral vectors and oncolytic viruses are widely used in cancer gene therapy research, these vectors suffer from several limitations. The first of these is the virus's inability to specifically seek out and target the tumour. The majority of therapies that utilize these vectors currently require intratumoural injection to elicit an effect. Whilst this approach may be beneficial in some cases, its uses are limited as many tumours are inaccessible and may have already spread to other areas of the body at the time of diagnosis and treatment, making them difficult to locate and treat. Another deficiency of viral vectors is their lack of capacity to efficiently penetrate and kill every cell within the tumour mass. This results in non-tumour stromal cells being unaffected thus having the ability to regrow into another tumour. Finally, the tumours hypoxic microenvironment also reduces the effectiveness of the viral vector.

Hypoxia is a prevalent feature found within most solid tumours. When a tumour grows to and exceeds about 2mm in diameter, the local vasculatures of the surrounding normal tissues become inadequate to support the growing mass[40]. This results in a increase in angiogenesis within the tumour resulting in the tumour becoming more vascularised. However, the normal efficient vascular architecture is disturbed and chaotic inside the growing tumour mass which leads to areas of tumour hypoxia, acidity, nutrient deficiency and cell death. These hypoxic regions have the ability to reduce the effectiveness of viral vectors thereby decreasing gene expression and proliferation leaving a proportion of the tumour mass unaffected, which may result in tumour regrowth.

4.1 Oncolytic clostridia

Solid tumours account for approximately 90% of all diagnosed cancer. Our current understanding of the unique microenvironment of solid tumours has highlighted the deficiencies of both traditional therapies and new viral gene therapies and now requires a rethink in the design of vectors. As mentioned, this hypoxic core provides a barrier for current gene therapy vectors; however, it is also the perfect environment for anaerobic bacteria.

Class	Species	Features	Advantages	Disadvantages
Class I:	*B. longum*	Gram+ non-motile	Non-pathogenic present in common intestinalflora,	No obvious oncolytic effect
Bifido-bacteria	*B. adolescentis*	obligate anaerobes	Have been used in human for many years	Non-spore former
	B. infantis		Probiotic bacteria	More susceptible to non-
			Can be used for intravenous or oral administration	permissive conditions
			Expression of recombinant protein	More difficult to store and handle
Class II:	*Salmonella*	Gram- facultative	Attenuated vaccine strain has been proved safe	Intracellular bacteria, thus may have difficulty to
Facultative	*S. typhimurium*	anaerobes	clinically in human,	infect and lyse quiescent
intracellular	*S. choleraesuis*	Agent for	Biochemistrypathway s and	cell
bacteria		intestine infection	genomes are well characterized	Have a tumour to normal tissue ratio of 1000:1,
			Auxotrophic isolates for	therefore a significant
			solid tumours have intrinsic antitumour activity	number of bacteria colonize normal organs
				Cell wall components are immunogenic
	Listeria	Gram+, facultative	Grow under aerobic and anaerobic conditions, thus	Virulence factors exist, especially LPS in the
	L. monocytogenes	anaerobes	can target both large and	bacterial cell wall, thus
	E. coli	Gram-,	small tumours, enter	safety is an issue

Class	Species	Features	Advantages	Disadvantages
		facultative	professional antigen	when large amount of bacteria
		anaerobes	presenting cells and induce strong innate immune response Have the potential as a vaccine vector for tumour therapy Biology is well studied and known	are delivered
Class III:	*Clostridium*	Gram+, strictly	Spore former	Some strains are
Strictly	Proteolytic	anaerobes	Spores are stable, easy to	pathogenic
Anaerobic	*C. sporogenes*	normal habitat in the soil,	produce and economic to use	Some strains are difficult to manipulate genetically
bacteria	Saccharolytic	aquatic sediments,	Clostridialspores can be delivered non-invasively	Only colonize in large tumours with area of
	C. novyi	and intestinal tract of both	and systemically, i.e. intravenous injection	hypoxia/necrosis
	C. butyricum	animals and humans	Have shown extensive oncolytic ability	Oncolysis interrupted at the rim causing incomplete
	C. acetobutylicum		Spores are non-immunogenic and can be	tumour lysis
	C. oncolyticum		repeatedly delivered	
	C. beijerinckii		Oncolysis occurs irrespective of tumour cells' heterogeneity or growth status	

Table 3. Types of aerobic and facultative anaerobes used in cancer gene therapy (*adapted from* [41]).

Both facultative and obligate anaerobic bacteria have several advantages over traditional viral vector systems as they have been shown to selectively target, colonise and regerminate into vegetative cells in the hypoxic microenvironment of solid tumours when delivered systemically (Table 2)[41]. One such bacterium, the strictly anaerobic *Clostridia*, have also been shown to cause tumour lysis and destruction even without any genetic modification. A number of non-pathogenic strains of *Clostridia* have also shown plausible safety when used in humans. However, these vectors also have limitations. As these bacterium require an anaerobic environment to survive, oncolysis is almost always stalled at the proliferative outer rim of the tumour mass. More recently, combinational approaches have to be implemented to deal with these limitations and a number of trials have commenced to test these protocols.

The intrinsic property of *Clostridia* to specifically target and colonise only within the hypoxic core of the tumour enables them to serve as perfect vectors for the delivery of genes for cancer therapy. Already, clostridial spores have been genetically manipulated to deliver genes for cancerstatic factors, prodrug converting enzymes, or cytokines with the aim of improving their innate oncolytic activity. Furthermore, when used in combination with conventional chemotherapy or radiation therapies these vectors often perform better then *Clostridia* alone. Another advantage of clostridial spores is their seemingly unlimited capacity to carry exogenous genes. This remarkable characteristic will allow for the development of novel ways to equip *Clostridia* with gene combinations that may have the ability to break immune suppression, overcome the limitation of tumour lysis in the outer rim or cause a strong anti-tumour response with the ability to eliminate tumour metastases, the ultimate cause of cancer death.

It is obvious that a major step towards the development of an effective cancer therapy will be to construct a vector that targets the tumour alone, and is capable of spreading to and throughout the tumour found in tissues. Clostridial spores fit into this equation very well. Clostridia are strictly anaerobic. They are gram-positive, rod-shaped, and form spores under unfavourable conditions. There are about 80 species and several of these have been tested in solid tumours. All known species require anaerobic conditions to grow but do vary in their oxygen tolerance and their biochemical profile. Clostridial spores have been administered intravenously and showed a distinct advantage for use in cancer therapy as they are easy to produce and store. Germination of spores will only occur when they encounter the requisite anaerobic conditions. Spontaneous colonization of tumours in cancer patients and the apparent selectivity of Clostridia for tumours were noticed more than 50 years ago. The first experiment in 1947 showed that direct injection of spores of *C. histolyticum* into mouse sarcoma caused oncolysis (liquefaction) and tumour regression[42]. Later experiments proved this selectivity by injecting mice *i.v.* with spores of C. tetani, the causative agent of tetanus. Injected non-tumour bearing animals remained healthy. However, tumour bearing mice died within 48 h because of *C. tetani* colonisation and tetanus production. This provided evidence that the *C. tetani* were able to germinate/replicate selectively in the anaerobic environment found within tumours, and released their toxins systemically[6]. Obviously, it would not be appropriate to use pathogenic strains of Clostridia for clinical therapy in humans. A non-pathogenic strain of *C. butyricum* M-55 has been isolated[43]. M-55 was later reclassified as *C. oncolyticum* and taxonomic studies have now clearly established that it is a *C. sporogenes* strain (ATCC13732). This is a proteolytic species causing liquefaction of colonised tumours. This was later verified by testing more isolates.

Saccharolytic clostridia, such as *C. beijerinckii* NCIMB8052 spores administered intravenously to EMT6 tumour-bearing mice germinated in the necrotic tumour regions while the oxygenated tumour areas remained free of spores[44]. Equally, intravenous injection of rhabdomyosarcoma-bearing rats with at least 107 spores of *C. beijerinckii* ATCC17778, C. acetobutylicum DSM792 (= ATCC824) or *C. acetobutylicum* NI-4082

(reclassified as *C. saccharoperbutylacetonicum*) showed tumour colonisation without complete tumour lysis[45].
C. sporogenes was the first *Clostridium* to be gene modified and this was performed with the E. coli Colicin E3 gene. Colicin E3 encodes a bacteriocin shown to have canceriostatic properties[46]. However, the overall anti-tumour efficacy of this bacteriocin was limited. This may have resulted from poor gene modification methodologies which were improved with the application of electroporation. In 2002 Prof. Brown's group introduced *E. coli* cytosine deaminase (CD) into *C. sporogenes* NCIMB10696 by electroporation[47]. Intravenous injection of the recombinant spores followed by the systemic administration of the prodrug 5-FC inhibited tumour growth which was more pronounced than the use of prodrug alone. Unfortunately, for reasons unknown this inhibition in tumour growth did not persist. However, it was clear that *C. sporogenes* has a great capacity to colonise the tumour. At least 10e8 CFU/g of tumour was obtained following the intravenous injection of the spores.
Saccharolytic Clostridia strains including *C. beijerinckii* ATCC17778, *C. acetobutylicum* DSM792 (ATCC824) or *C. acetobutylicum* NI4082 (reclassified as *C. saccharoperbutylacetonicum*) and *C. butyricum* are non-pathogenic and their development has been industry funded. Therapeutic genes, encoding the cytokine tumour necrosis factor *alpha* (TNF-α), CD or nitroreductase (NTR) have been introduced into these strains[48, 49]. Following transformation of *C. acetobutylicum* using strain-specific electroporation protocols, CD expression was monitored in lysates and supernatants of early logarithmic growth phase cultures of recombinant *C. acetobutylicum* (pKNT19closcodA)[50]. A considerable amount of heterologous protein was expressed and efficiently secreted. Also, *C. acetobutylicum* strains NI4082 and DSM792 engineered to produce cytosine deaminase were able to express and secrete this enzyme at the tumour site[48, 49]. Functional CD enzyme was detected in the tumour of rhabdomyosarcoma-bearing WAG/Rij rats that were injected with the recombinant *C. acetobutylicum*, but not in control animals. Animals, concomitantly treated with antivascular chemical agent, CombreAp, showed higher incidence of CD-positive tumours (100 versus 58%). Moreover, the level of active CD in these tumour specimens was considerably higher (mean conversion efficiency of 5-FC to 5-FU ~11%) as compared to tumours not treated with the vascular targeting drug (mean conversion efficiency of 5-FC to 5-FU ~11%) when compared to untreated tumours (mean conversion efficiency of 5-FC to 5-FU ~3%)[49]. However, when these recombinant strains were used in solid tumour models *in vivo*, there was a consistent lack of significant tumour regression observed. Factors that may have contributed to this lack of efficacy include a low level of bacterial colonisation of the tumour or insufficient recombinant gene expression and secretion at the tumour site[51]. Recent studies have reported the development of vectors utilising super tumour coloniser *Clostridial* strains *C. sporogenes* or *C. novyi-NT*. Recombinant *C. sporogenes* and *C. novyi-NT* overexpressing NTR showed significant *in vivo* anti-tumour effects[52] when used with prodrug demonstrating the clinical potential of these vectors.

5. Advantages of clostridial spores for cancer gene therapy

At present, there are various gene therapy vector systems under development against cancer. However, due to the complexity of the solid tumours involving angiogenesis, hypoxia, stromal cell, tumour cell heterogeneity and the emergence of de-differentiated stem cells, none of the existing vectors are holding any real promises. The clostridial spore-based vector system is not infectious, and has gained renewed interest, because of the following true advantages.

5.1 Preferentially growing within the unique tumour microenvironment

The biological properties of virus-based vectors, in particular the ability to enter and replicate (in the case of replication-competent viral vectors) within a tumour cell and then spread from cell to cell are highly relevant for effective cancer therapy. However, recent understanding of tumour pathology has revealed that several features of the tumour environment may not be conducive for viral replication[40, 53]. Hypoxia is an important feature of solid tumours and the ability of viruses to enter and replicate in hypoxic cells may be a critical determinant for the success or failure of viral vector-mediated cancer gene therapy. Turning off protein translation is a central process in the cellular adaptation to many types of stress, including viral infection and hypoxia. The hypoxic cells, the apoptotic cells, the quiescent cells are all refractory to viral entry and replication[54]. This is a major problem for virus-based vectors because if the vector can't reach a tumour cell, it can't act or deliver a therapeutic gene. On the contrary, clostridial spores are able to home in on these niche environments because of their own unique metabolic need, which enable them to utilise the tumour micro milieu and respective tissues for their own proliferation. Both wild-type and genetically modified Clostridia have been demonstrated to specifically colonise and destroy solid tumours. "Trojan horse" vectors have further created improved features that enable them to kill tumour cells through multimodality mechanisms.

5.2 Easy production

All of the viral vector systems need sophisticated cell culture systems, expensive culture media, rounds of filtrations and purifications and dedicated centrifugation and storages. On the contrary, clostridial spores can be easily and inexpensively produced from anaerobic bacterial culture. There are only a few steps involved and the spores, once produced can be stored at room temperature for at least 3–6 months.

5.3 Easy administration

While most viral vectors have to be intratumourally injected, intravenous injection of resuspended clostridial spores are possible and sufficient as they will be leaked out of the incomplete vessels in the solid tumour, thus specifically targeting to and colonising the hypoxic regions of the tumours.

5.4 Safety

Safety is always a concern when live vector systems are used for human gene therapy. Some of the hurdles of using viral vectors include: (1) whether the vector is sufficiently targeted to tumour alone; (2) whether the vector expresses low levels of viral genes that may lead to increased toxicity and immunogenicity[55]; (3) possible immunogenicity of the transgene that may be reduced with a reduction in the duration of gene expression[56]; and (4) whether viral particles are sequested within the target cells or secreted into body fluid such as urine and subsequently spread into environment. We postulate that the use of clostridial spore based vectors may be a safer option to using viral vectors. Clostridia are strictly anaerobic, are tumour targeted and would be unable to live in non-hypoxic environments. A recent experiment with *C. novyi-NT* has demonstrated that the strain was unable to colonise artificially created infarcted heart where the level of hypoxia was inadequate to support the replication of the Clostridia[7]. Early trials of non-pathogenic Clostridia strains in patients have demonstrated safety. In the unlikely event of an adverse effect, clostridia can be eliminated from the blood stream with the use of readily available antibiotics such as metronidazole which showed total spore clearance from the blood stream after 9 days of treatment[4].

6. Indiscriminant destruction of all cell types within the tumour

Solid tumours comprise not only malignant cells, but also extracellular matrix and many other non-malignant cell types, including stromal cells such as fibroblasts, endothelial cells and inflammatory cells. The mechanisms of clostridial vector-mediated tumour killing consist of several aspects: one is from its transgene that encodes prodrug converting enzymes for suicide-gene therapy or cytokines for immuno-gene therapy. These are essentially the same as the viral vectors. However, there is another side of the tumour killing effect that is resulting from the consequences of an innate antitumour effect of the clostridial strain due to production of hydrolytic enzymes including proteases, lipases, and nuclease. Furthermore, there is also a nutrients competition between the clostridia and cells surrounding them (including tumour cells, stromal cells and stem cells), where the clostridia multiplied much faster than the mammalian cells. The cumulative multiplications and the combined events of energy and substance metabolism effectively depleted the limited nutrient source and deprive the tumour cells, causing starvation and death. More recently, there were observations that indicate the germination of the clostridial spores, the transformation from spores to vegetative rods, and the continue multiplications of the vegetative rods inside the tumour activated the immune system, assisting the antitumour effects[57]. These tumour killing mechanisms destroy not only tumour cells, but also any other cells in their vicinity. These are characteristics that viral vectors are not so well equipped, nor any existing convectional cancer therapies.

6.1 Extracellular agent

While viral vectors need access to viable target cells and their cellular machinery to achieve transgene delivery and expression, this goal is often difficult to fulfil as some tumour cells are not viable at the time of gene delivery. Furthermore, none of the existing vector systems efficiently transfer genes to every tumour cell which subsequently allows for tumour regrowth. On the other hand clostridial spore replication is not tumour cell dependent and occurs via rod multiplication extra-cellularlly. Furthermore, the tumour killing mechanism of clostridial spores may operate independently of the requirement for gene transfer. Without the requirement for gene integration into the host cell genome removes the possibility of insertional mutagenesis when using Clostridia. Therefore, Clostridia may show tumour killing irrespective of the tumour cell heterogeneity found within the tumour environment.

6.2 No restrictions on accommodating therapeutic genes

One of the primary limitations of most viral vectors has been the small size of the virion, which only permits the packaging of very limited sizes (usually a few kilobases) of exogenous DNA that includes the promoter, the polyadenylation signal and any other enhancer elements that might be desired. However, for clostridia size limitations are far less restricted, not only because the plasmids used can harbour much larger DNA fragments, but in case the foreign gene is integrated in the host chromosome there is in fact unlimited capacity for insertion of therapeutic genes, forecasting the promising future for the development of ever powerful vectors.

7. Other developments for cancer gene therapy

Another potential direction for cancer gene therapy has come from the discovery of small non-coding RNAs that can significantly interfere with gene expression levels at the post-transcriptional level. RNA interference (RNAi) is an evolutionary conserved mechanism for specific gene silencing that can result in the degradation or inhibition of homologous mRNA. The most widely studied types of RNAi include both micro-RNA (miRNA) and short interfering RNA (siRNA).

Post-transcriptional gene silencing by RNAi represents an essential part of endogenous gene regulation, with much evidence to suggest that RNAi regulates more than one third of all cellular mRNAs, and that each RNAi can control hundreds of gene targets in both normal and diseased conditions. More recently mutations or aberrant expression patterns in RNAi have been shown to correlate with various diseases, including cancer, and indicate that some RNAi may have a tumour suppressor function or operate as oncogenes. It is now believed that RNAi may prove to be a beneficial factor in the treatment of cancer by either altering the endogenous levels of these RNAi or by the introduction of new RNAi to alter the expression of cancer causing genes.

RNAi therapy has already been trialled in a number of different models, however, several critical limitations must first be overcome. These limitations include non-specific effects in non-tumour tissue, potential toxicity due to interactions with endogenous RNAi, half-life of silencing, and inability to specifically target only the tumour mass. One possible approach, to overcome many of these limitations, is to use RNAi in combination with *Clostridia* as a gene delivery system to the hypoxic core of the tumour.

8. Conclusion

The unique pathophysiology of solid tumours presents a huge problem for the conventional therapies. Thus, the outcomes of current therapies are so far disappointing. Several new approaches aiming at developing effective treatments are on the horizon. These include a variety of virus-based therapy systems[2, 58, 59]. Amongst all these, replication-competent viral vector-mediated cancer therapy is most promising[60, 61]. However, even this system suffers from several deficiencies: First, the vectors currently have to be injected intratumourally to elicit an effect. This is far from ideal as many tumours are inaccessible and spread to other areas of the body making them difficult to detect and treat. Second, because of the heterogeneity within a tumour, the vector does not efficiently enter and spread to sufficient numbers of tumour cells. Third, hypoxia, a prevalent characteristic feature of most solid tumours, reduces the ability of the viral vector to function and decrease viral gene expression and production. Consequently, a proportion of the tumour mass is left unaffected and capable of re-growing. Fourth, pre-existing immunity pose a problem for the efficacy of viral vectors. Therefore, there have rarely been any cures with the use of the system.

The strictly anaerobic clostridia, on the other hand, have been shown to selectively colonise in solid tumours when delivered systemically and has resulted in high percentage of "cures" of experimental tumours. A phase I clinical trial combining spores of a non toxic strain (*C. novyi-NT*) with an antimicrotubuli agent has been initiated[62]. Genetic manipulation of clostridia to make them into "Trojan horse" vectors will provide further tumour killing mechanisms and amplifying antitumour effects. Clearly, it is just a matter of time that a "Trojan horse" type of clostridium will become a clinical reality, especially if we can further improve upon the system by providing additional features, ideally including (i) targeting tumours only and not anywhere else, (ii) able to effective kill primary tumours as well as metastases. Current technologies are in place to achieve these goals. Newer and effective therapies for solid tumours based on the "Trojan horse" will be a reality in a very near future.

9. References

[1] Toloza, E.M., *Gene therapy for lung cancer.* Thoracic Surgery Clinics, 2006. 16(4): p. 397-419, vii.

[2] Kasono, K., et al., *Selective gene delivery to head and neck cancer cells via an integrin targeted adenoviral vector.* Clinical Cancer Research, 1999. 5(9): p. 2571-9.

[3] Heppner, F. and J.R. Mose, *The liquefaction (oncolysis) of malignant gliomas by a non pathogenic Clostridium.* Acta Neurochirurgica, 1978. 42(1-2): p. 123-5.

[4] Nuyts, S., et al., *Clostridium spores for tumor-specific drug delivery.* Anti-Cancer Drugs, 2002. 13(2): p. 115-25.

[5] Wei, M.Q., et al., *Clostridial spores as live 'Trojan horse' vectors for cancer gene therapy: comparison with viral delivery systems.* Genetic Vaccines & Therapy, 2008. 6: p. 8.

[6] Malmgren, R.A. and C.C. Flanigan, *Localization of the vegetative form of Clostridium tetani in mouse tumors following intravenous spore administration.* Cancer Res. , 1955. 15: p. 473–8.

[7] Diaz, L.A., Jr., et al., *Pharmacologic and toxicologic evaluation of C. novyi-NT spores.* Toxicological Sciences, 2005. 88(2): p. 562-75.

[8] Raty, J.K., et al., *Gene therapy: the first approved gene-based medicines, molecular mechanisms and clinical indications.* Current Molecular Pharmacology, 2008. 1(1): p. 13-23.

[9] Colombo, F., et al., *Combined HSV-TK/IL-2 gene therapy in patients with recurrent glioblastoma multiforme: biological and clinical results.* Cancer Gene Therapy, 2005. 12(10): p. 835-48.

[10] Seth, P., *Vector-mediated cancer gene therapy: an overview.* Cancer Biology & Therapy, 2005. 4(5): p. 512-7.

[11] Rein, D.T., M. Breidenbach, and D.T. Curiel, *Current developments in adenovirus-based cancer gene therapy.* Future Oncology, 2006. 2(1): p. 137-43.

[12] Peng, Z., *Current status of gendicine in China: recombinant human Ad-p53 agent for treatment of cancers.* Human Gene Therapy, 2005. 16(9): p. 1016-27.

[13] Wang, X.Y., et al., *Preclinical evaluation of a prostate-targeted gene-directed enzyme prodrug therapy delivered by ovine atadenovirus.* Gene Therapy, 2004. 11(21): p. 1559-67.

[14] Matthews, Q.L., et al., *Genetic incorporation of a herpes simplex virus type 1 thymidine kinase and firefly luciferase fusion into the adenovirus protein IX for functional display on the virion.[Erratum appears in Mol Imaging. 2007 Jan-Feb;6(1):72].* Molecular Imaging: Official Journal of the Society for Molecular Imaging, 2006. 5(4): p. 510-9.

[15] Flotte, T.R., *Gene therapy progress and prospects: recombinant adeno-associated virus (rAAV) vectors.* Gene Therapy, 2004. 11(10): p. 805-10.

[16] Urabe, M., et al., *Scalable generation of high-titer recombinant adeno-associated virus type 5 in insect cells.* Journal of Virology, 2006. 80(4): p. 1874-85.

[17] Young, L.S., et al., *Viral gene therapy strategies: from basic science to clinical application.* Journal of Pathology, 2006. 208(2): p. 299-318.

[18] Ram, Z., et al., *Therapy of malignant brain tumors by intratumoral implantation of retroviral vector-producing cells.* Nature Medicine, 1997. 3(12): p. 1354-61.

[19] Tai, C.-K., et al., *Single-shot, multicycle suicide gene therapy by replication-competent retrovirus vectors achieves long-term survival benefit in experimental glioma.* Molecular Therapy: the Journal of the American Society of Gene Therapy, 2005. 12(5): p. 842-51.

[20] Buchholz, C.J. and K. Cichutek, *Is it going to be SIN?: a European Society of Gene Therapy commentary. Phasing-out the clinical use of non self-inactivating murine leukemia virus vectors: initiative on hold.* Journal of Gene Medicine, 2006. 8(10): p. 1274-6.

[21] Naldini, L., et al., *In vivo gene delivery and stable transduction of nondividing cells by a lentiviral vector.* Science, 1996. 272(5259): p. 263-7.

[22] Levine, B.L., et al., *Gene transfer in humans using a conditionally replicating lentiviral vector.* Proceedings of the National Academy of Sciences of the United States of America, 2006. 103(46): p. 17372-7.

[23] Metharom, P., et al., *Novel bovine lentiviral vectors based on Jembrana disease virus.* Journal of Gene Medicine, 2000. 2(3): p. 176-85.

[24] Metharom, P., et al., *The development of bovine lentiviral vectors based on the Jembana disease virus, an infectious agent of cattle.* Vet Microbiol, 2000. 80: p. 9-22.

[25] Harland, J., et al., *The herpes simplex virus (HSV) protein ICP34.5 is a virion component that forms a DNA-binding complex with proliferating cell nuclear antigen and HSV replication proteins.* Journal of Neurovirology, 2003. 9(4): p. 477-88.

[26] Derubertis, B.G., et al., *Cytokine-secreting herpes viral mutants effectively treat tumor in a murine metastatic colorectal liver model by oncolytic and T-cell-dependent mechanisms.* Cancer Gene Therapy, 2007. 14(6): p. 590-7.

[27] Lee, J.-S., et al., *Growth inhibitory effect of triple anti-tumor gene transfer using Semliki Forest virus vector in glioblastoma cells.* International Journal of Oncology, 2006. 28(3): p. 649-54.

[28] Izsvak, Z., Z. Ivics, and R.H. Plasterk, *Sleeping Beauty, a wide host-range transposon vector for genetic transformation in vertebrates.* Journal of Molecular Biology, 2000. 302(1): p. 93-102.

[29] Zhu, Z.B., et al., *Transport across a polarized monolayer of Caco-2 cells by transferrin receptor-mediated adenovirus transcytosis.* Virology, 2004. 325(1): p. 116-28.

[30] McIntosh, D.P., et al., *Targeting endothelium and its dynamic caveolae for tissue-specific transcytosis in vivo: a pathway to overcome cell barriers to drug and gene delivery.* Proceedings of the National Academy of Sciences of the United States of America, 2002. 99(4): p. 1996-2001.

[31] Pankhurst, Q.A. and et al., *Applications of magnetic nanoparticles in biomedicine.* Journal of Physics D: Applied Physics, 2003. 36(13): p. R167.

[32] Li, J., et al., *Genetic incorporation of HSV-1 thymidine kinase into the adenovirus protein IX for functional display on the virion.* Virology, 2005. 338(2): p. 247-58.

[33] Kuruppu, D. and K.K. Tanabe, *Viral oncolysis by herpes simplex virus and other viruses.* Cancer Biology & Therapy, 2005. 4(5): p. 524-31.

[34] Voroshilova, M.K., *Potential use of nonpathogenic enteroviruses for control of human diseases.* Progress in medical virology 1989. 36 p. 191–202.

[35] Pond, A.R. and E.E. Manuelidis, *Oncolytic effect of poliomyelitis virus on human epidermoid carcinoma (HeLa tumor) heterologously transplanted to guinea pigs.* The American Journal of Pathology, 1964. 45 p. 233–49.

[36] Kunin, C.M., *Cellular susceptibility to enteroviruses.* Bacteriological reviews 1964. 28 p. 382-90.

[37] Meerani, S. and Y. Yao, *Oncolytic viruses in cnacer therapy.* European Journal of Scientific Research, 2010. 40(1): p. 156 - 171.

[38] Lamont, J.P., et al., *A prospective phase II trial of ONYX-015 adenovirus and chemotherapy in recurrent squamous cell carcinoma of the head and neck (the Baylor experience).* Annals of Surgical Oncology, 2000. 7(8): p. 588-92.

[39] Nemunaitis, J., et al., *Selective replication and oncolysis in p53 mutant tumors with ONYX-015, an E1B-55kD gene-deleted adenovirus, in patients with advanced head and neck cancer: a phase II trial.* Cancer Research, 2000. 60(22): p. 6359-66.

[40] Folkman, J., *What is the evidence that tumors are angiogenesis dependent?* Journal of the National Cancer Institute, 1990. 82(1): p. 4-6.

[41] Wei, M.Q., et al., *Facultative or obligate anaerobic bacteria have the potential for multimodality therapy of solid tumours.* European Journal of Cancer, 2007. 43(3): p. 490-6.

[42] Parker, R.C., et al., *Effect of hispolyticus infection and toxin on transplantable mouse tumours.* Proc Soc Exp Biol Med. , 1947. 66: p. 461–465.
[43] Möse, J.R. and G.Z. Möse, *Onkolyseversuche mit apathogen, anaerogen sporenbildern am Erhlich-Tumor der maus* Z Krebsforsch, 1959. 63: p. 63–74.
[44] Lemmon, M.J., et al., *Anaerobic bacteria as a gene delivery system that is controlled by the tumor microenvironment.* Gene Therapy, 1997. 4(8): p. 791-6.
[45] Lambin, P., et al., *Colonisation of Clostridium in the body is restricted to hypoxic and necrotic areas of tumours.* Anaerobe, 1998. 4(4): p. 183-8.
[46] Schlechte, H. and B. Elbe, *Recombinant plasmid DNA variation of Clostridium oncolyticum--model experiments of cancerostatic gene transfer.* Zentralblatt fur Bakteriologie, Mikrobiologie, und Hygiene - Series A, Medical Microbiology, Infectious Diseases, Virology, Parasitology, 1988. 268(3): p. 347-56.
[47] Liu, S.C., et al., *Anticancer efficacy of systemically delivered anaerobic bacteria as gene therapy vectors targeting tumor hypoxia/necrosis.* Gene Therapy, 2002. 9(4): p. 291-6.
[48] Theys, J., et al., *Clostridium as a tumor-specific delivery system of therapeutic proteins.* Cancer Detection & Prevention, 2001. 25(6): p. 548-57.
[49] Van Mellaert, L., S. Barbe, and J. Anne, *Clostridium spores as anti-tumour agents.* Trends in Microbiology, 2006. 14(4): p. 190-6.
[50] Theys, J., et al., *Specific targeting of cytosine deaminase to solid tumors by engineered Clostridium acetobutylicum.* Cancer Gene Therapy, 2001. 8(4): p. 294-7.
[51] Wei, M.Q., et al., *Bacterial targeted tumour therapy-dawn of a new era.* Cancer Letters, 2008. 259(1): p. 16-27.
[52] Theys, J., et al., *Repeated cycles of Clostridium-directed enzyme prodrug therapy result in sustained antitumour effects in vivo.* British Journal of Cancer, 2006. 95(9): p. 1212-9.
[53] Vaupel, P. and A. Mayer, *Hypoxia in cancer: significance and impact on clinical outcome.* Cancer & Metastasis Reviews, 2007. 26(2): p. 225-39.
[54] Hay, J.G., *The potential impact of hypoxia on the success of oncolytic virotherapy.* Current Opinion in Molecular Therapeutics, 2005. 7(4): p. 353-8.
[55] Raper, S.E., et al., *Fatal systemic inflammatory response syndrome in a ornithine transcarbamylase deficient patient following adenoviral gene transfer.* Molecular Genetics & Metabolism, 2003. 80(1-2): p. 148-58.
[56] Yang, Y., et al., *Cellular and humoral immune responses to viral antigens create barriers to lung-directed gene therapy with recombinant adenoviruses.* Journal of Virology, 1995. 69(4): p. 2004-15.
[57] Janssen, H.L., et al., *Hypoxia in head and neck cancer: how much, how important?* Head & Neck, 2005. 27(7): p. 622-38.
[58] Agrawal, N., et al., *Bacteriolytic therapy can generate a potent immune response against experimental tumors.* Proceedings of the National Academy of Sciences of the United States of America, 2004. 101(42): p. 15172-7.
[59] Huang, Q., et al., *A novel conditionally replicative adenovirus vector targeting telomerase-positive tumor cells.* Clinical Cancer Research, 2004. 10(4): p. 1439-45.
[60] Papanastassiou, V., et al., *The potential for efficacy of the modified (ICP 34.5(-)) herpes simplex virus HSV1716 following intratumoural injection into human malignant glioma: a proof of principle study.* Gene Therapy, 2002. 9(6): p. 398-406.
[61] Pipiya, T., et al., *Hypoxia reduces adenoviral replication in cancer cells by downregulation of viral protein expression.* Gene Therapy, 2005. 12(11): p. 911-7.
[62] *http://www.clinicaltrials.gov/ct.*

15

Differential Gene Expression and Its Possible Therapeutic Implications

Safdar Ali and Sher Ali
National Institute of Immunology
New Delhi,
India

1. Introduction

With improving technology and accumulation of knowledge, there has been a constant improvement in the understanding of various anomalies affecting the human population. Still, a lot is yet to be done. The prognosis of any aberration in the living system which may result in disease/syndromes/death is dependent on multiple variables. These include the overall parameters defining the health of an individual like age, nutrition and environment. Further, the family health scenario is suggestive of health status of an individual concerned. This is where the inherited factors constituting the genome are involved.

2. Differential gene expression and correlation with human diseases/syndromes

Alterations in the genome can be either inherited or acquired. These alterations may or may not lead to disease. Moreover, not all the acquired alterations are passed on to the next generation. We need to address a few questions to be able to comprehend the situation. What factors decide the fate of a gene as if to be expressed or not, how much and when? What alterations in genes lead to diseases? Which conditions are inherited? Are there ways by which the body tries to repair these aberrations? And finally, can the affected part of the genome be replaced in a way that the individual becomes healthy again?

The expression of a gene is a very tightly regulated process with reference to when, where and how much to be expressed. A detailed discussion of the same is beyond the scope of this article. However, it's worth mentioning that sequence and expression variations can sometimes be directly correlated to a diseased situation. The alterations in sequence may or may not be inheritable depending on whether the somatic or germline cells are getting affected, respectively. There are situations where the somatic cells may be having an altered genome but the germline genome is protected from the same and hence the mutations are restricted to the present generation. This happens primarily because of two reasons. First, the germ cells are very much isolated as compared to the somatic cells and hence are often shielded from the causing agents in the environment or within. Secondly, the repair mechanisms active at the germline level are possibly much more efficient and sensitive than the ones at somatic level. Thereby, the chances of the alterations getting repaired before

Disorder	Point Mutation/s	Aberration in gene/s	Chromosomal aberrations	Gene/s involved	Chromosome	Reference
Cri du chat			•	Semaphorine F, Delta catenin, hTERT	5	Rodrifuez-Caballero et al 2010
Fabry disease	•			α galactosidase A	X	Saito et al 2011
Cystic fibrosis		•		CFTR	7	Madry et al 2011
Di George syndrome		•		TBX1	22	Huh and Omitz 2010
De grouchy syndrome		•		MBP, Galanin receptor	18	Wilson et al 1979
Sickle cell anemia	•			Hemoglobin gene	11	Mousa and Qari, 2010
Siderius X-linked mental retardation syndrome		•		PHF8	X	Abidi et al 2007
Wolf-Hirschhorn syndrome			•	WHSC1, WHSC2	4	South et al 2008
Myotonic dystrophy DM1		•		DMPK	19	Magana and Cisneros 2010
Myotonic dystrophy DM2		•		ZNF9	3	Raheem et al 2010
Huntingtons disease		•		HTT	4	Warby et al 2011
CADASIL disease	•			Notch3	19	Valenti et al 2011
Lesch-Nyhan syndrome	•			HPRT	X	Gucev et al 2010
Crohns disease	•			CARD15	16	Raelson et al 2007
Down syndrome			•		Trisomy 21	Purvey et al 2010

Disorder	Point Mutation/s	Aberration in gene/s	Chromosomal aberrations	Gene/s involved	Chromosome	Reference
Turner syndrome			•		45, X	Lopes et al 2010
Klinefelters syndrome			•		47, XXY	Judith et al 2009

Table 1. Representative genetic disorders affecting human population along with the involved genes.

being packaged for the next generation are enhanced. Besides, not all genetic alterations lead to diseases. There are some which make the individual susceptible to certain conditions while the actual occurrence and progression of the disease is dependent on environmental factors and lifestyle. For instance, mutations in BRCA1 gene have been successfully used for epidemiological studies and predicting the risk of individuals to develop breast cancer. Precautions in lifestyle, drugs and environment thereon have helped in combating the disease. Similarly, about 8 susceptibility loci are known for occurrence of prostate cancer and their detailed analysis is currently being pursued. So, what exactly are the possible alterations in genes which may lead to diseases?

2.1 Involvement of genes in disease: mutations, deletions and translocations

Genetic alterations affecting the physiology of the individual, resulting in any disease or syndrome can be classified into three types. First of all, a point mutation (insertion/deletion) of a single gene results in the diseased phenotype. Secondly, multiple genes need to be affected for the diseased phenotype. Herein, the genes may be partly or fully deleted, translocated or their length may increase or decrease due to change in copies of repeat elements. Lastly, the disorders caused by complete/partial loss or gain of chromosome. Several examples of these anomalies along with their affected genes/chromosomes are mentioned in table 1. The frequency of occurrence of these disorders varies across the world depending on the environmental factors, gene pool, lifestyle and even availability of health care facilities. The inheritance pattern of these diseases is dependent upon dominant or recessive nature of the causative gene as well as its chromosomal localization. This has been discussed in detail in the next section.

2.2 Genes and diseases

2.2.1 Single gene disorders

The disorders caused by alterations in a single gene are called monogenic disorders. Over 6000 such disorders are known till date and one in every 200 individuals is affected by them. Some of the common examples include cystic fibrosis, sickle cell anemia and Marfan syndrome. These follow the Mendelian laws of inheritance. The responsible gene may be localized on autosome or sex chromosome. Further, the gene may be dominant or recessive in nature. Hence, the monogenic diseases can be classified as autosomal dominant, autosomal recessive, sex linked dominant and sex linked recessive. Their inheritance patterns have been explained in figures 1-4.

From the figures shown below, we can conclusively state that the inheritance pattern of a monogenic disorder is determined by three factors as follows

a. The gene being dominant or recessive in expression

b. Localization of the gene on autosomes or sex chromosomes
c. Status of the parents with reference to the causative gene.

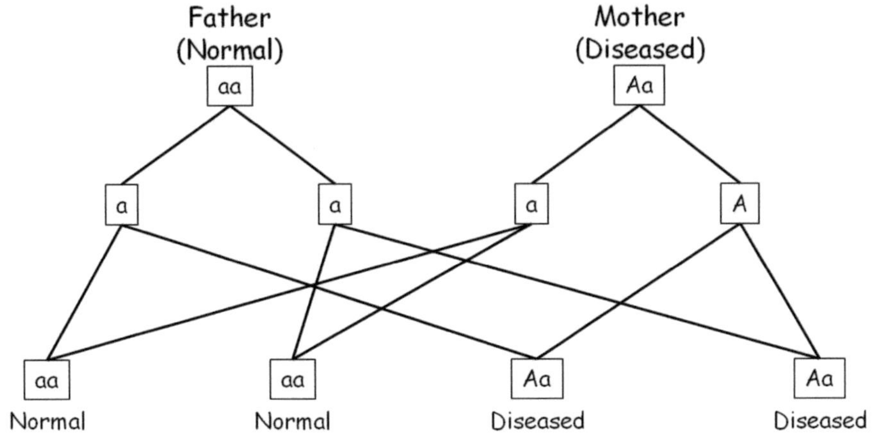

Fig. 1. The inheritance pattern of a monogenic autosomal dominant disorder. Here, the mother is diseased which leads to probability of an offspring getting affected to be ½ (50%). However, it should be noted that the inheritance pattern in such cases would be independent of the sex of the affected parent as well as that of offsprings getting affected. This means even if father was diseased and mother normal, the same pattern would be followed. The capital letter indicates affected allele while the small letter represents normal allele.

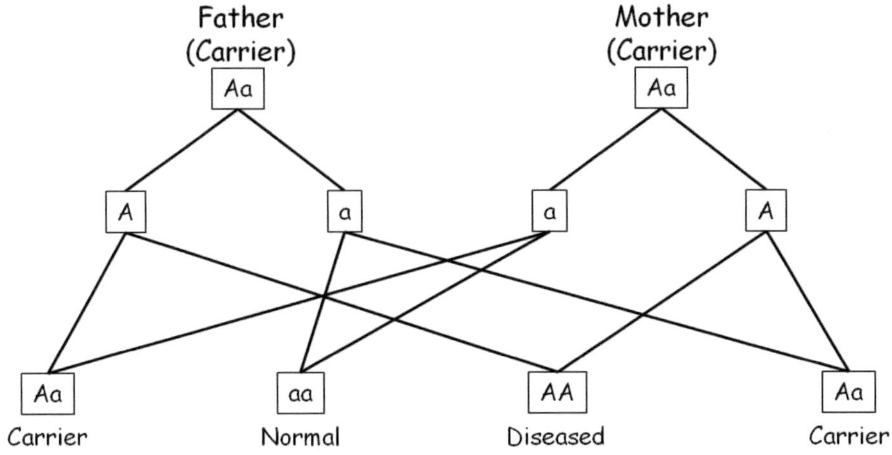

Fig. 2. The inheritance pattern of a monogenic autosomal recessive disorder. In the present example, both the parents are carriers for the gene which means they have one normal copy of the gene and one affected. In such a situation, the probability of the offsprings being carrier for the disease is ½, being normal is ¼ and that of being diseased is ¼. Here also the sex of the parents or offsprings is irrelevant. The capital letter indicates affected allele while the small letter represents normal allele.

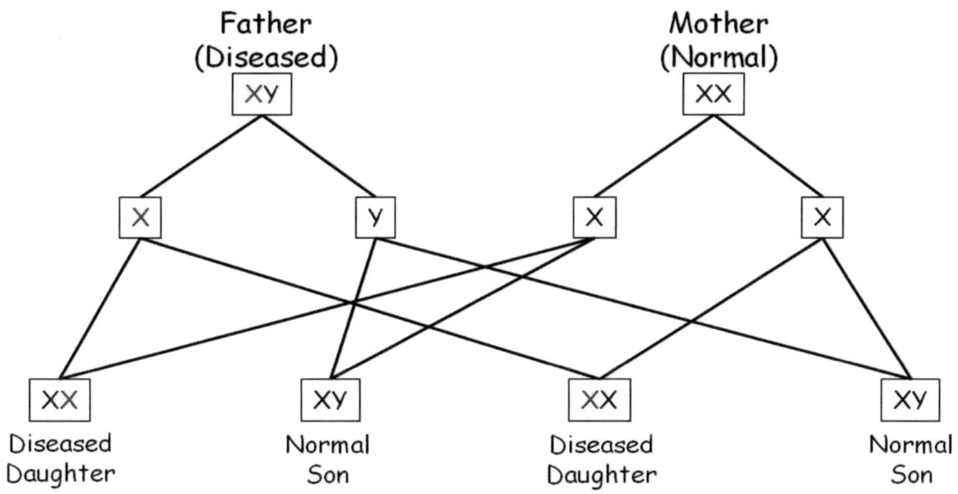

Fig. 3. The inheritance pattern of a X linked dominant disorder. The affected allele has been shown in blue. Herein, sex of both the affected parent as well as offsprings is relevant. For instance, in the above example, where father is diseased and mother is normal, all the daughters would be diseased while all the sons would be healthy.

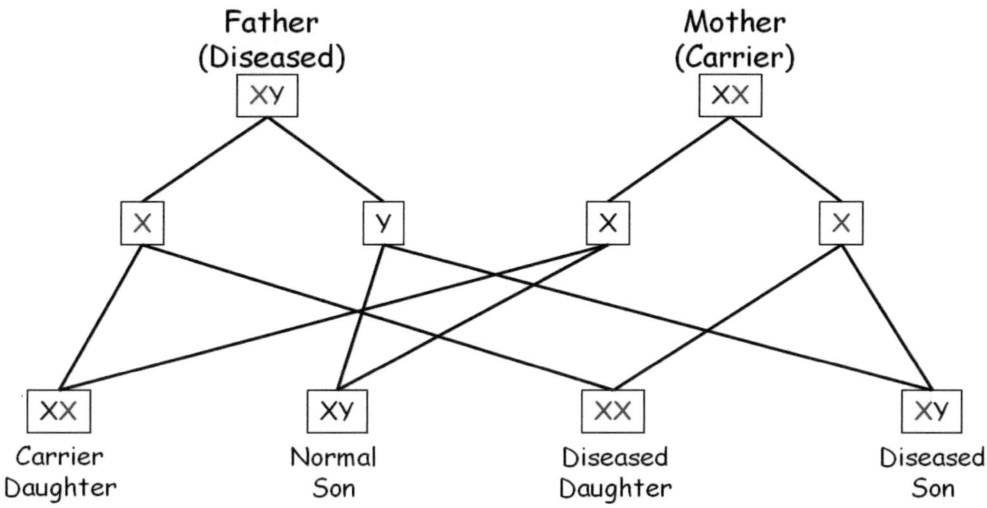

Fig. 4. The inheritance pattern of a X linked recessive disorder. The affected allele has been shown in blue. Here again, sex of affected parent and offsprings are important. In case of a diseased father and carrier mother, daughters have an equal chance of being diseased or carrier while the sons have an equal chance of being diseased or affected.

2.2.2 Multi-gene disorders

The total genes present in any organism's genome are often much less than the characteristics or traits in the phenotype of that organism. This led to the understanding that not every gene is responsible for an outcome in the phenotype. Thereon it has been established that many heritable traits such as eye colour, skin colour and height are determined by multiple factors. Similarly, all diseases cannot be attributed to a single gene defect. In most of the cases, more than one genetic element is involved, like in diabetes, cancer and obesity. These disorders do not follow a simple inheritance pattern as monogenic cases. Instead, the situation in the genome at multiple places needs to be monitored to understand the inheritance. Such cases have lead to the defining of susceptibility loci wherein there are genomic targets whose monitoring have helped us to evaluate the risk of an individual for getting the disease. Precautions at the lifestyle and genetic level (genetic counselling) have proved very useful in controlling and monitoring the disease.

2.2.3 Mitochondrial genetic disorders

Mitochondria are small circular or rod like organelles present in the eukaryotic cells cytoplasm and involved in the cellular respiration leading to the production of energy for the cell. The mitochondrial genome follows "cytoplasmic inheritance" or "maternal inheritance". At the time of fertilization, the cytoplasm (having mitochondria) of the zygote is contributed by ovum and hence the name. This has been illustrated in figure 5.

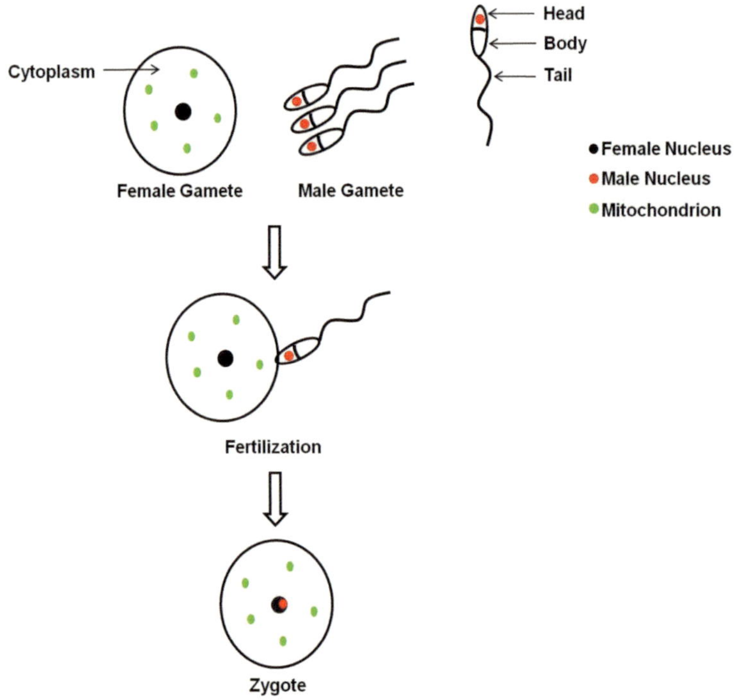

Fig. 5. Cytoplasmic inheritance of mitochondria. Formation of zygote (2n) requires the nucleic material from both the male and female gametes (1n each). However, the female gamete is the sole contributor of cytoplasm and hence that of mitochondrial DNA. Thus, the inheritance of mitochondrial genome is cytoplasmic or maternal.

Each mitochondrion may have several circular pieces of DNA and each cell may have several mitochondria depending upon the activity of the cell. Even within the same cell, different mitochondria would be differing in their genetic material (heteroplasmy). These

variations render uniqueness to every individual suffering from the same disease necessitating the need for personalized medicine. However, the most significant aspect of mitochondrial genetics lies in its contribution to a range of disorders from cancer, diabetes, Parkinson's disease, stroke to male infertility. Their exact involvement is still being explored.
So far, we have seen the possible means by which different genes can contribute to diseases either singly or in combination with others. Thereby, assessment of the expression level of the genes becomes significant to ascertain their roles at the functional level. The various techniques employed for the same have been discussed in the next section.

2.2.4 Y linked disorders

These are caused by alterations in genes located on the Y chromosome. The inheritance of Y chromosome is restricted to males being passed on from father to son and so on. Since, the Y chromosome doesn't have a concerned homologous chromosome, so all genes would have a dominant inheritance pattern. This means all the sons of affected a father would be affected and as expected the daughters would be unaffected from the same. One such attribute is the hypertrichosis pinnae or hair on the pinnae of ear.

3. Techniques for analyzing gene expression

Realizing the importance of gene expression profiles under various situations, techniques have been used for ascertaining the same. Northern blot has been one of the first approaches used for quantifying gene expression. Herein the RNA is blotted and hybridized before the final quantification. However, two factors radically changed this approach. First was the advent of polymerase chain reaction (PCR) and secondly, the discovery of reverse transcriptase.
Polymerase chain reaction (PCR), discovered by Kary Mullis, is based on thermal thermal cycling where specific DNA stretch is targeted by DNA oligo-nucleotides (primers) and amplification is carried out by thermo-stable Taq DNA polymerase. These steps result in manifold production of desired DNA sequence starting from relatively less template (Saiki et al 1985, 1988; Mullis 1990). Since its discovery, it has become an indispensable tool in genetics and molecular biology. It has been used successfully for a range of activities from clinical diagnostics, cloning, sequencing to carrying out site directed mutagenesis, besides others.
Till the discovery of reverse transcriptase, the central dogma of molecular biology was as shown in figure 6

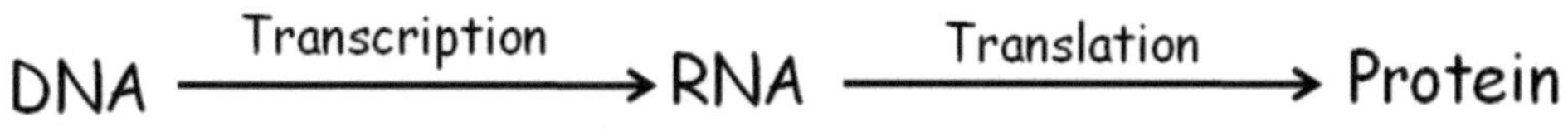

Fig. 6. The central dogma of molecular biology.

However, in 1970 Howard Temin and David Baltimore (Baltimore 1970; Temin 1964 a, b, c) independently discovered the existence of an enzyme which could reverse transcribe RNA to DNA. The enzyme was named "reverse transcriptase" for its action and both the scientists shared the 1975 Nobel Prize for the discovery. The central dogma was then modified as shown in figure 7.

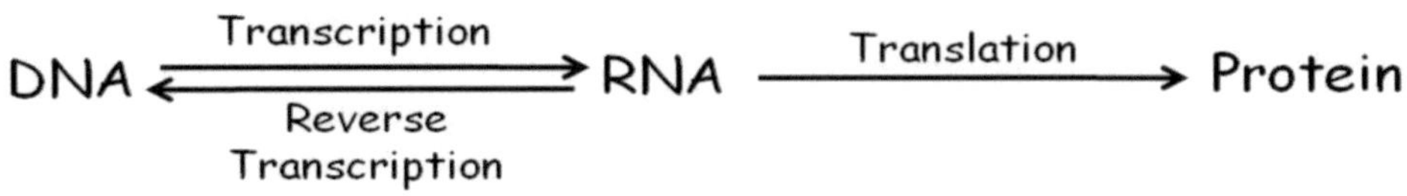

Fig. 7. The central dogma of molecular biology with discovery of reverse transcriptase.

This discovery has had far reaching consequences in the understanding of many aspects of RNA viruses in particular (Hurwitz and Leis 1972; Kulesh et al 1987, Rodgers et al 1995). Presently, we would be focussing on its significance in studying the expression of genes. Reverse transcriptase creates a single stranded DNA from RNA template. Thus, the RNA repertoire from a source can be reverse transcribed to cDNA wherein the relative levels of different genes would be a representation of their expression status. This has been discussed in the subsequent sections. Also, this enzyme made it possible to access the eukaryotic coding sequences without the introns. Hence, it has been immensely helpful in understanding and analyzing the splicing of different genes.

3.1 Reverse transcription

A combination of the above two approaches is being used exhaustively for the gene expression analysis. Herein, the total RNA is reverse transcribed to cDNA having repertoire of different transcribing genes in ratios comparable to their expression. These levels could then be estimated using labelled gene specific probes for hybridization and subsequently comparing the signal intensities. However, with advancements in technology and exhaustive information available about many genomes, more sensitive approaches are being used today. These include microarray and real time PCR which would be discussed in the coming sections.

3.2 Microarray analysis

The property of nucleotides to bind specifically (A-T; G-C) forms the essence of all hybridization experiments. Small specific probes (oligonucleotide) have been made radioactive and employed for ascertaining the presence of genes using southern hybridization. The same principle and the need for screening for fate of thousands of targets at the same time have driven the development of microarray technology. It began with the analysis of 378 bacterial lysates having different sequences and as of now over 30000 genes can be analyzed at one go. A flowchart for the microarray experiment has been shown in figure 8. Microarray has been used successfully for a range of applications including gene expression profiling, comparative genomic hybridization, detection of SNPs and analysis of splicing (Hacia et al 1999; Lashkari et al 1997; Nuwaysir et al 2002; Pollack et al 1999; Schena et al 1995; Shalon et al 1996) . A typical experiment for gene expression profiling involves hybridizing cDNA to an array of microscopic spots; each spot having a bound probe (oligonucleotide specific for a gene) and finally detection of hybridization using different fluorescence or chemiluminescence.

3.2.1 Sample

A microarray experiment for profiling gene expression would require at least two sets of cDNA as the final detection of signal intensities need a reference point to assess their fate (Wei et al 2004). For instance, the expression profile of genes in diseased individual would require a reference of a normal individual. Similarly, the profile in cells which have undergone any treatment can be compared with respect to untreated cells. The two or more sets of cDNA (of which one can be used as reference) hence constitutes the sample for microarray experiment.

The number of genes to be screened in an experiment varies. If no information is available regarding the targets to be screened, it's advisable to go for exhaustive screening of all possible genes. However, if preliminary information is available as to which pathways would be affected or which genes may be targeted in a particular situation; then, it makes sense to have multiple probes for those set of genes rather than assessing the whole transcriptome.

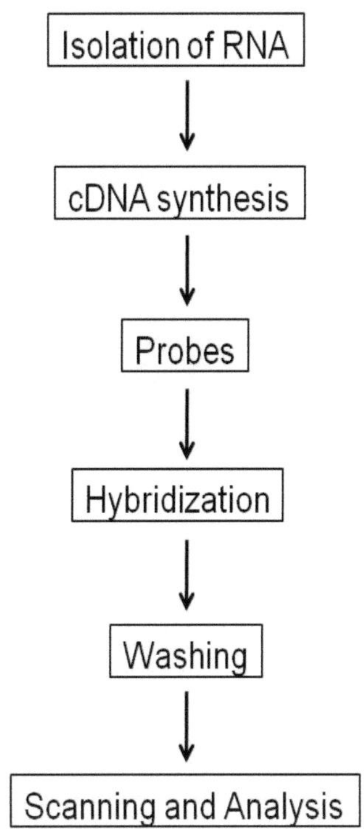

Fig. 8. Different steps in a microarray experiment.

3.2.2 Probes

The probes used in microarray experiment are short oligonucleotide sequences specific for a particular gene. In case some particular repertoire of genes needs to be focussed on, then multiple probes are designed on different regions of each gene to verify results.

3.2.3 Analysis

As mentioned earlier, the expression levels are indicated by post hybridization intensities, so an increase or decrease in intensities in relevance to the reference sample would give us the expression profile of the studied genes. Since equal amounts of samples are used for hybridization, an increase in intensity would correspond to an increase in expression and vice versa. It has been explained by an illustration in figure 9.

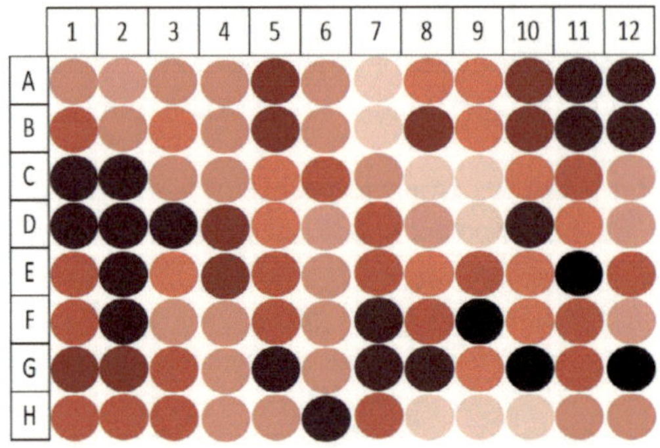

(A)

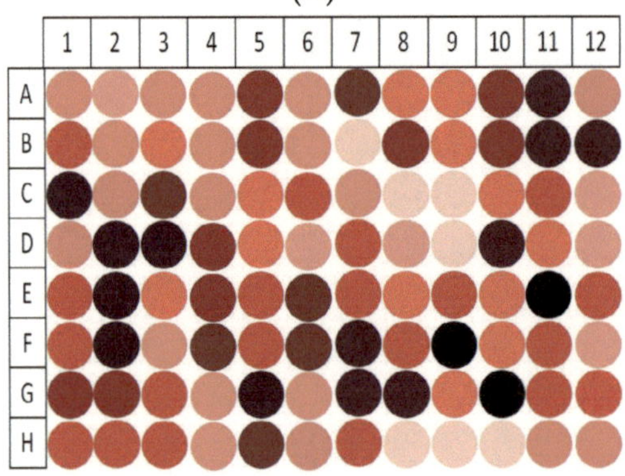

(B)

Fig. 9. The interpretation of microarray results. The above diagrammatic illustration represents microarray results. If (A) is taken to be the reference cDNA sample and (B) as that of the test sample then the final analysis shows comparative signal intensity of each spot. Since each spot is attached to a probe for a specific gene, the variations in intensities of the same well from two sets would indicate the fate of that gene. For instance, the intensities in spots A12, C2, D1 and G12 have gone down considerably in (B) as compared to (A). This reflects the reduction in corresponding genes expression. Contrastingly, positions A7 and H5 show an increase in the intensity in (B) as compared to (A) indicative of genes transcribing more in the situation.

3.2.4 Advantages and limitations

Thus, the microarray analysis helps us have an idea about the fate of genes in different circumstances. The greatest advantage of this approach lies in the ability to screen thousands of targets in a single experiment. This becomes particularly significant if we are to study a disease or response to any chemical/stress/radiations wherein the genetic targets are not known.

However, the variations in intensities are reflective of expression profiles and these intensities can be quantified as well but these quantifications are not the real representation of the relative expression of genes. This is primarily because the detection through fluorescence or chemiluminescence is an indirect approach. Though there have been improvements in detection but still a lot needs to be done (Tang et al 2007). Till date, microarray falls short in providing a numerical value with confidence as to how the expression levels were affected. Moreover, the approach can be applied to only those organisms where exhaustive information is available about both the genome and its corresponding transcriptome.

3.3 Real time PCR

In conventional PCR methods, the product is visualized at the end of the reaction. Since, amplification of target sequence from template takes place in an exponential manner, at the end of 20 amplification cycles the difference in intensities of products is not true representation of the difference at the beginning. This difference is all the more critical if we have to decide on the gene expression levels from cDNA leading to diseased or affected phenotypes. Under such circumstances, the initial level of the target gene in cDNA needs to be determined. This has lead to the development of real time PCR wherein the actual PCR reaction can be monitored with the help of fluorescence dyes. Hence, the initial template can be quantified. It has been used successfully for estimating the relative expression of genes, copy number variations and allelic profiling besides others (Mackay et al 2002; Nailis et al 2006; Nolan et al 2006; Spackman et al 2008). This article would focus on use of relative quantification (RQ) for ascertaining gene expression levels.

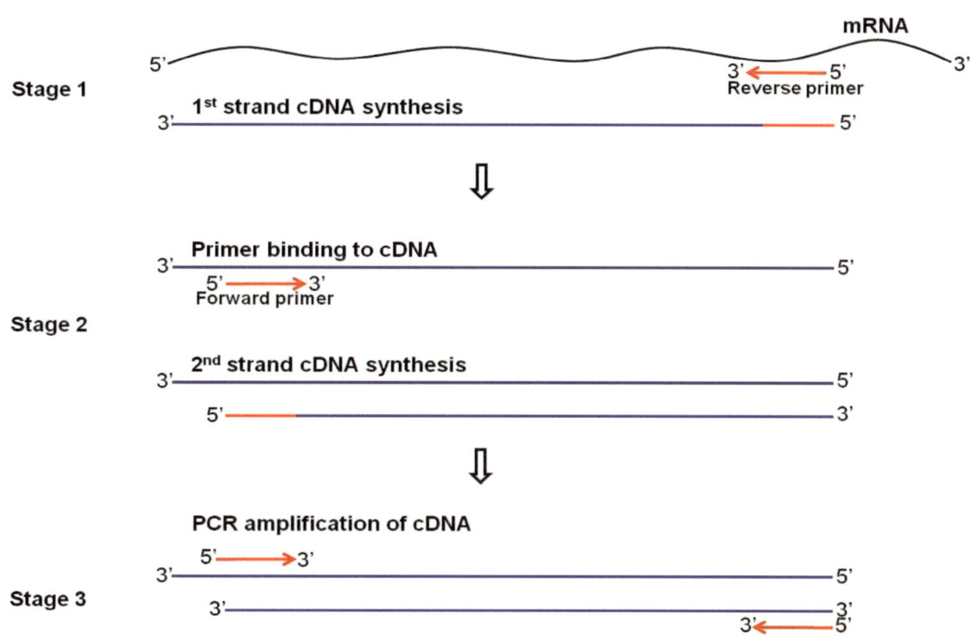

Fig. 10. Different steps in real time PCR. The real time PCR reactions can be performed in two ways: single step and two step. In single step approach all the 3 stages shown above take place in a single tube whereas in two step approach, stage 1 (cDNA preparation) takes place in one tube while the subsequent target specific PCR takes place in another tube.

The relative expression studies require two things: cDNA preparation from RNA and PCR amplification using gene specific primers. An overview of the same has been provided in figure 10. There are two established approaches involved in real time reactions for detection of PCR: SYBR green and Taqman.

3.3.1 SYBR green assays

SYBR green (SG) is a dye which binds to any double stranded DNA. The DNA dye complex absorbs blue light (λ_{max}=488nm) and emits green light (λ_{max}=522nm), hence the name (Zipper et al 2004). Its chemical structure has been shown in figure 11.

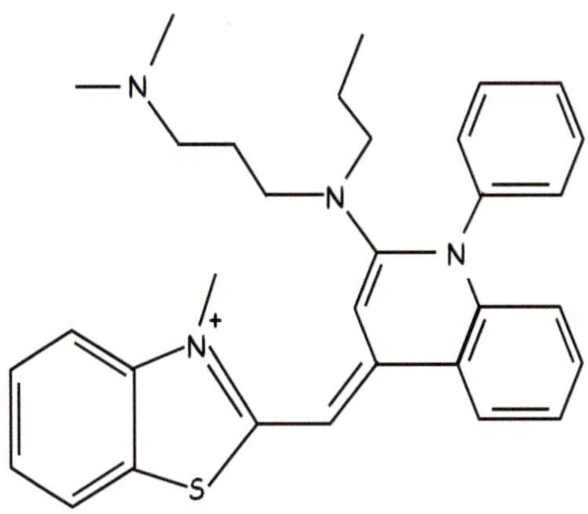

Fig. 11. The chemical structure of SYBR green. Its IUPAC nomenclature is N',N'-dimethyl-N-[4-[(E)-(3-methyl-1,3-benzothiazol-2-ylidene)methyl]-1-phenylquinolin-1-ium-2-yl]-N-propylpropane-1,3-diamine.

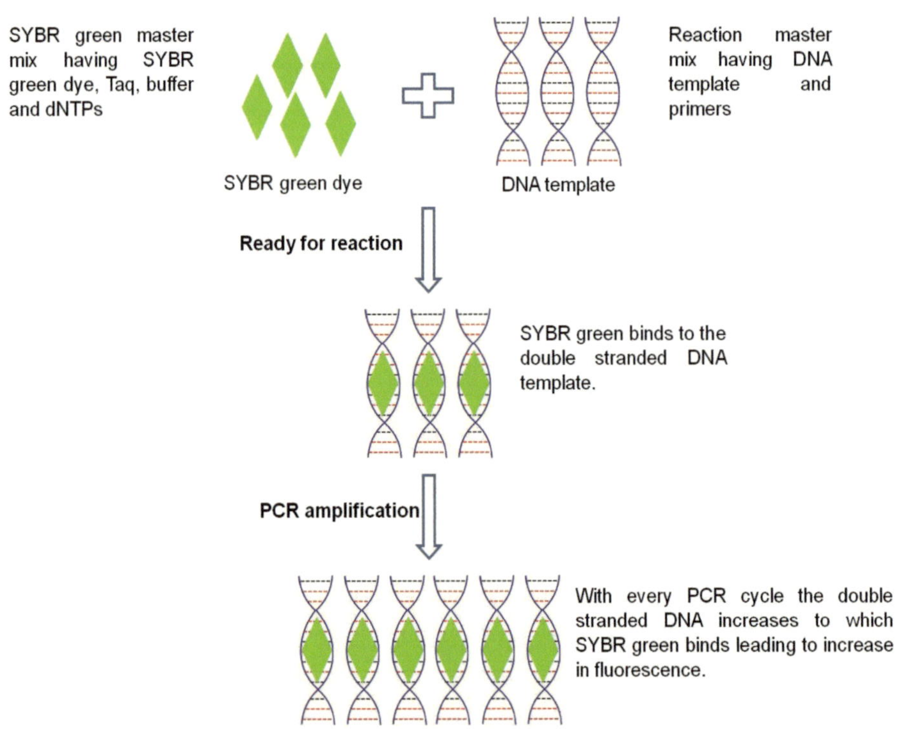

Fig. 12. A real time PCR assay using SG dye. As amount of DNA increases with every cycle more SG is bound to it corresponding to increase in fluorescence.

An overview of real time PCR reaction using SG dye has been shown in figure 12. The SG dye has no binding specificity of its own and would bind to any dsDNA present. It even binds to ssDNA, though with a much lower affinity. Hence, while carrying out the reaction, any additional DNA source would lead to false signal. To ensure that the signal we are observing as amplification is specific to the target from our template source we follow the following steps

a. Check for dissociation curve
b. Reaction controls

Dissociation curve is the calculation of Tm of product after the reaction is over. A single peak would be indicative of specific amplification while multiple peaks would refer to non specific detection. A reaction can be used for analysts only if the corresponding dissociation curve is having a single peak. Moreover, to check for any DNA/RNA contamination two controls are required. First, template where reverse transcription has not taken place and secondly, no template control (NTC) wherein water is added as template. Any amplification in the first signifies impurity of RNA whereas in second it would refer to nucleic acid contaminated water being used for reaction. Owing to the sensitivity of the reaction, all these steps must be ensured for accurate results.

3.3.2 Taqman assays

The real time PCR assays employing taqman chemistries differ from those with SG primarily in two aspects. First, in addition to the target specific primers employed for amplification, a probe is present located between the two primers. Secondly, the fluorescence comes from labelled probe (5′ end) and hence is target specific unlike SG binding to any DNA present. A representation of real time PCR using taqman chemistry is shown in figure 13.

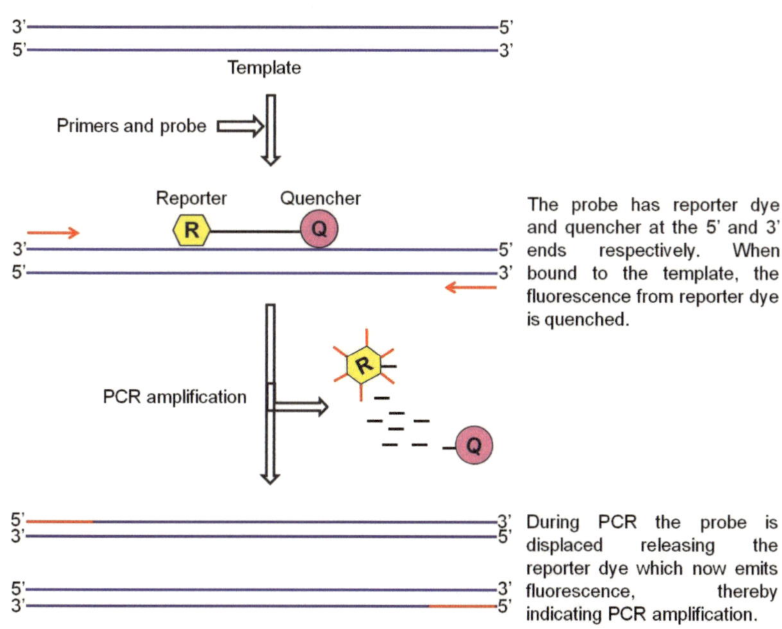

Fig. 13. A real time PCR assay employing taqman chemistry.

There are multiple options for labelling the probe like FAM and VIC. Since the probe is responsible for specificity, hence multiplex reactions can be carried out using taqman approach. This is not feasible when employing SG assays.

3.3.3 Analysis

In order to understand the expression level of a target gene between 2 or more samples two terms need to be introduced: Endogenous control and Calibrator. Endogenous control is a gene whose expression level is known to be fairly constant. These include the various housekeeping genes such as β-actin, and GAPDH. The expression of control needs to be ascertained in all the samples. The calibrator is the sample in reference to which the expression levels needs to be calculated for other samples. For example, if the purpose is study the variations in expression level of androgen receptor (AR) in patients suffering from prostate cancer, then a normal person should be taken as calibrator. When a real time PCR assay is performed it gives us the cycle in which the particular sample reaches threshold level. How this information is corroborated to give relative expression levels is explained below (Pfaffll 2001).

If,
X_0 = number of target molecules at cycle number 0
X_n = number of target molecules at cycle number "n"
E_x = Efficiency of PCR amplification
Then, the equation for target amplification is as follows

$$X_n = X_0 \times (1+E_x)^n \tag{1}$$

Similarly, for endogenous control, equation for amplification can be written as

$$R_n = R_0 \times (1+E_R)^n \tag{2}$$

The threshold cycle (C_t) is the cycle number at which the amplification crosses the threshold fluorescence. This amplification would be constant for the target as well as endogenous control. Hence the equations 1 and 2 can be written as

$$X_T = X_0 \times (1+E_x)^{Ctx} \tag{3}$$

And

$$R_T = R_0 \times (1+E_R)^{Ctr} \tag{4}$$

Where,
Ctx = threshold cycle number for target
Ctr = threshold cycle number for endogenous control
Taking the ratios

$$X_0 \times (1+E_x)^{Ctx} / R_0 \times (1+E_R)^{Ctr} = K \text{ (constant)} \tag{5}$$

Let's assume both the amplifications are occurring with same efficiency. Thereby,

$$E_x = E_r = E \tag{6}$$

Substituting 6 in 5 we get

$$K = X_0 \times (1+E)^{Ctx} / R_0 \times (1+E)^{Ctr} \tag{7}$$

Normalizing the target with control the equation becomes

$$K= X_N \times (1+E)^{\Delta Ct} \tag{8}$$

Where,

$$X_0 / R_0 = X_N \text{ (Normalized target)} \tag{9}$$

And

$$\Delta Ct = Ctx - Ctr \tag{10}$$

Rearranging equation 8,

$$X_N = K \times (1+E)^{-\Delta Ct} \tag{11}$$

Finally, comparing the value of X_N for nay sample X_{NS} with reference to the chosen calibrator X_{NC}, relative quantification is given by

$$Q = X_{NS} / X_{NC} = K \times (1+E)^{-\Delta CtS} / K \times (1+E)^{-\Delta CtC} = (1+E)^{-\Delta\Delta Ct} \tag{12}$$

Where,

$$\Delta\Delta Ct = \Delta CtS - \Delta CtC \tag{13}$$

Considering the efficiency for both reactions to be 1, equation 12 for relative quantification becomes as follows

$$RQ = 2^{-\Delta\Delta Ct} \tag{14}$$

Let's take a hypothetical example to understand the same. Relative expression assays were done to ascertain the levels of AR expression in prostate cancer patients with reference to normal males. B-actin was taken as endogenous control. The C_T values obtained and subsequent calculations have been shown in table 2. From the table, it can be observed that with reference to calibrator (expression level 1), the patients are showing up to 272 folds higher expression of AR.

Similarly, expression profile can be obtained for n number of genes across different sample sets. Since the approach doesn't quantify expression in absolute terms so it's also known as relative quantification method. Further as the expression level is determined by value of ΔΔCT the approach is often also referred to as ΔΔCT method.

3.3.4 Advantages and limitations

The first and foremost advantage that real time has over other conventional methods is assigning a numerical value to expression levels with great accuracy. The assays are relatively easy to perform and design. However, there are few limitations as well. Though housekeeping genes have been used successfully as controls for long, several reports suggest that even their expression may be affected in certain cases. The way forward is to use multiple controls and select the one exhibiting least variations (Dhanasekaran et al 2010). Further, designing assays wherein sufficient information is not available about the organism's genome/transcriptome is very difficult. This is so because the specificity of the primers/probes cannot be ascertained conclusively. Moreover in case of genomes very rich

Sample	AR C_T	Avg. C_T AR	β-actin C_T	Avg. C_T β-actin	ΔC_T (AR-βactin)	$\Delta\Delta C_T$ (sampleΔC_T - calibratorΔC_T)	Relative expression ($2^{-\Delta\Delta Ct}$)
Patient 1	24.34	24.39	8.45	8.47	15.92	-5.77	54.56
	24.45		8.43				
	24.39		8.53				
Patient 2	26.89	26.91	9.76	9.77	17.17	-4.52	22.94
	27.01		9.88				
	26.85		9.67				
Patient 3	22.12	22.15	8.55	8.55	13.6	-8.09	272.48
	22.09		8.48				
	22.24		8.61				
Patient 4	28.67	28.59	8.98	8.92	19.67	-2.02	4.06
	28.49		8.88				
	28.60		8.91				
Patient 5	24.52	24.38	9.98	10.03	14.35	-7.34	162
	24.39		10.08				
	24.24		10.1				
Patient 6	25.31	25.25	9.58	9.55	15.7	-5.99	63.6
	25.19		9.46				
	25.24		9.61				
Normal (Calibrator)	30.12	30.06	8.43	8.37	21.69	0	1
	29.89		8.36				
	30.18		8.32				

Table 2. An experimental result illustrating the calculation of relative expression using $\Delta\Delta C_T$ method.

in GC content designing primers and probes with required taqman specifications has often proved difficult. Since each gene needs a specific assay to be designed, therein we can use real time PCR only when we have candidate targets. It doesn't give us exhaustive data indicative of potential targets; instead it helps us explore candidate targets once known through other approaches. All these limitations notwithstanding, real time PCR would continue is a very effective and accurate approach for studying gene expression.

4. Targets for "Gene Therapy"

The identification of genetic basis of diseases would be significant only if we are able to use that information to be able to cure or at least manage the disease. There are many approaches that have been used for treatment and management of different diseases mostly at the protein level. These include vaccination, antibiotics, hormones and a wide range of drugs. Recently, the focus has been to "modify" or rather "correct" the gene alteration which caused the disease in its first place. This approach can be broadly described as what constitutes "gene therapy". In principle gene therapy refers to the replacement of an affected gene with a normal gene. This can be achieved primarily by two approaches:

a. Ex-vivo: Cells are removed from the tissue where the affected gene needs to be expressing normally and a normal copy of the gene is introduced in these cells.

Subsequently, these cells having a normal expression of the target gene are re-introduced in the body.

b. In-vivo: A normal copy of the gene is directly introduced in the body through viral vectors or liposome mediated approach.

There are various challenges which need to be considered while using gene therapy as a treatment option. Presently, we would focus on choosing a target for gene therapy rather than the approach itself.

a. The first and foremost requirement for any gene to be targeted for gene therapy is that the defect in the gene should be responsible for the disease. When a gene is affected it may either stop expressing or express an altered non-functional protein. This protein may need to be addressed. This situation is often referred to as dominant negative. In such cases, besides introduction of a normal copy of the gene, the altered copy needs to be removed as well. If it cannot be removed there are two options, either silence the gene and introduce a normal copy or repair the gene itself. Both the approaches have been used.
b. Secondly, it should be known that the introduction of a normal expressing gene in the system successfully cures the diseased situation. This is relatively easy to determine in case of monogenic disorders. However, gene therapy can also be used in multi-factorial disorders. In such cases, it's required to identify the gene which has a dominant functional role. This should enable to control the multiple elements through one.
c. Thirdly, the expression profile of the target gene needs to be available. This would include the various tissues where the gene is expressed. If its differential expression in any particular tissue is leading to the disease that tissue needs to be targeted.
d. Fourthly, the feasibility of the target gene to be introduced to the concerned tissue needs to be explored. The gene has to be present in the body such that it expresses only in the desired tissues otherwise it may lead to complications.
e. Lastly, the patient needs to be monitored for certain duration after successful expression of the introduced gene.

5. Conclusions

There has been a constant increase in our understanding of the genetic aspect of diseases, particularly in the last decade or so. This can be attributed to two reasons. First, the pace of technology advancements has been the highest in this period. This has resulted in faster, more sensitive and efficient generation as well as dispersal of data. Secondly, during this period there has been tremendous increase in public awareness and participation in health programmes. This has made the analysis as well as predictions statistically significant. Moreover, awareness has lead to better diagnosis and management of diseases. Though situation has improved but globally there are still many areas where lots need to be done. Unless a disease and its pathogen are completely eradicated from the world, the evolution of the pathogen may lead to more potent variants of the disease.

The chances of an individual getting diseased while living in a safe suitable environment and having a balanced diet are very low. Primarily, it is our life style which is responsible for our diseased body. Various socioeconomic and environmental factors are equally responsible for the life we live. However, awareness and precautions would be the best approach to stay healthy.

The cause of diseases at the physiological level is the imbalance between the three pillars of life; DNA, RNA and protein. Since DNA is the storehouse of all information, mostly, the cause can be traced back to it. DNA is a sequence of nucleotides which governs life. There are several mechanisms which ensure that DNA remains uncorrupted. However if it does get affected there are means to get it repaired. These machineries act as barrier for any wrongful transmission of the genetic material across generations. Still, genetic diseases are inherited possibly contributing not only to the evolution of the species but also to that of the disease.

Hypothetically, it should be possible to cure a disease which is caused by an alteration in gene by giving the body a normal copy of the gene. Even the body on its own tries to do the same which often leads to gene duplications resulting in copy number variations. This thought has formed the basis of gene therapy. To achieve this in reality however, involves exhaustive information about the pathogenesis of the disease; genes involved; their sequence variations and expression profiles. Though the idea is very promising but for it to be successful it needs to be used cautiously and in combination with other approaches.

6. References

Abidi, F.E., Miano, M.G., Murray, J.C. & Schwartz, C.E. (2007) A novel mutation in the PHF8 gene is associated with X-linked mental retardation with cleft lip/cleft palate. *Clinical Genetics*, Vol. 72, No. 1, pp. 19-22.

Baltimore, D. (1970). Viral RNA dependent DNA polymerase in virions of RNA tumor viruses. *Nature*, Vol. 226, pp. 1209-1211

Dhanasekaran, S., Mark Doherty, T., Kenneth, T., & TB Trials Study Group. (2010). Comparison of different standards for real-time PCR-based absolute quantification. *Immunology Methods*, Vol. 354, No. 1-2, pp. 34–9.

Gucev, Z., Koceva, S., Marinaki, A., Fairbanks, L., Kirovski, I. & Tasic, V. (2010) Lesch-Nyhan syndrome: a novel complex mutation with severe phenotype.*Clinical Genetics* Vol. 78, No. 3, pp. 296-7.

Hacia, J.G., Fan, J.B., Ryder, O., Jin, L., Edgemon, K., Ghandour, G., Mayer, R.A., Sun, B., Hsie, L., Robbins, C.M., Brody, L.C., Wang, D., Lander, E.S., Lipshutz, R., Fodor, S.P., & Collins, F.S. (1999). Determination of ancestral alleles for human single-nucleotide polymorphisms using high-density oligonucleotide arrays. *Nature Genetics*, Vol. 22, pp. 164–167.

Huh, S.H. & Ornitz, D.M. (2010). Beta-catenin deficiency causes DiGeorge syndrome-like phenotypes through regulation of Tbx1. *Development*, Vol. 137, No. 7, pp. 1137-47.

Hurwitz, J. & Leis, J.P. (1972). RNA-dependent DNA polymerase activity of RNA tumor viruses. I. Directing influence of DNA in the reaction. *J. Virology*, Vol. 9, No. 1, pp. 116–29.

Judith, L.R., Martha, P.D., Harvey, Kushner., Andrew, R.Z. &, and David P. R. (2009). An extra X or Y chromosome: contrasting the cognitive and motor phenotypes in childhood in boys with 47,XYY syndrome or 47,XXY Klinefelter syndrome. *Dev Disabil Res Rev*. Vol. 15, No. 4, pp. 309–317.

Kulesh, D.A., Clive, D.R., Zarlenga, D.S. & Greene, J.J. (1987). Identification of interferon-modulated proliferation-related cDNA sequences. *PNAS USA*, Vol. 84, No. 23, pp. 8453–8457.

Lashkari, D.A., DeRisi, J.L., McCusker, J.H., Namath, A.F., Gentile, C., Hwang, S.Y., Brown, P.O. & Davis, R.W. (1997). Yeast microarrays for genome wide parallel genetic and gene expression analysis. *PNAS USA*, Vol. 94, No. 24, pp. 13057–13062.

Lopes, A.M., Burgoyne, P.S., Ojarikre, A., Bauer, J., Sargent, C.A., Amorim, A. & Affara, N.A.(2010). Transcriptional changes in response to X chromosome dosage in the mouse: implications for X inactivation and the molecular basis of Turner Syndrome. *BMC Genomics*, Vol. 11, pp. 82.

Mackay, I.M., Arden, K.E. & Nitsche, A. (2002). Real-time PCR in virology. *Nucleic Acids Research, Vol.* 30, No. 6, pp. 1292–305.

Mądry, E., Fidler, E., Sobczyńska-Tomaszewska, A., Lisowska, A., Krzyżanowska, P., Pogorzelski, A., Minarowski, L., Oralewska, B., Mojs, E., Sapiejka, E., Marciniak, R., Sands, D., Korzon-Burakowska, A., Kwiecień, J. & Walkowiak, J. (2011). Mild CFTR mutations and genetic predisposition to lactase persistence in cystic fibrosis. *European J Human Genetics*, [Epub ahead of print].

Magaña, J.J. & Cisneros, B. (2010). Perspectives on gene therapy in myotonic dystrophy type 1.*J Neurosci Res*. [Epub ahead of print]

Mousa, S.A.& Qari, M.H. (2010). Diagnosis and management of sickle cell disorders. *Methods Mol Biol., Vol.* 663, pp. 291-307.

Mullis, K. (1990). The unusual origin of the polymerase chain reaction. *Scientific American*, Vol. 262, No. 4, pp. 56–61.

Nailis, H., Coenye, T., Van Nieuwerburgh, F., Deforce, D. & Nelis, H.J. (2006). Development and evaluation of different normalization strategies for gene expression studies in *Candida albicans* biofilms by real-time PCR. *BMC Molecular Biology*, Vol. 7, pp. 25.

Nolan, T., Hands, R.E. & Bustin, S.A. (2006). Quantification of mRNA using real-time RT-PCR. *Nature Protocols*, Vol. 1, No. 3, pp. 1559–1582.

Nuwaysir, E.F., Huang, W., Albert, T.J., Singh, J., Nuwaysir, K., Pitas, A., Richmond, T., Gorski, T., Berg, J.P., Ballin, J., McCormick, M., Norton, J., Pollock, T., Sumwalt, T., Butcher, L., Porter, D., Molla, M., Hall, C., Blattner, F., Sussman, M.R., Wallace, R.L., Cerrina, F. & Green, R.D. (2002). Gene expression analysis using oligonucleotide arrays produced by maskless photolithography. *Genome Research*, Vol. 12, No. 11, pp. 1749–1755.

Pfaffl, M.W. (2001) A new mathematical model for relative quantification in real-time RT-PCR. *Nucleic* Acids Research, Vol. 29, No. 9, e45.

Pollack, J.R., Perou, C.M., Alizadeh, A.A., Eisen, M.B., Pergamenschikov, A., Williams, C.F., Jeffrey, S.S., Botstein, D. & Brown, P.O. (1999). Genome-wide analysis of DNA copy-number changes using cDNA microarrays. *Nature Genetics*, Vol. 23, No. 1, pp. 41–46.

Purvey, S., Hanna, M., Shaib, W. & Saif, M.W. (2010). A case of Down syndrome who developed pancreatic cancer: a case report and review of literature. *J Pancreas online*, Vol. 11, No. 3, pp. 285-7.

Raelson, J.V., Little, R.D., Ruether, A., Fournier, H., Paquin, B., Van Eerdewegh, P., Bradley, W.E., Croteau, P., Nguyen-Huu, Q., Segal, J., Debrus, S., Allard, R., Rosenstiel, P., Franke, A., Jacobs, G., Nikolaus, S., Vidal, J.M., Szego, P., Laplante, N., Clark, H.F., Paulussen, R.J., Hooper, J.W., Keith, T.P., Belouchi, A. & Schreiber, S. (2007) Genome-wide association study for Crohn's disease in the Quebec Founder Population identifies multiple validated disease loci. *PNAS USA*, Vol. 104, No. 37, pp. 14747-52.

Raheem, O., Olufemi, S.E., Bachinski, L.L., Vihola, A., Sirito, M., Holmlund-Hampf, J., Haapasalo, H., Li, Y.P., Udd, B.& Krahe, R. (2010). Mutant (CCTG)n expansion causes abnormal expression of zinc finger protein 9 (ZNF9) in myotonic dystrophy type 2. *Am J Pathol.* Vol. 177, No. 6, pp. 3025-36.

Rodgers, D.W., Gamblin, S.J., Harris, B.A., Ray, S., Culp, J.S., Hellmig, B., Woolf, D.J., Debouck, C. & Harrison, S.C. (1995). The structure of unliganded reverse transcriptase from the human immunodeficiency virus type 1. *PNAS U.S.A.*, Vol. 92, No. 4, pp. 1222–1226.

Rodríguez-Caballero, A., Torres-Lagares, D., Rodríguez-Pérez, A., Serrera-Figallo, M.A., Hernández-Guisado, J.M. & Machuca-Portillo G. (2010) Cri du chat syndrome: a critical review. *Med Oral Patol Oral Cir Bucal.* Vol. 15, No. 3, pp. 473-478.

Schena, M., Shalon, D., Davis, R.W. & Brown, P.O. (1995). Quantitative monitoring of gene expression patterns with a complementary DNA microarray. *Science,* Vol. 270, No. 5235, pp. 467–470.

Shalon, D., Smith, S.J. & Brown, P.O. (1996). A DNA microarray system for analyzing complex DNA samples using two-color fluorescent probe hybridization. *Genome Research,* Vol. 6, No. 7, pp. 639–645.

Saiki, R.K., Scharf, S., Faloona, F., Mullis, K.B., Horn, G.T., Erlich, H.A. & Arnheim, N. (1985). Enzymatic amplification of beta-globin genomic sequences and restriction site analysis for diagnosis of sickle cell anemia. *Science,* Vol. 230, No. 4732, pp. 1350–1354.

Saiki, R.K., Gelfand, D.H., Stoffel, S., Scharf, S.J., Higuchi, R., Horn, G.T., Mullis, K.B. & Erlich, H.A. (1988). Primer-directed enzymatic amplification of DNA with a thermostable DNA polymerase. *Science,* Vol. 239, No. 4839, pp. 487–91.

Saito, S., Ohno, K., & Sakuraba, H. (2011). Fabry-database.org: database of the clinical phenotypes, genotypes and mutant α-galactosidase A structures in Fabry disease. *J Human Genetics,* [Epub ahead of print].

Spackman, E. & Suarez, D.L. (2008). Type A influenza virus detection and quantitation by real-time RT-PCR. *Methods Molecular Biology,* Vol. 436, pp. 19–26.

South, S.T., Hannes, F., Fisch, G.S., Vermeesch, J.R. & Zollino, M. (2008) Pathogenic significance of deletions distal to the currently described Wolf-Hirschhorn syndrome critical regions on 4p16.3. *Am J Med Genet C Semin Med Genet.* Vol. 15, No. 148C(4), pp. 270-4.

Tang, T., François, N., Glatigny, A., Agier, N., Mucchielli, M.H., Aggerbeck, L. & Delacroix. H. (2007). Expression ratio evaluation in two-colour microarray experiments is significantly improved by correcting image misalignment. *Bioinformatics,* Vol. 23, No. 20, pp. 2686–2691.

Temin, H. M. (1964a). Malignant transformation in cell culture. *Health Lab. Sci.,* Vol. 1, pp. 79-83.

Temin, H. M. (1964b). The participation of DNA in Rous sarcomavirus production. *Virology,* Vol. 23, pp. 486-494.

Temin, H. M. (1964c). Homology between RNA from Rous sarcoma virus and DNA from Rous sarcoma virus-infected cells. *PNAS USA,* Vol. 52, pp. 323-329.

Valenti, R., Bianchi, S., Pescini, F., D'Eramo, C., Inzitari, D., Dotti, M.T. & Pantoni, L. (2011) First report of a pathogenic mutation on exon 24 of the NOTCH3 gene in a CADASIL family. *J Neurology,* [Epub ahead of print].

Warby, S.C., Visscher, H., Collins, J.A., Doty, C.N., Carter, C., Butland, S.L., Hayden, A.R., Kanazawa, I., Ross, C.J. & Hayden, M.R. (2011). HTT haplotypes contribute to differences in Huntington disease prevalence between Europe and East Asia. *European J Human Genetics* [Epub ahead of print].

Wei, C., Li, J. & Bumgarner, R.E. (2004). Sample size for detecting differentially expressed genes in microarray experiments. *BMC Genomics,* Vol. 5, No. 1, pp. 87.

Wilson, M.G., Towner, J.W., Forsman, I. & Sims, E. (1979). Syndromes associated with deletion of the long arm of chromosome 18[del(18q)]. *Am. J. Med. Genet.* Vol. 3, pp. 155-174

Zipper, H., Brunner, H., Bernhagen, J. & Vitzthum, F. (2004). Investigations on DNA intercalation and surface binding by SYBR Green I, its structure determination and methodological implications. *Nucleic Acids Research,* Vol. 32, No.12, e103.

16

Engineered Drug Resistant Cell-Mediated Immunotherapy

Anindya Dasgupta and H. Trent Spencer
Emory University
U.S.A

1. Introduction

In principle, gene therapy is the introduction of a nucleic acid sequence(s) into target cells to prevent or cure a wide range of diseases. Such a therapeutic approach was initially directed toward the correction of inherited disorders. For example, one strategy involves introduction of a corrected gene into cells followed by transplantation of the genetically modified cells into patients. But technological hurdles such inadequate transfer of genetic materials into cells, thus leading to low transgene integration, and safety concerns with gene transfer methodologies have limited the use of gene therapy. However, significant improvements in gene delivery systems that are both efficient and safe have now directed the growth of gene therapy, as evidenced by several hundred gene therapy-based clinical trials being conducted worldwide. Advancements in all areas of gene therapy now allow for the development of genetically engineered immunocompetent cell-based therapies for cancer.

The therapeutic role of immune cells to control malignancies has been well established. For example, immunocompetent hosts frequently reject transplanted tumors while tumors can easily be established in immunosuppressant hosts. In vitro studies have demonstrated that immunocompetent cells exhibit powerful cytotoxicity toward a broad range of cancer cells and tumorigenic animal models have shown that these cells can infiltrate tumors resulting in tumor regression. Tumor infiltration by immunocompetent cells indicates favorable prognosis in various cancers, such as melanoma, colon, ovarian cancer, basal cell carcinoma, and lung cancer (Haanen et al., 2006; Halliday et al., 1995; Inoue et al., 2000; Kerr et al., 1998; Pages et al., 2005; Zhang et al., 2003). These observations have led to the development of cell based immunotherapy strategies to target cancer.

However, intensive chemotherapy regimens, the frontline therapy to treat patients with advanced cancer, frequently lead to non-specific cellular toxicity to adoptively transferred immunocompetent cells and to hematopoietic stem cells. One strategy to combat drug-induced toxicity is to genetically engineer immune cells to make them drug resistant. Several genes, such as methylguanine methyltransferase (MGMT), dihydrofolate reductase (DHFR), cytidine deaminase (CD), and multidrug resistant protein (MDR-1) have been identified that can confer drug resistance to anti-cancer immune cells, and advances in gene therapy techniques have made it possible to test the feasibility of using the cDNAs encoding these sequences in drug resistant gene therapy studies. The ability to generate chemo-resistant immune cells can be exploited to test novel anti-cancer therapies, such as "Drug

Resistant Immunotherapy" (or DRI) whereby drug resistant immunocompetent cells can be administered in conjunction with chemotherapy. Such a treatment modality can significantly enhance the generation of anti-tumor immunity that is quantitatively and qualitatively superior to that achieved by either cellular immunotherapy or chemotherapy alone. DRI can also benefit from the ability to selectively expanding the modified cells in vivo by administering specific chemotherapeutic agents thereby mitigating the problem of inefficient gene transfer to these cells. The anti-cancer effectiveness of DRI based therapy has been successfully demonstrated using either drug resistant bone marrow or immunocompetent cells with intrinsic cytotoxic capabilities. The therapeutic benefits afforded by a DRI based strategy can potentially be enhanced by the synergistic effects between chemotherapy and immunotherapy. For example, chemotherapy mediated lymphodepletion prior to adoptive transfer of drug resistant immunocompetent cells can mitigate immunosuppressive mechanisms that are advantageously exploited by progressive tumor cells to evade immune recognition. With the recent advances in *ex vivo* gene transfer technology, drug resistant variants of i) tumor specific lymphocytes, and their genetically engineered counterparts such as those harboring transgenic αβ T cell receptor (TCR)/cancer antigen receptor (CAR) modifications, and ii) lymphocytes with non-specific cytotoxic potentials, can be bioengineered to treat various malignancies.

However such a gene therapy based approach can be limited by inadequate transfer of cDNA that encodes drug resistant genes. The ability to genetically engineer immune cells, specifically hematopoietic cells, has greatly advanced in recent years. It is generally accepted that recombinant retroviral vectors, specifically those based on HIV-1) are the most efficient gene transfer systems for the ex vivo modification of hematopoietic cells. Retroviral systems have the advantage that i) recombinant viruses are now relatively easy to generate and characterize, ii) most components for retroviral transfer systems are commercially available, iii) retroviral gene transfer results in stable integration of the transferred nucleic acid sequence into the genome of the target cell, and iv) depending on the target cells, the efficiency of gene transfer can approach 100%.

This chapter will discuss cancer immunotherapy with genetically engineered immune cells and the feasibility of employing drug resistant variants of these cells during chemotherapy that can potentially augment such a cell therapy based approach.

2. Combining drug resistant immune cell therapy with chemotherapy: A new paradigm in cancer treatment

Despite relentless efforts worldwide to improve upon conventional treatment modalities for cancer, chemotherapy remains a much needed frontline therapy. Several cytotoxic agents, such as anti-metabolites, alkylating agents, anthracyclines, DNA methylasetransferase inhibitors, platinum compounds and spindle poisons have been developed to kill cancer cells. However, they are not uniformly effective, and the introduction of these agents with novel state-of-the-art therapies, such as immunotherapies, is problematic. For example, these agents can be detrimental to the establishment of robust anti-tumor immunocompetent cells due to the non-specific cellular toxicity of many anti-cancer agents. Intensive chemotherapy frequently administered to treat patients with advanced cancer can result in lymphopenia, which decrease the numbers and function of potential anti-cancer T cells in the blood thereby blunting the anti-tumor immune responses (Liseth et al., 2010). Tumor drug resistance can also develop, resulting in ineffective chemotherapy treatment

(Michael & Doherty, 2005). In addition, induced secondary cancers and long-term survivorship issues limit the effectiveness of some cytotoxic chemotherapy agents (Perry et al., 1998). If the chemotherapy regimens that are transiently effective can be combined with immunocompetent cell therapies, then it is predicted that a significant improvement of anti-neoplastic therapy can be achieved. However, because chemotherapy regimens are toxic to immunocompetent cells, the co-administration of these treatments reduces or eliminates the effectiveness of the immunocompetent cells.

One strategy to combat drug-induced toxicity is to genetically engineer immunocompetent cells to make them drug resistant. This strategy facilitated the development of a DRI-based anti-cancer technology that combines the therapeutic effectiveness afforded by drug resistant immunocompetent cells with conventional chemotherapy. This strategy involves 1) the use of lentivirus mediated applications to introduce cDNAs that encode for drug resistant genes into immunocompetent cells, and 2) administration of the genetically-modified immunocompetent cells in conjunction with chemotherapy to enhance tumor cell clearance. The novel features of such a strategy are 1) it can be more potent in tumor elimination than the individual administration of chemotherapy or immunotherapy, 2) it can easily be integrated with other conventional treatment modalities, such as surgery and antibody/vaccine based immunotherapy, 3) it is applicable to patients with any disease stages, and, 4) less aggressive chemotherapy can be applied during DRI therapy applications, thereby reducing the development of tumor drug resistance and induction of secondary cancers. Several strategies have been identified that can be used to confer drug resistance to targeted cells, and advances in gene therapy techniques have made it possible to test the feasibility of using the cDNA encoding proteins that confer resistance in drug resistance gene therapy studies. A number of proteins have been identified that confer drug resistance, but this chapter will focus on four that have already been used to confer resistance specifically to hematopoietic cells.

2.1 Drug resistant genes

DHFR regulates folate homeostasis by controlling the synthesis of purines and pyrimidines. Anti-folate drugs such methotrexate and trimetraxte, are inhibitors of DHFR. Gene therapy strategies have exploited the use of DHFR mutants that can confer resistance to antifolates. For example, bioengineered hematopoietic stem cells (HSCs) harboring a mutated DHFR transgene protects mice from an antifolate dose that is lethal to non-modified HSCs. (Allay et al., 1997, 1998a; Spencer et al., 1996,). However, HSCs bypass drug induced toxicity by increased nucleoside transport. To circumvent such effects, nucleoside transport inhibitors have been co-administered with antifolate drugs to significantly increase the population of cells modified with DHFR mutants, specifically L22Y (Allay et al., 1998b; Warlick et al., 2002).

The therapeutic efficiency of a single drug resistant based gene therapy can be significantly enhanced by genetically engineering dual drug resistant anti-cancer cells. Such a strategy can be particularly effective in treating tumors that respond to drug combinations that exhibit synergistic (or additive) effects. The combination of methotrexate and a cytosine nucleotide analog, cytosine arabinoside (Ara-C) has been successfully used in patients with Non-Hodgkins lymphoma (Fisher et al., 1993; Khouri et al., 1998). Ara-C is inactivated by CD which is involved in the salvage of pyrimidine compounds and in pyrimidine metabolism. The feasibility of bioengineering cells resistant to both an antifolate and Ara-C have led to the development of gene therapy strategies based on the generation of dual drug resistant cells (Sauerbrey et al., 1999). Transplantation of dual drug resistant bone marrow cells generated by the retroviral transfer of a fusion construct: mutDHFR-CD encoding for mutant DHFR and CD genes, into myoablated mice significantly reduced the growth of established leukemia, while protecting hematopoietic cells (Budak-Alpdogan et al., 2004).

During cancer progression, the tumor acquires resistance to multiple natural products by the expression of the MDR-1 gene. This gene encodes a membrane glycoprotein, known as P-glycoprotein (P-GP) involved in the transport of metabolic byproducts across the cell membrane. The P-GP protein displays broad specificity towards several structurally unrelated chemotherapy agents. Thus, pleitropic drug resistance can be conferred to cells by the transfer of nucleic acid sequence that encodes for MDR-1. MDR-1 gene was one of the first candidate genes to be exploited in the context of drug resistant gene therapy to confer protection to bone marrow cells. (Abonour et al., 2000; Bunting et al, 2000; Cowan et al, 1999; Moscow et al., 1999; Sellers et al., 2001; Sorrentino et al, 1992). These initial studies, and others, led to the development of the field of drug resistance gene therapy for cancer. One strategy is to harvest HSCs from cancer patients and genetically modify them to express the MDR-1 gene followed by transplantation into patients. During engraftment, chemotherapy is administered to selectively enrich for modified cells in vivo, which leads to lower cytotoxicity upon repeated chemotherapy treatments.

Among the drug resistant genes studied, MGMT is among the most promising. This gene encodes for human alkyl guanine transferase (hAGT), a DNA repair protein that confers resistance to the cytotoxic effects of alkylating agents, such as BCNU and temozolomide (Davis et al., 1997; Liu et al., 2002; Maze et al., 1996). Tumor cells have been shown to express high levels of AGT, which can be an effective mechanism of tumor cell drug resistance. To circumvent AGT-mediated resistance, alkylating agents have been administered in combination with inhibitors of AGT, namely 6-Benzyl Guanine (6-BG) (Dolan et al., 1989). Although 6-BG sensitizes tumor cells to alkylating agents, drug induced toxicities such as myelosuppression severely limit the use of these combined agents. To overcome this limitation, several BG-resistant variants of AGT have been generated and used in gene transfer studies. Among them, the P140KMGMT variant has been well characterized with respect to drug resistant gene therapy. (Gerull et al., 2007; Larochelle et al., 2009; Neff, et al., 2005; Pollok et al., 2003; Sawai et al., 2001; Zielske et al., 2003).

2.2 Evaluation of drug resistant immunotherapy (DRI)

The development of drug resistant genes along with the advancements in gene delivery systems has allowed for the chemoprotection of immunocompetent cells. Genetic engineering of drug resistant hematopoietic cells has been well documented (Allay et al, 1998a, 1998b; Davis et al, 1997; Maze et al, 1996; Zhao et al, 2008). Transplantation of modified HSCs has been shown to protect the hematopoietic system from chemotherapy-induced toxicity, and this strategy has been used to enrich the percentage of circulating gene-modified cells. The advantages to the establishment of such chemo-resistant bone marrow cells are two-fold. First, chemotherapy can be administered, possibly at a higher frequency and at higher doses. For example, transplantation of the DHFR mutant L22Y-modified HSCs allowed for the administration of the antifolate drug, trimetrexate (TMTX) at concentrations that are lethal to animals not receiving the genetically altered bone marrow cells (Allay et al., 1997, 1998; May et al., 1995; Spencer et al., 1996). Secondly, tumor targeting T lymphocytes can be expanded during chemotherapy challenges, leading to increased tumor infiltration and potentially increased tumor clearance

The anti-cancer effectiveness of combining drug resistant HSCs, immune-modulating agents, and chemotherapy was evaluated by combining the administration of an antifolate based chemotherapy, trimetrexate (TMTX), along with anti-CD137-based immunotherapy in mice transplanted with anti-folate resistant HSCs (McMillin et al., 2006). Mice were initially transplanted with L22Y-DHFR-modified bone marrow and were allowed to reconstitute with drug resistant hematopoietic cells. The reconstituted mice were implanted with sarcoma cells, i.e. the AG104 sarcoma cell line. The tumor bearing animals were exposed to treatments comprising of either anti-CD137, TMTX, or the combination of anti-CD137 and TMTX. Chemotherapy alone mediated tumor regressions only during the treatment phase. However, once this treatment ended all animals in this treatment group experienced rapid growth of their tumor. Similarly, administration of immunotherapy alone regressed tumors in the majority of animals, but only 40% of the animals achieve long-term tumor clearance. However, all animals treated with chemotherapy along with immunotherapy resulted in complete tumor regressions. Such an observation confirmed the existence of possible synergism between immunotherapy and chemotherapy in the context of a drug resistant immunotherapy strategy. Importantly, application of the DRI based strategy by combining chemo-and immunotherapies can lead to the induction of immunological memory. Such an effect was demonstrated by infusing splenocytes isolated from mice in the combined treatment group into untreated tumor bearing animals. The adoptive transfer of potential immunocompetent cell populations led to reductions in tumor burdens and extension of survival of the recipient mice. These studies have important implications in designing treatment modalities to generate a robust antitumor response that may lead to eradicate residual tumor. Such a strategy will involve the co-administration of chemo-protected immunocompetent cells with chemotherapy that mediate a fast antitumor response to reduce tumor burden followed by the induction of immune memory cells that are sustained over a long time to eliminate any persistent cancer cells.

Although initial studies focused on immunotherapy driven by HSCs, which is the source of all immune cells, other proof-of-concept studies were directed toward the evaluation of specific immunocompetent cells as mediators of DRI. For example, one study exploited the use of genetically engineered drug resistant variants of the anti-cancer immune cells, NK92 and T-ALL104 cells, in combination with temozolomide (Dasgupta, et al., 2010). These cells were selected based on their direct immunotherapeutic properties to mediate robust anti-tumor properties without the requirement of MHC presentation (Gong et al., 1994; Tam et al., 1999; Tonn et al., 2001). TALL-104 cells represent a leukemic T cell line that has surface markers typical of both cytotoxic T lymphocytes and natural killer cells and adoptive immunotherapy with TALL-104 cells has induced long-term complete or partial remissions in tumor bearing animals (Cesano et al., 1998; Geoerger et al., 2000). In this study, a SIV-based lentiviral system was employed to deliver the drug resistant variant P140KMGMT into the immunocompetent cell lines NK-92 and TALL-104, and in the myelogenous leukemia cell line, K562, which is a target for both NK-92 and TALL-104 cells. Using in vitro survival and cytotoxicity assays it was demonstrated that 1) the genetically-modified cells developed significant resistance to the alkylating drug temozolomide when compared to the untransfected wild type cells, 2) genetic modification of the immune effector cells did not alter their ability to kill target cells, and 3) genetically altered cells were active in killing target cells after drug treatments, while the killing effectiveness of the unmodified effector cells is significantly diminished after a chemotherapy challenge. However, genetically modified drug resistant cells killed virtually all of un-modified K562 target cells in the presence of drug, which was significantly higher compared to the killing effectiveness of the non-modified effector cells.

These in vivo and in vitro proof-of-concept studies demonstrate that drug resistant immunocompetent effector cells are superior cytotoxic effectors during a chemotherapy challenge. This is a significant finding which can potentially be combined with current cell-based and adoptive immunotherapies. Regression of large, vascularized tumors has been shown in patients with refractory metastatic melanoma. However, for maximum effectiveness a lympho-depleting regimen is necessary prior to autologous lymphocyte cell transfer (Rosenberg & Dudley, 2004). Generation and expansion of drug-resistant lymphocytes ex vivo can allow, in this setting, for the administration of immunocompetent cell-based therapy concurrently with chemotherapy, potentially improving tumor clearance while anti-tumor immunity is established and maintained. In this scenario, non-transduced lymphocytes can continually be depleted using a selective chemotherapy treatment, which could be repeatedly applied during the administration of adoptive immunotherapy. The co-administration of chemo- and immunotherapies could then lead to long-term tumor clearance. Thus, it is anticipated that the T lymphocytes with memory phenotypes are suitable candidates to be incorporated into future DRI studies to target advanced cancer.

3. Synergism between chemotherapy and immunotherapy can benefit drug resistant immunotherapy

Combining chemotherapy with immunotherapy is an attractive strategy to enhance the effectiveness of both treatments, but initial combination strategies consisting of high-dose chemotherapy combined with interleukin-2 (IL-2) were no better than chemotherapy alone (Pollera et al., 1994; Rinehart et al., 1992). However, studies in the last decade have demonstrated potential synergistic effects between chemotherapy and immunotherapy (Fridlender et al., 2010; Lake et al., 2005; Ramakrishnan et al., 2011). Conventional chemotherapy can augment immunotherapy in several ways: 1) induction of chemotherapy mediated-lymphodepletion leading to i) enhanced persistence of the tumor reactive T lymphocytes, ii) increase in tumor trafficking by the tumor responsive T cells (Dudley et al, 2002a, 2005), iii) modulation of immunosuppressive factors (Cui et al., 2009), and iv) promotion of differentiation of central memory effector cells (to augment vaccine based strategies) (Badovinac et al., 2005; Wrzesinski et al., 2007), and 2) chemotherapy induced sensitization of tumor to the immunocompetent cells by i) the induction of stress responsive molecules on tumor surface and ii) increasing the availability of tumor antigens to "boost" the T cell response (Fridlender et al., 2010). Thus a DRI therapy approach that integrates both chemo- and drug resistant immune cell therapies can significantly benefit from such partnerships.

3.1 Chemotherapy induced lymphopenia

Several clinical trials with melanoma patients support the concept that adoptive transfer of genetically engineered T lymphocytes may not be sufficient to improve treatment outcomes without lymphodepletion. For example, in the treatment of patients with advanced melanoma, anti-tumor response rate was observed only after adoptive transfer of T lymphocytes (with or without engineered specificity towards melanoma antigens) with lymphodepleting regimens (Dudley, et al., 2001, 2002b, 2005; Hughes et al, 2005). Lymphodepletion is thought to provide space in the lymphoid compartment thereby allowing robust establishment of the transferred lymphocytes (Klebanoff et al., 2005) which resulted in the induction of faster and more efficient immune response with enhanced anti-tumor properties (Dudley et al., 2002; Rosenberg & Dudley, 2004; Wang et al., 2005a, 2005b). Lymphopenia also induces the rescue of memory T cells as shown in the treatment of mice with established melanoma. For example, the anti-tumor efficacy of an immunotherapy comprising an oncolytic vaccinia virus expressing CD137 T-cell costimulatory molecule is significantly enhanced when animals were lymphodepleted prior to vaccination (Kim et al., 2009). In addition, T regulatory cells (Tregs) have been implicated as having potent immune suppressive functions, and clinical trials have indicated that depleting or inhibiting such cells can increase anticancer efficacy (Phan et al., 2003). The number of Tregs can be reduced by chemotherapy and also by a combination of an adenoviral based immunogene therapy (Fridlender et al., 2010).

3.2 Chemotherapy induced upregulation of stress antigens on tumor surface

Chemotherapy can sensitize tumors to augment immunotherapy by the up-regulation of tumor specific antigens that are recognized by the activating receptors expressed by NK and γδ T cells, thereby leading to an increase in tumor clearance (Nausch & Cerwenka, 2008). It has been reported that various cancer cells exposed to drugs upregulate stress-associated molecules MIC-A, MIC-B, and UL-16 binding proteins which are recognized by immunocompetent NK and γδ T cells through their MHC-independent NKG2D/TCR pathways. Such innate HLA-independent interactions lead to the activation of anti-tumor properties of these cells, as has been demonstrated by γδ T cell mediated destruction of glioblastoma cells exposed to temozolomide, the frontline chemotherapy agent in the treatment of patients afflicted with glioblastoma multiforme (GBM) (Lamb, 2009). This mode of immune cell-activation opens the possibility of testing a treatment modality that can combine immunotherapy based on drug resistant variants of NK or γδ T cells and chemotherapy to target cancer types that express these activators during drug treatments. It was also demonstrated that in mouse models of colon and mammary cancer, applications of chemotherapeutic drugs upregulated the expression of a tumor cell surface receptor, mannose 6-phosphate receptor (Motyka et al, 2000). This receptor is implicated in the uptake of granzyme B released by CTLs upon contact with tumor cells, thereby establishing a synergy between chemotherapy and immunotherapy (Ramakrishnan et al, 2010).

3.3 Enhancement of tumor antigen presentation

Chemotherapy induced tumor cell apoptosis can liberate massive amounts of tumor specific antigens that are duly processed by antigen presenting cells and the processed antigens are presented, in association with MHC class I molecules, to CTLs leading to an increase in antigen presentation (Lake et al, 2005). Thus chemotherapy can augment immunotherapy by increasing antigen presentation, which can 1) lead to T lymphocyte expansion and increased lymphocyte infiltration of solid tumors and 2) mediate cancer vaccination effects. For example, it has been shown that chemotherapy can prime the host's immunity and enhance antitumor responses (Nowak et al., 2003a). Antitumor cytotoxic T lymphocytes (CTLs) showed increased proliferation because of increased tumor apoptosis when chemotherapy was administered, and incorporating immunotherapy with chemotherapy extended animal survival (Nowak et al., 2003b). Importantly, this study showed that the delivery of chemotherapy before immunotherapy is more effective than after immunotherapy (Nowak et al., 2003a).

4. Potential immunocompetent cell sources for implementing DRI

Our knowledge about the host immune response to cancer has led to the development of immunocompetent cell-based therapeutics. Two distinct classes of cells that are defined by their mechanism to invoke anti-tumor immunity have been exploited: i) the widely used tumor specific T lymphocytes, which must be primed prior to tumor cell killing, and ii) non-specific MHC-unrestricted effector cells with intrinsic tumor killing properties.

4.1 Tumor-directed T lymphocytes

T cells mediate their potent anti-tumor effectiveness by their ability to recognize a wide spectrum of antigens expressed on the tumor surface. These tumor associated antigens are processed by the antigen presenting cells, such as dendritic cells into smaller peptides which are presented to T cells in combination with MHC complexes. T cell activation occurs after the recognition of the peptide-MHC complex via their antigen specific receptor, i.e. TCR-CD3 complex. The T cell receptor is a heterodimer composed of either α and β or γ and δ polypeptide chains. Each chain of the TCR is composed of a variable region (V) and a constant region (C). The V region determines the antigen binding specificity of the TCR. The vast majority of peripheral blood T lymphocytes and TCR+ thymocytes have $\alpha\beta$ TCR while epithelial T cells contain the $\gamma\delta$ TCR. The TCR heterodimer is associated with the CD3 complex. The CD3 complex is necessary for i) the expression of TCR on the T cell surface and ii) activation of T cells by signal transduction when the TCR binds to its specific polypeptide primed MHC complex. Following the recognition of peptide-MHC, the CD3 complex initiates signal transduction pathways to mediate cell proliferation, cytokine secretion and activation of T cell anti-tumor properties (Chan et al.; 1992; Punt et al., 1994). Several tumor antigens such as melanoma/melanocyte differentiation antigens (MART-1 and gp100) and NY-ESO-1 cancer-testis antigen have been identified (Cormier et al., 1998; Morgan, et al., 2003; Zhao et al., 2005). The tumor antigens can activate a large number of T lymphocytes that can infiltrate the tumor (TIL). These immune cells have been widely employed during the administration of ACT to treat cancer. ACT involves i) the isolation of tumor infiltrating lymphocytes, either from a surgically removed tumor or from the peripheral blood, ii) ex vivo expansion of the selected cells in the presence of cytokines, and iii) infusion of the expanded cells back into the patient, typically after 'conditioning' of the patient with lymphodepleting regimens comprised of either chemotherapy or total body irradiation (TBI). It is now well established that ACT can establish or augment immunity and eradicate malignant cells.

Following the discovery of a large number of tumor antigens, TILs directed against such antigens have been successfully generated, mainly from melanoma but also from renal cell carcinoma and glioma (Dillman et al., 1991; Figlin et al., 1997; Kradin et al., 1989; Quattrocchi et al, 1999). TILs mediated tumor regression when transferred into tumor-bearing mice. ACT with TILs directed against melanoma antigens have proven successful since patients with melanoma are immunized against antigens expressed by their own tumors and melanoma tumors generate relatively higher quantities of melanoma antigen specific T lymphocytes. However, the use of TILs in the treatment of patients with cancer other than melanoma has met with limited success, possibly due to the presence of low number of cytotoxic T lymphocytes within TILs (Finke et al., 1994; Hom et al., 1993; Schwartzentruber et al., 1992). Therefore, improvements in the usefulness of TILs are needed, and DRI studies are in progress to determine if such modifications can improve the therapeutic potential of these cells.

4.1.1 Chimeric αβ TCR modified T cells

In general, αβ T lymphocytes display low affinity TCRs. Therefore, success with ACT with tumor directing αβ T lymphocytes is limited by the difficulty in isolating high affinity αβ T lymphocytes that exist in low numbers in vivo and in ex vivo expansion of these cells to generate adequate quantities for in vivo anti-tumor efficacy. Furthermore, tumor derived immunosuppression mechanisms reduce the number of tumor specific αβ T cells in circulation. As a means of enhancing the anti-cancer efficacy of αβ T lymphocytes, these cells can be genetically modified to express transgenic α and β TCR chains, which can be derived from T cell clones specific for tumor-associated antigens. These genetically engineered CTLs harboring a transgenic αβ TCR, in addition to their native αβ TCR, acquire the same antigen specificity as the high affinity T cells from which the TCR was cloned. Several CTLs harboring transgenic TCRs have now been developed that are directed specifically to tumor antigens, such as MART-1, gp100, NY-ESO-1 and CEA, resulting in tumor elimination in animal models (Abad, et al., 2008; Morgan, et al., 2003; 2006; Kessels et al., 2001; Stanislawski et al., 2001; Wargo et al., 2009; Xue et al., 2005). Bicistronic viral vectors encoding cDNA sequences for both α and β chains have been successfully incorporated into retroviral based strategies to transfer αβ transgenic TCR into T lymphocytes (Yang et al., 2008). The functional efficacies of the engineered CTLs have also been improved by codon optimizing α and β sequences that result in increased surface expression of the transgenic TCRs (Jorritsma et al., 2007; Scholten et al., 2006). The chimeric αβ T cells can be rapidly expanded ex vivo to produce sufficient quantities of tumor reactive cells and after adoptive transfer to patients display potent MHC-restricted cytotoxic activity against tumor cells expressing the specific epitope. ACT with tumor directed chimeric αβ T lymphocytes have been widely used to treat various malignancies, particularly melanoma, because of the ease of isolating and expanding melanoma reactive CTLs ex vivo.

However, the genetic engineering of CTLs that express the transgenic αβ TCR along with their endogenous TCR has inherent disadvantages. The endogenous TCR can compete with the transgenic αβ TCR to bind to the initiator CD3 molecule. Consequently, the chimeric αβ TCR-modified CTLs may suffer from reduced activation leading to a decrease in affinity of the transgenic αβ TCR towards specific tumor antigens. Furthermore rearrangements between the chimeric and the naïve TCR chains can induce new and unwanted reactivities. To combat such undesired consequences TCR negative lymphocytes have been modified to harbor αβ transgenic TCR while the sequences of such chimeric αβ TCRs have been redesigned to reduce cross competition within T lymphocytes harboring naïve TCR (Kuball et al., 2007; Robbins et al., 2008).

4.1.2 Cancer Antigen Receptor (CAR)-modified T cells

Adoptive immunotherapy for cancer utilizes additional bioengineering strategies adaptable to drug resistant immunotherapy whereby T lymphocytes are genetically modified to express chimeric antigen receptors. In contrast to chimeric αβ TCR, CAR combines antigen specificity derived from a tumor antigen specific monoclonal antibody fragment and T cell proliferation signal moieties. Upon infusion into patients, immunocompetent T cells genetically engineered to express CAR can specifically recognize and respond to soluble, immobilized and/or tumor antigens and, to date, a range of CARs targeting a variety of surface molecules expressed by many solid tumors and hematological malignancies, such as B cell malignancies and melanoma, have been developed (Kohn et al., 2011).

The potency of CAR modified CTLs have evolved through several generations of design changes (Cartellieri et al., 2010). First generation CARs are constructed by the fusion of the single-chain Fv (scFv) moiety, derived from the light and variable chains of a monoclonal antibody, directed against tumor associated antigens with the transmembrane and cytoplasmic signaling domains derived from the CD3 ζ chain. The CD3 domain provides activation signal to the CAR for the induction of cytotoxicity towards the tumor expressing the protein that is recognized by the scFV. Thus CAR integrates the antigen specificity of an antibody and anti-tumor properties of CTLs. However, bioengineered CTLs were poorly activated by the first generation CARs, possibly due to in sufficient co- stimulatory signaling as evident by low response rates in clinical trials in subjects with various malignancies, such as lymphoma, and ovarian cancer (Kershaw et al., 2006; Lamers et al., 2006). To circumvent this issue, various signaling domains from costimulatory molecules such as CD28, OX40, and CD137 (4-1BB) were fused to the cytoplasmic tail of the CAR which improved the anti-tumor efficacies of the CTLs modified with the second generation CAR in preclinical models (Kowolik et al, 2006). To further enhance the potency of the engineered CTLs, recent third generation CARs are designed to incorporate tripartite signaling domains, such as CD3ζ-CD28-41BB or CD3ζ-CD28-OX40. Several vector systems have been designed to introduce the chimeric receptors into T cells. Such systems include γ-retroviral vectors, lentiviral vectors and transposon based (sleeping beauty) constructs (Hackett et al., 2010; Westwood & Kershaw, 2010).

CAR based anti-neoplastic cellular therapy can be applicable to patients with any HLA type since CARs use antibodies as the component that recognize the target antigen and thereby the CAR-modified cells act in "HLA non-restricted" fashion to destroy their target. Thus CAR mediated cellular immunotherapy is refractory to the immune evasion strategies by tumors, such as downregulation of HLA class I molecules or failure to process or present proteins. However, CAR can be targeted only against extracellular (surface) antigens, which represent only a subset of potential tumor-associated antigens. To circumvent limitation, CARs have also been designed to recognize carbohydrates and glycolipids (Dotti et al, 2005; Sadelain et al., 2009). It should also be noted that currently, murine derived antibodies are employed to design the antibody components of most CARs, which raises the possibility of evoking immune responses against the CAR-engineered cells after infusion.

4.2 MHC-unrestricted immune cells

Conventional cell based immunotherapeutic strategies that are based on the activation of HLA-restricted lymphocytes have limited anti-tumor response. This is due to i) frequent down regulation of HLA on the tumor cell surface thereby mitigating the activity of adaptive immune responsive cells, ii) secretion of immunosuppressive factors by the tumors and iii) limited expression of tumor antigens in small subset of the tumor cells. Thus novel strategies that harness the anti-cancer responsive-innate immune cells, such as NK92 cells and a minor subclass in the T lymphocyte repertoire, γδ T cells present a promising alternative to conventional adaptive cell based therapy approaches to treat cancer.

4.2.1 Natural killer (NK) cells

NK cells comprise a unique subset of lymphocytes, distinct from T and B cells, and are members of the innate immune response cells with potent immunosurveillance properties. These cells do not require any prior immune sensitization by the host to lyze tumor cells

(Herberman et al., 1975; Kiessling et al., 1975; Klingemann, 2005). Early pioneering work demonstrated the therapeutic benefits of adopting innate immune responsive killer cell based strategies, specifically with LAK cells along with IL2, to target advanced metastatic renal cell carcinoma and melanoma (Rosenberg, et al., 1985). However, later studies found similar benefits with administrations of IL2 alone (Law et al., 1995). It was initially thought that NK cells exhibit potent cytotoxicity towards transformed cells that express altered MHC molecules (missing self recognition) while sparing normal cells that express unaltered MHC molecules (self recognition) via the activation of the inhibitory receptors. However, NK cells are able to efficiently attack some target cells that express normal levels of class I MHC molecules, while some other cells are not sensitive to NK cell-lysis despite low or absent class I MHC expression. It is now established that NK cells express NKG2D (natural killer group D) receptors that are activated by the recognition of ligands that are strongly upregulated in stressed tumor cells (Bauer et al., 1999; Cosman et al., 2001). Surprisingly, normal non-stressed cells of bone marrow activated peripheral blood T lymphocytes and even normal non-hematopoetitic cells express NKG2D ligands. The specific roles of NK cells towards each of these cell types are under investigation (Eagle et al, 2009). The use of autologous NK cells has met with limited success (Burns et al, 2003; Law et al, 1995; Rosenberg et al, 1985). Consequently, focus has shifted to the use of allogeneic NK cells to treat cancer (Miller, et al., 2005; Ljunggren & Malmberg, 2007).

Several NK cell lines have been developed that share functional and phenotypic characteristics of activated NK cells. Among these, the most promising is the NK92 cell line, an allogeneic cell line derived from a patient with non-Hodgkin's lymphoma (Gong et al., 1994; Tam et al., 1999; Tonn et al., 2001). There are several advantages to employing NK92 cells, or similar cell lines, in adoptive immunotherapy: i) they represent a well characterized immunophenotype with powerful anti-tumor properties that are independent of MHC restrictions, ii) these cells express activating receptors and lack most of the inhibitory killer immunoglobulin-like receptors, KIRs (Middleton et al., 2002), thus retaining their cytotoxicity against cancer cells that up-regulate MHC class I molecules and iii) the ease of culturing these cells to generate adequate quantities for clinical use. Currently, there are several clinical trials are underway to evaluate the efficacy of NK cell mediated cancer immunotherapy.

4.2.2 γδ T cells

γδ T cells are defined by their expression of T cell receptors (TCR) encoded by γ and δ loci. γδ T cells combine features of both innate and adaptive immune systems. These cells exhibit direct anti-tumor properties via MHC-independent NKG2D and TCR pathways. γδ T cell based immunotherapy strategies have been extensively tested to target GBM (Bryant et al., 2011; Lamb, 2009). Thus, γδ T cells that require no priming and mediate their cytotoxicity by direct recognition of chemotherapy induced antigens on the surface of GBM cells represent an attractive cellular immunotherapeutic candidate for GBM therapy. In this context, genetic engineering of γδ T cells that are resistant to temozolomide, the frontline chemotherapy agent to treat GBM, presents an attractive scenario whereby drug resistant γδ T cell based immunotherapy can be administered in combination with a traditional chemotherapeutic agent.

Freshly isolated and expanded γδ T cells from the peripheral blood of healthy donors can destroy neuroblastoma cells while adoptive transfer of γδ T cells, expanded under clinical grade conditions, in combination with immunocytokines are effective against disseminated neuroblastoma established in mice (Otto et al., 2005; Schilbach et al., 2000). Recently, a clinical study of 25 patients with advanced stages of various solid tumors demonstrated that γδ T cell based immunotherapy is beneficial and importantly, such a therapy did not induce any serious treatment related side effects (Noguchi et al., 2011). However, these cells comprise a minor fraction (1-5 %) of the peripheral blood lymphocytes and consequently γδ T cell based immunotherapy requires prior expansion ex vivo. Protocols to expand γδ T cells using therapeutic grade materials have been developed to facilitate the initiation of clinical trials to treat patients with cancer (Noguchi et al., 2011).

5. Conclusion

Although the combination of surgery and chemotherapy is effective for some types of cancer, there are obvious limitations to our current state-of-the-art treatment of cancer. Among the various potential therapeutic modalities being used to treat cancer, immunocompetent cell-based therapy is becoming an effective alternative, which is possible because of the advancements in technologies used to genetically engineer these cells. As described in this chapter, various engineering strategies have potentiated the acquired or intrinsic anti-tumor response of immunocompetent cells. It is now anticipated that bioengineered cell-based therapies, when partnered with conventional chemotherapies, can invoke an anti-tumor response that is superior to results achieved by the individual therapies. Both the chemotherapy and cellular therapy fields are focused on determining optimal strategies for combining these therapies, and many types of combination approaches are being evaluated. Several successes using combination strategies have already been reported. For example, administration of chemotherapy following vaccine based immunotherapy have shown therapeutic efficacies in patients with several types of cancer, such as small-cell lung cancer, prostate cancer and advanced stages of ovarian, breast, colorectal, renal and prostrate cancers (Antonia et al., 2006; Arlen et al, 2006; Gribben et al. 2005). Strikingly, when chemotherapy was added to tumor bearing mice previously administered with immunotherapy, both the percentage and potency of tumor specific immunocompetent cells were increased (Fridlender, et al., 2010), indicating that immunotherapy and chemotherapy can be combined, but combining the two treatment modalities is not straightforward. Although potential synergism exists between chemotherapy and immunotherapy, drug mediated myelosuppressive effects limits the employment of immune-effector cells during chemotherapy applications. DRI can allow for the administration of a dual therapy regimen, which combines genetically engineered drug resistant cell-based therapy with chemotherapy. Proof-of-concept studies evaluating DRI have yielded promising results, which show robust anti-tumor responses can be maintained during chemotherapy challenges. However, challenges remain as to i) the manipulation of the immune effector cells, ii) the timing of infusion of the bioengineered cells with chemotherapy, and iii) the long term safety profiles of such treatments. But the potential benefits afforded that can be accomplished by employing engineered immune cells, and specifically modified cells that have been engineered as drug resistant cells, warrants the continued development of such therapeutic approaches. The use of cDNA sequences that confer drug resistance to immunocompetent cells can eventually be directed toward a broad range of human malignant diseases that continue to have unmet medical needs.

6. References

Abad, J. D.; Wrzensinski, C.; Overwijk, W.; De Witte, M. A.; Jorritsma, A.; et al. (2008). T-cell receptor gene therapy of established tumors in a murine melanoma model. *J Immunother*, Vol. 31, No.1, (January), pp 1-6, ISSN 1524-9557

Abonour, R.; Williams, D.A.; Einhorn, L.; Hall, K.M.; Chen, J.; et al. (2000). Efficient retrovirus-mediated transfer of the multidrug resistance 1 gene into autologous human long-term repopulating hematopoietic stem cells. *Nat Med*, Vol. 6, No.6, (June) pp. 652-8, ISSN 1078-8956

Allay, J.A.; Spencer, H.T.; Wilkinson, S.L.; Belt, J.A.; Blakley, R.L.; et al. (1997). Sensitization of hematopoietic stem and progenitor cells to trimetrexate using nucleoside transport inhibitors. *Blood*, Vol.90, No.9, (November), pp. 3546-54, ISSN 0006-4971, ISSN 0006-4971

Allay, J.A.; Galipeau, J.; Blakley, R.L. & Sorrentino, B.P. (1998a). Retroviral vectors containing a variant dihydrofolate reductase gene for drug protection and *in vivo* selection of hematopoietic cells. *Stem Cells*, Vol.16 (Suppl. 1), pp. 223–233, ISSN 1066-5099

Allay, J.A.; Persons, D.A.; Galipeau, J.; Riberdy, J.M.; Ashmun, R.A.; et al. (1998b). In vivo selection of retroviraly transduced hematopoietic stem cells *Nat Med*, Vol.4, No.10, (October), pp. 1136-43, ISSN 1078-8956

Antonia, S.J.; Mirza, N.; Fricke, I.; Chiappori, A.; Thompson, P.; et al. (2006). Combination of p53 cancer vaccine with chemotherapy in patients with extensive stage small cell lung cancer. *Clin Cancer Res* Vol.12 (3 Pt 1), (February), pp. 878–887, ISSN 1078-0432

Arlen, P.M.; Gulley, J.L.; Parker, C.; Skarupa, L.; Pazdur, M.; Panicali, D. et al. (2006). A randomized phase II study of concurrent docetaxel plus vaccine versus vaccine alone in metastatic androgen-independent prostate cancer. *Clin Cancer Res*, Vol.12 No.4, (February), pp. 1260–1269, ISSN 1078-0432

Badovinac, V. P.; Messingham, K. A.; Jabbari, A.; Haring, J. S. & Harty, J. T. (2005). Accelerated CD8 T-cell memory and prime-boost response after dendritic-cell vaccination. *Nat Med*, Vol.11, No.7, (July 2005), pp. 748–756, ISSN 1078-8956

Bauer, S.; Groh V.; Wu J.; Steinle, A.; Phillips J.H.; Lanier L.L. & Spies, T. (1999). Activation of NK cells and T cells by NKG2D, a receptor for stress-inducible MICA. *Science*, Vol.285, No.5428, (July), pp. 727-729, ISSN 0036-8075

Bryant, N.L.; Gillespie, G.Y.; Lopez, R.D.; Markert, J.M;, Cloud, G.A.; et al. (2011) Preclinical evaluation of ex vivo expanded/activated γδ T cells for immunotherapy of glioblastoma multiforme. *J Neurooncol*, Vol.101, No.2, (January), pp. 179-88, ISSN 0167-594X

Budak-Alpdogan, T.; Alpdogan, O.; Banerjee, D.; Wang, E.; Moore, M.A. et al. (2004). Methotrexate and cytarabine inhibit progression of human lymphoma in NOD/SCID mice carrying a mutant dihydrofolate reductase and cytidine deaminase fusion gene. *Mol Ther*, Vol. 10, No.3, (September), pp. 574-84, ISSN 1525-0016

Bunting, K,D.; Zhou, S.; Lu, T. & Sorrentino, B.P. (2000). Enforced P-glycoprotein pump function in murine bone marrow cells results in expansion of side population stem cells in vitro and repopulating cells in vivo. *Blood*, Vol.96, No.3, (August), pp. 902-9, ISSN 0006-4971

Burns, L.J.; Weisdorf, D.J.; DeFor, T,E.; Vesole D.H.; Repka T.L.; et al. (2003). IL-2-based immunotherapy after autologous transplantation for lymphoma and breast cancer induces immune activation and cytokine release: a phase I/II trial. *Bone Marrow Transplant*, Vol.32, No.2, (July), pp. 177-86, ISSN 0268-3369

Cartellieri, M.; Bachmann, M.; Feldmann, A.; Bippes, C.; Stamova, S.; et al. (2010). Chimeric antigen receptor-engineered T cells for immunotherapy of cancer. *J Biomed Biotechnol*. Vol.2010, Article ID.956304, ISSN 1110-7243

Cesano, A.; Visonneau, S. & Santoli D. (1998). TALL-104 cell therapy of human solid tumors implanted in immunodeficient (SCID) mice. *Anticancer Res*, Vol.18, No.4A, (July-August), pp 2289-95, ISSN 0250-7005

Chan, A.C.; Irving, B.A. & Weiss, A. (1992). New insights into T-cell antigen receptor structure and signal transduction. *Curr Opin Immunol*, Vol.4, No.3, (June), pp. 246–251, ISSN 0952-7915

Cormier, J.N.; Abati, A.; Fetsch, P.; Hijazi, Y.M.; Rosenberg, S.A.; et al. (1998). Comparative analysis of the in vivo expression of tyrosinase, MART-1/Melan-A, and gp100 in metastatic melanoma lesions: implications for immunotherapy. *J Immunother*, Vol.21, No.1, (January), pp. 27-31, ISSN 1524-9557

Cosman, D.; Müllberg, J.; Sutherland, C.L.; Chin, W.; Armitage, R.; et al. (2001). ULBPs, novel MHC class I-related molecules, bind to CMV glycoprotein UL16 and stimulate NK cytotoxicity through the NKG2D receptor. *Immunity*, Vol.14, No.2, (February), pp. 123-33, ISSN 1074-7613

Cowan, K.H.; Moscow, J.A.; Huang, H.; Zujewski, J.A.; O'Shaughnessy, J.; et al. (1999). Paclitaxel chemotherapy after autologous stem-cell transplantation and engraftment of hematopoietic cells transduced with a retrovirus containing the multidrug resistance complementary DNA (MDR1) in metastatic breast cancer patients, *Clin Cancer Res*, Vol.5, No.7, (July), pp. 1619-1628, ISSN 1078-0432

Cui, Y.; Zhang, H.; Meadors, J.; Poon , R.; Guimond, M.; et al. (2009). Harnessing the physiology of lymphopenia to support adoptive immunotherapy in lymphodeplete hosts. *Blood*, Vol.114, No.18, (October 2009), pp. 3831-40, ISSN 0006-4971

Dasgupta, A.; McCarty, D. & Spencer H.T. (2010). Engineered drug-resistant immunocompetent cells enhance tumor cell killing during a chemotherapy challenge. *Biochemical and Biophysical Research Communications,* Vol.391, No.1, (January), pp. 170-17, ISSN 0006-291X

Davis, B.M.; Reese, J.S.; Koç, O.N.; Lee, K.; Schupp, J.E.; et al. (1997). Selection for G156A O6-methylguanine DNA methyltransferase gene-transduced hematopoietic progenitors and protection from lethality in mice treated with O6-benzylguanine and 1,3-bis(2-chloroethyl)-1-nitrosourea. *Cancer Res*, Vol.57, No.22, (November), pp. 5093-9, ISSN 0008-5472

Dillman, R.O.; Oldham, R.K.; Barth, N.M.; Cohen, R.J.; Minor, D.R.; et al. (1991). Continuous interleukin-2 and tumor-infiltrating lymphocytes as treatment of advanced melanoma. A national biotherapy study group trial. *Cancer*, Vol.68, No.1, (July), pp. 1–8

Dolan, M.E.; Larkin, G.L.; English, H.F. & Pegg, A.E. (1989) Depletion of O6-alkylguanine-DNA alkyltransferase activity in mammalian tissues and human tumor xenografts in nude mice by treatment with O6-methylguanine. *Cancer Chemother Pharmacol* , Vol.25, No.2, pp. 103-108, ISSN 0344-5704

Dotti G & Heslop H.E. (2005). Current status of genetic modification of T cells for cancer treatment. *Cytotherapy*, Vol.7, No.3, pp. 262–272, ISSN 1465-3249

Dudley, M. E.; Wunderlich, J.; Nishimura, M. I.; Yu, D.; Yang, J. C.; et al (2001). Adoptive transfer of cloned melanoma-reactive T lymphocytes for the treatment of patients with metastatic melanoma. *J Immunother*, Vol.24, No.4, (July-August), pp. 363-373, ISSN 1524-9557

Dudley, M.E.; Wunderlich, J.R.; Robbins, P.F.; Yang, J.C.; Hwu. P.; et al. (2002a). Cancer regression and autoimmunity in patients after clonal repopulation with antitumor lymphocytes. *Science*, Vol.298, No.5594, (October), pp. 850-854, ISSN 0036-8075

Dudley, M. E.; Wunderlich, J. R.; Yang, J. C.; Hwu, P.; Schwartzentruber, D. J.; et al. (2002b). A phase I study of nonmyeloablative chemotherapy and adoptive transfer of autologous tumor antigen-specific T lymphocytes in patients with metastatic melanoma. *J Immunother*, Vol. 25, No.3, (May-June), pp. 243–251, ISSN 1524-9557

Dudley, M.E.; Wunderlich, J.R.; Yang, J.C.; Sherry, R.M.; Topalian, S.L.; et al (2005). Adoptive cell transfer therapy following non-myeloablative but lymphodepleting chemotherapy for the treatment of patients with refractory metastatic melanoma. *J Clin Oncol*, Vol.23, No.10, (April), pp. 2346–2357, ISSN 0732-183X

Eagle, R.A.; Jafferji, I. & Barrow, A.D. (2009). Beyond Stressed Self: Evidence for NKG2D Ligand Expression on Healthy Cells. *Curr Immunol Rev*, Vol.5, No.1, (February), pp. 22-34, ISSN 1573-3955

Figlin, R.A.; Pierce, W.C.; Kaboo, R.; Tso, C.L.; Moldawer, N.; et al.; (1997). Treatment of metastatic renal cell carcinoma with nephrectomy, interleukin-2 and cytokine-primed or CD8(+) selected tumor infiltrating lymphocytes from primary tumor. *J Urol*, Vol.158, No.3, (September), pp. 740–745, ISSN 0022-5347

Finke, J.H.; Rayman, P.; Hart, L.; Alexander, J.P.; Edinger, M.G.; et al. (1994). Characterization of tumor-infiltrating lymphocyte subsets from human renal cell carcinoma: specific reactivity defined by cytotoxicity, interferon-gamma secretion, and proliferation. *J Immunother Emphasis Tumor Immunol*, Vol.15, No.2, (February), pp. 91–104, ISSN 1067-5582

Fisher, R.I.; Gaynor E.R.; Dahlberg S.; Oken M.M.; Grogan, T.M.; et al. (1993). Comparison of a standard regimen (CHOP) with three intensive chemotherapy regimens for advanced non-Hodgkin's lymphoma. *N Engl J Med*, Vol.328, No.14, (April), pp. 1002–1006, ISSN 0028-4793

Fridlender, Z. G.; Sun, J.; Singhal, S.; Kapoor, V.; Cheng, G.; et al. (2010). Chemotherapy Delivered After Viral Immunogene Therapy Augments Antitumor Efficacy Via Multiple Immune-mediated Mechanisms. *Mol Ther*, Vol.18, No.11, (November), pp. 1947-1959, ISSN 1525-0016

Geoerger, B.; Tang, C.B.; Cesano, A.; Visonneau, S.; Marwaha, S.; et al. (2000). Antitumor activity of a human cytotoxic T-cell line (TALL-104) in brain tumor xenografts. *Neuro Oncol*, Vol.2, No.2, (April 2000), pp. 103-13

Gerull, S.; Beard, B.C.; Peterson, L.J.; Neff, T. & Kiem, H.P. (2007). In vivo selection and chemoprotection after drug resistance gene therapy in a nonmyeloablative allogeneic transplantation setting in dogs, *Hum Gene Ther*, Vol.18, No.5, (May), pp. 451-456, ISSN 1043-0342

Gong, J.; Maki, G. & Klingemann H.G. (1994). Characterization of a human cell line (NK-92) with phenotypical and functional characteristics of activated natural killer cells. *Leukemia,* Vol.8, No.4, (April), pp. 652– 8, ISSN 0887-6924

Gribben, J.G.; Ryan, D.P.; Boyajian, R.; Urban, R.G.; Hedley, M.L.; et al. (2005). Unexpected association between induction of immunity to the universal tumor antigen CYP1B1 and response to next therapy. *Clin Cancer Res,* Vol.11, No.12, (June), pp. 4430–4436, ISSN 1078-0432

Haanen, J.B.; Baars, A.; Gomez, R.; Weder, P.; Smits, M.; et al. (2006). Melanoma-specific tumor-infiltrating lymphocytes but not circulating melanoma-specific T cells may predict survival in resected advanced-stage melanoma patients. *Cancer Immunol Immunother,* Vol.55, No.4, (April), pp. 451–458, ISSN 0340-7004

Hackett, P.B.; Largaespada D.A. & Cooper L.J. (2010). A transposon and transposase system for human application. Mol Ther, Vol.18, No.4, (April), pp. 674-83, ISSN 1525-0016

Halliday, G.M., Patel, A., Hunt, M.J., Tefany, F.J. & Barnetson, R.S. (1995). Spontaneous regression of human melanoma/nonmelanoma skin cancer: association with infiltrating CD4+ T cells. *World J Surg,* Vol.19, Vol.3, (May-June), pp. 352–358, ISSN 0364-2313

Herberman, R.B.; Nunn M.E. & Lavrin, D.H. (1975). Natural cytotoxic reactivity of mouse lymphoid cells against syngeneic acid allogeneic tumors. I. Distribution of reactivity and specificity. *Int J Cancer,* Vol.16, No.2, (August), pp. 216-29, ISSN 0020-7136

Hom, S.S.; Rosenberg, S.A. & Topalian, S.L. (1993). Specific immune recognition of autologous tumor by lymphocytes infiltrating colon carcinomas: analysis by cytokine secretion. *Cancer Immunol Immunother,* Vol.36, No 1, pp. 1–8, ISSN 0340-7004

Hughes, M.S.; Yu, Y.Y.; Dudley, M.E; Zheng, Z.; Robbins, P.F.; et al. (2005). Transfer of a TCR gene derived from a patient with a marked antitumor response conveys highly active T-cell effector functions. *Hum Gene Ther,* Vol.16, No.4, (April), pp. 457–472, ISSN 1043-0342

Inoue, T.; Yoneda, K.; Manabe, M. & Demitsu, T. (2000). Spontaneous regression of merkel cell carcinoma: a comparative study of TUNEL index and tumor-infiltrating lymphocytes between spontane ous regression and non-regression group. *J Dermatol Sci,* Vol.24, No.3, (December), pp. 203–211, ISSN 0923-1811

Jorritsma, A.; Gomez-Eerland, R.; Dokter, M.; van de Kasteele, W.; Zoet, Y.M.; et al. (2007). Selecting highly affinity and well-expressed TCRs for gene therapy of melanoma. *Blood, Vol.*110, No.10, (November), pp. 3564 –3572, ISSN 0006-4971

Kerr, K.M.; Johnson, S.K.; King, G.; Kennedy, M.M.; Weir, J. & Jeffrey, R. (1998). Partial regression in primary carcinoma of the lung: does it occur? *Histopathology,* Vol.33 No.1, (July), pp. 55–63, ISSN 0309-0167

Kershaw, M.H.; Westwood, J.A.; Parker, L.L.; et al. (2006). A phase I study on adoptive immunotherapy using gene-modified T cells for ovarian cancer. *Clin Cancer Res,* Vol.12 (20 Pt 1), (October), pp. 6106–6115, ISSN 1078-0432

Kessels, H.W., Wolkers, M.C., van den Boom, M.D., van der Valk, M.A. & Schumacher, T.N. (2001). Immunotherapy through TCR gene transfer. *Nat Immunol,* Vol.2, No. 10, (October) pp. 957–961, ISSN 1529-2908

Khouri, I.F.; Romaguera, J.; Kantarjian, H.; Palmer, J.L., Pugh, W.C.; et al. (1998). HyperCVAD and high-dose methotrexate/ cytarabine followed by stem-cell transplantation: an active regimen for aggressive mantle-cell lymphoma. *J Clin Oncol*, Vol.16, Vol.12, (December), pp. 3803–3809, ISSN 0732-183X

Kiessling, R.; Klein, E. & Wigzell, H. (1975). "Natural" killer cells in the mouse. I. Cytotoxic cells with specificity for mouse Moloney leukemia cells. Specificity and distribution according to genotype. *Eur J Immunol*, Vol.5, No.2, (February), pp. 112-7, ISSN 0014-2980

Kim, H.S.; Kim-Schulze, S.; Kim, D.W.; Kaufman, H.L. (2009). Host lymphodepletion enhances the therapeutic activity of an oncolytic vaccinia virus expressing 4-1BB ligand. *Cancer Res*, Vol. 69, No.21, (November), pp. 8516-8525, ISSN 0008-5472

Klebanoff, C.A., Khong, H.T.; Antony, P.A.; Palmer, D.C. & Restifo, N.P. (2005). Sinks, suppressors and antigen presenters: how lymphodepletion enhances T cell-mediated tumor immunotherapy. *Trends Immunol*, Vol.26, No.2, (February), pp. 111–117, ISSN 1471-4906

Klingemann, H.G. (2005). Natural killer cell-based immunotherapeutic strategies. *Cytotherapy, Vol.* 7, No.1, pp. 16-22, ISSN 1465-3249

Kohn, D.B.; Dotti, G.; Brentjens, R.; Savoldo, B.; Jensen, M.; et al. (2011). CARs on Track in the Clinic. *Mol Ther*, Vol.19, No.3, (March), pp. 432-8, ISSN 1525-0016

Kowolik, C.M.; Topp, M.S.; Gonzalez, S.; Pfeiffer, T.; Olivares, S.; et al. (2006). CD28 costimulation provided through a CD19-specific chimeric antigen receptor enhances in vivo persistence and antitumor efficacy of adoptively transferred T cells. *Cancer Res*, Vol.66, No.22, (November), pp. 10995-1004, ISSN 0008-5472

Kradin, R.L.; Kurnick, J.T.; Lazarus, D.S.; Preffer, F.I.; Dubinett, S.M.; et al. (1989).Tumour-infiltrating lymphocytes and interleukin-2 in treatment of advanced cancer. *Lancet*, Vol.1, No.8638, (March), pp. 577-80, ISSN 0140-6736

Kuball, J.; Dossett M.L.; Wolfl M.; Ho, W.Y.; Voss, R.H.; et al. (2007). Facilitating matched pairing and expression of TCR chains introduced into human T cells. *Blood*, Vol.109 No.6, (March), pp. 2331–2338, ISSN 0006-4971

Lake, R.A. & Robinson, B.W. (2005) Immunotherapy and chemotherapy—a practical partnership. *Nat Rev Cancer*, Vol.5, No.5, (May), pp. 397–405, ISSN 1474-175X

Lamb LS Jr. (2009). Gammadelta T cells as immune effectors against high-grade gliomas. *Immunol Res*, Vol.45, No.1, pp. 85-95, ISSN 0257-277X

Lamers, C.H.; Sleijfer, S.; Vulto, A.G, Kruit, W.H.; Kliffen, M.; et al. (2006).Treatment of metastatic renal cell carcinoma with autologous T-lymphocytes genetically retargeted against carbonic anhydrase IX: first clinical experience. *J Clin Oncol*, Vol.24, No.13, (May), pp. e20-2, ISSN 0732-183X

Larochelle, A.; Choi, U.; Shou, Y.; Naumann, N.; Loktionova, N.A.; et al. (2009). In vivo selection of hematopoietic progenitor cells and temozolomide dose intensification in rhesus macaques through lentiviral transduction with a drug resistance gene, *J Clin Invest*, Vol.119, No.7, (July), pp. 1952-63, ISSN 0021-9738

Law, T.M.; Motzer, R.J.; Mazumdar, M.; Sell, K.W.; Walther, P.J.; et al. (1995). Phase III randomized trial of interleukin-2 with or without lymphokine-activated killer cells in the treatment of patients with advanced renal cell carcinoma. *Cancer*, Vol.76, No.5, (September), pp. 824-32

Liseth, K.; Ersvaer, E.; Hervig, T. & Bruserud O. (2010) Combination of intensive chemotherapy and anticancer vaccines in the treatment of human malignancies: the hematological experience. *J Biomed Biotechnol,* 2010:692097, ISSN 1110-7243

Liu, L.; Schwartz, S.; Davis, B.M. & Gerson, S.L. (2002). Chemotherapy-induced O(6)-benzylguanine-resistant alkyltransferase mutations in mismatch-deficient colon cancer. *Cancer Res,* Vol.62, No.11, (June), pp. 3070-6, ISSN 0008-5472

Ljunggren, H.G. & Malmberg, KJ. (2007). Prospects for the use of NK cells in immunotherapy of human cancer. *Nat Rev Immunol,* Vol.7, No.5, (May), pp .329-39, ISSN 1474-1733

May, C.; Gunther, R. & Mc Ivor, R.S. (1995). Protection of mice from lethal dose methotrexate by transplantation with transgenic marrow expressing drug-resistant dihydrofolate reductase activity. *Blood, Vol.*86, No.6, (September), pp. 2439–2448, ISSN 0006-4971

Maze, R.; Carney, J.P.; Kelley, M.R.; Glassner, B.J.; Williams, D.A. & Samson L. (1996). Increasing DNA repair methyltransferase levels via bone marrow stem cell transduction rescues mice from the toxic effects of 1,3-bis(2-chloroethyl)-1-nitrosourea, a chemotherapeutic alkylating agent. *Proc Natl Acad Sci U S A,* Vol.93, No.1, (January), pp. 206-10, ISSN 0027-8424

McMillin, D.W.; Hewes, B.; Gangadharan, B.; Archer, D.R.; Mittler RS, Spencer HT. (2006). Complete regression of large solid tumors using engineered drug-resistant hematopoietic cells and anti-CD137 immunotherapy. *Hum Gene Ther,* Vol.17, No.8 (August), pp. 798-806, ISSN 1043-0342

Michael, M. & Doherty, M.M. (2005). Tumoral drug metabolism: Overview and its implications for cancer therapy. *J Clin Oncol,* Vol.23, No. 1, (January), pp. 205–229, ISSN 0732-183X

Middleton, D.; Curran, M. & Maxwell, L. (2002). Natural killer cells and their receptors. Transpl Immunol, Vol.10, No.2-3, (August), pp. 147-64, ISSN 0966-3274

Miller, J.S.; Soignier Y.; Panoskaltsis-Mortari A.; McNearney S.A.; Yun G.H.; et al. (2005). Successful adoptive transfer and in vivo expansion of human haploidentical NK cells in patients with cancer. *Blood,* Vol.105, No.8, (April), pp. 3051-7, ISSN 0006-4971

Morgan, R.A.; Dudley, M.E.; Yu, Y.Y.; Zheng, Z.; Robbins, P.F.; et al. (2003). High efficiency TCR gene transfer into primary human lymphocytes affords avid recognition of melanoma tumor antigen glycoprotein 100 and does not alter the recognition of autologous melanoma antigens. *J Immunol,* Vol.171, No.6, (September), pp. 3287-95, ISSN 0022-1767

Morgan, R. A.; Dudley, M. E.; Wunderlich, J. R.; Hughes, M. S.; Yang, J. C.; et al. (2006). Cancer regression in patients after transfer of genetically engineered lymphocytes. *Science,* Vol.314, No.5796, (October), pp. 126 –129, ISSN 0036-8075

Moscow, J.A.; Huang, H.; Carter, C.; Hines, K.; Zujewski, J.; et al. (1999). Engraftment of MDR1 and NeoR gene-transduced hematopoietic cells after breast cancer chemotherapy. *Blood,* Vol.94, No.1, (July), pp. 52–61, ISSN 0006-4971

Motyka, B.; Korbutt G.; Pinkoski M.J.; Heibein J.A.; Caputo A.; et al (2000). Mannose 6-phosphate/insulin-like growth factor II receptor is a death receptor for granzyme B during cytotoxic T cell-induced apoptosis. *Cell,* Vol.103, No.3, (October), pp. 491–500, ISSN 0092-8674

Nausch, N. & Cerwenka, A. (2008). NKG2D ligands in tumor immunity. *Oncogene*, Vol.27, No.45, (October), pp. 5944 - 5958, ISSN 0950-9232

Neff, T.; Beard, B.C.; Peterson, L.J.; Anandakumar, P.; Thompson, J. & Kiem, H.P. (2005). Polyclonal chemoprotection against temozolomide in a large-animal model of drug resistance gene therapy, *Blood*, Vol.105, No.3, (February), pp. 997-1002, ISSN 0006-4971

Noguchi, A.; Kaneko T.; Kamigaki T.; Fujimoto, K.; Ozawa, M.; et al. (2011). Zoledronate-activated Vgamma9gammadelta T cell-based immunotherapy is feasible and restores the impairment of gamma delta T cells in patients with solid tumors. *Cytotherapy*, Vol.13, No.1, (January), pp. 92–97, ISSN 1465-3249

Nowak, A.K.; Lake, R.A.; Marzo, A.L.; Scott, B.; Heath, W.R.; et al. (2003a). Induction of tumor cell apoptosis in vivo increases tumor antigen cross-presentation, cross-priming rather than cross-tolerizing host tumor-specific CD8 T cells. *J Immunol*, Vol.170, No.10, (May), pp. 4905–4913, ISSN 0022-1767

Nowak, A.K.; Robinson, B.W. & Lake, R.A. (2003b). Synergy between chemotherapy and immunotherapy in the treatment of established murine solid tumors. *Cancer Res*, Vol.63, No.15, (August), pp. 4490–4496, ISSN 0008-5472

Otto, M.; Barfield, R.C.; Chaleff, S.; Gillies, S.D.; Martin, W.J.; et al. (2005). Combination Immunotherapy with Clinical-Scale Enriched Human gammadelta T cells, hu14.18 Antibody, and the Immunocytokine Fc-IL7 in Disseminated Neuroblastoma. *Clin Cancer Res*, Vol.11, No.23, (December), pp. 8486-8491, ISSN 1078-0432

Pages, F.; Berger, A.; Camus, M.; Sanchez-Cabo, F.; Costes, A.; et al. (2005). Effector memory T cells, early metastasis, and survival in colorectal cancer. *N Engl J Med*, Vol.353, No.25, (December), pp. 2654–2666, ISSN 0028-4793

Perry, J.R.; Brown, M.T. & Gockerman, J.P. (1998). Acute leukemia following treatment of malignant glioma. *J Neurooncol*, Vol. 40, No.1, (October), pp. 39–46, ISSN 0167-594X

Phan, G.Q.; Yang J.C.; Sherry, R.M.; Hwu,, P; Topalian S.L.; et al. (2003). Cancer regression and autoimmunity induced by cytotoxic T lymphocyte-associated antigen 4 blockade in patients with metastatic melanoma. *Proc Natl Acad Sci USA* Vol.100, No.14, (July), pp. 8372–8377, ISSN 0027-8424

Pollera, C.F.; Calabresi, F.; Moreschi, M.; Ruggeri, E.M.; Giannarelli, D.; et al. (1994). High dose-intense chemotherapy alone or in combination with interleukin-2 for small cell lung cancer: A pilot study. *Cancer Invest*, Vol.12, No.6, pp. 574–587, ISSN 0735-7907

Pollok, K.E.; Hartwell J.R.; Braber, A.; Cooper R.J.; Jansen M.; et al. (2003). In vivo selection of human hematopoietic cells in a xenograft model using combined pharmacologic and genetic manipulations, *Hum Gene Ther*, Vol.14, No.18, (December), pp. 1703-14, ISSN 1043-0342

Punt, J.A.; Roberts J.L.; Kearse K.P. & Singer A. (1994) Stoichiometry of the T cell antigen receptor (TCR) complex: each TCR/CD3 complex contains one TCR alpha, one TCR beta, and two CD3 epsilon chains. *J Exp Med*, Vol.180, No.2, (August), pp. 587–593, ISSN 0022-1007

Quattrocchi, K.B.; Miller, C.H., Cush, S., Bernard, S.A., Dull, S.T. et al. (1999). Pilot study of local autologous tumor infiltrating lymphocytes for the treatment of recurrent malignant gliomas. *J Neurooncol*, Vol.45, No.2, pp. 141–157, ISSN 0167-594X

Ramakrishnan, R.; Assudani, D.; Nagaraj, S.; Hunter, T.; Cho, H.I.; et al. (2010) Chemotherapy enhances tumor cell susceptibility to CTL-mediated killing during cancer immunotherapy in mice. *J Clin Invest,* Vol.120, No.4, (April), pp. 1111–1124, ISSN 0021-9738

Ramakrishnan, R.; Dmitry I. & Gabrilovich DI. (2011). Mechanism of synergistic effect of chemotherapy and immunotherapy of cancer. *Cancer Immunol Immunother*, Vol.60, No.3, (March), pp. 419-23, ISSN 0340-7004

Rinehart, J.J.; Triozzi, P.L.; Lee, M.H.; Aldrich, W. & Young, D. (1992). Modulation of hematologic and immunologic effects of high dose chemotherapy by interleukin-2 in a murine tumor model. *Mol Biother*, Vol.4, No.2, (June), pp. 77–82, ISSN 0952-8172

Robbins, P.F.; Li, Y.F.; El-Gamil, M.; Zhao, Y.; Wargo, J.A.; et al. (2008). Single and dual amino acid substitutions in TCR CDRs can enhance antigen-specific T cell functions. *J Immunol*, Vol.180, No. 9, (May), pp. 6116–6131, ISSN 0022-1767

Rosenberg, S.A.; Lotze, M.T.; Muul, L.M.; Leitman S.; Chang A.E.; et al. (1985). Observations on the systemic administration of autologous lymphokine-activated killer cells and recombinant interleukin-2 to patients with metastatic cancer. *N Engl J Med*, Vol.313, No.23, (December), pp. 1485-92, ISSN 0028-4793

Rosenberg, S.A. & Dudley, M.E. (2004). Cancer regression in patients with metastatic melanoma after the transfer of autologous antitumor lymphocytes. *Proc. Natl. Acad. Sci. USA.*, Vol.101 (Suppl. 2), (October), pp. 14639-14645

Sadelain, M.; Brentjens, R. & Riviere, I. (2009). The promise and potential pitfalls of chimeric antigen receptors. *Curr Opin Immunol*, Vol.21, No. 2, (April), pp. 215–223, ISSN 0952-7915

Sauerbrey, A.; McPherson, J.P.; Zhao, S-C.; Banerjee, D. & Bertino, J.R. (1999). Expression of a novel double-mutant dihydrofolate reductase-cytidine deaminase fusion gene confers resistance to both methotrexate and cytosine arabinoside. *Hum Gene Ther*, Vol.10, No.15, (October), pp. 2495-504, ISSN 1043-0342

Sawai, N.; Zhou, S.; Vanin, E.F.; Houghton, P.; Brent, T.P.; et al. (2001). Protection and in vivo selection of hematopoietic stem cells using temozolomide, O(6)-benzylguanine and an alkyltransferase expressing retroviral vector, *Mol Ther*, Vol.3, No.1, (January), pp. 78-87, ISSN 1525-0016

Schilbach, K.E.; Geiselhart, A.; Wessels, J.T.; Niethammer, D. & Handgretinger, R. (2000). Human gammadelta gamma delta T Lymphocytes Exert Natural and IL-2–Induced Cytotoxicity to Neuroblastoma Cells. *J Immunother*, Vol.23, No.5, (September-October), pp. 536–548, ISSN 1524-9557

Scholten, K.B.; Kramer, D.; Kueter, E.W.; Graf, M.; Schoedl, T.; et al. (2006). Codon modification of T cell receptors allows enhanced functional expression in transgenic human T cells. *Clin Immunol*, Vol.119, No.2, (May), pp. 135–145, ISSN 1521-6616

Schwartzentruber, D.J.; Solomon, D.; Rosenberg, S.A. & Topalian, S.L. (1992) Characterization of lymphocytes infiltrating human breast cancer: specific immune reactivity detected by measuring cytokine secretion. *J Immunother*, Vol.12, No.1, (July), pp. 1–12, ISSN 1524-9557

Sellers, S.E.; Tisdale, J.F.; Agricola, B.A.; Metzger, M.E.; Donahue, R.E.; Dunbar, C.E. & Sorrentino, B.P. (2001). The effect of multidrug-resistance 1 gene versus neo transduction on ex vivo and in vivo expansion of rhesus macaque hematopoietic repopulating cells. *Blood*, Vol.97, No.6, (March), pp. 1888-91, ISSN 0006-4971

Sorrentino, B.P.; Brandt, S.J.; Bodine, D.; Gottesman M.; Pastan I.; et al. (1992). Selection of drug-resistant bone marrow cells in vivo after retroviral transfer of human MDR1. *Science*, Vol.257, No.5066, (July), pp. 99-103, ISSN 0036-8075

Spencer, H.T.; Sleep, S.E.; Rehg, J.E.; Blakley, R.L. & Sorrentino, B.P. (1996). A gene transfer strategy for making bone marrow cells resistant to trimetrexate. *Blood*, Vol.87, No. 6, (March), pp. 2579–2587, ISSN 0006-4971

Stanislawski, T.; Voss, R.H.; Lotz. C.; Sadovnikova, E.; Willemsen, R.A.; et al. (2001). Circumventing tolerance to a human MDM2-derived tumor antigen by TCR gene transfer. *Nat Immunol*, Vol.2, No.10, (October), pp. 962–970, ISSN 1529-2908

Tam Y.K.; Miyagawa, B.; Ho, V.C. & Klingemann, H.G. (1999). Immunotherapy of malignant melanoma in a SCID mouse model using the highly cytotoxic natural killer cell line NK-92. *J Hematother*, Vol.8, No.3, (June), pp. 281–290, ISSN 1061-6128

Tonn, T.; Becker, S.; Esser, R.; Schwabe, D. & Seifried, E. (2001). Cellular immunotherapy of malignancies using the clonal natural killer cell line NK-92. *J Hematother Stem Cell Res*, Vol.10, No.4, (August), pp. 535-44, ISSN 1525-8165

Wang, L. X.; Shu, S. & Plautz, G. E. (2005a). Host lymphodepletion augments T cell adoptive immunotherapy through enhanced intratumoral proliferation of effector cells. *Cancer Res*, Vol.65, No.20, (October), pp. 9547-9554, ISSN 0008-5472

Wang L.X.; Li R.; Yang G.; Lim M.; O'Hara A.; et al. (2005b). Interleukin-7-dependent expansion and persistence of melanoma-specific T cells in lymphodepleted mice lead to tumor regression and editing. *Cancer Res*, Vol.65, No.22, (November), pp. 10569-10577, ISSN 0008-5472

Wargo, J. A.; Robbins, P. F.; Li, Y.; Zhao, Y.; El-Gamil, M.; et al. (2009) Recognition of NY-ESO-1 tumor cells by engineered lymphocytes is enhanced by improved vector design and epigenetic modulation of tumor antigen expression. *Cancer Immunol Immunother*, Vol.58, No.3, (March), pp. 383–394, ISSN 0340-7004

Warlick, C.A.; Diers, M.D.; Wagner, J.E.; & McIvor, R.S. (2002). In vivo selection of antifolate-resistant transgenic hematopoietic stem cells in a murine bone marrow transplant model. *J Pharmacol Exp Ther*, Vol.300, No.1, (January), pp. 50-6

Westwood, J.A. & Kershaw, M.H. (2010). Genetic redirection of T cells for cancer therapy. *J Leukoc Biol*, Vol.87, No.5, (May), pp. 791-803, ISSN 0741-5400

Wrzesinski, C.; Paulos, C.M.; Gattinoni, L.; Palmer, D.C., Kaiser A.; et al. (2007). Hematopoietic stem cells promote the expansion and function of adoptively transferred antitumor CD8 T cells. *J Clin Invest*, Vol.117, No.2, (February), pp. 492–501, ISSN 0021-9738

Xue, S.A.; Gao, L.; Hart, D.; Gillmore, R.; Qasim, W.; et al. (2005). Elimination of human leukemia cells in NOD/SCID mice by WT1TCR gene-transduced human T cells. *Blood*, Vol.106, No.9, (November), pp. 3062–3067, ISSN 0006-4971

Yang, S.; Cohen C.J.; Peng P.D.; Zhao, Y.; Cassard, L.; et al. (2008). Development of optimal bicistronic lentiviral vectors facilitates high-level TCR gene expression and robust tumor cell recognition. *Gene Ther*, Vol.15, No.21, (November), pp. 1411–1423, ISSN 0969-7128